ERS HANDBOOK RESPIRATORY MEDICINE

FIRST EDITION

Editors
Paolo Palange
Anita Simonds

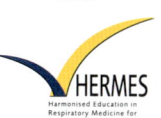

Visit www.ersnet.org/handbook to access exclusive online content using the code printed on the back cover of this book.

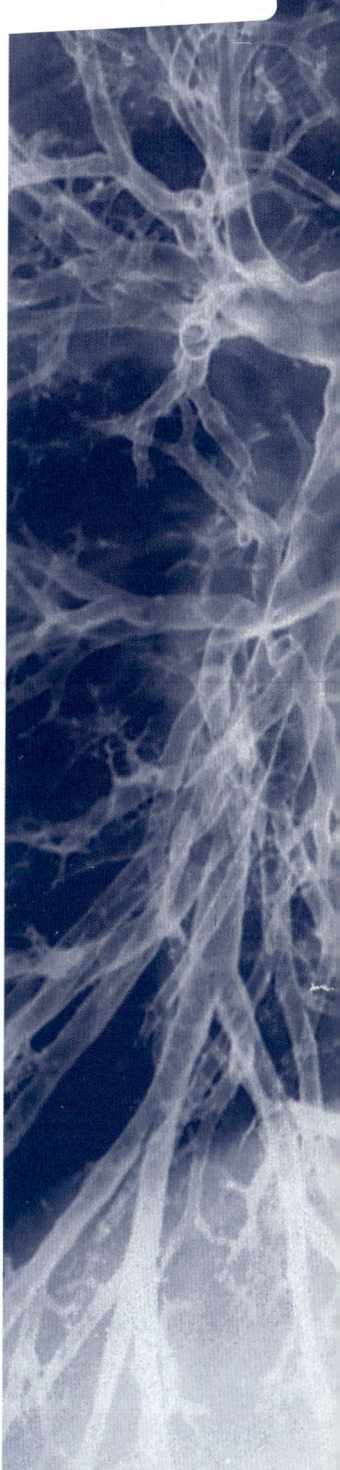

PUBLISHED BY
EUROPEAN RESPIRATORY SOCIETY

CHIEF EDITORS
Paolo Palange (Rome, Italy)
Anita Simonds (London, UK)

SCHOOL COMMITTEE

Mario Cazzola	Gilbert Massard
Johannes H. Wildhaber	Leif Bjermer
Enrico Clini	Paolo Pelosi
Thomas Geiser	Wilfried De Backer
Guy Joos	Bo E.J. Lundback
Ernst Eber	Annette Boehler
Geraldine Burge	Gernot Rohde
Johan Vansteenkiste	Konrad Bloch

MANAGING EDITORS
Matt Broadhead, Tania Séverin

SUPPORT STAFF
Sharon Mitchell, Veronica Pock, Claire Turner,
Victoria Morton, Matt Heald, Pippa Powell

FIRST EDITION 2010
© 2010 European Respiratory Society

Design by Ian Turpin
Typeset in China by Charlesworth Group
Printed in the UK by Latimer Trend & Co. Ltd
Indexed by Merrall-Ross International Ltd

All material is copyright to the European Respiratory Society.
It may not be reproduced in any way including electronically without the express permission of the society.

CONTACT AND PERMISSIONS REQUESTS:
European Respiratory Society, 442 Glossop Road, Sheffield, S10 2PX, UK
Tel: 44 114 2672860 Fax: 44 114 2665064 e-mail: info@ersj.org.uk

ISBN 978-1-904097-99-0

PREFACE

The mind is not a vessel to be filled but a fire to be kindled.
Plutarch

Why an ERS Handbook of Respiratory Medicine? Education is one of the pillars of the European Respiratory Society (ERS) and the fundamental aim of the ERS School is to provide excellence in education in the field of respiratory medicine. Five years ago, the School started a very ambitious project, to Harmonise Education in Respiratory Medicine for European Specialists (HERMES). A preliminary survey among 29 European countries showed considerable variation in post-graduate training. Based on these findings, the School developed a range of consensus documents: a core syllabus describing the competencies required, a curriculum of recommendations indicating how competencies should be taught and learned, an accreditation methodology for training centres, and a voluntary European examination to assess whether specialists have acquired the knowledge-based component of competence. Moreover, during the past few years, a vast array of educational material, such as lectures, articles published in two of the society's publications – *Breathe* and the *European Respiratory Monograph* – web lectures and courses, have been produced and made available on the School website (the ERS School maintains the biggest online resource in respiratory medicine, which functions both as an e-library and as an interactive education).

The School committee has now decided that the time is right to deliver the first edition of the ERS Handbook of Respiratory Medicine. We hope it will inform our trainees and provide an easily accessible, comprehensive update for medical, nursing and paramedical colleagues at all levels across the specialty.

The ERS Handbook consists of concise state-of-the art summaries which will be updated regularly in electronic and hard copy versions. Hard copy users will have access to electronic updates and further CME questions. Our contributors are all clinical experts in the field. We are particularly indebted to the ERS School Committee, Managing Editor Matt Broadhead who curated the contents of the handbook, Tania Séverin who oversaw the project, and all the contributors.

Paolo Palange, Anita Simonds
CHIEF EDITORS

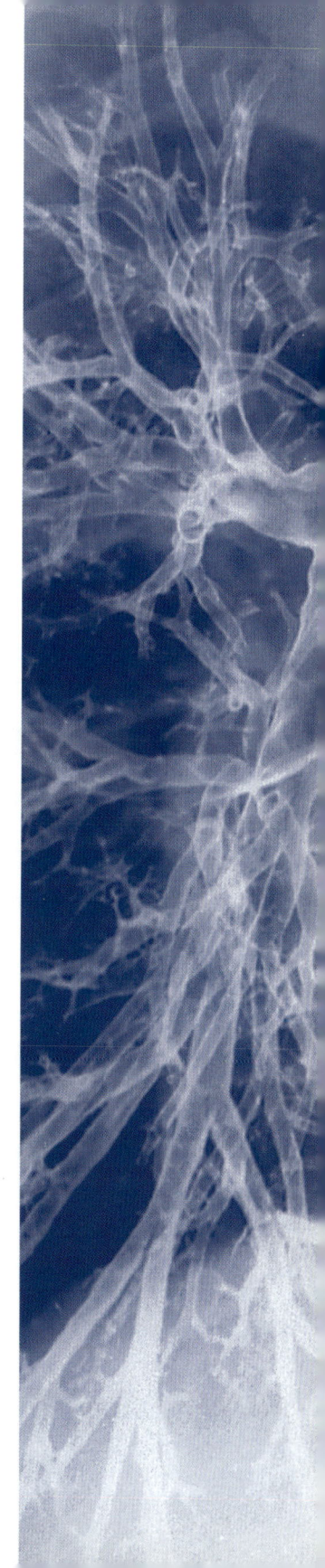

CONTENTS

1. STRUCTURE AND FUNCTION OF THE RESPIRATORY SYSTEM

GENETICS — 2
G. Zissel

MOLECULAR BIOLOGY OF THE LUNG — 7
M. Königshoff and O. Eickelberg

ANATOMY OF THE RESPIRATORY SYSTEM — 11
P.L. Shah

RESPIRATORY PHYSIOLOGY — 15
S.A. Ward

IMMUNOLOGY AND DEFENCE MECHANISMS — 26
B. Balbi, C. Vicari and A. Di Stefano

2. SIGNS AND SYMPTOMS

COUGH AND SPUTUM — 34
A.H. Morice

DYSPNOEA — 41
G. Scano and P. Laveneziana

CHEST PAIN — 49
M. Hind

PHYSICAL EXAMINATION IN RESPIRATORY MEDICINE — 51
MR. Partridge

3. PULMONARY FUNCTION TESTING

STATIC AND DYNAMIC LUNG VOLUMES — 58
R. Pellegrino and A. Antonelli

RESPIRATORY MECHANICS — 63
D. Navajas and R. Farré

GAS TRANSFER ($T_{L,CO}$) — 68
J.M.B. Hughes

CONTROL OF VENTILATION — 72
B.J. Whipp

ARTERIAL BLOOD GAS ASSESSMENT	77
P. Palange, A. Ferrazza and J. Roca	
EXERCISE TESTING	83
P. Palange	
BRONCHIAL PROVOCATION TESTING	88
K-H. Carlsen	
SPUTUM AND EXHALED BREATH ANALYSIS	92
O. Toungoussova, S. Dragonieri, A. Zanini, and A. Spanevello	

4. OTHER DIAGNOSTIC TESTS

BRONCHOSCOPY	98
P.L. Shah	
BRONCHOALVEOLAR LAVAGE	103
P.L. Haslam	
FINE-NEEDLE BIOPSY	110
S. Gasparini	
MEDICAL THORACOSCOPY/PLEUROSCOPY	112
R. Loddenkemper	
THORACENTESIS	115
E. Canalis and M.C. Gilavert	
INTERVENTIONAL PULMONOLOGY	118
M. Noppen	

5. LUNG IMAGING

CHEST X-RAY AND FLUOROSCOPY	126
W. De Wever	
LUNG CT AND MRI	130
J.A. Verschakelen	
NUCLEAR MEDICINE OF THE LUNG	135
A. Palla	
TRANSTHORACIC ULTRASOUND	138
F. Von Groote-Bidlingmaier, C.F.N. Koegelenberg and C.T. Bolliger	

CONTENTS

6. LUNG INJURY AND RESPIRATORY FAILURE

LUNG INJURY — 146
B. Schönhofer

RESPIRATORY FAILURE — 148
N. Ambrosino and F. Guarracino

OXYGEN THERAPY AND VENTILATORY SUPPORT — 151
A.K. Simonds

INTENSIVE CARE AND HIGH-DEPENDENCY UNIT — 154
S. Nava and P. Navalesi

ASSESSMENT FOR ANAESTHESIA/SURGERY — 156
M.M. Schuurmans, C.T. Bolliger and A. Boehler

7. RESPIRATORY INFECTIONS

MICROBIOLOGY TESTING AND INTERPRETATION — 162
M. Ieven

UPPER RESPIRATORY TRACT INFECTIONS — 168
G. Rohde

INFECTIVE EXACERBATIONS OF COPD — 172
M. Miravitlles

PNEUMONIA — 176
M. Woodhead

HOSPITAL-ACQUIRED PNEUMONIA — 180
F. Blasi

PNEUMONIA IN THE IMMUNOCOMPROMISED HOST — 183
S. Ewig

PLEURAL INFECTION AND LUNG ABSCESS — 186
C. Hooper and N. Maskell

INFLUENZA, PANDEMICS AND SARS — 191
W.S. Lim

8. TUBERCULOSIS

PULMONARY TUBERCULOSIS 200
G. Sotgiu, C. Lange and G.B. Migliori

EXTRAPULMONARY TUBERCULOSIS 209
A. Bossink

TUBERCULOSIS IN THE IMMUNOCOMPROMISED HOST 212
M. Sester

LATENT TUBERCULOSIS 215
J-P. Zellweger

NONTUBERCULOUS MYCOBACTERIAL DISEASES 218
C. Piersimoni

9. AIRWAY DISEASES

CHRONIC RHINITIS 224
A. Bourdain and P. Chanez

ASTHMA 227
B. Beghé and L.M. Fabbri

VOCAL CORD DYSFUNCTION 236
A.H. Mansur

BRONCHITIS 240
G. Rohde

GASTRO-OESOPHAGEAL REFLUX 242
L. Dupont

COPD AND EMPHYSEMA 246
E.G. Tzortzaki, K.D. Samara and N.M. Siafakas

BRONCHIECTASIS 252
N. Ten Hacken

CYSTIC FIBROSIS 256
A. Bush, J. Davies

CONTENTS

10. OCCUPATIONAL AND ENVIRONMENTAL LUNG DISEASES

WORK-RELATED AND OCCUPATIONAL ASTHMA E. Zervas and M. Gaga	268
RESPIRATORY DISEASES CAUSED BY ACUTE INHALATION OF GASES, VAPOURS AND DUSTS B. Nemery	273
HYPERSENSITIVITY PNEUMONITIS T. Sigsgaard and A. Rask-Andersen	278
PNEUMOCONIOSIS R.D. Stevenson	282
INDOOR AND OUTDOOR POLLUTION G. Viegi, M. Simoni, S. Maio, S. Cerrai, G. Sarno and S. Baldacci	285
SMOKING-RELATED DISEASES Y. Martinet and N. Wirth	291
TREATMENT OF TOBACCO DEPENDENCE L. Clancy and Z. Kabir	295
HIGH-ALTITUDE DISEASE Y. Nussbaumer-Ochsner and K.E. Bloch	298
DIVING-RELATED DISEASES E. Thorsen	302
RADIATION-INDUCED DISEASE R.P. Coppes and P. Van Luijk	304

11. INTERSTITIAL LUNG DISEASE

SARCOIDOSIS U. Costabel	308
IDIOPATHIC INTERSTITIAL PNEUMONIAS D. Olivieri, S. Chiesa and P. Tzani	311
EOSINOPHILIC DISEASES A. Menzies-Gow	319
DRUG-INDUCED RESPIRATORY DISEASE Ph. Camus	322

12. PULMONARY VASCULAR DISEASES

PULMONARY EMBOLISM 332
M. Pistolesi

PULMONARY VASCULITIS 336
A.U. Wells

PULMONARY HYPERTENSION 340
M. Humbert and G. Simonneau

13. PLEURAL, MEDIASTINAL AND CHEST WALL DISEASES

PLEURAL EFFUSION 348
R. Loddenkemper

PNEUMOTHORAX AND PNEUMOMEDIASTINUM 352
P. Schneider

MEDIASTINITIS 358
P-E. Falcoz, N. Santelmo and G. Massard

NEUROMUSCULAR DISORDERS 361
A. Vianello

CHEST WALL DISORDERS 366
P-E. Falcoz, N. Santelmo and G. Massard

14. THORACIC TUMOURS

LUNG CANCER 372
J. Vansteenkiste and S. Derijcke

CHEMOTHERAPY AND OTHER ANTI-TUMOUR THERAPY FOR THORACIC MALIGNANCIES 377
A. Tufman and R.M. Huber

PRINCIPLES OF SURGICAL TREATMENT FOR EARLY-STAGE NONSMALL CELL LUNG CANCER 382
G. Massard, N. Santelmo and P-E. Falcoz

CONTENTS

METASTATIC TUMOURS E. Quoix	**388**
PLEURAL AND CHEST WALL TUMOURS A. Scherpereel	**392**
MEDIASTINAL TUMOURS P.E. Van Schil, P. Lauwers, J.M. Hendriks	**399**

15. SLEEP-RELATED DISORDERS

OBSTRUCTIVE SLEEP APNOEA/ **HYPOPNOEA SYNDROME** W. De Backer	**404**
CENTRAL SLEEP APNOEA K.E. Bloch and T. Brack	**410**
HYPOVENTILATION SYNDROMES J-F. Muir	**414**

16. IMMUNODEFICIENCY DISORDERS AND ORPHAN LUNG DISEASE

PULMONARY DISEASES IN PRIMARY **IMMUNODEFICIENCY SYNDROMES** I. Quinti, C. Milito, L. Bonanni and F. La Marra	**420**
HIV-RELATED DISEASE M.C.I. Lipman and R.F. Miller	**423**
GRAFT *VERSUS* HOST DISEASE I. Quinti, C. Milito, L. Bonanni and F. La Marra	**430**
AMYLOIDOSIS H.J. Lachmann	**433**
PULMONARY ALVEOLAR PROTEINOSIS M. Luisetti	**435**
ADULT PULMONARY LANGERHANS' **CELL HISTIOCYTOSIS** J-F. Cordier and V. Cottin	**438**
LYMPHANGIOLEIOMYOMATOSIS J-F. Cordier and V. Cottin	**441**

17. PULMONARY REHABILITATION

RESPIRATORY PHYSIOTHERAPY 446
J. Bott

PULMONARY REHABILITATION 451
T. Troosters, H. Van Remoortel, D. Langer and C. Burtin

SELF-ASSESSMENT 458

INDEX 462

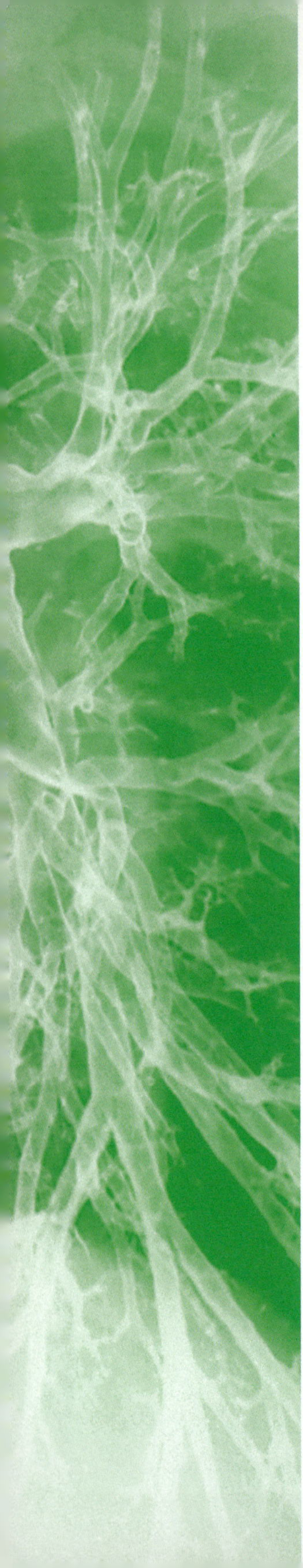

CHAPTER 1:

STRUCTURE AND FUNCTION OF THE RESPIRATORY SYSTEM

GENETICS G. Zissel	2
MOLECULAR BIOLOGY OF THE LUNG M. Königshoff and O. Eickelberg	7
ANATOMY OF THE RESPIRATORY SYSTEM P.L. Shah	11
RESPIRATORY PHYSIOLOGY S.A. Ward	15
IMMUNOLOGY AND DEFENCE MECHANISMS B. Balbi, C. Vicari and A Di Stefano	26

GENETICS

G. Zissel
Dept of Pneumology, Medical University Hospital Freiburg, Freiburg, Germany
E-mail: gernot.zissel@uniklinik-freiburg.de

Genetics addresses the composition, function and transmission of inherited entities (genes). Generally, the term "gene" is understood as a unit coding for a single RNA that gives rise to a single and specific protein. However, due to alternative splicing, one gene may code for different proteins and in addition there are also genes coding for catalytic RNA (tRNA, rRNA) or regulatory (micro)RNAs (miRNA). The genotype is the specific composition of genes of an individual; it influences the phenotype of an individual. However, in contrast to the genotype, which is simply inherited, a phenotype is shaped by epigenetic phenomena, environment, climate, nutrition and other external factors.

It is, in some respect, worthwhile to stress that genes code for proteins, and not for "diseases". Every genetic disease is based on an altered or missing protein. Because we are all equipped with a double set of chromosomes, in the vast majority of cases, a dysfunctional gene is corrected by its counterpart gene with normal function. A deficiency occurs only when the respective gene is dysfunctional on both chromosomes, or the gene product is either missing or does not exert its task.

Diseases caused by the alteration of a single gene that pulmonologists are most frequently faced with are cystic fibrosis (CF) and α_1-proteinase inhibitor (PI) deficiency (formerly α_1-antitrypsin (AT) deficiency; see below). In other diseases, such a clear-cut relationship between a gene and a disease is not evident, although facts such as geographical distribution or familial clusters indicate a genetic background to the disease. This is the case in asthma, sarcoidosis, pulmonary fibrosis and primary pulmonary hypertension. Table 1 shows mutated genes involved in respiratory disorders.

There are also a number of gene variations that are regarded as neutral variation of the human gene pool. These variations are not harmful *per se* but, together with distinct external stimuli, they foster the development of certain diseases. Glutamine at position 69 in the human leukocyte antigen (HLA)-DPB1 gene is not considered as an illness; however, when in contact with beryllium dust, carriers of Glu69+ HLA-DPB1 are at an increased risk of developing chronic beryllium disease (CBD). Up to 97% of CBD patients are Glu69+ HLA-DPB1 positive. Another example is the lack of functional receptors for interferon-γ or interleukin-12. In this case, individuals grow up normally and reach

Key points

- A few respiratory diseases, such as CF and α_1-PI deficiency, are single-gene conditions.
- A large range of respiratory diseases, including asthma, sarcoidosis and primary pulmonary hypertension, have a genetic background.
- Non-harmful gene variants can nonetheless confer susceptibility to conditions such as chronic beryllium disease.
- The role of epigenetic regulatory mechanisms in respiratory disease is likely to be very significant.

Table 1. Mutated genes involved in respiratory disorders

Disease	Gene	Mutation(s)
Cystic fibrosis	Cystic fibrosis transmembrane conductance regulator (CFTR)	>1,500
Emphysema	Serpin peptidase inhibitor, clade A (α_1-antiproteinase, antitrypsin)	SNP at position 342 G→A (glycine to lysine) >90% of cases
Chronic beryllium disease	HLA-DPB1	Glutamine at position 69
Sarcoidosis	Butyrophilin-like 2	SNP G→A causing alternative splicing and premature stop codon
Sarcoidosis	Annexin A11	SNP C→T, arginine to cysteine
Cancer	c-myc	Promoter translocation

HLA: human leukocyte antigen; SNP: single nucleotide polymorphism.

adolescence; however, after BCG vaccination or when they encounter environmental mycobacteria (*e.g. Mycobacterium fortuitum*, *Mycobacterium chelonae*), these patients develop severe and sometimes fatal diseases.

Epigenetics and regulatory genes

In additon to these classical forms of genetics, coded in the sequence of the four bases A/T and C/G, additional mechanisms of genetic regulation – epigenetics and regulatory genes – have been discovered in recent years.

The term epigenetics describes a wide field of DNA and histone modifications that contribute to the regulation of gene transcription. One of these modifications is the methylation of the nucleobase cytosine. Cytosine is methylated only in CG islands; single cytosines are not methylated. Cytosine methylation inhibits binding of RNA polymerases to the gene, which is subsequently not translated. Cytosine methylation is important in promoter silencing and inactivation of the X chromosome.

Histone modifications are an additional form of epigenetic regulation. Histones are protein spheres that bind DNA; there are four different histones, and two of each histone together with the bound DNA make up a nucleosome, the core of a chromosome. Histones can be modified, mainly by acetylation, methylation and various other mechanisms. Generally, acetylation of histones opens the nucleosome structure and the gene becomes accessible for transcription. In contrast, histone methylation leads to the accumulation of other proteins leading to a compacted nucleosome, which inhibits gene transcription.

miRNAs are short, highly conserved, noncoding RNAs binding to 5′-untranslated regions (5′-UTR) of messenger RNAs. Incomplete binding leads to silencing, and complete binding to degradation of the RNA. In fact, miRNAs are powerful regulators. Activation of transcription factors such as nuclear factor-κB leads to transcription of a variety of immune mediator genes. Simultaneous activation of miRNAs suppresses certain mediators giving rise to a specific pattern of mediator activation. This area of research is at an early stage, and novel aspects of gene regulation might be expected.

Genetics in CF

As mentioned above, CF is caused by the dysfunction of the cystic fibrosis transmembrane conductance regulator (CFTR) gene, which codes for a chloride channel. However, although in all CF patients the CFTR is dysfunctional, there are >1,500 different mutations known to affect CFTR and lead to a dysfunctional chloride channel. CF is inherited in an autosomally recessive fashion: the disease becomes manifest only when the CFTR genes on both chromosomes are mutated, although not necessarily by the same mutation. The most common defect is the deletion of a phenylalanine at position 508 (ΔF508), which is responsible for up to 70% of all CF cases. Interestingly, there is a marked difference in the frequency of this disease in different populations. With a frequency of 1:2,000, CF is most common in Caucasians (being highest in Scotland and the Faroe Islands). Populations of African descent have a risk of 1:15,000; populations of Asian descent have the lowest risk (1:30,000). CFTR mutations can be grouped into classes based on their functional consequences on the CFTR within the cell: CFTR is either not synthesised, inadequately processed, not regulated, shows abnormal conductance, discloses partially defective production, or shows accelerated degradation.

Genetics in PIs

The PI α_1-AT belongs to a family of serine PIs (serpins) and blocks serine proteases such as neutrophil elastase, cathepsin G and proteinase 3, all released by neutrophils. Because more than one proteinase is blocked by this inhibitor, it is more precisely named α_1-PI. The lack of α_1-PI leads to an incomplete or absent containment of proteinases resulting in severe organ damage (emphysema), mostly in the lung. In the USA, α_1-PI deficiency causes 7.6% of lung transplantations.

There are several known mutations in the α_1-PI gene, such as base substitutions, in-frame deletions, frame shift mutations and exon deletions. >90% of the cases are caused by single amino acid exchange at position 342 (glycine to lysine), which is called Z mutation. The Z mutation results in a structural alteration, which inhibits post-translational modifications and secretion. Patients bearing the Z allele disclose <15% of the normal α_1-PI level in serum, which, additionally, seems to be nonfunctional.

The gene frequency of the Z allele is rather common in Europe, with up to 4% of the population being heterozygotic. However, the frequency declines to <1% in southern Europe. The lowest frequency is found in African-Americans (0.4%).

Genetics in interstitial lung diseases

There is some indication that interstitial lung diseases such as sarcoidosis, CBD, or idiopathic pulmonary fibrosis (IPF) are based on a specific genetic background. In sarcoidosis and IPF, familial clusters are seen. In Europe, sarcoidosis frequency increases from South to North. This might also be a matter of climate, as the same distribution is seen in Japan. However, the Ainu, a minority distinct from the Japanese population in northern Japan, exhibit a markedly lower frequency. The Swedish population encounters the highest prevalence in Europe (55–64 per 100,000); in contrast, the Finnish population live at the same latitude but the prevalence is just half that of the Swedish (28 per 100,000). These differences point to a strong genetic background in the pathogenesis of sarcoidosis.

The contribution of an inherited predisposition to the aetiology of sarcoidosis is indicated by an increased risk of sarcoidosis in close relatives of patients. The percentage of patients with a positive family history ranges from 2.7% in Spain to 17% in African-Americans. Analysis of familial sarcoidosis suggests that multiple small or moderate genetic effects cause a predisposition for sarcoidosis.

Genes of interest have been HLA class II antigens. Although some of these linkages are largely dependent on the population investigated, several associations do seem to be preserved, *e.g.* HLA-DRB1*03 associates with spontaneous resolution and mild disease, as demonstrated in Swedish, Polish, Croatian and Czech populations.

Using genome-wide association scans, two additional candidate genes were identified, the butyrophilin-like 2 gene (BTNL2) and Annexin A11 (ANXA11) gene. The BTNL2 disease-associated splice site (rs 276530) introduces a premature stop resulting in truncated nonfunctional protein. Because BTNL2 is necessary for the down-regulation of T-cell activation, the dysfunctional gene product contributes to the exaggerated T-cell activation in sarcoidosis.

Annexin A11 exerts complex and essential functions in several biological pathways, including apoptosis and proliferation.

There is a large body of studies analysing the association of cytokine genes with sarcoidosis. With exception of the association of Löfgren's syndrome and a variant of the tumour necrosis factor (TNF)-α gene related to higher cytokine production (TNFA2), these studies did not reveal conclusive results.

Angiotensin-converting enzyme (ACE) is often used in the diagnosis and clinical monitoring of sarcoidosis. However, serum levels of ACE (sACE) are highly variable, which impairs the clinical use of ACE. The variability of sACE is based on a deletion/insertion in intron 16 of the ACE gene. The homozygote deletion variant is associated with higher sACE, whereas homozygote insertion is associated with lower levels. Heterozygotes exhibit intermediate values. Therefore, in populations of Caucasian origin, the knowledge of the zygosity of the deletion/insertion variants allows the application of genotype-corrected reference values of sACE, which leads to an improvement of the clinical application of this marker. However, this is not applicable in populations of African origin: the ACE gene in these populations is much more polymorphic and sACE levels are not linked with the deletion/insertion polymorphism.

Familial pulmonary fibrosis is linked with two mutations in the surfactant protein C (SP-C) gene. The first mutation causes a change from guanine to adenine at the starting point of exon 4, resulting in a splice deletion of exon 4 and subsequently a final protein lacking 37 amino acids. This shortened protein is misfolded and accumulates in a perinuclear pattern in the cells. The misfolded SP-C protein aggregates with the normal SP-C, which subsequently leads to a lack of mature SP-C in the alveolar lumen. This phenomenon provides an explanation for the dominant autosomal heredity of this mutation.

The second mutation causes a change from thymidine to adenine in exon 5 that results in the substitution of glutamine (position +188) by leucine. This variant of SP-C cannot be processed and accumulates as pro-SP-C in the cell. The pathological pattern of fibrosis is in both forms consistent with nonspecific interstitial pneumonitis in younger patients and usual interstitial pneumonia in the elderly.

CBD is largely linked with Glu69+ HLA-DPB1, as 97% of CBD patients bear this HLA variant. However, the frequency of Glu69+ HLA-DPB1 is also increased in beryllium-sensitised healthy individuals. Interestingly, Glu69+ HLA-DPB1 homozygosity was higher in CBD patients compared with beryllium-sensitised individuals. Therefore, Glu69+ HLA-DPB1 is a risk marker of beryllium sensitisation and homozygote Glu69+ HLA-DPB1 increases the risk for the progression from beryllium sensitisation to CBD; however, there is a large variation in the time course for this conversion. This, together with the fact that Glu69+ HLA-DPB1 heterozygotes also develop CBD, implies that additional genes may add to the predisposition to CBD.

Genetics in asthma

There is a plethora of work related to the genetics of asthma. The idea of a genetic basis for asthma is supported by the fact that there are familial clusters of asthma and differences of asthma frequency in different populations (with the highest being >20% of the population of the South Atlantic island Tristan da Cunha). However, no single gene is responsible for the development or the clinical course of asthma; instead, several genes are regarded as risk genes for developing asthma. The gene products of these genes are involved in T-cell activation, cytokine release and balance, epithelial function and repair or smooth muscle contractility.

As methods in association studies improve rapidly, new candidate genes will be added to this list in future.

Nevertheless, although there are predisposing genes in asthma, the influence of lifestyle on the development of asthma is also evident. There is a clear increase in asthma incidences in developing countries. Therefore, asthma might be an elucidating example for the complex genotype/phenotype relationship.

Genetics in cancer

Mutations and epigenetic modifications are passed to the offspring as far as the germ cells are concerned. However, there are also mutations outside the germline – so-called somatic mutations. As these mutations accumulate over years, a growing organism resembles a genetic mosaic rather than a unique clone of the germ cell it is derived from.

Most of these somatic mutations are silent and either do not cause any defect or are corrected by its respective counterpart. However, there is a variety of somatic mutations that finally cause tumour genesis. An example of such a somatic mutation involved in cancer is a mutation in the MYC gene, leading to the overexpression of c-myc. c-myc is a regulatory protein inducing histone acetylation (see above). Overexpression of c-myc leads to histone hyperacetylation and subsequently to the transcription of a variety of genes. Overexpression of c-myc is an important factor in the pathogenesis genesis of small cell lung cancer (SCLC). However, no single event, like the mutation of c-myc, is responsible for tumour genesis. In general, tumours like SCLC or nonsmall cell lung cancer present with a large variety of genetic alterations, like DNA methylation, alternative splicing, or histone modifications, which all might be involved in oncognesis.

As genetic tools become more common, the analysis of the individual pathways involved in the individual cancer pathogenesis might help to develop individual targets for therapy.

Conclusion

Genetic aspects have to be considered in all areas of pulmonary medicine. As physicians are faced with phenotypes, the underlying degree of genetic influence is not always obvious. The knowledge of the genotype causing a respective phenotype might be a promising tool to predict outcome or therapeutic options, and would enable individual genotype/phenotype-based therapies.

References

- Al-Muhsen S, Casanova JL. The genetic heterogeneity of mendelian susceptibility to mycobacterial diseases. *J Allergy Clin Immunol* 2008; 122: 1043–1051.
- Biller H, *et al.* Genotype-corrected reference values for serum angiotensin-converting enzyme. *Eur Respir J* 2006; 28: 1085–1090.
- Bogunia-Kubik K, *et al.* HLA-DRB1*03, DRB1*11 or DRB1*12 and their respective DRB3 specificities in clinical variants of sarcoidosis. *Tissue Antigens* 2001; 57: 87–90.
- Coakley RJ, *et al.* Alpha1-antitrypsin deficiency: biological answers to clinical questions. *Am J Med Sci* 2001; 321: 33–41.
- Maier LA, *et al.* Influence of MHC class II in susceptibility to beryllium sensitization and chronic beryllium disease. *J Immunol* 2003; 171: 6910–6918.
- Postma DS, Koppelman GH. Genetics of asthma: where are we and where do we go? *Proc Am Thorac Soc* 2009; 6: 283–287.
- Rowe SM, *et al.* Cystic fibrosis. *N Engl J Med* 2005; 352: 1992–2001.
- Selroos O. Differences in sarcoidosis around the world: what they tell us. *In:* Baughman RP, ed. Sarcoidosis. New York, Informa, 2006; pp. 47–64.
- Thomas AQ, *et al.* Heterozygosity for a surfactant protein C gene mutation associated with usual interstitial pneumonitis and cellular nonspecific interstitial pneumonitis in one kindred. *Am J Respir Crit Care Med* 2002; 165: 1322–1328.
- Turcios NL. Cystic fibrosis: an overview. *J Clin Gastroenterol* 2005; 39: 307–317.

MOLECULAR BIOLOGY OF THE LUNG

M. Königshoff and O. Eickelberg
Comprehensive Pneumology Center, Ludwig-Maximilians-University and Helmholtz Zentrum München
E-mail: oliver.eickelberg@helmholtz-muenchen.de

Understanding of lung disease on the cellular and molecular level is crucial to develop new approaches for the diagnosis, treatment and prevention of lung disease. Although our knowledge on the molecular level is steadily increasing, we still have a limited understanding of the molecular events underlying the diseases, which is reflected by the fact that very few therapies target specific defects.

The field of molecular biology focuses on the interactions between various systems of a cell and between cells, and particularly includes:

- gene structure, expression, replication, and recombination

- structure, function, chemistry, and *in vivo* modification and processing of proteins and nucleic acids

- cellular and developmental biology

- genetics, structure and growth cycles of viruses, bacteria, and bacteriophages.

This article focuses on selective (signal) molecules and structures, all of which are altered in various lung diseases and are important topics in the field of molecular biological research.

The extracellular matrix

Components of the extracellular matrix (ECM) surround and support the cell and cell–cell interaction. In the lung, the ECM around the conducting airways, alveolar cells and the vascular system has a major impact on lung architecture and function, in particular gas exchange. All lung cell types interact and signal through the ECM *via* adhesive molecules, surface receptors or growth factors.

The lung fibroblast is the main producer of pulmonary ECM, which consists of collagens, elastins and proteoglycans. The interstitium of the lung parenchyma contains mostly collagen type I and III, which are mainly responsible for tensile strength.

The pulmonary ECM is subjected to a continuous turnover of >10% of the total ECM per day. Thus, a dynamic equilibrium between synthesis and degradation of the pulmonary ECM maintains the physiological balance. This balance is tightly controlled by three regulatory mechanisms: 1) *de novo* synthesis and deposition of ECM components such as collagens, mainly by interstitial fibroblasts; 2) proteolytic degradation of existing ECM by matrix metalloproteinases (MMPs), a family of zinc enzymes; and 3) inhibition of MMP activity by specific endogenous antiproteases, the tissue inhibitors of metalloproteinases (TIMPs).

> **Key points**
>
> Major features of lung diseases are:
>
> - altered deposition of extracellular matrix
> - impaired surfactant metabolism
> - distorted endogenous defence mechanisms

Excessive or inappropriate expression of MMPs is related to the pathogenesis of tissue destructive processes in many of lung diseases, such as MMP-12 in emphysema, or MMP-7 in lung fibrosis.

The surfactant system

The maintenance of normal lung function throughout the life of an organism is ensured largely by alveolar epithelial cells, which form a tight functional barrier essential for gas exchange. The alveolar epithelium is composed of alveolar type I (ATI) and type II (ATII) cells. ATII and ATI cells produce and secrete components of the extracellular matrix and growth factors thereof, which facilitates restoration of the interstitium and, subsequently, functional alveolar structure. ATII cells are cuboidal secretory cells mainly responsible for surfactant secretion.

Pulmonary surfactant is a complex mixture of phospholipids and proteins, with surfactant proteins (SP)-A, -B and -C constituting 10% of surfactant. Its main role is to reduce surface tension in the alveoli following the onset of breathing, thereby leading to lung expansion. Mechanical stretching of the lung forces the secretion of lamellar bodies, the intracellular storage granules of surfactant, which form tubular myelin. The surfactant film stabilises the alveolar–air interface with a low surface tension and prevents lung collapse. Following secretion, both surfactant proteins and lipids are recycled by the respiratory epithelium.

Surfactant abnormalities have been described in many infant and adult lung diseases, such as respiratory distress syndrome, bronchiolitis, chronic obstructive pulmonary disease (COPD) or interstitial lung disease.

Defence and clearance mechanisms

From the above-mentioned proteins, surfactant proteins SP-A and SP-D are primarily involved in the innate host defence of the lung. In addition, antimicrobial peptides (AMPs), such as defensins, cathelicidins or lactoferrin, are present in the airways to prevent infection. Moreover, cellular defence mechanisms include macrophage- and neutrophil-mediated release of cytokines, such as interleukins 1 and 8, tumor necrosis factor (TNF)-α, or granulocyte macrophage colony-stimulating factor (GM-CSF).

Pulmonary alveolar proteinosis is caused by disruption of GM-CSF signalling. Loss of GM-CSF signalling in macrophages results in an impaired ability to catabolise surfactant proteins. Abnormal surfactant accumulation leads to respiratory insufficiency.

Mucociliary clearance represents the primary physiological defense mechanism. The ciliated airway cells clear the mucus, which is produced by secretory cells, by forcing the mucus toward the larynx for elemination. An impaired mucociliary clearance is the main feature of cystic fibrosis.

Transforming growth factor-β

The transforming growth factor (TGF)-β superfamily is critically involved in embryonic development, organogenesis and tissue homeostasis. TGF-β superfamily members act as multifunctional regulators of cell growth and differentiation. The TGF-β superfamily comprises more than 40 members, including TGF-βs themselves. Three TGF-β isoforms have been characterised so far: TGF-β1, TGF-β2 and TGF-β3. TGF-β1 is the most important isoform in the cardiopulmonary system, as it is ubiquitously expressed and secreted by several cell types, such as endothelial, epithelial and smooth muscle cells, as well as fibroblasts and most cells of the immune system. TGF-β is secreted in covalent association with the latent TGF-β binding protein (LTBP), thus providing a reservoir in the ECM. For active signalling, TGF-β needs to dissociate from the complex by a mechanism that involves proteases, such as plasmin or matrix metalloproteinases, as well as interaction with integrins. Active TGF-β ligands bind to the type II TGF-β receptor, which binds to the type I TGF-β receptors. Subsequent transphosphorylation of the type I receptor results in recruitment of specific intracellular signals mediators, called Smad proteins. Smad2 and Smad3 have been shown to be phosphorylated by the type I receptor, followed by complex formation with Smad4 and, finally, nuclear translocation and regulation of gene transcription (fig. 1). The receptor-regulated Smad2 or Smad3, in combination with the co-Smad Smad4, positively regulate TGF-β-induced effects, while the inhibitory Smads (Smad6 and Smad7) negatively regulate TGF-β signalling.

Increased TGF-β signalling is the key pathophysiological mechanism that leads to fibrotic lung disease, which is characterised by an increase in activated (myo)fibroblasts and excessive deposition of ECM.

There is emerging interest in the role of TGF-β in the pathogenesis of COPD, particularly

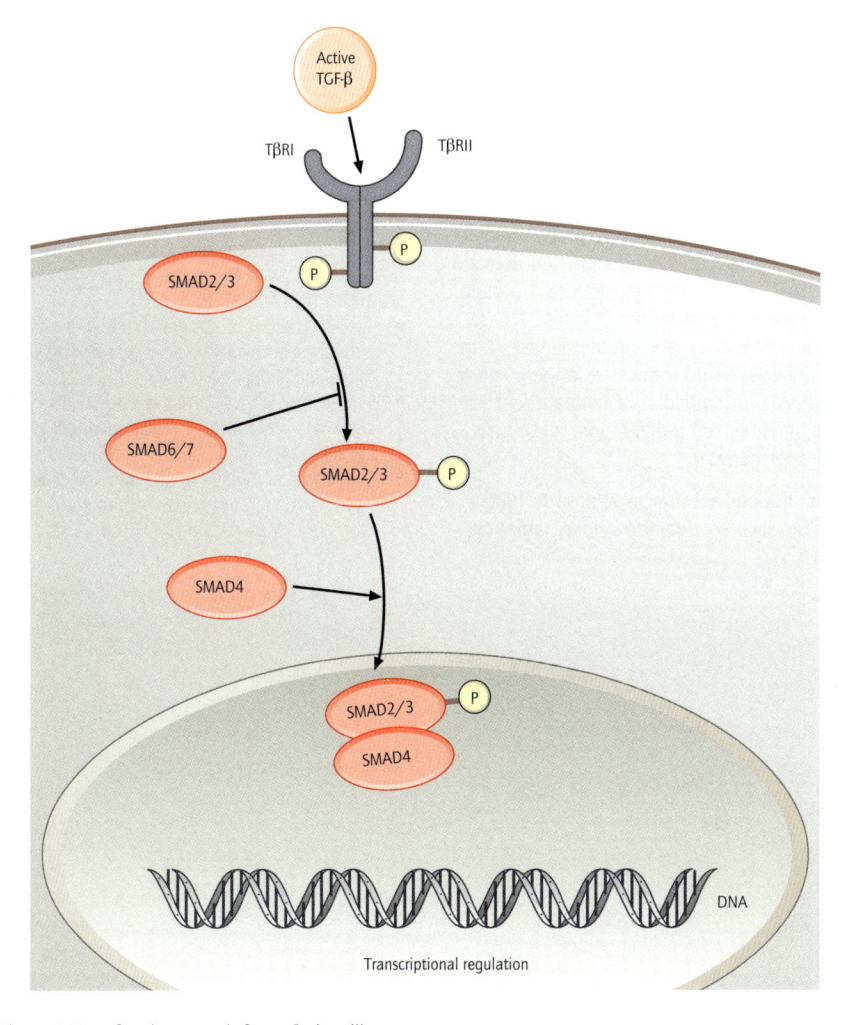

Figure 1. Transforming growth factor-β signalling.

since genetic studies have demonstrated an association of gene polymorphisms of the TGF-β superfamily with COPD. In addition, increased expression of TGF-β1 in COPD has been reported, suggesting an impact of TGF-β signalling in the development and progression of COPD.

Nuclear factor-κB

Nuclear factor (NF)-κB is a ubiquitous transcription factor present in all cell types. In its resting stage, this factor resides in the cytoplasm as a heterotrimer consisting of p50, p65 and the inhibitory protein IκBα. Upon activation, the IκBα protein undergoes phosphorylation, ubiquitination and degradation. p50 and p65 are then released to be translocated to the nucleus, where they bind specific DNA sequences present in the promoters of various genes and initiate transcription. IκBα kinase or IKK is responsible for the initial phosporylation. Several kinases have been shown to activate IKK, such as AKT, mitogen-activated protein/extracellular signal-regulated kinase kinase kinase 1 (MEKK1), and protein kinase C. In the nucleus, NF-κB induces a range of gene expression, in particular of mediators of inflammation, cell proliferation, metastasis and angiogenesis.

Many noxious substances related to lung disease, such as cigarette smoke, radiation, chemotherapeutic agents, or cytokines and growth factors, activate NF-κB, and increased NF-κB signalling has been associated with COPD or asthma.

References

- Bartram U, Speer CP. The role of transforming growth factor beta in lung development and disease. *Chest* 2004; 125: 754-765.
- Edwards MR, *et al.* Targeting the NF-κB pathway in asthma and chronic obstructive pulmonary disease. *Pharmacol Ther* 2009; 121: 1-13.
- Herzog EL, *et al.* Knowns and unknowns of the alveolus. *Proc Am Thorac Soc* 2008; 5: 778-782.
- Königshoff M, *et al.* TGF-beta signaling in COPD: deciphering genetic and cellular susceptibilities for future therapeutic regimen. *Swiss Med Wkly* 2009; 139: 554-563.
- Marraro GA. Surfactant in child and adult pathology: is it time to review our acquisitions? *Pediatr Crit Care Med* 2008; 9: 537-538.
- Oikonomidi S, *et al.* Matrix metalloproteinases in respiratory diseases: from pathogenesis to potential clinical implications. *Curr Med Chem* 2009; 16: 1214-1228.
- Suki B, Bates JH. Extracellular matrix mechanics in lung parenchymal diseases. *Respir Physiol Neurobiol* 2008; 163: 33-43.
- Sun SC, Ley SC. New insights into NF-κB regulation and function. *Trends Immunol* 2008; 29: 469-478.
- Suzuki T, *et al.* Role of innate immune cells and their products in lung immunopathology. *Int J Biochem Cell Biol* 2008; 40: 1348-1361.

ANATOMY OF THE RESPIRATORY SYSTEM

P.L. Shah
Royal Brompton Hospital, London, UK
E-mail: pallav.shah@ic.ac.uk

The thoracic structures include the vital organs for respiration and circulation. This anatomical section will focus on the pleura, lungs, mediastinum and the diaphragm. The anatomy of the heart is not discussed.

Pleura

The lungs are covered by a fine membrane known as the pleura. The parietal pleura is the outer layer and the visceral pleura is adherent to the lungs. The two are in continuity with each other and there is a very fine space between the two, the pleural cavity. The parietal pleura is described according to the surface that it is adjacent to: costo-vertebral, diaphragmatic, cervical and mediastinal. There are also pleural recesses where the two different pleural surfaces are situated next to each other without any intervening lung in normal respiration. The costo-diaphragmatic recesses are a thin area between the costal and diaphragmatic pleura. The costo-mediastinal recess is between the costal and mediastinal pleura and is found behind the sternum and costal cartilages.

The pleura is supplied by its regional blood vessels. Hence, the cervical pleura is supplied by branches of the subclavian artery, the costo-vertebral pleura by the intercostal arteries, and the diaphragmatic pleura from the vascular plexus from the surface of the diaphragm. The venous drainage occurs into the corresponding veins, which then drain into the vena cava. The lymphatic drainage is into the corresponding lymph nodes, *e.g.* the intercostal lymphatics drain into the posterior lymph nodes and then into the thoracic duct. The visceral pleura is supplied by the bronchial vessels and the lymphatics drain into the intercostal and peri-bronchial lymphatics. The parietal pleura is supplied by the regional nerves and contains the pain fibres. The costal and peripheral aspects of the diaphragmatic pleura are supplied by the corresponding intercostal nerves, whereas the diaphragmatic and mediastinal pleura are supplied by the phrenic nerves.

Lungs

The apex of the lung extends into the thoracic inlet and on the anterior aspect lies above the first costal cartilage. On the posterior aspect, the apex of the lung is level with the neck of the first rib. At its highest position it is ~2.5 cm above the clavicle. The base of the lung is a concave structure and lies over the diaphragm. The main surface of the lung is the costal surface, which is smooth and shaped according to the chest wall. The

> **Key points**
>
> - The anatomy of the thorax can be divided broadly into the pleura, lungs, mediastinum, diaphragm and heart.
>
> - The lungs can be further sub-divided into lobes, segments, trachea and bronchi and hila.
>
> - The mediastinal space contains structures including the thymus gland, thoracic lymph nodes, thoracic duct, vagus nerve and autonomic nerve plexus.

medial surface of the lung is shaped posteriorly according to the vertebral column and medially by the heart. The lungs are also indented by the numerous vascular structures, such as the aorta, that are in contact with them.

The right lung consists of upper, middle and lower lobes. The left lung is composed of an upper and lower lobe. In the right lung there are two fissures. The oblique fissure separates the lower lobe from the upper and the middle lobe. The smaller horizontal fissure separates the upper and middle lobes. In the left lung, the oblique fissure separates the upper lobe from the lower lobe.

Bronchopulmonary segments

The main bronchi divide into lobar bronchi that in turn divide into segmental bronchi. Each divides into a structurally and functionally independent unit of tissue. The right lung consists of 10 bronchopulmonary segments, three in the upper lobe, two in the middle lobe and five in the lower lobe.

The left lung comprises nine segments, five in the upper lobe, including two within the lingula, and four in the lower lobes. There is no true medial segment in the left lower lobe as this area is occupied by the heart.

Each bronchus continues to subdivide into smaller narrower airways until they finally form terminal bronchioles and then respiratory bronchioles, which are devoid of cartilage. These in turn lead to several alveolar ducts, which in turn end in several alveoli. The collective structure is termed an acinus. The secondary pulmonary lobule is the smallest part of the peripheral lung bounded by connective tissue and usually consists of six bronchi forming a hexagonal pattern with a central artery, lymphatic and peripheral veins.

Trachea and bronchi

The trachea (fig. 1) is 100 mm long and made up of anterolateral cartilage rings with a fibro-muscular posterior wall. The trachea divides at the level of the fourth vertebral body (level with the aortic arch) into the right and left bronchi. The right main bronchus is ~25 mm long and divides into the right upper lobe at the level of the fifth thoracic vertebra. It then continues as the bronchus intermedius, which is ~20 mm in length. The right main bronchus is wider, shorter and more vertical than the left main bronchus and hence foreign bodies tend to lodge more frequently into the right main bronchus. The bronchus intermedius then branches into the middle and lower lobes. The right middle lobe is formed on the anterior aspect of the bronchus intermedius. The right lower lobe bronchus gives off a branch to the superior segment and continues to descend postero-laterally giving off branches to the medial, anterior, lateral and posterior segments of the lower lobe.

The left main bronchus is longer, measuring ~40 mm in length, and enters the hilum of the left lung at approximately the level of the sixth thoracic vertebra. It divides into the left upper lobe and left lower lobe bronchus; the left upper lobe bronchus in turn gives off the superior division and supplies the apical posterior and anterior branches of the left

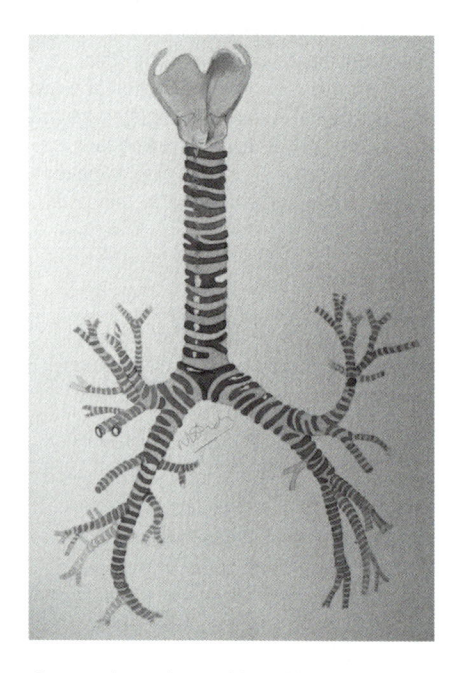

Figure 1. The trachea and bronchi. ©P.L. Shah.

upper lobe and the inferior division, which supplies the superior segment of the lingula and inferior segment of the lingula. The left lower lobe descends postero-laterally and first gives off a posteriorly located branch to the apical segment of the lower lobe and then gives branches to antero-medial, lateral and posterior basal bronchi.

The trachea is supplied superiorly by branches of the inferior thyroid arteries and more inferiorly by branches of the bronchial arteries. The venous drainage tends to be towards the inferior thyroid venous plexus and the lymphatic drainage to the pre-tracheal and para-tracheal lymph nodes. The bronchi and the airways are supplied by the bronchial arteries, which originate from the systemic circulation and arise either directly from the descending thoracic aorta or indirectly via the intercostal arteries. The venous drainage of the airways is more complicated and consists of deep bronchial veins that communicate with pulmonary veins that drain back into the left atrium. There are also superficial bronchial veins that drain into the azygos or the intercostal veins. The innervation of the endobronchial tree is via the anterior and posterior pulmonary plexus, which include branches from the vagus, recurrent laryngeal and sympathetic nerves.

Hila

The pulmonary hila join the medial aspect of the lung to the heart and the trachea. In each hilum there are a number of structures either entering or leaving the structure. They include the main bronchi, pulmonary artery, superior pulmonary vein, inferior pulmonary vein, bronchial artery, bronchial vein, pulmonary autonomic neural plexus, lymphatics and loose connective tissue.

Pulmonary vasculature and lymphatic drainage

The pulmonary artery carries deoxygenated blood to the alveoli and the oxygenated blood then returns via the pulmonary veins to the left atrium. The pulmonary arteries lie anterior to the carina and the corresponding main bronchi. The artery then enters the lung via the hilum. On the right side the upper lobe branch of the pulmonary arteries is anterior and lateral to the right upper lobe whereas the inferior branch of the pulmonary artery passes laterally and posterior to the lower lobe bronchus. On the left side, both upper and lower lobe pulmonary artery branches are lateral and posterior to the corresponding airways. The descending branch of the left pulmonary artery passes behind the left upper lobe and travels laterally and inferior to the left lower lobe bronchi.

There are two pulmonary veins on each side (superior and inferior pulmonary veins) that pass anterior and inferior to the pulmonary artery and bronchi. The lymphatic vessels drain into the hilar and subsequently into the tracheo-bronchial lymph nodes.

Mediastinum

The mediastinum is the space between the two lungs. The superior extent of the mediastinum is the thoracic inlet and the inferior extent the diaphragm. The anterior border is the sternum and the posterior border is the vertebral column. It is divided into the superior, anterior, middle and posterior mediastinum. The mediastinum contains numerous structures, such as the thymus gland, thoracic lymph nodes, thoracic duct, vagus nerve and the autonomic nerve plexus.

The thymus gland lies in the superior and anterior mediastinum. The lower border is down to the fourth costal cartilage. Its blood supply is derived from a branch of the internal thoracic artery and the inferior thyroid artery. The thymic veins drain into the left brachial cephalic vein and internal thoracic veins. The lymphatic drainage is into the trachea-bronchial lymph nodes.

The mediastinum lymph nodes have special significance in the staging of lung cancer. They are found in the pre-tracheal, paratracheal, subcarinal and para-oesophageal positions. They are classified according to the International Association for the Study of Lung Cancer (IASLC) lymph node map into lymph node stations, *e.g.* station 4 is the right paratracheal lymph node. The thoracic duct starts at the lower level of the 12th thoracic vertebra and enters the mediastinum through the aortic opening of the diaphragm. It runs in the posterior aspect of the mediastinum just right of the mid line between the aorta and the azygos vein. In the superior mediastinum, it ascends onto the left side adjacent to the oesophagus. It finally terminates into one of the subclavian veins or the internal jugular vein.

The vagus nerve on the right side is found lateral to the trachea and posterior medial to the right brachial cephalic vein and super vena cava. It then passes behind the right main bronchus and continues to the posterior aspect of the right atrium. Here it divides into braches, which form the pulmonary autonomic plexus. The left vagus nerve is found between the left common carotid and subclavian artery and behind the left brachiocephalic vein. It crosses the aortic arch and passes behind the left hilum. Here it divides and forms the pulmonary plexus. The autonomic nervous plexus in the mediastinum is formed from the vagus nerve, thoracic sympathetic chain and the autonomic plexus (cardiac, oesophageal and pulmonary plexus).

The right phrenic nerve descends lateral to the super vena cava anterior to the pulmonary hilar and then along the pericardium (over the right atrium) before reaching the diaphragm. The left phrenic nerve runs antero-medial to the vagus nerve above the aortic arch and then anterior to the left hilum. It then runs along the pericardium (covering the left ventricle) before supplying the diaphragm.

Diaphragm

This is a musculo-fibrous sheet that separates the thorax and abdomen. The diaphragm has an important role in the mechanism of breathing and coughing. It is a convex upper surface and is circumferentially attached to the lower aspect of the thorax with muscle fibres that converge to a central tendon. The diaphragm has three openings within it through which pass the inferior vena cava (at the level of eighth thoracic vertebra, T8), the oesophagus (T10) and the aorta (T12). Its blood supply is from the lower five intercostal arteries, the subcostal artery and phrenic arteries. The venous drainage is from the phrenic nerves, which drain into the inferior vena cava. The diaphragm is supplied by the phrenic nerve, which primarily originates from C4, C5 and C6 cervical nerve root (the course of which is described above).

Development

The development of the respiratory system occurs at ~26 days of gestation with proliferation of a diverticulum that originates from the foregut. The larynogotracheal tube and main bronchi are formed first. Over the next 10 weeks, the lower conducting airways develop and finally the acinar structures develop. The alveoli and interstitial tissue is then formed. Alveolar development occurs from 28 weeks gestation and continues during early childhood.

References

- Shah PL. Pleura, lungs, trachea and bronchi. *In*: Standring S., ed. Gray's Anatomy. 40th Edn. Churchill Livingstone, London, 2008; pp. 989–1006.
- Shah PL. Diaphragm and phrenic nerve. *In*: Standring S., ed. Gray's Anatomy. 40th Edn. Churchill Livingstone, London, 2008; pp. 1007–1012.
- Shah PL, Spratt J. Mediastinum. *In*: Standring S., ed. Gray's Anatomy. 40th Edn. Churchill Livingstone, London, 2008; pp. 939–957.

RESPIRATORY PHYSIOLOGY

S.A. Ward
Human Bio-Energetics Research Centre, Crickhowell, UK
E-mail: saward@dsl.pipex.com

The appropriateness of the ventilatory (V'_E) response to a challenge such as hypoxia or altered metabolic rate depends not on the level of V'_E achieved but whether the pulmonary gas-exchange and acid–base requirements are achieved: *i.e.* regulating arterial CO_2 tension (P_{a,CO_2}), pH (pHa) and O_2 tension (P_{a,O_2}) within the relatively narrow range that provides optimal functioning. This regulation involves a cascade of mechanisms: airflow and volume generation, pulmonary O_2 uptake (V'_{O_2}) and CO_2 output (V'_{CO_2}), and V'_E control with its associated respiratory perceptions. Each of these mechanisms can be adversely affected in pulmonary disease, with impaired respiratory-mechanical and gas-exchange function increasing the V'_E demands of a particular task and, in turn, the costs of meeting these demands in terms of respiratory-muscle work, perfusion and O_2 consumption.

Ventilatory requirements

Alveolar, and hence arterial, CO_2 and O_2 tension (P_{A,CO_2}, P_{A,O_2}, P_{a,CO_2} and P_{a,O_2}, respectively) can only be regulated if alveolar ventilation (V'_A) increases in an appropriate proportion to V'_{CO_2} and V'_{O_2}, respectively. With respect to CO_2 exchange (Fick's principle):

$$V'_A = 863 \cdot V'_{CO_2} / P_{A,CO_2} \quad (1)$$

where 863 is the constant that corrects for the different conditions of reporting gas volumes (*i.e.* standard temperature and pressure, dry, body temperature and pressure, saturated) and the transformation of fractional concentration to partial pressure.

Similarly, for O_2:

$$V'_A = 863 \cdot V'_{O_2} / [P_{I^*,O_2} - P_{A,O_2}] \quad (2)$$

where P_{I,O_2} is the inspired P_{O_2}, and * is a relatively small correction factor ($= F_{A,N_2}/F_{I,N_2}$, where F_{A,N_2} and F_{I,N_2} are the alveolar and inspired nitrogen fractions, respectively) that takes account of inspired ventilation normally being slightly greater than expired ventilation. This is a consequence of the body's metabolic processes releasing less CO_2 relative to the O_2 used for a normal western diet, for which the respiratory quotient (RQ = metabolic CO_2 production/metabolic O_2 consumption) is normally ≈0.85.

As V'_A is common to equations 1 and 2, then:

$$[863 \cdot V'_{CO_2}]/P_{A,CO_2} \leftarrow V'_A \rightarrow [863 \cdot V'_{O_2}]/[P_{I^*,O_2} - P_{A,O_2}] \quad (3)$$

Thus, if V'_{CO_2} and V'_{O_2} are equal (*i.e.* respiratory exchange ratio (RER) = 1), both P_{A,CO_2} and P_{A,O_2} can be regulated. However,

Key points

- The mechanical work of breathing comprises elastic (or volume - related) and resistive (flow related) components.

- With expiratory efforts that cause intrapleural pressure to become positive, the presence of an "equal pressure point" results in expiratory flow limitation.

- Arterial hypoxaemia can result from alveolar hypoventilation, diffusion limitation, ventilation - perfusion maldistribution and/or right-to-left shunt. Only the latter three mechanisms also lead to a widened alveolar-to-arterial P_{O_2} difference (*i.e.* inefficient pulmonary O_2 exchange).

both cannot be regulated if $V'{CO_2}$ and $V'{O_2}$ differ, as is the case when: 1) RQ changes as a result of dietary- or activity-related alterations in the metabolic substrate utilisation profile or 2) there are transient variations in body gas stores (particularly the CO_2 stores) that occur as metabolic rate changes. Under such conditions $V'A$ changes in closer proportion to $V'{CO_2}$ than to $V'{O_2}$, with P_{A,CO_2} consequently being the more closely regulated variable and P_{A,O_2} consequently being allowed to change. However, as these P_{O_2} changes are normally within the range in which the O_2 dissociation curve is relatively flat, arterial O_2 content (C_{a,O_2}) will not be affected to any great extent. The regulatory outcome becomes more complex if, for example, significant arterial hypoxaemia develops when $V'A$ increases out of proportion to $V'{CO_2}$ (hyperventilation) in order to constrain the fall in P_{A,O_2} or with metabolic acid–base disturbances that evoke respiratory compensatory responses to ameliorate the pHa change.

However, it is the total $V'E$ rather than $V'A$ that is controlled to effect these regulatory functions. Account can be taken of the influence of the physiological dead space volume (V_D) by substituting $V'E \cdot (1-V_D/V_T)$, where V_T is the tidal volume, for $V'A$ in equation 1 (where V_D/V_T is the physiological dead space fraction of the breath), and P_{A,CO_2} being assumed equal to P_{a,CO_2}, i.e.

$$V'E = [863 \cdot V'{CO_2}]/[P_{a,CO_2} \cdot (1-V_D/V_T)] \quad (4)$$

Thus, the $V'E$ requirement is determined by P_{a,CO_2}, $V'{CO_2}$ and V_D/V_T. Furthermore, the influence of metabolic acid–base disturbances can be accommodated by substituting for P_{a,CO_2} from equation 4 into the Henderson–Hasselbalch equation, i.e.

$$pHa = pK' + \log([HCO_3^-]a/\alpha \cdot P_{a,CO_2}) \quad (5)$$

where α is the CO_2 solubility coefficient which relates P_{a,CO_2} to CO_2 content. This yields:

$$pHa = pK' + [\log([HCO_3^-]a/25.6)] \cdot [V'E/V'{CO_2}] \cdot [1-V_D/V_T] \quad (6)$$

⇓   ⇓   ⇓

set-point   control   efficiency

Respiratory mechanics

A particular $V'E$ requirement can, in theory, be accomplished with an infinite combination of V_T and breathing frequency (f_R). The V_T-f_R combination, in turn, will influence the inspiratory-muscle pressure (P_{MUS}) needed to effect inspiration:

$$P_{MUS} = E \cdot V + R \cdot v' + I \cdot v'' \quad (7)$$

where V, v' and v'' are volume, air (and pulmonary tissue) flow and acceleration, respectively, and E, R and I are the pulmonary elastance, resistance and inertance, respectively. Normally, the inertance-related term does not make a significant contribution, i.e. although the acceleration of the air can be large, its mass is small, and while the mass of the thorax is relatively large, its acceleration is small (c.f. conditions such as obesity where the mass of the thorax can be abnormally increased). Thus, P_{MUS} typically has a static, or volume-related, component (i.e. with no associated air flow) and a resistive, or flow-related, component.

The static component of P_{MUS} equals the increment in transpulmonary pressure (P_{TP}) required to effect the required degree of lung distension under static conditions, i.e.

$$P_{TP} = P_{ALV} - P_{IP} = V/C \quad (8)$$

where P_{ALV} and P_{IP} are the alveolar and intrapleural pressures, respectively; and C is lung compliance. C is determined by the elastic properties of the lung parenchyma and also by the surface-active forces operating at the alveolar air–liquid interface; the latter being offset by the influence of surfactant.

The static V-P_{TP} relationship (fig. 1, line 2) shows C to be largely independent of V over the tidal range; however, C decreases progressively as total lung capacity (TLC) is approached. A decreased compliance (e.g. restrictive lung disease) requires a greater than normal increase in P_{TP} to effect a given lung inflation (fig. 1, line 1), while a reduced compliance (e.g. emphysema) requires a smaller P_{TP} increment (fig. 1, line 3). Also, as forced residual capacity (FRC) and the

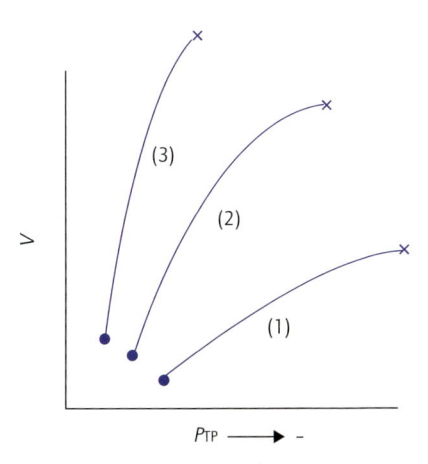

Figure 1. Lung compliance curve between forced residual capacity (●) and total lung capacity (×) for increased (1) and decreased (3) lung recoil relative to normal (2). The slope at any point represents compliance, i.e. change in lung volume (V) induced by change in transpulmonary pressure (P_{TP}).

associated P_{IP} are determined by the magnitude of the opposing chest wall and lung recoil forces, FRC is smaller and P_{IP} more subatmospheric under conditions of increased recoil (fig. 1, line 1) than when recoil is reduced (fig. 1, line 3).

The resistive or flow-related component of P_{MUS} is the increment in "driving" pressure required to effect air flow, i.e. the difference between P_{ALV} and pressure at the airway opening (atmospheric pressure, P_{ATM}):

$$P_{ALV}\text{-}P_{ATM} = v' \cdot R = k_1 \cdot v' + k_2 \cdot v'^2 \quad (9)$$

The major site of this resistance lies in the segmental bronchi and larger-sized small bronchi; because of their very large number, the bronchioles, which individually constitute sites of high resistance because of their very small radius, collectively contribute relatively little to the overall resistance (only ~10–20% of the airway resistance being related to airways <2 mm in diameter). The term $k_1 \cdot v'$ reflects the "laminar" component of airflow, with $k_1 = 8\eta l/r^4$ where l is airway length, r is airway radius and η is gas viscosity. The term $k_2 \cdot v'^2$ reflects the "turbulent" component, which imposes a greater demand on pressure generation because of the v'^2 term. Turbulent flow develops when the "Reynolds" number (Re) exceeds a value of ~2,000. As Re = $v \cdot 2r \cdot \rho/\eta$, where v is the linear velocity and ρ is gas density, it is readily apparent that turbulent flow predominates when v is high, or at branch points, or across constricted regions. Hence, reducing ρ, e.g. by breathing high concentrations of helium instead of nitrogen ("heliox"), makes turbulence less likely.

The thoracic expansion that occurs during inspiration causes P_{ALV} to become negative (i.e. below P_{ATM}) and flow to occur, until the end of inspiration when P_{ALV} again equals P_{ATM} (fig. 2a). Thus, the pressure requirements for inspiratory flow and volume generation are reflected in P_{IP}: under static conditions, volume changes are simply related to changes in P_{IP} through the static lung compliance relationship (as P_{ALV} is zero) while, during a normal inspiration, the additional muscular force needed to overcome R causes a greater negativity of P_{IP} at any given lung volume. The difference between the P_{IP} change needed to provide v' and that required to distend the lung statically is represented by the blue area in figure 2a, and is consequently greatest when v' is greatest. The respiratory-muscle work (W) performed in producing the inspiration can thus be calculated as: $\Delta V \cdot \Delta P_{IP}$ (fig. 2b), i.e. the sum of the elastic work required to overcome the static lung recoil forces (red area) and the resistive work (blue area). When breathing is stimulated (e.g. in exercise), the greater P_{ALV} required to generate the increased v' amplifies the dynamic component of the V–P relationship (fig. 2a, right) and therefore increases W. A similar effect is seen in patients with an abnormally increased R, in whom a greater P_{ALV} is required to achieve a particular v'. Expressing W relative to time yields the power output (W') of the inspiratory muscles which, when related to their O_2 consumption ($Q'O_2$), allows considerations of overall respiratory muscle efficiency. It is only at very high levels of $V'E$ (e.g. at peak exercise in highly fit endurance athletes) or when

Respiratory physiology

17

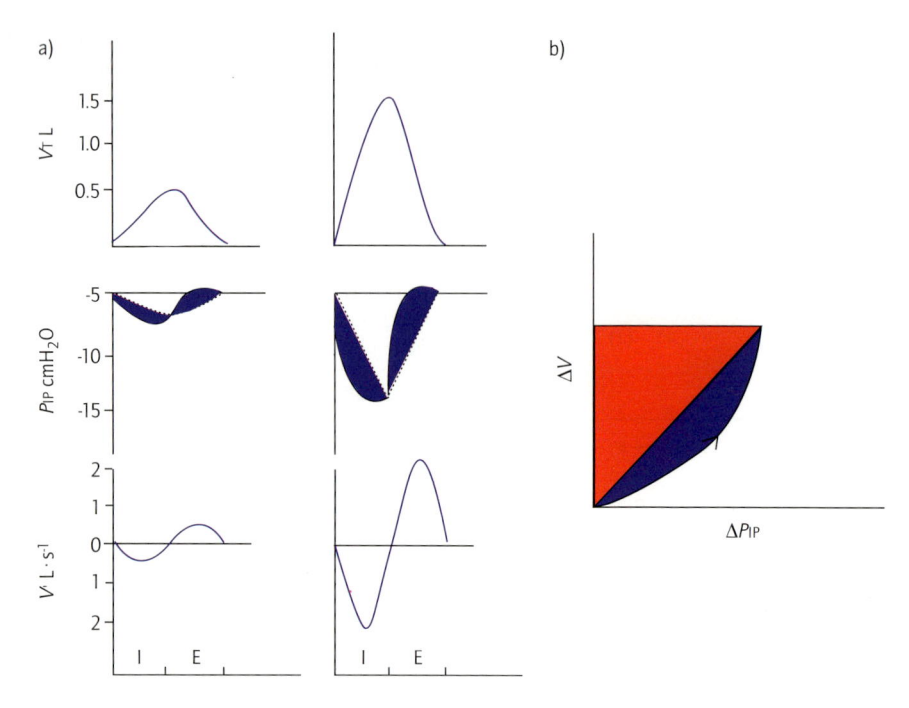

Figure 2. a) Tidal volume (VT), intrapleural pressure (PIP) and flow (v') changes for normal resting and exercising breaths. The dashed line on the PIP curve represents pressure needed to produce lung inflation statically. The shaded area is the extra PIP required to generate flow. b) Dynamic inspiratory volume (V)–PIP curve. The stippled area represents static inspiratory work of breathing; the shaded area is the dynamic component. I: inspiration; E: expiration.

respiratory impedance is abnormally high (as in pulmonary disease) that W, W' and Q'O₂ are anything other than insignificant in magnitude; this can lead to respiratory muscle fatigue.

When V'E is low, expiration can be achieved entirely through the recoil pressure (PREC) generated in the elastic structures of the lungs during the previous inspiration, i.e. providing the necessary driving pressure by increasing PALV (fig. 2a, left):

$$P_{TP} = P_{REC} = P_{ALV}\text{-}P_{IP} = R \cdot v' \quad (10)$$

Flow at any point in expiration is thus determined by the interplay between static lung recoil, PIP and resistance:

$$v' = P_{REC} + P_{IP}/R \quad (11)$$

Furthermore, the equality for PREC deriving from equations 8 and 9 yields:

$$V/C = R \cdot v'$$

which can be rearranged as:

$$v'/V = 1/R \cdot C \quad (12)$$

The term $R \cdot C$ is the "mechanical time constant" (τ) of the respiratory system, and has the unit of time, i.e. $(cmH_2O \cdot L^{-1} \cdot s) \cdot (L \cdot cmH_2O^{-1}) = s$. Thus, if R or C (or, of course, both) are large, then v' will be low for a given lung volume. Complete passive emptying (i.e. down to FRC) for a spontaneous expiration requires expiratory duration to be sufficiently long (i.e. effectively four time constants for an exponential process). Considering a normal τ of ~0.4 s (R and C being ~2 $cmH_2O \cdot L^{-1} \cdot s$ and 0.2 $L \cdot cm\ H_2O^{-1}$, respectively), this minimum period is ~1.6 s and translates to a total breath duration (t_{tot}) of ~3 s, assuming an "inspiratory duty cycle" (t_I/t_{tot}, where t_I is inspiratory duration) of ~0.4. Thus, if f_R exceeds ~20 min^{-1}, complete emptying requires expiratory flow to be augmented by expiratory muscle action; without this, end-expiratory lung volume will be greater than FRC. Such "dynamic hyperinflation" is a hallmark of the exercising chronic obstructive pulmonary disease (COPD) patient (fig. 3, right), where disease-related increases in R and/or C can lower this limiting f_R quite considerably.

That the maximal volitionally generated expiratory v' is greater at high lung volumes than when lung volume is low (fig. 3) is, of course, implicit in equation 11. That is, R and P_{REC} are each volume-dependent: at high volumes, R is relatively low reflecting a modest degree of airway distension (whose effect is amplified through the r^4 term) while P_{REC} is relatively high. Indeed, for a given τ, v' decreases as a linear function of V (equation 12), accounting for the descending limb of the maximal expiratory flow–volume curve normally being so linear (fig. 3, left).

In COPD, however, the lower maximal v' at TLC, despite the higher absolute lung volume (fig. 1, line 3), is indicative of an increased R and, for emphysema, decreased P_{REC} (fig. 3, right), and thus v' at a particular lung volume is lower than normal. In contrast, for restrictive lung disease, while maximal v' at TLC is low owing to poor dispensability (fig. 1, line 1), v' at a particular lung volume can be even slightly higher than normal owing to an increased P_{REC}. Furthermore, when there is regional nonuniformity of τ, as in COPD, for example, this can contribute to the typically "scooped" maximal expiratory v' profile (fig. 3, right).

The effects of P_{IP} on expiratory v' are not quite as straightforward, however, as those of R and P_{REC} (equation 12). P_{IP} is an index of the effort transmitted from the respiratory muscles to the lungs *via* the chest wall. During expiration, P_{IP} can become positive as a function of the applied expiratory effort, *i.e.* the chest wall volume decreases faster than the lungs' intrinsic recoil. This results in a compressive force being applied to the intrapleural space. As $P_{ALV} = P_{IP} + P_{REC}$ (equation 10), P_{ALV} will be more positive than P_{IP} by an amount equal to P_{REC}. Airway pressure (P_{AW}) declines from the alveolar value down to zero at the mouth as a result of frictional losses along the airways. At the point at which $P_{AW} = P_{IP}$ (*i.e.* the transmural pressure across the airway is zero) (fig. 4), an "equal pressure point" (EPP) results.

In normal subjects, the EPP occurs in the large airways (lower trachea or mainstem bronchi), which, despite the tendency to become compressed, are prevented from collapsing by their cartilaginous support. Thus, the EPP becomes the limiting point for expiratory flow generation, dictating the maximum expiratory flow (v'_{max}):

$$v'_{max} = P_{REC}/R_{us} \quad (13)$$

where R_{us} is the resistance of the "upstream segment" of the airways (between the alveolus and the EPP) (fig. 4). This explains why progressively greater expiratory efforts, although leading to a progressively more positive P_{IP}, do not lead to a progressively greater v'; greater expiratory effort simply compresses the airways more, raising downstream resistance in proportion to the

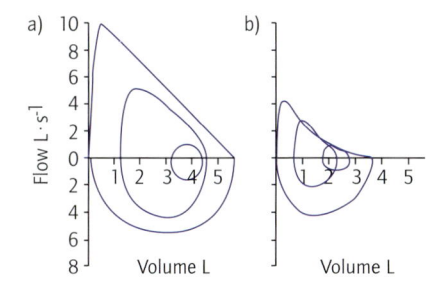

Figure 3. Inspiratory (downwards) and expiratory (upwards) flow–volume curves at rest, maximal exercise and with maximal volitional effort for a) a normal subject and b) a patient with chronic obstructive pulmonary disease. Reproduced from KLAS (1989), with permission from the publisher.

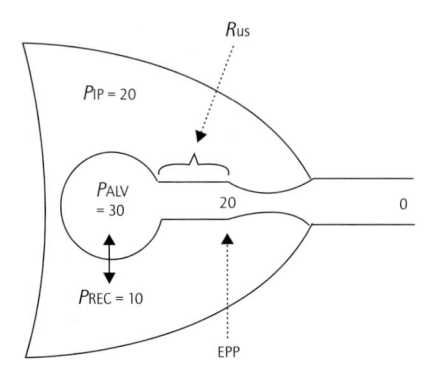

Figure 4. Airflow limitation in expiration. An equal pressure point (EPP) results when airway pressure declines to a value equal to the recoil pressure (P_{REC}); R_{us} is the resistance of the "upstream segment" of the airways. P_{IP}: intrapleural pressure; P_{ALV}: alveolar pressure.

increased effort. v' therefore becomes maximised at a constant value (at that lung volume), independent of effort.

With loss of lung recoil and/or increases in small airways resistance, however, the EPP migrates upstream. If it encroaches into the small unsupported airways, airways collapse occurs – with, consequently, profound effects on v'max (equation 13).

Pulmonary gas exchange

The effectiveness of pulmonary O_2 exchange is conventionally judged by the magnitude of the alveolar–arterial O_2 tension difference (P_{A-a,O_2}) where P_{Ai,O_2} is considered the P_{A,O_2} of the "ideal lung", which hypothetically exchanges gases ideally. P_{Ai,O_2} thus circumvents the difficulty of providing a single representative value for P_{A,O_2} when there are regional variations in gas-exchange efficiency, and can be derived as follows (*i.e.* by re-arranging and amalgamating equations 1 and 2: V'_{CO_2}/V'_{O_2} = RER = {$V'_A \cdot [(P_{I,O_2} \cdot F_{A,N_2}/F_{I,N_2})-P_{Ai,O_2}]$}/($V'_A \cdot P_{A,CO_2}$):

$$P_{Ai,O_2} = P_{I,O_2}\text{-}P_{a,CO_2}/R + [P_{a,CO_2} \cdot F_{I,O_2} \cdot (1\text{-}R)/R]$$

It is common practice to neglect the term in the square brackets, as it only contributes a few mmHg or so when $R \neq 1$ and is zero when $R = 1$, yielding:

$$P_{Ai,O_2} = P_{I,O_2}\text{-}P_{a,CO_2}/R \quad (14)$$

Impairments of pulmonary gas exchange typically result in arterial hypoxaemia and, in some instances, arterial hypercapnia. Six mechanisms can be identified as independent causes of arterial hypoxaemia: three of these affect P_{A,O_2} (ambient hypoxia as occurs on ascent to altitude, reduced RQ and alveolar hypoventilation) and three affect P_{A-a,O_2} (diffusion limitation, increased right-to-left shunt and ventilation–perfusion (Q') maldistribution (V'_A/Q')).

Reduced RQ Recalling that V'_E normally operates to regulate P_{a,CO_2}, by responding in a proportional fashion to V'_{CO_2}, when the RQ of the dietary substrate is reduced (*i.e.* by ingestion of a high-fat diet), the associated reduction in metabolic CO_2 production will require less ventilation to maintain a stable P_{a,CO_2} (equation 3). This leads to hypoventilation relative to O_2, *i.e.* V'_E is normal relative to V'_{CO_2} but low relative to V'_{O_2}. Thus, P_{A,O_2} and P_{a,O_2} will fall.

Alveolar hypoventilation Alveolar hypoventilation can occur in diseases or with drugs that affect the medullary respiratory-integrating centres or respiratory neuromuscular function and therefore reduce the level of respiratory motor output. It may also be seen in severe COPD, consequent to the abnormally increased small-airways resistance and high resistive work of breathing. Arterial hypoxaemia and hypercapnia result (equations 2 and 1, respectively), with the fall of P_{a,O_2} being related to the rise of P_{a,CO_2} by R (equation 14). Thus, when $R = 1$, the increase in P_{A,CO_2} and the fall in P_{A,O_2}, which result from a reduction in V'_A, are numerically equal, as notionally are the corresponding changes in P_{a,CO_2} and P_{a,O_2}. However, as R is normally ~0.8 at rest, for each 10 mmHg decrease in P_{a,O_2} that results from a fall of V'_A, P_{a,CO_2} will increase by ~8 mmHg. It should be noted that the hypoxaemia can be offset by administration of supplementary O_2.

Diffusion impairment Fick's law indicates that impairments in the pulmonary diffusive flux of O_2 (or CO_2) can result from 1) a reduction in the "driving pressure" (for O_2, ΔP_{O_2}); 2) a reduction in the available surface area for diffusion (A); and/or 3) an increased path length for diffusion (l):

$$V'_{O_2} = A/l \cdot d \cdot \Delta P_{O_2} \quad (15)$$

where d is the diffusion coefficient for O_2 which is inversely proportional to gas molecular weight (MW) in the gas phase ($d = 1/\sqrt{MW}$), while directly proportional also to gas solubility (s) in the blood phase ($d = s/\sqrt{MW}$). Hence, as O_2 is lighter than CO_2, it diffuses 18% more rapidly in the gas phase for the same partial pressure gradient. In the blood phase, however, CO_2 is 20 times more diffusible than O_2, owing to its greater solubility.

During inspiration, O_2 is transported down the tracheobronchial tree by convective or bulk flow. At the level of the alveolar ducts, owing to the large overall cross-sectional area of the airways and the resulting reduction in the linear velocity of the inspired gas, movement to the alveolar–capillary membrane relies on diffusion. Diffusion through the alveolar gas space does not normally limit gas transfer into pulmonary capillary blood. Thus, as the average alveolar diameter is normally only ~100 μm, diffusion equilibrium (*i.e.* $\Delta P_{O_2} = 0$) throughout the alveolus is attained rapidly: this is normally 80% complete within ~ 0.002 s, which is several orders of magnitude less than the time for which the pulmonary capillary blood is exposed to the alveolar gas-exchange surface (*i.e.* the pulmonary–capillary transit time (t_{TR}), which is ~0.8 s at rest). In conditions such as emphysema, air-sac enlargement increases intra-alveolar diffusion distances, predisposing to less efficient O_2 and CO_2 exchange.

More commonly, however, diffusion limitation reflects exchange impairments between alveolar gas and pulmonary capillary blood. The rate of diffusive uptake of O_2 into blood is given by:

$$V'_{O_2} = A/1 \cdot d \cdot (P_{A,O_2} - P_{\bar{c},O_2})$$

where A is the alveolar surface area in contact with perfused pulmonary capillaries; l is the diffusion pathlength which extends from the alveolar surface fluid lining to the erythrocyte interior to include the alveolar epithelium, interstitial space, capillary endothelial cells, plasma, the erythrocyte cell membrane and, for a reactive gas species such as O_2, its chemical combination with haemoglobin (Hb); and $P_{\bar{c},O_2}$ is the mean pulmonary capillary P_{O_2}. It is conventional to combine A, l and d into a single term, the pulmonary diffusing capacity of the lung for O_2 (D_{L,O_2}) or transfer factor:

$$V'_{O_2} = D_{L,O_2} \cdot (P_{A,O_2} - P_{\bar{c},O_2}) \quad (16)$$

D_{L,O_2} can be usefully subdivided into its functional components, *i.e.* the "membrane" component (D_{M,O_2}) and that due to chemical combination:

$$1/D_{L,O_2} = 1/D_{M,O_2} + 1/\theta \cdot V_c \quad (17)$$

where θ is the reaction rate coefficient for chemical combination of O_2 with haemoglobin (Hb), and V_c is the pulmonary capillary blood volume. Because of technical limitations associated with estimating $P_{\bar{c},O_2}$, it is conventional to determine diffusing capacity of the lung and membrane in terms of carbon monoxide ($D_{L,CO}$, $D_{M,CO}$) as the high affinity of Hb for CO ensures that the pulmonary capillary CO tension (P_{CO}) is effectively zero (see Chapter 3, Gas transfer).

The initial driving pressure across the alveolar–capillary membrane (*i.e.* at the entrance to the capillary bed) is given by the difference between P_{A,O_2} (normally ~100 mmHg) and the mixed venous P_{O_2} ($P_{\bar{v},O_2}$, normally ~40 mmHg at rest, although the latter decreases as in exercise). The rate at which O_2 is taken up into the blood decreases from this point as blood traverses the capillary, reflecting the increasing $P_{\bar{c},O_2}$ (and consequent decrease in P_{A,O_2}), which in turn reduces the instantaneous ΔP_{O_2}. Diffusion equilibrium is normally reached within 0.25–0.3 s (*i.e.* well before the blood reaches the end of the capillary), such that pulmonary end-capillary PO_2 (Pc',O_2)=PA,O_2. This large safety margin becomes compromised, however, when t_{TR} is shortened to a degree that there is insufficient time for the attainment of diffusion equilibrium, *i.e.* $Pc',O_2 < PA,O_2$. As $t_{TR} = Vc/Q'$ (where Q' is pulmonary blood flow), an increase in Q' (*e.g.* high-intensity exercise) predisposes to lack of diffusion equilibrium resulting in arterial hypoxaemia. However, the decrease in t_{TR} with increases in Q' is less than expected because Qc actually increases with Q', consequent to distension of already-perfused capillaries and recruitment of previously unperfused capillaries; this serves to protect against diffusion disequilibrium.

A lowered PA,O_2, as occurs with ascent to high altitude, or when a subject breathes an hypoxic inspirate or with hypoventilation, will slow the Pc,O_2 rise time. This is because the initial driving pressure ($PA,O_2 - P\bar{v},O_2$) is smaller, as the operating slope of the O_2 dissociation curve (β) is steeper, with the arterio-venous O_2 content difference expressing a smaller arterio-venous PO_2 difference.

A useful expression relating to the interplay of factors which dictate whether or not diffusion equilibrium will actually be attained (*i.e.* whether $Pc',O_2 = PA,O_2$) is:

$$(PA,O_2 - P\bar{c},O_2) = (PA,O_2 - P\bar{v},O_2) \cdot e^{-DL,O_2/Q' \cdot \beta} \quad (18)$$

The term $DL,O_2/Q' \cdot \beta$ has been termed the "equilibrium coefficient" by PIIPER and SCHEID (1980) and the "diffusive–perfusive conductance" ratio by WEST and WAGNER (1998). Thus, diffusion equilibrium is less likely to be attained if DL,O_2 is low, and Q' and β are high. For example, an increased path length (*e.g.* alveolar proteinosis, pulmonary oedema) and/or a reduced surface area for exchange (*e.g.* pulmonary embolism, restrictive lung disease) slow the diffusive flux of O_2 because of their effects on DL,O_2. With very high levels of Q' (*e.g.* highly fit endurance athletes exercising at or close to maximum) or very high linear velocities (*e.g.*

pulmonary embolism, where there are fewer participating capillaries), the reduction in t_{TR} can lead to a widening of the $PA-a,O_2$ and arterial hypoxaemia. Supplemental O_2 can, through its effects on PA,O_2 and therefore driving pressure, speed the increase of Pc,O_2 and thus ameliorate the degree of gas-exchange impairment.

Even though severe degrees of arterial hypoxaemia can result from diffusion impairment, CO_2 retention is rarely a problem. This is because any increase in Pa,CO_2 that might occur tends to be corrected by ventilatory control mechanisms, which are considered to be exquisitely sensitive to CO_2 (*i.e.* central and carotid body chemoreflexes); in contrast, hypoxic ventilatory stimulation only becomes appreciable when Pa,O_2 falls below ~ 60 mmHg (see Chapter 3, Control of ventilation). Hence, moderate diffusion impairment is accompanied by a decreased Pa,O_2, a widened $PA-a,O_2$ and a relatively normal Pa,CO_2; more severe impairment which leads to hypoxic ventilatory stimulation will evidence more marked arterial hypoxaemia, greater widening of $PA-a,O_2$ and a low Pa,CO_2.

Right-to-left shunt A right-to-left shunt (Q's) occurs when venous blood by-passes the pulmonary capillary circulation, thus providing a degree of venous admixture with blood from the exchanging alveolar units. It normally reflects venous drainage from the larger airways (which enters the pulmonary veins) and from coronary venous blood (which enters the left ventricles *via* the thebesian veins). This represents only a small percentage of the cardiac output (Q') and therefore amounts to a reduction in PA,O_2 of only a few mmHg below Pc',O_2. However, $Q's/Q'$ can be markedly increased in patients with congenital heart disease (*e.g.* atrial or ventricular septal defects; pulmonary arterio-venous fistulae), leading to significant arterial hypoxaemia and widening of the $PA-a,O_2$.

The $Q's/Q'$ relationship derives from the recognition that the rate of O_2 delivery into the systemic arterial circulation can be viewed as being made up of a homogeneous "ideal" pulmonary capillary component and a "pure" shunt component. Reverting again to the Fick principle, but now for the "blood" side, and using the simple equality $Q'=Q'c+Q's$:

$$Q' \cdot C_{a,O_2} = Q'c \cdot C_{c',O_2} + Q's \cdot C_{\bar{v},O_2}$$

which rearranges to yield:

$$Q's/Q' = (C_{c',O_2} - C_{a,O_2})/(C_{c',O_2} - C_{\bar{v},O_2}) \quad (19)$$

where $C_{\bar{v},O_2}$ and C_{c',O_2} are mixed-venous and pulmonary end-capillary O_2 content, respectively. C_{a,O_2} and $C_{\bar{v},O_2}$ can be measured directly from blood samples, while C_{c',O_2} is derived through the standard O_2 dissociation curve, assuming $P_{c',O_2} = P_{Ai,O_2}$ (equation 14). It should be noted that this equation also assumes that all the shunted blood is of mixed-venous composition, which may not necessarily be the case for bronchial venous blood. This estimate of $Q's/Q'$ thus provides an overestimate of the true shunt, as it incorporates a fraction of the perfusion draining from units having poorly functional capillaries (with low V'_A/Q' values), i.e. creating a "shunt-like" effect.

A right-to-left shunt must therefore result in arterial hypoxaemia, i.e. even a small contribution from nonarterialised blood will depress the resulting C_{a,O_2}, owing to the influence of the nonlinear O_2 dissociation curve. The severity of the hypoxaemia will depend both on $Q's/Q'$ and $C_{\bar{v},O_2}$, being more marked when the former is larger and the latter is lower. A hallmark feature of a pure right-to-left shunt is that the response of P_{a,O_2} to administration of 100% O_2 is appreciably less than expected. This is because the shunt flow cannot "see" the elevated P_{A,O_2} in the exchanging alveoli, and also that further increases in P_{A,O_2} will have little effect on the C_{c',O_2} because the blood is already essentially fully saturated; it is only the dissolved component of the O_2 content that can be increased, and this will be relatively small because of the low solubility of O_2 in plasma.

A right-to-left shunt also has the potential to cause CO_2 retention, but this is rarely observed owing to the normally small venous-to-arterial CO_2 tension (P_{CO_2}) difference (~6 mmHg at rest; c.f. ~60 mmHg for O_2) and also (see above) the mechanisms of ventilatory control can normally restore an increased P_{a,CO_2} back to normal. Again, however, should P_{a,O_2} fall sufficiently to cause hypoxic stimulation of the carotid chemoreceptors, then P_{a,CO_2} will fall (see Chapter 3, Control of ventilation); but, without this, P_{a,CO_2} will rise. Thus, a moderate right-to-left shunt leads to a reduced P_{a,O_2}, a widened P_{A-a,O_2}, but a relatively normal P_{a,CO_2}. Severe right-to-left shunts cause a markedly reduced P_{a,O_2} and a markedly widened P_{A-a,O_2}, with the possibility of a lowered P_{a,CO_2}.

V'_A/Q' maldistribution Although overall V'_A may be approximately equal to overall Q' in the lung, there may nonetheless be regions with high, normal and low V'_A/Q' ratios. This has important implications for regional alveolar gas and pulmonary end-capillary blood composition, and therefore for overall arterial blood-gas status. That is, gas and blood from low V'_A/Q' regions will reflect hypoventilation (i.e. low P_{O_2}, high P_{CO_2}) and, in the extreme, alveolar shunt ($V'_A/Q'=0$) (see above); gas and blood from normal V'_A/Q' regions will have a normal P_{O_2} and P_{CO_2}; and gas and blood from high V'_A/Q' regions will reflect hyperventilation (i.e. high P_{O_2}, low P_{CO_2}) with alveolar dead space in the extreme ($V'_A/Q'=\infty$).

An analogous formulation to that for estimation of $Q's/Q'$ can be applied to the estimation of V_D/V_T (recalling that V_D reflects the sum of the anatomical and alveolar dead spaces). That is, the assumption is made that the volume of CO_2 cleared in exhalation originates solely from a homogeneous exchanging alveolar compartment (Bohr technique):

$$V_T \cdot F_{\bar{E},CO_2} = V_A \cdot F_{A,CO_2}$$

where $F_{\bar{E},CO_2}$ is the mixed expired CO_2 fraction and V_A is the volume of exchanging alveoli. Rearranging and substitution yields:

$$V_D/V_T = (P_{a,CO_2} - P_{\bar{E},CO_2})/P_{a,CO_2} \quad (20)$$

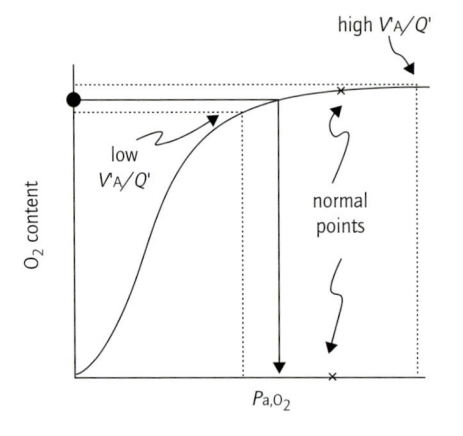

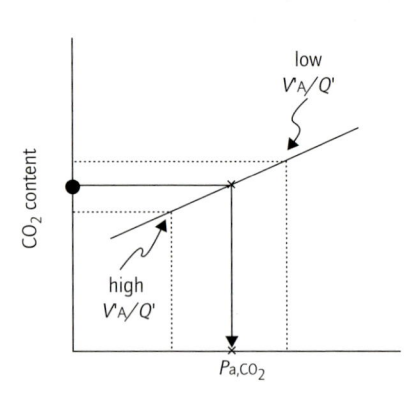

Figure 5. Influence of altered ventilation-to-perfusion ratios on mean arterial oxygen ($\bar{P}a,O_2$) and carbon dioxide ($\bar{P}a,CO_2$) tensions. The nonlinear O_2 dissociation curve results in hypoxaemia ($\downarrow$) compared with "normal" ($\times$); this effect is not evident for CO_2, because the CO_2 dissociation curve is linear. $V'A/Q'$: alveolar ventilation–perfusion ratio. Reproduced from Whipp (2002) with permission from the publisher.

(The shift from PA,CO_2 to Pa,CO_2 is attributable to Enghoff.)

Even in the normal lung, there is evidence of mild $V'A/Q'$ maldistribution. Owing to the influence of gravity, Q' is distributed preferentially to the dependent regions of the lung (i.e. towards the base in the upright posture). A similar, gravitationally induced effect is also seen for $V'A$, though it is less striking. Thus, the alveoli in the dependent regions of the lung adopt a smaller volume, with a greater hydrostatic pressure in the alveolar interstitium. They are therefore constrained to operate over the steeper, lower portion of the lung compliance curve, in contrast to the larger apical units. Thus, the smaller basal units undergo a greater volume increase for a given increase of P_{TP} during inspiration, and are therefore better ventilated than are the apical units. Taking these effects together, the apical units have a relatively high $V'A/Q'$ while the basal units have a low $V'A/Q'$. Naturally, the degree of $V'A/Q'$ maldistribution is considerably more marked in many pulmonary disease states (e.g. COPD, diffuse interstitial fibrosis, pulmonary vascular occlusive disease), and its topographical location is not predictable.

In the presence of $V'A/Q'$ maldistribution, the overall (or mean) PA,O_2 and PA,CO_2 will result from an averaging of the respective gas concentrations from each individual gas "stream", in proportion to the local $V'A$. Likewise, the overall (or mean) Pa,O_2 and Pa,CO_2 will result from a flow-weighted averaging of the respective gas contents from each individual blood "stream". However, it is important to recognise in this regard that account has also to be taken of the shape of the O_2 and CO_2 dissociation curves in order to derive these $\bar{P}a,O_2$ and $\bar{P}a,CO_2$ values (fig. 5).

Owing to the sigmoid shape of the O_2 dissociation curve, low $V'A/Q'$ regions lead both to low PO_2 and low O_2 content in pulmonary end-capillary blood; in contrast, while high $V'A/Q'$ regions lead to a high Pc',O_2, Cc',O_2 is only slightly increased above normal value because the O_2 dissociation curve is relatively flat in this range (fig. 5). Mixing blood from low $V'A/Q'$ regions with blood from high $V'A/Q'$ regions will therefore result in an average Pa,O_2 that is "weighted" towards low $V'A/Q'$ blood values (fig. 5). The $\bar{P}a,O_2$ will also depend on the volumes of blood from each "region" contributing to the mixed arterial blood. Thus, the high $V'A/Q'$

regions (even if Hb is completely saturated) are unable to "compensate" for the low $V'A/Q'$ regions, as their perfusion is usually less. Consequently, even though the overall $V'A/Q'$ may be normal, $V'A/Q'$ maldistribution results in arterial hypoxaemia, with mean Pa,O_2 being lower than the actual mean PA,O_2 or its "ideal" representation; *i.e.* $PA\text{-}a,O_2$ is widened.

In contrast, the CO_2 dissociation curve is essentially linear in the physiological range (fig. 5). This therefore allows the hyperventilatory effects of the high $V'A/Q'$ regions to better counterbalance the hypoventilatory effects of the low $V'A/Q'$ regions on the resulting mean Pa,CO_2 (fig. 5). It should be noted, however, that the high $V'A/Q'$ regions exert a proportionally greater influence on mean PA,CO_2 than do the low $V'A/Q'$ regions. Hence, $PA,CO_2 < Pa,CO_2$.

The pattern of arterial blood and alveolar gas tensions in $V'A/Q'$ maldistribution is such that with mild or moderate maldistribution, Pa,O_2 is low, $PA\text{-}a,O_2$ is widened, with Pa,CO_2 being normal or low depending on the degree of ventilatory stimulation consequent to the hypoxaemia. In severe $V'A/Q'$ impairment associated with severe airways obstruction, hypoventilation can ensue owing to the increased work of breathing, and therefore cause an increased Pa,CO_2. This, of course, reduces Pa,O_2 even more.

References

- D'Angelo E. Dynamics. *In*: Milic-Emili J, ed. Respiratory Mechanics. *Eur Respir Mon* 1999; 12: 54-67.
- Farhi LE. Ventilation-perfusion relationships. *In*: Farhi LE, Tenney SM, eds. Handbook of Physiology. The Respiratory System, Mechanics of Breathing, vol. IV. Bethesda, MD, American Physiological Society, 1986; pp. 199-215.
- Hughes JMB. Diffusive gas exchange. *In*: Whipp BJ, Wasserman K, eds. Pulmonary Physiology and Pathophysiology of Exercise. New York, Dekker, 1991; pp. 143-171.
- Klas JV, Dempsey JA. Voluntary *versus* reflex regulation of maximal exercise flow: volume loops. *Am Rev Respir Dis* 1989; 139: 150-156.
- Maina JN, West JB. Thin and strong! The bioengineering dilemma in the structural and functional design of the blood-gas barrier. *Physiol Rev* 2005; 85: 811-844.
- Mead J, Agostoni E. Dynamics of breathing. *In*: Fenn WO, Rahn H, eds. Handbook of Physiology, Respiration, vol. 1. Washington DC, American Physiological Society, 1964; pp. 411-427.
- Nunn JF. Applied Respiratory Physiology, 4th Edn. Oxford, Butterworth-Heinemann, 1993.
- Otis AB. The work of breathing. *In*: Fenn WO, Rahn H, eds. Handbook of Physiology, Respiration, vol. 1. Washington DC, American Physiological Society, 1964; pp. 592-607.
- Piiper J, Scheid P. Boold gas equilibration in lungs. *In*: West JB, ed. Pulmonary Gas Exchange, Vol. II. New York, Academic Press, 1998: 132-161.
- Pride NB, Macklem PT. Lung mechanics in disease. *In*: Macklem PT, Mead J, eds. Handbook of Physiology. The Respiratory System, Mechanics of Breathing, vol. III, part 2. Bethesda, MD, American Physiological Society, 1986; pp. 659-692.
- Riley RL, Cournand A. "Ideal" alveolar air and the analysis of ventilation-perfusion relationships in the lung. *J Appl Physiol* 1949; 1: 825-847.
- Rodarte JR, Rehder K. Dynamics of respiration. *In*: Macklem PT, Mead J, eds. Handbook of Physiology. The Respiratory System, Mechanics of Breathing, vol. III, part 1. Bethesda, MD, American Physiological Society, 1986; pp. 131-144.
- Weibel ER. Pathway for Oxygen. Cambridge, MA, Harvard University Press. 1984.
- West JB. Ventilation/Blood Flow and Gas Exchange. Oxford, Blackwell, 1990.
- West JB, Wagner PD. Pulmonary gas exchange. Am J Respir Crit Care Med 1998; 157: S82-S87.
- Whipp BJ. The physiology and pathophysiology of gas exchange. *In*: Bittar EE, ed. Pulmonary Biology in Health and Disease. New York, Springer-Verlag, 2002; pp. 189-217.

IMMUNOLOGY AND DEFENCE MECHANISMS

B. Balbi, C. Vicari and A. Di Stefano
Fondazione Salvatore Maugeri, I.R.C.C.S., Veruno, Italy
E-mail: bbalbi@fsm.it

Each day, 10,000–15,000 L of air is inhaled by the respiratory system. This air contains micro-organisms and pollutant gases and particles. It is conceivable therefore that adequate and efficient immunological and defence mechanisms exist inside the respiratory system to avoid damage to its structure, and to limit the number, extent and severity of upper and lower respiratory tract (URT and LRT) infections.

The first line of defence against pathogens is represented by the epithelial barrier of the airways. Additional protection comes from polypeptide mediators of the innate, non-antibody-mediated host defence and by professional phagocytes. Once the innate host defence system is activated, also by the cytokine and chemokine pathways, acquired antibody-mediated immune responses and subsequent tissue repair and remodelling following infection are orchestrated by immunocompetent cells and mediators.

Anatomical barriers

The density of microbes is greater in the URT than in the LRT. In fact, it is usually considered that only a small number of bacteria are present in the LRT of healthy individuals. This process of exclusion of bacteria is also due to mechanical barriers and reflex mechanisms. The nose itself can be considered a first-line barrier. Its vibrissae, present on the vestibular region of the nasal cavity, are able to filter the largest particles contained in inhaled air. Nasal mucosa is a type of respiratory mucosa able to trap other smaller particles by means of its mucus layer. Nasal cilia are able to transport the mucus

Key points

- An integrated system of innate, intrinsic and adaptive acquired defences protects the lungs from injury by inhaled pathogens or substances.

- The components of the system range from mechanical barriers and reflexes to antimicrobial molecules, professional phagocytes and acquired immune reactions.

- Impairments of the system underly a range of respiratory disorders.

toward the oro-pharynx to be swallowed. LRT airways represent a system with a physical barrier that is difficult to overcome. Dichotomous branching and angulation of airways favour the impact of inhaled particles on to the bronchial mucosa surface. At points of impact, bronchial-associated lymphoid tissue (BALT) is able to interact with inhaled airborne microbes and particles, and to start clearance processes *via* phagocytes and immune reactions by immunocompetent cells.

Reflex mechanisms

A number of reflex mechanisms may help the defence of the respiratory tract. They are made possible by the presence of irritant and stretching receptors on the mucosa of the airways of the URT and of the larger LRT. Sneezing is a complex reflex initiated by the irritant receptors in the nose, usually triggered by inhaled particles, followed by itching, mucus secretion and ultimately leading to a forceful and sudden expiration through the nose, preceded by a deep and fast inspiration, able to eliminate the potentially harmful inhaled particles. In the tracheobronchial tree, the cough reflex plays a similar role in eliminating foreign inhaled particles (see the article on Cough and sputum). Dyspnoea can also be considered, at least under certain circumstances, to be a defence mechanism, as it can result from both hypersecretion of mucus and/or bronchospasm. By reducing the airway calibre, both are able to impair the ability of inhaled harmful particles to reach the LRT.

Mucociliary clearance and fluid homeostasis

The constant mechanical clearance of mucus from the airways is considered a primary airway defence mechanism. The airway epithelial surface is able to act through ciliary function and mucus secretion with proper salt/water components in order to maintain the mucociliary clearance with a mucus "escalator" from the lower airways to the top. With a mucus layer at the top containing different types of mucins and a largely aqueous layer at the bottom, the airway secretions are, under normal conditions, able to entrap the vast majority of inhaled foreign particles and microbes on the mucus layer and to transport the mucus up to the larger airways to be swallowed or eliminated by coughing. More recent studies have emphasised the role of a "chemical shield" from inhaled bacteria. This view underlines the importance of the production and secretion into the airway lumen by the airway epithelia of two components: salt-sensitive defensins (see below) and low-salt liquid able to activate defensins.

Innate defence molecules

The epithelial lining fluid in the airways and in the lung contains myriad molecules, peptides and proteins exerting innate antimicrobial activities, not only against bacteria and viruses but also, in some cases, against fungi and parasites. As a whole, although these innate antimicrobial molecules have many differences depending on the site and cell types producing them, secretory stimuli, and direct and indirect activities (table 1), they provide an evolutionarily highly conserved and powerful screen against infections in the naive host. They also trigger more specific and targeted immune reactions taking place in the airways and alveolar structures. In addition, the same molecules have a role as immune-modulators, and as antioxidants and antiproteases. Not surprisingly, attempts have been made to use some of these "natural antibiotics" for therapeutic purposes.

Professional phagocytes

Microbial pathogens activate pattern recognition cell receptors (*e.g.* toll-like receptors, scavenger receptors, *etc*.) on phagocytes, namely macrophages and neutrophils, and also epithelial cells, mast cells, eosinophils and natural killer cells. This is followed by the release of several mediators and factors with effector functions and inflammatory cascades, such as the complementary acute phase reactant proteins, oxidative and nitrosative stress molecules, prostaglandins, interferons, cytokines and chemokines. Macrophages are the resident respiratory phagocytes. Although they are present throughout the airways and interstitium, their major roles are played in the alveolar spaces, as alveolar macrophages (AMs). In normal people, the vast majority of cells recovered through bronchoalveolar lavage (BAL) are AMs. These cells initiate and orchestrate the immune reactions against pathogens and chemicals inhaled by the host (*e.g.* mineral particles). In a hypothetical model of infection by a bacterial species, a pathogen that has reached the alveolar space, eluding URT and LRT first-line defences, represents a risk for the host as its replication and associated alveolar inflammation may damage respiratory structures. This invader microorganism will ultimately be enmeshed with the epithelial lining fluid and thus be coated with opsonins. The latter can be either nonimmune (see previous paragraph) or

Table 1. Key antimicrobial factors in epithelial lining fluid and their activities

Factors, structures	Cell origin	Antimicrobial activities	Main immuno-modulatory activities
Defensins, peptides	Phagocytic cells, lymphocytes, airway epithelial cells	BC, BS, AV, AF, AP	Mitogenic, CT, degranulate MC
Cathelicidins, pro-peptides	Neutrophils, monocytes, MC, lymphocytes, airway epithelial cells	BC, BS, AV, AF	Downregulation of TNF-α, CT
SLPI, protein	Macrophages, neutrophils, airway epithelial cells	BC, BS, AV	Antiprotease
SPA, SPD lipoproteins	Alveolar type II cells, Clara cells	BC, BS, AV, AF	Opsonin, modulate leukocyte functions, structural barrier
Lactoferrin, glyco-protein	Neutrophils, airway epithelial cells	BC, BS, AV, AF, inhibits biofilm formation	Antioxidant, binds LPS
Lysozyme, enzyme	Neutrophils, airway epithelial cells	BC, BS	Unknown
Lactoperoxidase, enzyme	Airway epithelial cells	BC, AV, AF	Antioxidant?

BC: bactericidal; BS: bacteriostatic; AV: anti-viral; AF: anti-fungal; AP: anti-parasitic; CT: chemotaxis; MC: mast cells; TNF: tumour necrosis factor; LPS: lipopolysaccharide.

immune, *i.e.* specific immunoglobulins (Ig) originated by previous immunisation of the host against the pathogen. Opsonins facilitate AM phagocytosis and subsequent bacterial clearance by the intracellular killing systems of AMs. The size of the bacterial inoculum, their virulence and resistance and possibly deficits in the local immune mechanisms of the host may alternatively cause the failure, at least in a first round, of host defences. This will cause recruitment of additional phagocytes, as neutrophils, at sites of infection and sustain an immune and inflammatory reaction.

Acquired immune reactions with Ig, cytokine and chemokine production

Lymphoid tissue is present in the respiratory tract in different forms: tonsils and adenoids in the URT, lymph nodes in the mediastinum and hila, submucosal aggregates in branching points of the airways (BALT) and immunocompetent cells free on the airways and alveolar surface. BALT is also considered to be part of a lymphoid network common to other types of mucosa. In this model, an immunisation can occur at a distant site (*e.g.* gastrointestinal mucosa) and, by the recirculation of lymphocytes, protection can also be provided to the respiratory system. Acquired immune reactions also start in the lung, with the interaction between antigens and antigen-presenting cells (APC). In the lung, at least two types of APC exist: macrophages and dendritic cells. Dendritic cells are present in the bronchi, representing roughly 1% of epithelial cells, in the alveolar septa and in the interstitium. Together with a phagocytic function, they share with AMs the ability to process microbial proteins into small peptide fragments that are then transported on the cell surface together with major histocompatibility complex molecules. The complex between the major histocompatibility complex and antigenic epitopes is then presented to T-lymphocytes. Antigen

Table 2. Integrated host defence system in the respiratory tract

Intrinsic and innate host defences		Adaptive and acquired immune defences
Anatomical barriers and defence reflexes		S-IgA and other immune opsonins and antigen recognition and presentation
Mucociliary clearance and fluid homeostasis	**Pathogens and particles**	Cellular immunity and T- and B-lymphocytes
Innate defence molecules and nonimmune opsonins		Cytokine/chemokine production and networking
Professional phagocytes		Chemotactic influx of inflammatory, immunoeffector cells

S-IgA: secretory-IgA.

presentation is made through the T-cell receptor on the T-lymphocyte surface.

The antigen presentation initiates the production of immuno-enhancing cytokines and chemokines. Apart from the interleukins (ILs) and other mediators associated with the T-helper type I or II immune reactions, IL-17 is a pro-inflammatory cytokine mainly produced by T-lymphocytes with an important role in induction of the neutrophil-mediated protective immune response against bacteria or fungal pathogens. IL-17 seems to be an example of the crossroads between different host defence mechanisms, as it regulates cell-mediated immunity and induction of antimicrobial peptides, such as defensins.

The process of specific immune reaction described above also promotes adaptive B-lymphocyte proliferation and specific Ig production. The relative proportions of different Igs in the URT and LRT differ, and also differ compared with the blood. In the URT, IgA represents the vast majority of Igs, the latter as a whole being roughly 10% of the total proteins in airway secretions. Airway IgA is predominantly polymeric. Secretory IgA comprises two IgA monomers held together by a joining chain and by another glycoprotein, the secretory component produced by serous and epithelial cells. In contrast with the airways, IgG is predominant in the lung, as detected by BAL, representing roughly 5% of the total protein content in BAL fluid from normal individuals. IgM is present only in trace amounts, due to its large size.

Conclusions

The complex, integrated host defence system described and depicted in table 2 represents a superb model of how the human body is able to efficiently interact with the external environment in order to preserve its structure and function.

Conversely, impairment and/or dysfunction of each of the different and variously acting components of this system represents the pathogenetic basis for the development of many respiratory disorders. As an example, primary ciliary dyskinesia results in recurrent airway infections; cystic fibrosis is associated with dysfunction of mucociliary clearance and fluid homeostasis; while in chronic colonisation and/or infection of the airways and in inflammatory airway disorders, many different mechanisms undergo changes, enhancement or impairment.

To summarise, the respiratory system is exposed to a variety of microbiological, physical and chemical insults through inhaled air. Innate intrinsic and adaptive acquired host and immune defences cooperate in lowering the risk of being damaged for the respiratory structures in an integrated host defence system. In diseased states, one or more of these complex mechanisms can be impaired and/or dysfunctional.

References

- Bals R, Hiemstra PS. Innate immunity in the lung: how epithelial cells fight against respiratory pathogens. *Eur Respir J* 2004; 23: 327-333.
- Di Stefano A, *et al*. T helper type 17-related cytokine expression is increased in the bronchial mucosa of stable chronic obstructive pulmonary disease patients. *Clin Exp Immunol* 2009; 157: 316-324.
- Knowles MR, Boucher RC. Mucus clearance as a primary innate defense mechanism for mammalian airways. *J Clin Invest* 2002; 109: 571-577.
- Martin TR, Frevert CW. Innate immunity in the lungs. *Proc Am Thorac Soc* 2005; 2: 403-411.
- Matsuzaki G, Umemura M. Interleukin-17 as an effector molecule of innate and acquired immunity against infections. *Microbiol Immunol* 2007; 51: 1139-1147.
- McCormack FX, Whitsett JA. The pulmonary collectins, SP-A and SP-D, orchestrate innate immunity in the lung. *J Clin Invest* 2002; 109: 707-712.
- Oppenheim JJ, *et al*. Roles of antimicrobial peptides such as defensins in innate and adaptive immunity. *Ann Rheum Dis* 2003; 26: ii17-ii21.
- Pignatti P, *et al*. Tracheostomy and related host-pathogen interaction are associated with airway inflammation as characterised by tracheal aspirate analysis. *Respir Med* 2009; 103: 201-208.
- Reynolds HY. Integrated host defense against infections. *In:* Crystal RG, *et al.*, eds. The Lung: Scientific Foundation. Philadelphia, Lippincott-Raven Publishers, 1997; pp. 2353-2365.
- Rogan MP, *et al*. Antimicrobial proteins and polypoptides in pulmonary innate defence. *Respir Res* 2006; 7: 29-40.
- Whitsett JA. Intrinsic and innate defenses in the lung: intersection of pathways regulating lung morphogenesis, host defense, and repair. *J Clin Invest* 2002; 109: 565-569.
- Yang D, *et al*. Participation of mammalian defensins and cathelicidins in antimicrobial immunity: receptors and activities of human defensins and cathelicidin (LL-37). *J Leuk Biol* 2001; 69: 691-697.
- Zanetti M. The role of cathelicidins in the innate host defenses of mammals. *Curr Issues Mol Biol* 2005; 7: 179-196.

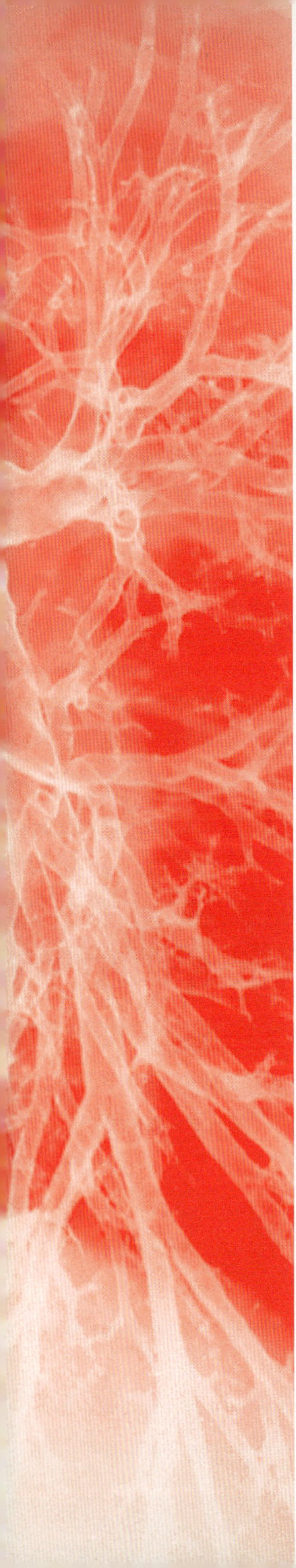

CHAPTER 2:

SIGNS AND SYMPTOMS

COUGH AND SPUTUM   **34**
A.H. Morice

DYSPNOEA   **41**
G. Scano and P. Laveneziana

CHEST PAIN   **49**
M. Hind

PHYSICAL EXAMINATION IN   **51**
RESPIRATORY MEDICINE
M.R. Partridge

COUGH AND SPUTUM

A.H. Morice
Hull York Medical School, University of Hull, Hull, UK
E-mail: a.h.morice@hull.ac.uk

Cough is a vital protective mechanism defending the airways from inhalation and aspiration. Patients with a defective cough reflex, such as those with stroke or Parkinson's disease, have an increase in mortality and morbidity caused by the increased propensity for aspiration. However, in lung disease, cough is often not helpful. Thus, in the commonest form of cough, that due to upper respiratory tract infection, coughing serves no useful purpose from the sufferer's point of view, but is useful for the virus aiding its transmission to the next victim. In chronic cough, the frequency and severity of coughing bouts may cause serious disruption to the patient's life. Quality-of-life instruments have indicated that patients with chronic cough may have a similar decrement to that seen with conditions such as cancer and chronic obstructive pulmonary disease. Cough may have significant comorbidity. 50% of the females attending cough clinics are incontinent and cough syncope is thought to be responsible for a number of driving fatalities.

Acute cough

Acute cough due to one of the myriad upper respiratory tract viruses places an enormous demand on the healthcare community. It is the commonest new presentation to primary care, accounting for 50% of consultations. In temperate regions there is a marked seasonal variation with autumn and winter epidemics. Viral transmission requires person-to-person contact, either through airborne droplet infection or the manual passage of secretions. Superimposed on this seasonal pattern are peaks caused by socialisation, *e.g.* return to school for the autumn term and Christmas family gatherings. Apart from general health measures, such as hand washing and avoidance of contact, there is no specific treatment for upper respiratory tract infection-induced cough. The demonstrable effect of the many cough remedies is likely to be due to a physicochemical (demulcent) effect rather than through a specific pharmacological action of any particular agent.

Chronic cough

Chronic cough is one of the commonest presentations to the respiratory physician. A survey in Yorkshire, UK, indicated that 12% of the normal population complain of a chronic cough and 7% of these thought it interfered with activities of daily living. Many reports from specialist cough clinics point to a particular syndrome in patients with chronic cough. The average patient is middle-aged and female. The cough appears to have no pattern to it but a careful history will often reveal many features in common with other patients' presentation. It has been traditional to divide this group of patients who have chronic cough without radiographic abnormalities and no obvious other lung disease into a triad of diagnoses, namely asthmatic cough, post-nasal drip syndrome

---

Key points

- Cough is characterised by irritant receptor hypersensitivity.
- Nonacid reflux into the airways frequently precipitates cough.
- Clinical history followed by therapeutic trials is the management strategy of choice.

Table 1. Early reports from cough clinics illustrating the variety of cough diagnosis dependent on criteria used

First author, year	Mean age yrs	Patients n (female n)	Diagnosis (% of total)		
			Asthma syndrome	GOR	Rhinitis
Irwin 1981	50.3	49 (27)	25	10	29
Poe 1982	-	109 (68)	36	0	8
Poe 1989	44.8	139 (84)	35	5	26
Irwin 1990	51	102 (59)	24	21	41
Hoffstein 1994	47	228 (139)	25	24	26
O'Connell 1994	49	87 (63)	6	10	13
Smyrnios 1995	58	71 (32)	24	15	40
Mello 1996	53.1	88 (64)	14	40	38
Marchesani 1998	51	92 (72)	14	5	56
McGarvey 1998	47.5	43 (29)	23	19	21
Palombini 1999	57	78 (51)	59	41	58
Brightling 1999	-	91 (-)	31	8	24

The typical patient is a middle-aged female. These diagnoses are now thought to represent phenotypes of the cough hypersensitivity syndrome. GOR: gastro-oesophageal reflux. Studies can be found in Morice et al. (2004).

and reflux cough (table 1). These subdivisions have recently been called into question. For example, asthmatic cough is unlike classic atopic asthma in that it is of late onset without obvious precipitants and often without evidence of bronchoconstriction. In the form known as eosinophilic bronchitis there is even an absence of bronchial hyperreactivity. Similar caveats apply to the post-nasal drip syndrome and reflux cough, which does not conform to the criteria for heartburn-related gastro-oesophageal reflux disease. Because of the commonality of the clinical history (see table 2), it has been suggested that there is a single unifying diagnosis in chronic cough of the cough hypersensitivity syndrome with the other diagnoses representing different phenotypes of the condition. The risk factors for chronic cough suggest that nonacid reflux may be an important precipitant (see table 3).

Virtually all patients presenting with a chronic cough complain of increased sensitivity to a wide range of environmental stimuli. This hypersensitivity can be objectively demonstrated in the laboratory using cough

Table 2. Areas of enquiry in chronic cough

Hoarseness or a problem with your voice
Clearing your throat
The feeling of something dripping down the back of your nose or throat
Retching or vomiting when you cough
Cough on first lying down or bending over
Chest tightness or wheeze when coughing
Heartburn, indigestion, stomach acid coming up or do you take medications for this?
A tickle in your throat, or a lump in your throat
Cough with eating (during or soon after meals)
Cough with certain foods
Cough when you get out of bed in the morning
Cough brought on by singing or speaking (for example, on the telephone)
Coughing more when awake rather than asleep
A strange taste in your mouth

Responses may either lead to further questioning or be scored 0-5 and used as a diagnostic tool to demonstrate the presence of cough hypersensitivity syndrome. A questionnaire version in various languages is available at www.issc.info

challenge. Thus patients cough with ethanol inhalation, whereas normal subjects do not. There is a wide variation in cough reflex sensitivity in normal subjects, with females being more sensitive than males. Sensitivity is accentuated in cough patients. Inhalation of capsaicin, the pungent extract of peppers, is typically used to demonstrate cough reflex responsiveness (fig. 1). Capsaicin works by stimulating one of a family of nociceptors of the transient receptor potential group (fig. 2). The capsaicin sensitive "hot" receptor (TRPV1) is up-regulated in patients with cough. This is due to pro-inflammatory mediators increasing expression of TRPV1, either on the neurones or in other airway tissues. Rather than directly causing a cough, angiotensin-converting enzyme inhibitors alter cough sensitivity by a TRPV1-dependent mechanism explaining the continued irritation long after drug withdrawal. Another transient receptor potential (TRP) receptor, TRPA1 is highly reactive to a wide range of environmental irritants and causes cough in man. Up-regulation of this receptor provides a mechanism the hypersensitivity in patients to agonist such as acreolin, the pro-tussive ingredient in smoke.

Management of chronic cough

All patients presenting with chronic cough should have a chest radiograph. The clinical history should indicate the most likely treatment options. The European Respiratory Society guidelines recommend therapeutic trials based on clinical judgement. Thus, in patients with episodes of wheezing and evidence of eosinophilic inflammation a trial of asthmatic medication may well be beneficial (fig. 3). Where available, exhaled nitric oxide fraction may be a useful screening tool. Bronchoconstriction may not be a major

Table 3. Risk factors for chronic cough

Variable	With cough n (%)	Unadjusted OR	95% CI	p-value
Sex				
Male	78/1704 (4.6)	1.0	1.03–1.86	0.028
Female	135/2179 (6.2)	1.38		
Heartburn				
No	148/2990 (4.9)	1.0	1.10–2.06	0.009
Yes	65/889 (7.3)	1.51		
Regurgitation				
No	158/3314 (4.8)	1.0	1.49–2.92	<0.0001
Yes	54/568 (9.5)	2.10		
IBS				
No	111/2914 (3.8)	1.0	2.27–4.09	<0.0001
Yes	98/909 (10.8)	3.05		
BMI category				
Normal	74/1547 (4.8)	1.0		
Overweight	72/1448 (5.0)	1.04	0.74–1.47	0.86
Obese	60/776 (7.7)	1.67	1.15–2.41	0.006

Nonacid reflux symptoms in the form of regurgitation are more closely associated with cough than acid reflux. OR: odds ratio; CI: confidence interval; IBS: irritable bowel syndrome.

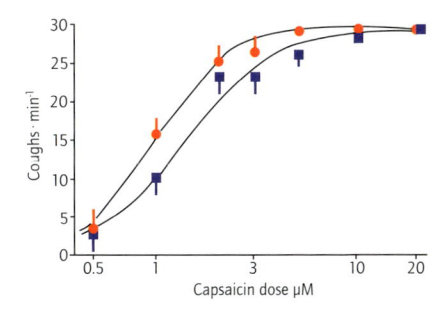

Figure 1. Capsaicin cough challenge in normal subjects. The effect of capropril increasing cough reflex sensitivity. ■: placebo; ●: captopril.

Sputum

In subjects with chronic cough, production of moderate amounts of sputum does not alter the diagnostic profile. The separation from individuals with excessive sputum production is arbitrary, but is generally regarded as a cup of sputum per day. Above this limit a diagnosis of bronchiectasis becomes increasingly likely. The presence of sputum purulence indicates a greater likelihood, but does not seem to predict the degree of anatomical damage to the airway. Indeed the diagnosis of bronchiectasis, relying as it does on the dilation and destruction of the airways, will not include many patients with functional abnormalities of the bronchi.

component of this phenotype of the cough hypersensitivity syndrome and consequently long-acting β-agonists may be less effective than anti-eosinophilic medication such as leukotriene antagonists. Reflux disease may be very problematical since much airway reflux is nonacidic and therefore not amenable to blockade by proton pump inhibitors. Pro-motility agents such as metoclopramide and domperidone may be used. Other motility agents such as erythromycin and magnesium have also been advocated. Finally, operative treatment *via* Nissan fundoplication can be effective in intractable coughing. An alternative strategy is to use cough suppression in the form of anti-tussive agents such as low-dose morphine. This has been demonstrated to ameliorate cough in a third of patients with otherwise intractable symptoms.

In conditions characterised by sputum hypersecretion, there is usually a change in the composition of the mucus. Several mechanisms are responsible for this change. Thus in cystic fibrosis the increase in sodium reabsorption leads to a reduction in the sol phase of airway surface liquid. Airway inflammation, particularly caused by release of enzymes such as myeloperoxidase (which produces the characteristic green colour) and neutral endopeptidase and from polymorphs causes alteration of MUC gene expression through proteinase activated receptors. The death of inflammatory cells and bacteria lead to a soup of DNA which cross-links with filamentous actin-producing gelatinous plugs which increases ventilation/perfusion ratio mismatch with resulting systemic hypoxia.

HOT					COLD
55°C	43°C	33°C	30°C	25°C	17°C
TRPV2	TRPV1	TRPV3	TRPV4	TRPM8	TRPA1
VRL1	VR1 capsaicin protons	VRL3	VR-OAZ OTRPC4 osmotic	CMR1 cold/menthol	Coexpressed with VR1 acreolin cinnamaldehyde etc.

Figure 2. The thermosensitive transient receptor potential (TRP) channels important in cough reflex sensitivity.

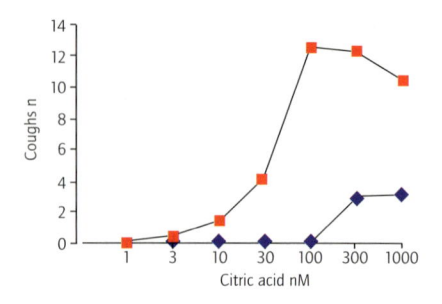

Figure 3. Cough challenge with citric acid in eosinophilic bronchitis and the response to inhaled steroids. ■: number of coughs off budesonide; ◆: number of coughs on budesonide.

The treatment of mucus hyper-secretion may be challenging. In the presence of purulent sputum, every effort should be made to identify the causative organism. Eradication with appropriate high-dose antibiotic therapy may lead to sustained remission. More frequently there is rapid relapse indication the need for maintenance antibiotics either orally or via the nebulised route. The advantage of this latter strategy is that side-effects may be minimised by using agents with high local potency but poor oral bioavailability such as colomycin or tobramycin. Antioxidant mucolytics are widely prescribed but evidence of efficacy is limited. The largest study of N-acetylcysteine over 3 yrs showed no effect on decline in lung function or exacerbation rate.

Haemoptysis

Haemoptysis presents in two clinical scenarios. First, the patient may present with de novo haemoptysis without pre-existing lung disease. Any mucosal lesion may cause haemoptysis of small amounts of blood mixed with sputum. Since a common presentation of this is lung cancer, chest radiography is obligatory in patients when presenting with haemoptysis. Aspergiloma and tuberculosis may similarly cause a blood-stained bronchitis. More peripheral lung pathology, such as lobar pneumonia, gives rise to sputum that is frequently described as 'rusty'. Haemoptysis of frank blood is a common sign of pulmonary embolism or infarction.

Obviously recurrent haemoptysis initially presents with acute haemoptysis. Typically, bronchiectasis leads to recurrent, sometimes massive and occasionally fatal haemoptysis. The bronchial blood supply arises from the aorta and, in contrast to the pulmonary circulation, is at systemic pressure. In bronchiectasis there is hypertrophy of the bronchial arteries as a consequence of recurrent infection. When the patient presents with life-threatening haemoptysis, percutaneous bronchial artery embolisation is the treatment of choice. Vasculitis is a common and frequently missed cause of recurrent haemoptysis and diffuse alveolar haemorrhage. Whilst the systemic connective tissue diseases, such as systemic lupus erythematosus, may produce small vessel haemoptysis, the commonest cause is microcytic polyangiitis. The perinuclear anti-neutrophil cytoplasmic antibody (pANCA) is positive in ~70% of cases. Finally, haemoptysis may be the result of alveolar haemorrhage. Disease of the vascular or alveolar wall, such as Goodpasture's syndrome or alveolar haemosiderosis, may present with recurrent haemoptysis. Clearly, disorders of coagulation, such as warfarin therapy or thrombocytopenia, will predispose to haemoptysis.

References

- Birrell MA, et al. TRPA1 agonists evoke coughing in guinea-pig and human volunteers. Am J Respir Crit Care Med 2009; 180: 1042–1047.
- Decramer M, et al. Effects of N-acetylcysteine on outcomes in chronic obstructive pulmonary disease (Bronchitis Randomized on NAC Cost-Utility Study, BRONCUS): a randomised placebo-controlled trial. Lancet 2005; 365: 1552–1560.
- Ford AC, et al. Cough in the community: a cross sectional survey and the relationship to gastrointestinal symptoms. Thorax 2006; 61: 975–979.
- Millqvist E, et al. Inhaled ethanol potentiates the cough response to capsaicin in patients with airway sensory hyperreactivity. Pulm Pharmacol Ther 2008; 21: 794–797.

- Mitchell JE, *et al.* Expression and characterization of the intracellular vanilloid receptor (TRPV1) in bronchi from patients with chronic cough. *Exp Lung Res* 2005; 31: 295-306.
- Morice AH. The cough hypersensitivity syndrome: a novel paradigm for understanding cough. *Lung* 2010; 188: 87-90.
- Morice AH, *et al.* Opiate therapy in chronic cough. *Am J Respir Crit Care Med* 2007; 175: 312-315.
- Morice AH, *et al.* The diagnosis and management of chronic cough. *Eur Respir J* 2004; 24: 481-492.
- Palombini BC, *et al.* A pathogenic triad in chronic cough: asthma, postnasal drip syndrome, and gastroesophageal reflux disease. *Chest* 1999; 116: 279-284.
- Rogers DF. Physiology of airway mucus secretion and pathophysiology of hypersecretion. *Respir Care* 2007; 52: 1134-1146.

DYSPNOEA

G. Scano and P. Laveneziana
Dept of Pulmonary Rehabilitation, Fondazione Don C. Gnocchi, and Dept of Internal Medicine, Section of Immunology and Respiratory Medicine, University of Florence, Florence, Italy
E-mail: pier_lav@yahoo.it

Key points

- Dyspnoea is a subjective experience of breathing discomfort that consists of qualitatively distinct sensations that vary in intensity.

- Its aetiology can be elucidated to some degree by taking a medical history and physical examination.

- The mechanisms of dyspnoea are complex and multifactorial – there is no unique central or peripheral source of this symptom.

- The sense of heightened inspiratory effort is an integral component of exertional dyspnoea and is pervasive across health and disease.

- The neuroventilatory dissociation (NVD) theory of dyspnoea states that the symptom arises when there is a disparity between the central reflexic drive (efferent discharge) and the simultaneous afferent feedback from a multitude of peripheral sensory receptors throughout the respiratory system. The feedback system provides information about the extent and appropriateness of the mechanical response to central drive.

- Despite the diversity of causes, the similarity of described experiences of dyspnoea suggests common underlying mechanisms.

Dyspnoea is the major reason for referral to pharmacological treatment and respiratory rehabilitation programmes in patients with chronic obstructive pulmonary disease (COPD). Dyspnoea is a subjective experience of breathing difficulty that consists of qualitatively distinct sensations that vary in intensity. This definition underlines the importance of the different qualities (cluster descriptors) covered by the term dyspnoea, the involvement of integration of multiple sources of neural information about breathing and the physiological consequences.

Aetiology

Dyspnoea has many pulmonary, cardiac and other causes, which vary by acuity of onset (tables 1 and 2).

Different causes of dyspnoea are associated with derangements of a number of functions and apparatus:

- Alveoli
- Ventilatory pump
- Upper and lower airways
- Pulmonary vasculature
- Cardiac pump
- Red blood cells
- Peripheral circulation
- Skeletal muscles

It is important to remember that the most common cause of dyspnoea in patients with chronic pulmonary or cardiac disorders is an exacerbation of their underlying disease.

Table 1. Some common causes of acute (within minutes) and subacute (within hours or days) dyspnoea

	Suggestive findings
Acute cause	
Pulmonary causes	
Pneumothorax	Abrupt onset of sharp chest pain, tachypnoea, diminished breath sounds, and hyperresonance to percussion. May follow injury or occur spontaneously (especially in tall, thin patients and in those with COPD).
Pulmonary embolism	Abrupt onset of sharp chest pain, tachypnoea and tachycardia. Often risk factors for pulmonary embolism (*e.g.* cancer, immobilisation, deep venous thrombosis, pregnancy, use of oral contraceptives or other oestrogen-containing drugs, recent surgery or hospitalisation, family history).
Asthma, bronchospasm, or reactive airway disease	Wheezing and poor air exchange that arise spontaneously or after exposure to specific stimuli (*e.g.* allergen, upper respiratory infection, cold, exercise). Possibly pulsus paradoxus. Often a pre-existing history of reactive airway disease.
Foreign body inhalation	Sudden onset of cough or stridor in a patient (typically an infant or young child) without upper respiratory infection or constitutional symptoms.
Cardiac causes	
Acute myocardial ischaemia or infarction	Substernal chest pressure with or without radiation to the arm or jaw, particularly in patients with risk factors for CAD.
Heart failure	Crackles, S_3 gallop and signs of central or peripheral volume overload (*e.g.* elevated neck veins, peripheral oedema). Orthopnea or appearing 1–2 h after falling asleep (paroxysmal nocturnal dyspnoea).
Other causes	
Diaphragmatic paralysis	Sudden onset after trauma affecting the phrenic nerve. Frequent orthopnoea.
Anxiety disorder-hyperventilation	Situational dyspnoea often accompanied by psychomotor agitation and paresthesias in the fingers or around the mouth. Normal examination findings and pulse oximetry measurements.
Subacute cause	
Pulmonary causes	
Pneumonia	Fever, productive cough, dyspnoea, sometimes pleuritic chest pain. Focal lung findings, including crackles, decreased breath sounds and egophony.
COPD exacerbation	Cough, productive or nonproductive. Poor air movement. Accessory muscle use or pursed lip breathing.
Cardiac causes	
Angina or CAD	Substernal chest pressure with or without radiation to the arm or jaw, often provoked by physical exertion, particularly in patients with risk factors for CAD.
Pericardial effusion or tamponade	Muffled heart sounds or enlarged cardiac silhouette in patients with risk factors for pericardial effusion (*e.g.* cancer, pericarditis, systemic lupus erythematosus). Possibly pulsus paradoxus.

COPD: chronic obstructive pulmonary disease; CAD: coronary artery disease; S_3: 3rd heart sound.

Table 2. Some common causes of chronic (hours to years) dyspnoea

	Suggestive findings
Pulmonary causes	
Obstructive lung disease	Extensive smoking history, barrel chest and poor air entry and exit.
Restrictive lung disease	Progressive dyspnoea in patients with known occupational exposure or neurological condition.
Interstitial lung disease	Fine crackles on auscultation.
Pleural effusion	Pleuritic chest pain and lung field that is dull to percussion with diminished breath sounds. Sometimes history of cancer, heart failure, rheumatoid arthritis, systemic lupus erythematosus, or acute pneumonia.
Cardiac causes	
Heart failure	Crackles, S_3 gallop and signs of central or peripheral volume overload (*e.g.* elevated neck veins, peripheral oedema). Orthopnea or paroxysmal nocturnal dyspnoea.
Stable angina or CAD	Substernal chest pressure with or without radiation to the arm or jaw, often provoked by physical exertion, particularly in patients with risk factors for CAD.
Other causes	
Anaemia	Dyspnoea on exertion progressing to dyspnoea at rest. Normal lung examination and pulse oximetry measurement. Sometimes systolic heart murmur due to increased flow.
Physical deconditioning	Dyspnoea only on exertion in patients with sedentary lifestyle.

CAD: coronary artery disease; S_3: 3rd heart sound.

Medical history

It is important to ask patients how long they have had dyspnoea and in what situations it occurs. Therefore, clinical history should cover the duration, temporal onset (*e.g.* abrupt, insidious), and provoking or exacerbating factors (*e.g.* allergen exposure, cold, exertion, supine position). Severity of dyspnoea can be determined by assessing the activity level required to produce dyspnoea (*i.e.* dyspnoea at rest is more severe than dyspnoea only with climbing stairs). For this purpose, the Medical Research Council dyspnoea scale can be used (table 3), along with other scales such as the Baseline Dyspnoea Index (BDI). For patients with baseline dyspnoea, the physician should note how much dyspnoea has changed from the patient's usual state. Dyspnoea can also be evaluated during a physical task, such as cardiopulmonary exercise testing. For this purpose, the 10-point Borg scale can be used (table 3). In the Borg scale, the end-points are anchored such that zero represents "no breathlessness at all" and 10 is "the most severe breathlessness that one had ever experienced or could imagine experiencing". By pointing to the Borg scale, subjects rate the magnitude of their perceived breathing discomfort during exercise. Most patients with dyspnoea, not just those with heart failure, feel worse when they lie down (orthopnea).

The physician should seek symptoms of possible causes, including chest pain (pulmonary embolism, myocardial ischaemia, pneumonia); dependent oedema, orthopnea and paroxysmal nocturnal dyspnoea (heart failure); fever, chills, cough and sputum production (pneumonia); black, tarry stools or heavy menses (occult bleeding possibly causing anaemia); and weight loss or night sweats (cancer or chronic lung infection). Past medical history should cover disorders known to cause dyspnoea, including asthma, COPD

Table 3. The Medical Research Council (MRC) dyspnoea scale and the Borg scale

MRC Grade	Description
1	Not troubled by breathlessness except with strenuous exercise
2	Troubled by shortness of breath when hurrying on the level or walking up a slight hill
3	Walks slower than people of the same age on the level because of breathlessness or has to stop for breath when walking at own pace on the level
4	Stops for breath after walking ~90 m or after a few minutes on the level
5	Too breathless to leave the house or breathlessness when dressing or undressing
Borg scale	**Severity**
0	No breathlessness at all
0.5	Very very slight (just noticeable)
1	Very slight
2	Slight breathlessness
3	Moderate
4	Somewhat severe
5	Severe breathlessness
6	
7	Very severe breathlessness
8	
9	Very very severe (almost maximum)
10	Maximum

and heart disease, as well as risk factors for the different aetiologies:

- smoking history for cancer, COPD and heart disease.
- family history, hypertension and high cholesterol levels for coronary artery disease.
- recent immobilisation or surgery, recent long-distance travel, cancer or risk factors for or signs of occult cancer, prior or family history of clotting, pregnancy, oral contraceptive use, calf pain, leg swelling and known deep venous thrombosis for pulmonary embolism.

Occupational exposures (*e.g.* gases, smoke and asbestos) should also be investigated.

Physical examination

The history and physical examination often suggest a cause and guide further testing. Physical examination focuses on the cardiovascular and pulmonary systems. A full lung examination is done, particularly including adequacy of air entry and exit, symmetry of breath sounds, and presence of crackles, rhonchi, stridor and wheezes. Wheezing suggests asthma or COPD. Stridor suggests extrathoracic airway obstruction (*e.g.* foreign body, epiglottitis, vocal cord dysfunction). In-drawing of the lower ribcage towards the end of inspiration (Stock or Hoover's sign) suggests (but does not prove) the presence of chronic lung hyperinflation from COPD. Paradoxical inspiratory inward motion of the abdomen is seen in bilateral diaphragm paralysis (easier to see when the patients are lying down and/or when they sniff). The presence of contraction of the accessory muscles when the patient is at rest could make the physician think of a more generalised muscle or nerve problem which has affected the diaphragm and the intercostals and parasternal muscles.

Inspiratory squeaks usually mean extrinsic allergic alveolitis, although sometimes they are heard in bronchiectasis. Crackles suggest left heart failure, interstitial lung disease or, if accompanied by signs of consolidation (*e.g.* egophony, dullness to percussion), pneumonia. The cervical, supraclavicular and inguinal areas should be inspected and palpated for lymphadenopathy. Neck veins should be inspected for distension (suggestive of heart failure, pulmonary embolism or pulmonary hypertension), and the legs and presacral area should be palpated for pitting oedema (suggesting heart failure). Heart sounds should be auscultated with notation of any extra heart sounds, muffled heart sounds, or murmur. It should be remembered, however, that signs and symptoms of life-threatening conditions, such as myocardial ischaemia and pulmonary embolism, can be nonspecific. Furthermore, the severity of symptoms is not always proportional to the severity of the cause (*e.g.* pulmonary embolism in a fit, healthy person may cause only mild dyspnoea). Thus, a high degree of suspicion for these common conditions is prudent. It is often appropriate to rule out these conditions before attributing dyspnoea to a less serious aetiology. A clinical prediction rule can help estimate the risk for pulmonary embolism. Note that a normal oxygen saturation does not exclude pulmonary embolism. Hyperventilation syndrome is a diagnosis of exclusion. Because hypoxia may cause tachypnoea and agitation, it is unwise to assume every rapidly breathing, anxious young person merely has hyperventilation syndrome.

Physiology

To gain more insight into our understanding of dyspnoea, a case can be made for answering the following questions: 1) what is the role of mechanical factors and ventilatory constraints in dyspnoea?; 2) what are the neurophysiological underpinnings of the most selected cluster descriptors that define the qualitative dimension of dyspnoea in patients?; 3) do obstructive and restrictive lung diseases share some common underlying mechanisms?

Dyspnoea is perceived as a sense of effort During voluntary increase in ventilation, the motor cortex increases the outgoing motor signal to respiratory muscles and conveys a copy (central corollary discharge) through cortical interneurones to the sensory/association cortex, which is informed of the voluntary effort to increase ventilation. It is also likely that the sense of the respiratory effort arises from the simultaneous activation of the sensory cortex and muscle contraction: a variety of muscle receptors provides feedback to the central nervous system about force and tension, and information from these receptors may conceivably underlie the sense of effort. For clinical purposes the perceived magnitude of respiratory effort is expressed by the ratio of the tidal oesophageal pressure (P_{oes}) to the maximal pressure generation capacity of the respiratory muscles ($P_{I,max}$). In healthy subjects, volitional respiratory effort is matched with lung/chest wall displacement (i.e. change in tidal volume percentage vital capacity) via concurrent afferent proprioceptive information, transmitted via vagal, glossopharyngeal, spinal and phrenic nerves, that monitors displacement and is processed and integrated in the sensory cortex. The result is a harmonious neuromechanical coupling (NMC) with avoidance of respiratory discomfort or distress.

Dyspnoea is perceived as a sense of air hunger Under some clinical and experimental circumstances the relationship between dyspnoea and effort is less apparent. If normal subjects suppress their ventilation to a level below that dictated by chemical drive (CO_2), dyspnoea increases without corresponding increases in indices of respiratory effort. Likewise, in experimental and clinical conditions where peripheral stretch receptors are inhibited, the sensory cortex is not informed of the ventilatory response. In these circumstances, dyspnoea is perceived as a sensation of air hunger whose intensity depends on a mismatching between the level of chemical stimulated drive and ongoing inhibition from pulmonary mechanosensors signalling the current level of ventilation. In turn, dyspnoea arises and may qualitatively change when peripheral afferent feedback is altered and inspiratory motor output either increases or stabilises.

Pathophysiology

COPD Two clusters of dyspnoea are commonly selected by patients with COPD during physical activity.

The cluster respiratory effort is commonly selected by patients with COPD. Acute mechanical loading and functional respiratory muscle weakness decrease $P_{I,max}$, and further increase P_{oes} percentage $P_{I,max}$. Furthermore, because of the limbic system activation, the corollary discharge may be sensed as abnormal, thus evoking a sensation of distress.

The other cluster is unsatisfied inspiration. Structural abnormalities (chronic bronchitis and emphysema) *via* their physiological negative consequences, *i.e.* expiratory flow limitation and dynamic hyperinflation, result in dyspnoea. A patient's physical activity is indeed characterised by a mismatch between increase in neural output to the respiratory muscles and lung/chest wall displacement. We call this mismatch neuroventilatory dissociation (NVD). In a clinical setting, the slope that defines NVD (*i.e.* effort *versus* displacement) is steeper and shifted upward compared with healthy subjects. The steeper the slope, the greater the intensity of dyspnoea (fig. 1). In particular, patients experience intolerable dyspnoea during exercise because tidal volume expansion is constrained from below (by the effects of dynamic lung hyperinflation) as there is no space to breathe. This so-called dyspnoea threshold seems to be at the level at which the inspiratory reserve volume approaches 0.5 L. In turn, unsatisfied inspiration reflects a discrepancy between high ventilatory drive and ventilation less than that dictated by the respiratory drive. The data support the central importance of mechanical restriction in causing dyspnoea in COPD patients.

Neuromuscular disorders (NMD) Patients with NMD exhibit heightened neuromotor output, which is sensed as increased respiratory muscle effort and, as such, is likely to be the principal mechanism of dyspnoea in NMD. Nonetheless, a significant positive relationship between increased dyspnoea per unit increase in ventilation and dynamic elastance affects the coupling between respiratory effort and displacement (fig. 2).

Interstitial lung disease (ILD) One of the characteristic features of ILD is a reduction in lung compliance and lung volumes. The mechanical response of the respiratory system is similarly restricted in patients with ILD as in those with COPD: tidal volume expansion is constrained from above (reflecting the reduced total lung capacity and inspiratory reserve volume), which results in greater reliance on an increase in breathing frequency to increase ventilation. Differences in dynamic ventilatory mechanics, including possible expiratory flow limitation in some patients, account for distinct qualitative perception in ILD patients, namely inspiratory difficulty and

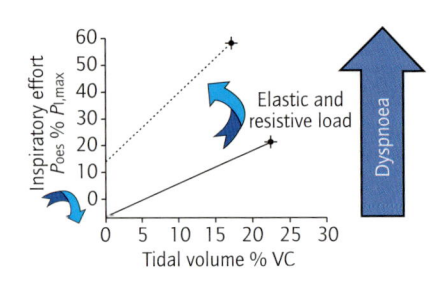

Figure 1. Neuroventilatory dissociation. The slope that defines the mismatch between increase in neural output (inspiratory effort, *i.e.* P_{oes} %$P_{I,max}$) and lung/chest wall displacement (tidal volume, %VC) is steeper and shifted upwards in patients with COPD (- - - -) compared with healthy subjects (——). P_{oes}: tidal oesophageal pressure; $P_{I,max}$: maximal pressure generation capacity of the respiratory muscles.

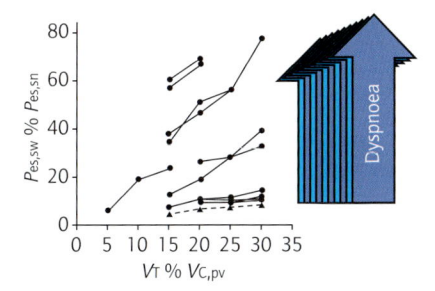

Figure 2. A mismatch between inspiratory effort ($P_{oes,sw}$ % $P_{oes,sn}$) and lung/chest wall displacement (V_T %$V_{C,pv}$) in patients with NMD (—) as compared with average data from controls (- - - -). The steeper the slopes the greater the perception of dyspnoea. $P_{oes,sw}$: swing in oesophageal pressure; $P_{oes,sn}$: oesophageal pressure during a sniff manoeuvre; V_T: tidal volume; $V_{C,pv}$: predicted values of vital capacity.

rapid shallow breathing. Because of increase in both dynamic elastance and efferent respiratory drive, inspiratory difficulty may have its psychophysical basis in the conscious awareness of a dissociation between respiratory effort and the mechanical response, *i.e.* inability to expand tidal volume appropriately in the face of an increased drive to breathe. In turn, the possibility has also been put forward that intensity of exertional dyspnoea in ILD is more closely linked to mechanical constraints on volume expansion than to indexes of inspiratory effort *per se*.

Chronic heart failure (CHF) The key message that has emerged from therapeutic intervention studies in patients with CHF is that exertional dyspnoea alleviation is consistently associated with reduced excessive ventilatory demand (secondary to reduced central neural drive), improved respiratory mechanics and muscle function and, consequently, enhanced neuromechanical coupling of the respiratory system during exercise. Pressure support is reported to reduce the tidal inspiratory pleural pressure–time slope without affecting submaximal dyspnoea ratings but allows patients to exercise for additional minutes without experiencing any significant rise in dyspnoea.

The available data suggest that increased ventilatory demand, abnormal dynamic ventilatory mechanics and respiratory muscle dysfunction are instrumental in causing exertional dyspnoea in patients with severe cardiac impairment.

Obesity An increase in respiratory neural drive is deemed to be the reason for the similar increase in dyspnoea in obese and lean subjects. However, different underlying mechanisms may affect dyspnoea in obese subjects. Exercise performance is impaired compared with healthy normal-weight subjects when corrected for the increased lean body mass, but normal when expressed as a percentage of predicted for ideal body weight in subjects who hyperinflate the lungs to the same extent as those obese subjects who deflate the lungs, with both volume subgroups reaching similar dyspnoea scores. In "hyperinflators", dynamic hyperinflation along with a decrease in inspiratory reserve volume increases respiratory muscle loading, respiratory drive and perception of respiratory discomfort. In contrast, "deflators" exhibit a negative relationship between resting end-expiratory lung volume (EELV) and perceptual respiratory response during exercise: the lower the EELV the greater the Borg score. A low resting EELV has three important consequences linked together during exercise: 1) decrease in expiratory reserve volume, 2) dynamic airway compression, and 3) changes in transmural airway pressure resulting in airway dynamic compression. Thus, an alteration in the central drive to the respiratory muscles in response to afferent activity from upper airway mechanoreceptors may also contribute to the unpleasant respiratory sensation in obese subjects.

Diabetes A study on respiratory muscle effort and load has helped elucidate the pathophysiology of dyspnoea during hypoxic stimulation of ventilation in type I diabetes mellitus. The study shows that because of an increase in dynamic elastance, the greater perception of dyspnoea is associated with changes in inspiratory effort, which is out of proportion with changes in tidal volume in patients with no smoking history.

Conclusions

We are still a long way from understanding the symptom of dyspnoea. Although mechanical factors are important contributors to dyspnoea, the precise mechanisms of dyspnoea remain obscure. One approach to the study of this symptom is to identify the major qualitative dimensions of the symptom in an attempt to uncover different underlying neurophysiological mechanisms. The remarkable similarity in choices of qualitative descriptors (work/effort, inspiratory difficulty/ unsatisfied inspiration, air hunger, rapid breathing) for exertional dyspnoea in patients with restrictive and obstructive syndromes raises the intriguing possibility that they share some common underlying mechanisms.

References

- DeLorey DS, et al. Mild to moderate obesity: implications for respiratory mechanics at rest and during exercise in young men. *Int J Obes (Lond)* 2005; 29: 1039-1047.
- Killian KJ, Campbell EJM. Dyspnoea. *In*: Roussos C, ed. The Thorax, part B. New York, Dekker, 1995; pp. 1709-1747.
- Lanini B, et al. Perception of dyspnea in patients with neuromuscular disease. *Chest* 2001; 120: 402-408.
- Laveneziana P, et al. Effect of biventricular pacing on ventilatory and perceptual responses to exercise in patients with stable chronic heart failure. *J Appl Physiol* 2009; 106: 1574-1583.
- O'Donnell DE, et al. Pathophysiology of dyspnea in chronic obstructive pulmonary disease. *Proc Am Thorac Soc* 2007; 4: 145-168.
- O'Donnell DE, et al. Qualitative aspects of exertional breathlessness in chronic airflow limitation: pathophysiologic mechanisms. *Am J Respir Crit Care Med* 1997; 155: 109-115.
- O'Donnell DE, et al. Qualitative aspects of exertional dyspnoea in patients with interstitial lung disease. *J Appl Physiol* 1998; 84: 2000-2009.
- O'Donnell DE, et al. Sensory-mechanical relationships during high intensity, constant-work-rate exercise in COPD. *J Appl Physiol* 2006; 101: 1025-1035.
- O'Donnell DE, et al. Ventilatory assistance improves exercise endurance in stable congestive heart failure. *Am J Resp Crit Care Med* 1999; 160: 1804-1811.
- Ofir D, et al. Ventilatory and perceptual responses to cycle exercise in obese females. *J Appl Physiol* 2007; 102: 2217-2226.
- Romagnoli I, et al. Role of hyperinflation vs deflation on dyspnea in severely to extremely obese subjects. *Acta Physiol* 2008; 193: 393-402.
- Scano G, et al. Dyspnoea, peripheral airway involvement and respiratory muscle effort in patients with type I diabetes mellitus under good metabolic control. *Clin Sci* 1999; 96: 499-506.
- Scano G, et al. Understanding dyspnoea by its language. *Eur Respir J* 2005; 25: 380-385.

CHEST PAIN

M. Hind
NIHR Advanced Lung Diseases Unit, Royal Brompton and Harefield NHS Foundation Trust, London, UK
E-mail: M.Hind@rbht.nhs.uk

Chest pain is a frequent symptom of illness and a common reason for seeking medical attention. Rapid assessment is crucial so that life-threatening disease, such as cardiac chest pain, aortic dissection and oesophogeal rupture, can be identified and managed appropriately. A basic history often points to the cause and is used in triage of patients attending emergency rooms. Questions are typically asked about the character, location, radiation, severity, exacerbating and relieving factors of the pain, and its relationship to movements such as breathing or coughing. Objective assessment using a questionnaire, such as the McGill Pain score can be useful. Occasionally, it is difficult to tease out differences between cardiac, gastrointestinal and respiratory causes of pain.

The pathophysiology of chest pain is complex and not completely understood but involves peripheral noiciceptors, either small Aδ myelinated or unmyelinated C afferent fibres that project *via* sympathetic and para-sympathetic nerves into the dorsal horn of the spinal cord. These neurones synapse with spinothalamic fibres which ascend, cross the spinal cord and terminate in the contralateral ventero-posterior thalamic nucleus. Thalamo-cortical neurons project *via* the posterior limb of the internal capsule to the somatosensory cortex. The diaphragm has dual noiciceptive sensory innervation from both the phrenic nerve and the lower six intercostal nerves, therefore diaphragmatic irritation can present with pain referred to the shoulder or upper abdomen. The trachea and large airways have afferent fibres that project along the vagus nerve. Respiratory chest pain can therefore originate from the chest wall, pleura, large airways and mediastinum, but visceral "lung" pain is unusual.

> **Key points**
>
> - Chest pain can be a feature of a wide range of pathology
> - An accurate history is essential to direct appropriate investigation of patients presenting with chest pain

Pleural pain is often described as sharp, stabbing and made worse by movement such as deep respiration. The pain is often unilateral, reflecting the site of the disease. A pleural rub may be heard. Pleuritic pain with sudden onset prompts a diagnosis of pulmonary emboli, infarction or pneumothorax, whereas pleuritic pain building over a few hours may suggest infection such as pneumonia or pleurisy. Onset over days suggests empyema, malignancy or tuberculosis.

Tracheobronchitis can present with a midline burning pain made worse with respiration. Massive mediastinal lymphadenopathy can cause an indistinct, heavy central chest pain. Similarly, chest pain associated with pulmonary hypertension can be difficult to distinguish from cardiac chest pain. Nondescript, heavy chest pain is quite common in exacerbations of bronchiectasis.

Chest wall pain is usually well localised, reproduced with movement and associated with tenderness. Costo-condritis and Tietze's syndrome are inflammatory disorders of thoracic joints that present with chest wall pain and tenderness. Bornholm disease (epidemic pleurodynia or devil's grip), often associated with Coxsackie B virus, can present with epidemics of chest wall pain of sudden onset.

Neuralgic pain can be sharp and knife-like or dull and heavy, and there may be associated sensory symptoms. Pain in a dermatomal distribution requires examination of overlying skin for the characteristic vesicular rash of herpes zoster.

ECG is essential for immediate assessment of cardiac chest pain. Further investigation may include exercise ECG, stress echocardiography or myocardial perfusion scan. Angiography offers the opportunity for therapeutic angioplasty and stent insertion.

Chest radiographs are useful to identify consolidation, pneumothorax, pleural effusion, and bony abnormalities such as vertebral fractures. Contrast computed tomography scanning has made identification of pulmonary emboli, aortic dissection and oesophogeal rupture straightforward, and can identify abnormalities often missed on plain radiographs. Nuclear medicine scans have a role in both diagnosis and management of pulmonary emboli. Bone scintigraphy is useful in evaluation of 'bony' pain. Magnetic resonance examination is of particular use in visualising nerve roots. Direct endoscopic visualisation of either the upper gastointestinal tract (oesophagogastroduodenoscopy) or major airways (bronchoscopy) allows epithelial inspection and offers the opportunity for direct microbiological, cytological and histological sampling.

Reference

- Melzack R, The McGill Pain Questionnaire: major properties and scoring methods. *Pain* 1975; 1: 277–299.

PHYSICAL EXAMINATION IN RESPIRATORY MEDICINE

M.R. Partridge
Imperial College, London, UK
E-mail: m.partridge@imperial.ac.uk

Physical findings in the context of the history

The purpose of clinical assessment is to make an accurate diagnosis. Making an accurate diagnosis in cases of respiratory disease can be challenging not only because of the diversity of respiratory ill-health, but also because symptoms of respiratory disease are shared with disorders of other body systems.

Breathlessness (a sensation of difficult, laboured or uncomfortable breathing) may have a physiological or psychological explanation but it is extremely important that every time we are faced with a patient complaining of shortness of breath we consider the following points.

Is this patient breathless because of:

- Heart disease?
- Lung disease?
- Pulmonary vascular disease?
- A systemic disorder (anaemia, obesity or hyperthyroidism), or
- Respiratory muscle weakness

It is vital that we go through this checklist both with new presentations of the symptom of breathlessness and also in those with established disease, and we need to bear this list in mind when examining the patient. The patient with chronic obstructive pulmonary disease might this time be breathless, not because of an exacerbation, but because they have gone into atrial fibrillation; or the patient with known heart failure may this time be breathless because of a complicating pneumonia.

Asking specifically about the onset of the symptom of breathlessness can be helpful in the differential diagnostic process and this is summarised in table 1.

Cough

A practical approach to the assessment of cough and breathlessness is summarised in fig. 1.

Physical examination

In the vast majority of cases, the taking of the medical history should lead to the

Key points

- It is essential to bear in mind that breathlessness can have a variety of causes.
- Physical examination should follow the taking of the medical history and differential diagnoses, and is an opportunity to confirm normality or discover abnormality.
- Physical examination comprises inspection, palpation, auscultation and percussion.
- The respiratory physician must not forget that other systems may also be the cause of the symptoms and that comorbidity is common.

Table 1. Breathlessness: differential diagnosis according to onset

Within minutes	Think: pulmonary embolus, pneumothorax, myocardial infarction, cardiac rhythm disturbance, dissecting aneurysm, acute asthma
Over hours or days	Think: pneumonia, pleural effusion, LVF (LV dysfunction or valve dysfunction or septal rupture post-MI), asthma, blood loss, lobar collapse, respiratory muscle weakness (Guillain-Barré syndrome)
Over weeks	Think: infiltration (malignancy, sarcoidosis, fibrosing alveolitis, extrinsic allergic alveolitis, eosinophilic pneumonia), respiratory muscle weakness (motor neurone disease), main airway obstruction, anaemia, valvular dysfunction (SBE)
Over months	Think: same as for weeks plus obesity, muscular dystrophy, asbestos-related conditions.
Over years	Think: COPD, chest wall deformity, heart valve dysfunction, obesity.

LVF: left ventricular failure; MI: myocardial infarction; SBE: subacute bacterial endocarditis; COPD: chronic obstructive pulmonary disease.

construction of a list of differential diagnoses. The examination is then an opportunity either to confirm normality or to discover abnormalities consistent with one or other of one's differential diagnoses. Key features, as with all clinical examination, depend upon inspection, palpation, auscultation and percussion.

Inspection

On inspection the key points to observe are:

- General appearance (breathlessness? cachetic?)
- Respiratory rate
- Appearances of the hand (finger clubbing? tremor? tobacco staining? flapping tremor suggestive of CO_2 retention?)
- Does the chest wall move symmetrically?
- Are there any chest wall deformities (scoliosis, pectus excavatum) or scars?
- Any abnormal vessels suggestive of superior vena cava obstruction (fig. 2)?
- Nasal stuffiness or obstruction should be noted.
- A note should be made of the neck/collar size and also of obvious jaw abnormalities and oropharyngeal abnormalities.

Palpation

This involves the following:

- Assessment of chest expansion, where we may be able to elicit reduced expansion symmetrically suggestive of hyperinflation, or reduced movement on one side suggesting localised pathology on that side.
- Determining the position of the trachea by inserting the index and middle fingers in the supra sternal notch.
- Examining the cervical and supra clavicular lymph nodes for enlargement.
- Assessing vocal fremitus by asking the patient to loudly and deeply repeat the words '99' whilst you compare both sides of the chest. Voice sounds are better transmitted through consolidated lung than normal lung and poorly transmitted through pleural effusions.

Percussion

Percussion is often poorly undertaken and the key features are to make the movement of your finger as a stroke from the wrist and strike firmly at right angles upon the finger of the other hand which lies along the intercostal space, and to do so in a symmetrical manner systematically comparing both sides of the chest at a point equidistant

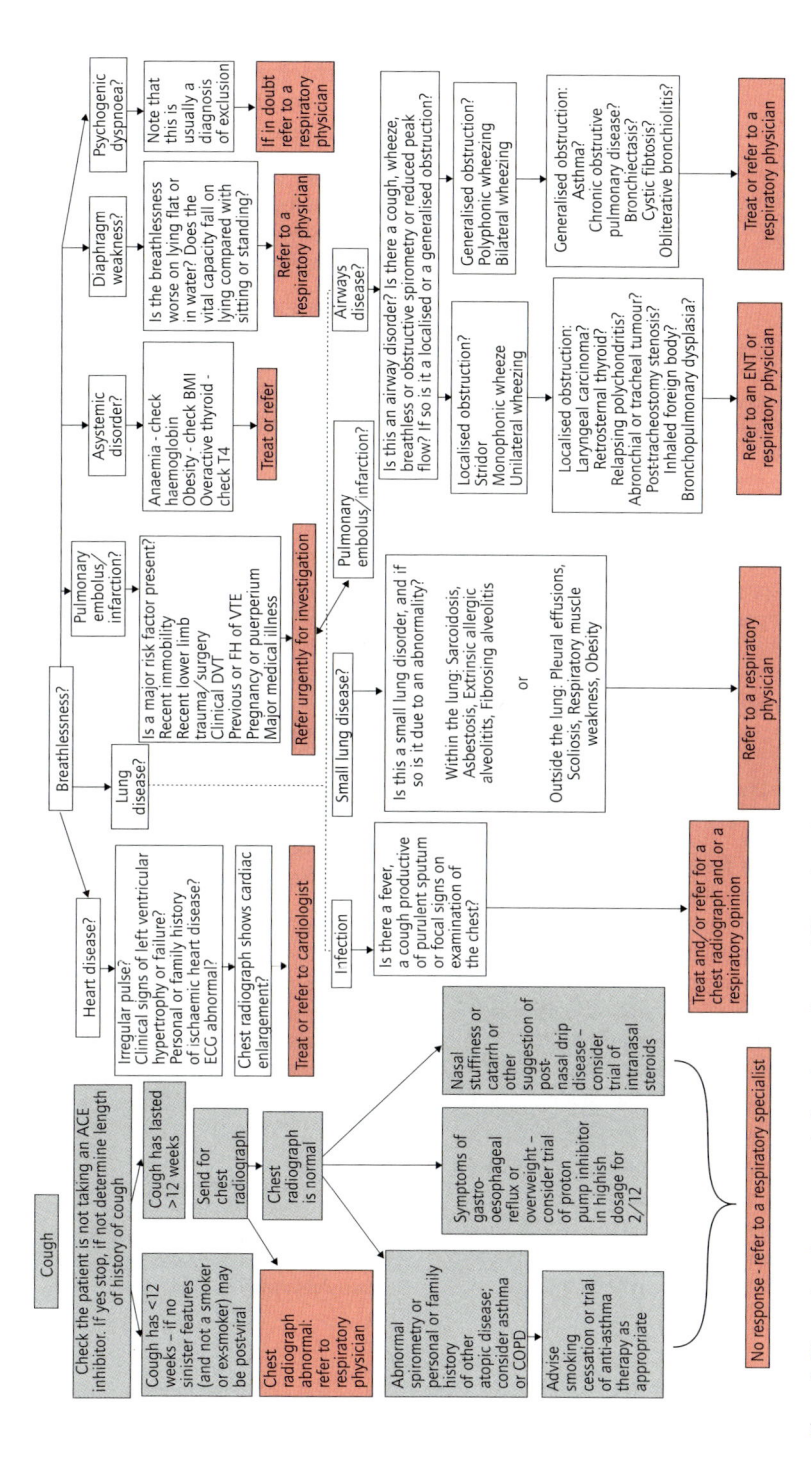

Figure 1. Diagnosis and management of respiratory disease. ACE: angiotensin-converting enzyme; DVT: deep vein thrombosis; FH: family history; VTE: venous thromboembolism; BMI: body mass index; COPD: chronic obstructive pulmonary disease; ENT: ear-nose-throat.

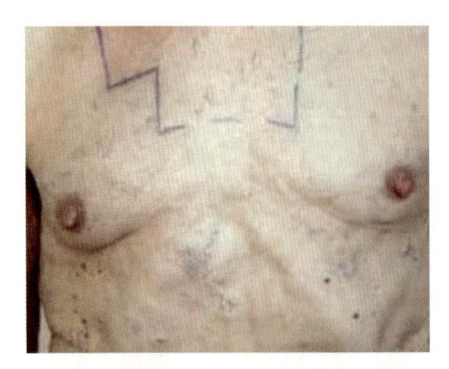

Figure 2. Dilated vessels over the anterior chest wall are often the most obvious pointer to superior vena cava obstruction, with the other features being a raised jugular venous pressure, which is nonpulsatile.

from the midline. The percussion note may be hyper-resonant symmetrically in patients with underlying hyperinflated lungs or asymmetrically in a large pneumothorax, or may be dull in cases of consolidation or pleural effusion.

Auscultation

Listening to the breath sounds involves the following:

- Checking for the presence of bronchial breathing, which is the presence of breath sounds that are similar to those heard over the large central airways in a more peripheral location. Bronchial breathing is classically heard over a consolidated lung (and in association with dullness to percussion), but is also sometimes heard over the upper aspect of a pleural effusion and sometimes over a collapsed lung.
- Determining whether there are or are not any abnormal added sounds, which may be musical sounds (wheezing) or crackles. In cases of wheezing, it is important to determine whether the wheezing is *poly-phonic and bilateral*, as in asthma or COPD, or *monophonic and localised*, as may be found in cases of lung cancer or bronchial stenosis or inhaled foreign bodies.
- Crackles may be *fine* and occur in cases of interstitial lung disease or acutely in cases of pulmonary oedema, or *coarse*, as often heard in patients with bronchiectasis.
- Pleural rubs sound like a squeaky noise, are usually localised and clearly vary in intensity with respiration. Care in interpreting a noise as a pleural rub is necessary in very thin patients where the diaphragm of the stethoscope may move over the ribs.
- Vocal resonance is found under the same circumstances as vocal fremitus, and when found in conjunction with bronchial breathing is highly suggestive of consolidation. Some physicians find detection of whispering pectoriloquoy (WP) a more definite sign; to elicit WP, one asks the patient to whisper '99' and, when it is present, for example, in cases of consolidation, the whispered sound is heard clearly over the chest wall when transmitted through consolidated lung whereas a normally air-filled lung would muffle the whispered sound and make it indistinct.

Finally, one should remember that disorders of other systems may coexist and, whilst examining the chest, one should especially look for evidence of heart and pulmonary vascular disease, noting signs of peripheral oedema and elevation of the jugular venous pressure.

References

- Gibson GJ, *et al.* Respiratory Medicine. Saunders Elsevier Science Ltd, 2002.
- Partridge MR. Understanding Respiratory Medicine: a Problem-Orientated Approach. Manson Publishing Ltd, 2006.

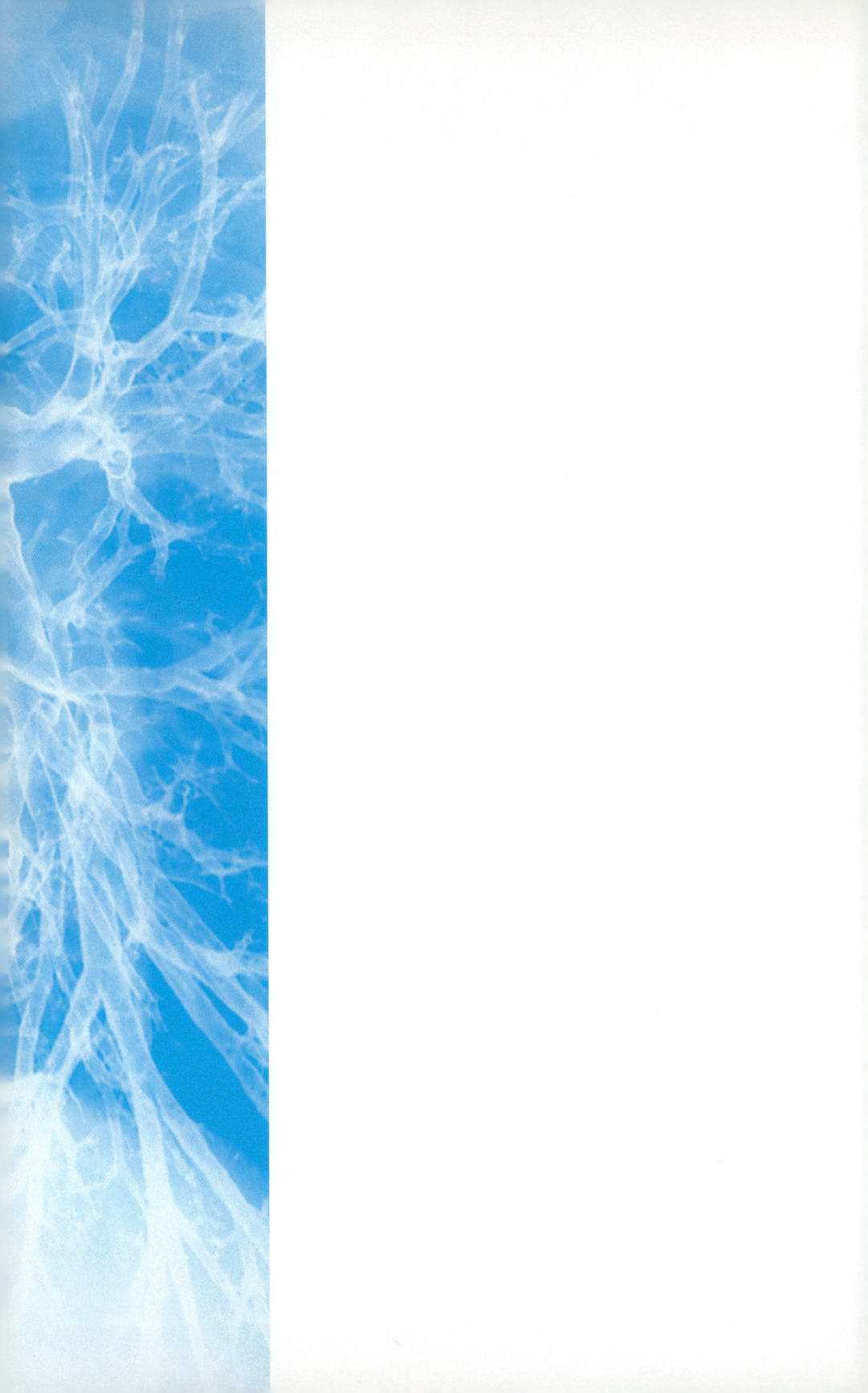

CHAPTER 3:

PULMONARY FUNCTION TESTING

STATIC AND DYNAMIC LUNG VOLUMES — 58
R. Pellegrino and A. Antonelli

RESPIRATORY MECHANICS — 63
D. Navajas and R. Farré

GAS TRANSFER ($T_{L,CO}$) — 68
J.M.B. Hughes

CONTROL OF VENTILATION — 72
B.J. Whipp

ARTERIAL BLOOD GAS ASSESSMENT — 77
P. Palange, A. Ferrazza and J. Roca

EXERCISE TESTING — 83
P. Palange

BRONCHIAL PROVOCATION TESTING — 88
K-H. Carlsen

SPUTUM AND EXHALED BREATH ANALYSIS — 92
O. Toungoussova, S. Dragonieri, A. Zanini and A. Spanevello

STATIC AND DYNAMIC LUNG VOLUMES

R. Pellegrino and A. Antonelli
Allergologia e Fisiopatologia Respiratoria, ASO S. Croce e Carle, Cuneo, Italy
E-mail: pellegrino.r@ospedale.cuneo.it

Ventilation is constrained by the mechanical properties of the airways, lung and chest wall. The latter two set up the volume at which the movement of gas is accomplished at rest and with daily activities, such as exercise, phonation, laughing, changes in body posture and others. However, with the occurrence of cardiopulmonary diseases, lung volumes may also be modified as a result of dynamic mechanisms within the airways and changes in breathing pattern in addition to static changes in lung and chest wall properties.

Determinants of lung volumes in health and disease

Tidal volume (V_T) is the volume of gas inspired during each breath (fig. 1) necessary to preserve gas exchange. In healthy subjects, inspiration is switched off by neural reflexes, whereas expiration is terminated near the relaxation volume (V_r) as a result of static or dynamic mechanisms (see section dedicated to functional residual capacity). Except during exercise, when a lack of increase in V_T with ventilation is a functional marker of ventilatory limitation, and perhaps in patients undergoing assisted ventilation, V_T has little clinical usefulness in clinical practice.

Total lung capacity (TLC) is the volume of gas contained in the lungs after a deep breath. It is determined by the maximum force exerted by the inspiratory muscles to balance lung and chest wall elastic recoils (figs 1 and 2).

In healthy conditions, TLC tends to remain fairly stable with ageing, presumably because the natural decrease of the force of the inspiratory muscles and/or the increase in chest wall stiffness are balanced by the progressive loss of lung elastic recoil.

In contrast, TLC tends to increase in emphysema and sometimes in chronic bronchitis and severe asthma. Though the decrease in lung elastic recoil is presumably the most important mechanism of the increase in TLC under these conditions, an increased force of the inspiratory muscles and chest wall remodelling may also play a role. Surprisingly, for the same level of airflow obstruction, TLC tends to increase during spontaneous long-lasting but not acutely induced bronchospasm. This is presumably because of the different time course necessary to produce airflow obstruction and hyperinflation. That this may be so is shown by a study documenting that when a resistive valve was implanted in the dog trachea, it took time for TLC to increase. Thus it is

---

Key points

Measurement of lung volumes in clinical practice has been proven to be important to assist in the following.

- Diagnosis of pulmonary defects.
- Evaluation of candidates for lung volume resection surgery.
- prognosis of COPD and interstitial lung diseases.
- Evaluation of the bronchomotor response to constrictor and dilator agents as well as to physical exercise.

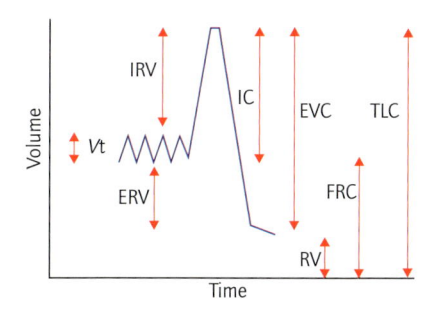

Figure 1. Lung volume plotted *versus* time. V_T: tidal volume; EVC: slow expiratory vital capacity; IRV and ERV: inspiratory and expiratory volume reserves, respectively; IC: inspiratory capacity; RV: residual volume; FRC: functional residual capacity; TLC: total lung capacity.

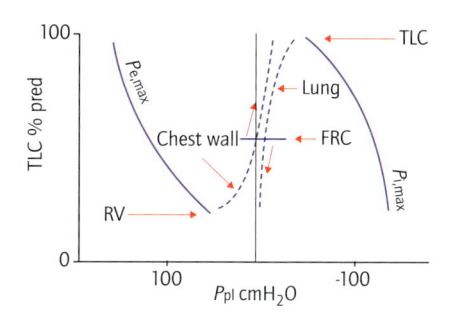

Figure 2. Quasi-static pressure–volume curves of the chest wall and the lung (dashed lines) related to pleural pressure (P_{pl}) generated during maximum inspiratory and expiratory static efforts ($P_{i,max}$ and $P_{e,max}$, respectively; continuous lines). Volume is expressed as % of total lung capacity (TLC). TLC is the volume at which $P_{i,max}$ equals the inward elastic recoils of both lung and chest wall. Residual volume (RV) is the volume at which $P_{e,max}$ overcomes the outward elastic recoil of the chest wall. Functional residual capacity (FRC) is the volume at which inward lung recoil equals outward chest wall recoil (arrows with opposite direction). % pred: % predicted.

possible that breathing at high lung volumes for long periods of time as a result of severe chronic airflow obstruction may also contribute to the increase in TLC.

TLC decreases in all conditions characterised by an increase in lung elastic recoil (*e.g.* pulmonary fibrosis, cardiac failure), chest wall stiffness (*e.g.* neuromuscular diseases, obesity, ascitis and pregnancy) or thoracic space competition (*e.g.* pleural effusions, pneumothorax).

Measuring TLC is of great importance in clinical practice as it allows identification of the restrictive pulmonary defects. In addition, TLC is also useful in the evaluation of an emphysematous patient as a candidate for lung volume resection surgery or for follow-up of interstitial lung diseases.

Residual volume (RV) is the volume of gas that remains in the lungs after a complete expiration. In young healthy individuals, RV is mostly determined by the balance between the force of the expiratory muscles and the outward recoil of the chest wall (figs 1 and 2). In the elderly, it increases as a result of airway closure.

In restrictive diseases, RV decreases in proportion to the increase in lung elastic or chest wall recoils and/or loss of lung parenchyma.

In obstructive pulmonary diseases, RV is higher than predicted because of premature airway closure, loss of lung elastic recoil, and stiffness of chest wall. Additional mechanisms may dynamically contribute to elevate RV in obstructive lung diseases. For instance, in patients with acutely induced or chronic airflow obstruction, RV achieved after a forced expiration is always higher than after a slow expiration. This is mainly because of two mechanisms. First, during forced expiration in airflow obstruction, expiratory flow limitation (EFL) occurs soon after initiation of the manoeuvre, especially within the airways that are already narrowed. In contrast, during a slow expiration, pleural pressure will exceed the critical pressure necessary to generate maximal flow, and thus EFL late on expiration and at a lower lung volume. Secondly, some airways could close near TLC early on expiration as a result of the disease, thus preventing the subtending alveolar units from emptying and contributing to increased RV.

Also, the effects of volume history of the manoeuvre preceding the expiration may

Static and dynamic lung volumes

affect RV. For instance, in healthy subjects or mild-to-moderate asthmatics exposed to a bronchoconstrictor agent, a manoeuvre initiated from TLC will generate greater flow and lower RV than a manoeuvre initiated from end-tidal inspiration. The opposite occurs in chronic airflow obstruction. This suggests that RV is also modulated through the changes in airway calibre caused by large lung inflations. How the deep inspiration manoeuvre affects lung and airways mechanics is still a matter of debate. When a deep breath is taken, the inflating stimulus is transmitted to the lung as well as the airways through the elastic network of lung parenchyma. According to FROEB and MEAD (1968), the effects of volume history on airway size depend on the mechanical characteristics of lung parenchyma and airways. Both tissues may lose energy or pressure and deform with stretching, a phenomenon named hysteresis. Since lung elastic recoil and transmural pressure are the forces that determine airway size, any change relative to one of these will necessarily entail a change in flow and RV. As shown in figure 3, if airway hysteresis exceeds parenchymal hysteresis, airway volume will be greater during deflation than inflation and RV will be achieved at a lower lung volume. This generally occurs when constriction is mostly limited to the airways and little affects lung parenchyma, such as with induced airway narrowing. In contrast, when lung parenchyma hysteresis is larger than airway hysteresis, airway volume will be reduced on expiration compared with inspiration and RV

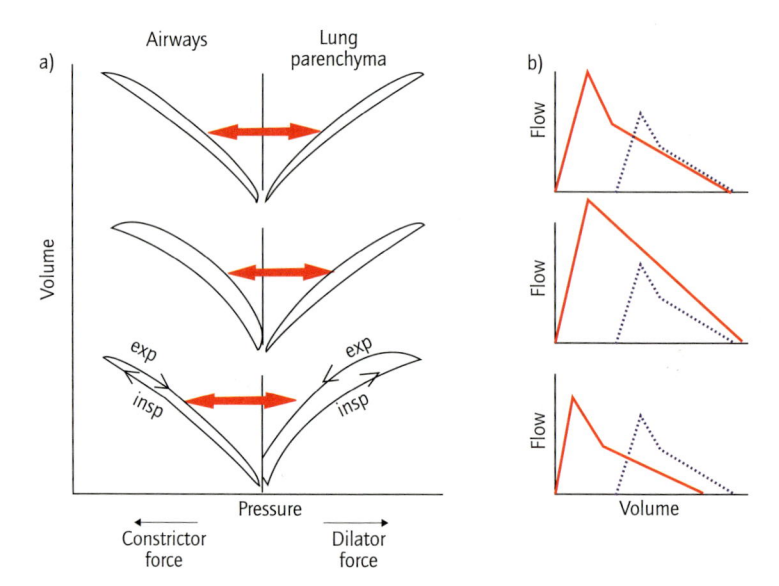

Figure 3. Effects of deep breath on maximum expiratory flow and residual volume according to the relative hysteresis theory of FROEB and MEAD (1968). a) Pressure–volume loops of lung parenchyma and airways on inspiration and expiration. The area inside the loop is called hysteresis. b) Partial and maximal flow–volume loops (dotted and continuous lines, respectively). Upper panels of a) and b): both hystereses are similar, so that the constrictor and dilator forces after the deep breath remain equal compared to before inflation. As a result, forced flow and residual volume during the maximum forced expiratory manoeuvre are the same of the partial manoeuvre. Central panels of a) and b): airway hysteresis prevails over lung hysteresis, so that the constrictor force is reduced after the large inflation. Consequently, for a given lung volume, maximum flow will exceed partial flow and residual volume will decrease more after a maximal compared to partial manoeuvre. Lower panels of a) and b): lung parenchyma hysteresis prevails over airway hysteresis, so that the dilator force will decrease after the deep breath. Under these conditions, forced expiratory flow and residual volume after a maximal manoeuvre will decrease and increase, respectively, compared to a partial manoeuvre. exp: expiration; insp: inspiration.

achieved at a higher volume. This is what presumably occurs in chronic airflow obstruction or severe ASM shortening. Finally, when airway and lung parenchyma hystereses change by similar extent, airway size will be similar before and after a deep breath and so will RV. The effects of volume history may be easily assessed *in vivo* by comparing forced expiratory manoeuvres initiated from total lung capacity and a volume below it (fig. 3b), or by changes in airflow resistance soon after taking a deep breath.

Vital capacity (VC) is the difference between TLC and RV. Because RV is dependent on volume and flow histories in addition to airway, parenchyma, and/or chest wall components of the diseases as discussed above, VC will depend on the type of respiratory manoeuvre from which it is taken and the underlying disease. In general, the largest VC is that obtained during a full inflation from RV (achieved after a slow expiration from end-tidal inspiration) to TLC (inspiratory vital capacity), followed by the slow expiratory vital capacity from TLC to RV (EVC), and the VC measured during a forced expiratory manoeuvre (forced vital capacity). A decrease of VC does not allow differentiation between restriction and obstruction, as it may be due to a decrease in TLC or an increase in RV, or both.

In clinical practice, VC is of central importance for the diagnosis of obstructive pulmonary defects.

Functional residual capacity (FRC) is the volume of gas remaining in the lungs at the end of a tidal expiration in a seated or upright position (fig. 1). Its mechanical determinants are the inward elastic recoil of the lung balancing the outward recoil of the chest wall (fig. 2). In supine position, the abdominal content is displaced towards the chest cavity, thus reducing FRC. Also during speech, singing, laughing or exercise FRC tends to decrease to favour these activities.

In obstructive pulmonary diseases, FRC tends to increase for a series of reasons. For instance, an increase in breathing frequency or in time constant of the respiratory system as a result of either an increase in airflow resistance or a decrease in lung compliance, will lead to an expiratory time relatively too short to allow the respiratory system to empty fully. Presumably, the occurrence of EFL during tidal expiration may also contribute to an increase in FRC to a lung volume where EFL is minimal. Under these circumstances, the dynamic compression of the airways downstream from the flow limiting segment may evoke neural reflexes that prematurely activate the inspiratory muscles to avoid breathing for too long a time under EFL conditions. On the one hand the increase in FRC in airflow obstruction is beneficial as it allows breathing at a volume where the airways are larger, thus decreasing the resistive work of breathing. On the other hand, however, breathing at high lung volume is associated with an increase in the elastic work of breathing and causes dyspnoea.

A decrease in FRC occurs in restrictive respiratory diseases due to an increase in lung elastic recoil (*e.g.* in pulmonary fibrosis, atelectasis, lung resection, alveolar liquid filling, cardiac diseases) or in chest wall elastance (*e.g.* in chest wall and pleural diseases, respiratory muscle paralysis, obesity).

Inspiratory capacity (IC) is the volume difference between TLC and FRC. In pulmonary diseases, it tends to decrease as a result of an increase in FRC (obstructive conditions) or a decrease in TLC (restrictive diseases), or both. In clinical practice, changes in IC with acute interventions on airway calibre, such as bronchoprovocation or reversibility tests, or during exercise, reflect mirror-like changes in FRC, assuming that TLC remains unmodified.

IC has no role in the diagnosis of ventilatory defects.

Expiratory and inspiratory reserve volumes are the volumes available to V_T to expand when necessary (fig. 1). Though of little interest at rest, they play a critical role during exercise. For instance, in healthy subjects the increase in V_T with exercise is achieved at the expenses of a decrease in end-expiratory lung volume

(EELV) and an increase in end-inspiratory lung volume (EILV). In contrast, in airflow obstruction, the increase in V_T is limited by the premature and sustained increase in EELV that may eventually contribute to cause dyspnoea.

Measurements of lung volumes in clinical practice: technical aspects

VC, V_T, IC, EILV and EELV can be measured by simple spirometry. In contrast, TLC, RV and FRC need to be measured with special techniques described below.

Gas dilution techniques (nitrogen washout and helium dilution) are based on the principle of the conservation of mass, that is the amount of gas resident in the lungs at the beginning of the test can be calculated as the product of concentration and volume of eliminated nitrogen or diluted helium. Both methods yield measurements of lung volumes that communicate with open airways only. In severely obstructed patients, an underestimation of the true lung volume may be a result of some regions with long time constants.

Body plethysmography allows rapid and reproducible measurements of absolute lung volumes. The test is based on Boyle's law, in that lung volume can be calculated from the relationship between changes in mouth pressure (assumed equal to alveolar pressure) and box pressure (constant-volume plethysmography) or volume (constant-pressure plethysmography) during gentle panting manoeuvres against a closed shutter. As opposed to gas dilution techniques, plethysmography measures the whole intrathoracic gas, thus including nonventilated and/or poorly ventilated lung regions. This method may overestimate lung volumes in cases of severe airflow obstruction if the panting frequency >1 Hz.

Conclusions

Measuring lung volumes is now an integrative part of lung function assessment. In addition to assist in the diagnosis of the ventilatory defects, it helps explain the presence of respiratory symptoms and hypoxia in cardiopulmonary diseases, has clinical prognostic implications in both obstructive and restrictive diseases, and plays an integral role in the functional evaluation for lung volume reduction surgery in emphysema.

References

- Agostoni E, Hyatt RE. Static behaviour of the respiratory system. *In*: Macklem PT, Mead J, eds. Handbook of Physiology. The Respiratory System. Mechanics of breathing. Section 3, Vol. III, part 1. Bethesda, American Physiological Society, 1986; pp. 113-130.
- Brusasco V, *et al*. Vital capacities during acute and chronic bronchoconstriction. Dependence of flow and volume histories. *Eur Respir J* 1997; 10: 1316-1320.
- Casanova C, *et al*. Inspiratory-to-total lung capacity ratio predicts mortality in patients with chronic obstructive pulmonary disease. *Am J Respir Crit Care Med* 2005; 171: 591-597.
- Criner GJ, Sternberg AL, for the National Emphysema Treatment Trial Research Group, A clinician's guide to the use of lung volume reduction surgery. *Proc Am Thorac Soc* 2008; 5: 461-467.
- Froeb HF, Mead J. Relative hysteresis of the dead space and lung *in vivo*. *J Appl Physiol* 1968; 25: 244-248.
- King TE, Jr, *et al*. Predicting survival in idiopathic pulmonary fibrosis. Scoring system and survival model. *Am J Respir Crit Care Med* 2001; 164: 1171-1181.
- Olive JT, Hyatt RE. Maximal expiratory flow and total respiratory resistance during induced bronchoconstriction in asthmatic subjects. *Am Rev Respir Dis* 1972; 106: 366-376.
- Pellegrino R, *et al*. Expiratory flow limitation and regulation of end-expiratory lung volume during exercise. *J Appl Physiol* 1979; 74: 2552-2558.
- Pellegrino R, *et al*. Interpretative strategies for lung function tests. Official statement of the American Thoracic Society and the European Respiratory Society. *Eur Respir J* 2005; 26: 948-968.
- Pellegrino R, *et al*. Lung mechanics during induced bronchoconstriction. *J Appl Physiol* 1996; 81: 964-975.
- Pride NB, Macklem PT. Lung mechanics in disease. *In*: Macklem PT, Mead J, eds. Handbook of Physiology. The Respiratory System. Mechanics of breathing. Section 3, Vol. III, part 2. Bethesda, American Physiological Society, 1986; pp. 659-692.
- Vinegar A, *et al*. Dynamic mechanisms determine functional residual capacity in mice, *Mus musculus*. *J Appl Physiol* 1979; 46: 867-871.

RESPIRATORY MECHANICS

D. Navajas[1,2,3] and R. Farré[1,2,4]
[1] Unitat de Biofisica i Bioenginyeria, Facultat de Medicina, Universitat de Barcelona
[2] CIBER Enfermedades Respiratorias
[3] Institut de Bioenginyeria de Catalunya
[4] Institut de Investigacions Biomèdiques August Pi Sunyer, Barcelona, Spain
E-mail: rfarre@ub.edu

Pulmonary ventilation is determined by the resistive and elastic properties of the lungs and chest wall and by the driving pressure of the respiratory muscles. Both the lungs and chest wall are elastic structures. The lungs have a very small resting volume. Above this volume the lungs are distended, exerting an inward elastic recoil pressure (P_L) that rises markedly with lung volume (V_L). The chest wall has a much higher resting volume, exhibiting outward and inward elastic recoil pressure (P_{CW}) below and above its resting volume, respectively.

At end-expiratory volume during quiet breathing (functional residual capacity (FRC)) in a healthy subject the respiratory muscles are relaxed and the lungs and chest wall reach the combined resting state (fig. 1). In this situation, the inward P_L is counterbalanced by the outward P_{CW} and the alveolar pressure (P_{alv}) equals atmospheric pressure. Inspiration is produced by activation of inspiratory muscles. The outward muscular pressure (P_{mus}) expands the chest wall, thereby lowering pleural pressure (P_{pl}). This drop in P_{pl} expands the lung and decreases P_{alv} to subatmospheric values. The mouth–alveolar pressure gradient drives inspiratory flow. During quiet breathing in a normal subject, expiration is achieved by relaxing inspiratory muscles. The net inward elastic recoil of the total respiratory system ($P_{RS} = P_L + P_{CW}$) tends to return the system to the overall equilibrium volume, increasing P_{alv} to above mouth pressure (P_{mo}) and driving expiratory flow. The activation of the expiratory muscles results in a faster expiration.

Airway resistance

The airflow generated by the pressure gradient between the mouth and the alveoli is determined by airway resistance (R_{aw}), defined as

$$R_{aw} = (P_{mo} - P_{alv})/V'$$

> **Key points**
>
> - Alveolar pressure is lower and higher than pressure at the airway opening during inspiration and expiration, respectively.
> - The lungs exert inward elastic recoil that increases with lung volume.
> - Body plethysmography allows the measurement of both airway resistance and lung volume.
> - The forced oscillation technique allows the measurement of respiratory resistance during spontaneous breathing with minimum patient collaboration.
> - Respiratory mechanics can be monitored in sedated mechanically ventilated patients performing post-inspiratory and post-expiratory pauses.

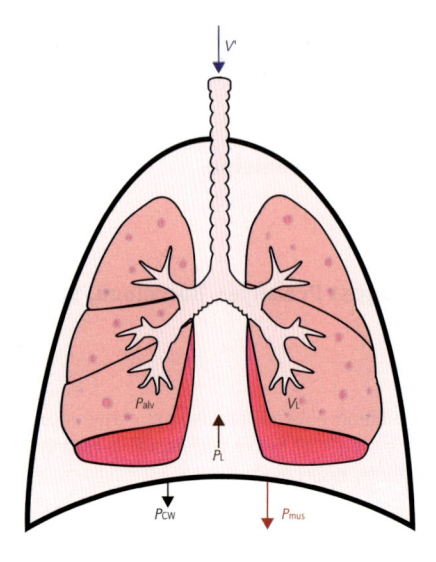

Figure 1. Mechanial behaviour of the respiratory system. V': gas flow; P_{alv}: alveolar pressure; V_L: lung volume; P_L: lung elastic recoil pressure; P_{CW}: chest wall elastic recoil pressure; P_{mus}: outward muscular pressure.

where V' is the gas flow.

In healthy adults, R_{aw} measured at FRC is about 2 $hPa·s·L^{-1}$. Intrathoracic airway calibre increases as lungs expand, resulting in a hyperbolic dependence of R_{aw} on lung volume. Therefore, an approximately linear relationship is obtained by computing airway conductance ($G_{aw} = 1/R_{aw}$). Since large lungs have wider airways, the specific airway resistance computed as

$$sR_{aw} = R_{aw} · FRC$$

provides a resistance measurement normalised for differences in lung size. Similarly, specific conductance is defined as

$$sG_{aw} = G_{aw}/FRC.$$

Body plethysmography

Measurement of R_{aw} requires the recording of airflow and driving pressure. Airflow can be recorded with a pneumotachograph connected to the mouth. Mouth pressure is simply atmospheric pressure or, alternatively, it can be readily measured with a pressure transducer. As the alveolar airspace is not directly accessible, P_{alv} can be estimated by means of a whole-body plethysmograph (fig. 2). This technique involves the subject sitting inside a closed cabin breathing the gas from the box. The mouth can be occluded with a shutter coupled to the mouthpiece. First, the shutter is opened and the ratio between V' and the pressure within the box (P_{box}) is measured during breathing (V'/P_{box}).

During inspiration the air moves from the box to the lung. The inspired gas takes on a higher volume in the lungs than in the box due to the decrease in pressure ($P_{alv} < P_{box}$), the increase in temperature (37°C) and the addition of water vapour. The calibration ratio of the plethysmograph ($k = P_{alv}/P_{box}$) is experimentally determined by closing the shutter at FRC and recording P_{mo} and P_{box} during gentle respiratory efforts against the occlusion. Under zero airflow conditions, $P_{alv} \approx P_{mo}$ and

$$k = P_{alv}/P_{box}$$

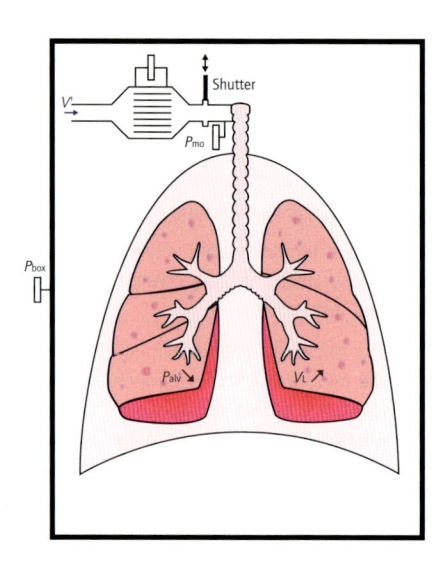

Figure 2. Measurement of airway resistance by body plethysmography. V': gas flow; P_{mo}: mouth pressure; P_{alv}: alveolar pressure; V_L: lung volume; P_{box}: pressure within the box.

Therefore,

$R_{aw} = P_{alv}/V' = k \cdot P_{box}/V'$

Body plethysmography measurements of R_{aw} are usually computed at low respiratory flows (<0.5 L) recorded during shallow panting to minimise the effects of temperature changes during inspiration and expiration. Alternatively, measurements can be made during quiet breathing after computer correction for changes in the physical conditions of the gas.

Whole-body plethysmography is the procedure most commonly used to measure R_{aw}. An added advantage of this technique is that it provides a FRC measurement for the computation of sR_{aw}. However, the device is bulky and expensive and is not suited to measurement in supine patients.

Interrupter technique

Airway resistance can also be measured outside the box with a pneumotacograph–shutter system. The subject breathes at rest through the pneumotacograph. When airflow reaches a given threshold the mouth is briefly (~0.1 s) occluded with the shutter. During flow interruption the pressure is equilibrated within the different lung compartments. Therefore, R_{aw} can be computed as the ratio between the flow just before occlusion and the mouth pressure recorded during flow interruption. R_{aw} is usually computed as the mean of flow interruptions performed in several breathings.

The interrupter technique can be implemented in handy devices and requires only minimal patient cooperation. However, due to progressive equilibration between mouth and alveolar pressure the computed value of R_{aw} depends on the time lag between the start of occlusion and P_{mo} measurement. Slow pressure equilibration in patients with airflow obstruction results in an underestimation of R_{aw}.

Forced oscillation technique

In addition to the airflow resistance of the airways, lung and chest wall tissues also exhibit resistive load because of internal frictional resistance to motion. Resistance of the total respiratory system (R_{rs}) is the sum of airway and tissue resistance. The tissue component of R_{rs} is generally small in comparison with R_{aw}.

R_{rs} can be measured during quiet breathing by the forced oscillation technique (FOT). This technique is based on applying a small amplitude (± 1 hPa) pressure oscillation to the patient's mouth or nose with a loudspeaker or a small pump. R_{rs} is computed as the ratio of forced pressure oscillation and in-phase flow. The ratio between forced pressure and the out-of-phase flow defines the reactance (X_{rs}) that provides a combined measurement of the inertial and elastic properties of the respiratory system. Forced oscillation is applied at frequencies (>4 Hz) higher than the breathing rate to facilitate the separation of forced oscillation from tidal breathing. The use of multifrequency oscillation (usually 4–32 Hz) provides a measurement of the frequency dependence of respiratory mechanics.

Current FOT devices are portable and easy to use. The technique does not require any special collaboration from the patient and measurements can be performed in supine. Changes in R_{rs} during the breathing cycle can be precisely monitored. Moreover, FOT can be coupled to mechanical ventilators. Therefore, FOT is especially useful for epidemiological studies, measurements in infants and monitoring respiratory mechanics in patients during sleep and mechanical ventilation.

Lung compliance

The elastic behaviour of the lung is described by the P_L-V_L relationship. Lung deformability is measured as lung compliance (C_L), defined as the change in volume divided by the change in pressure.

$C_L = \Delta V_L/\Delta P_L$

The change in volume can readily be measured with a spirometer connected to the mouth. The measurement of ΔP_L requires the simultaneous recording of P_{pl} and P_{alv}. Pleural pressure is usually estimated from the oesophageal pressure (P_{soe}) recorded with a small balloon attached to the tip of a catheter introduced through the nose into the lower oesophagus. Alveolar pressure is estimated in the mouth during brief flow interruptions. In practice, the subject performs a full inspiration followed by a very slow expiration to FRC. A shutter attached to the spirometer performs successive brief (~1 s) occlusions during expiration. The P_L-V_L relationship is curvilinear, with C_L decreasing markedly with volume. C_L is habitually computed in the range of tidal volume at rest (between FRC and FRC+0.5 L). In the normal adult, C_L is about 0.2 $L \cdot hPa^{-1}$. The elastic behaviour of the lung can also be characterised by lung elastance (E_L), defined as the reciprocal of C_L ($E_L = 1/C_L$).

Chest wall compliance is computed as

$$C_{CW} = \Delta V_L / \Delta P_{CW}$$

In healthy subjects, the value of C_{CW} is comparable to that of C_L. Since the elastic pressure of the respiratory system is $P_{rs} = P_L + P_{CW}$, the compliance of the respiratory system (C_{rs}) is related to the compliance of the lungs and chest wall components as

$$1/C_{rs} = 1/C_L + 1/C_{CW}$$

C_{rs} or C_{CW} can only be measured during complete respiratory muscle relaxation, which is extremely difficult to achieve in conscious patients.

Measurement of respiratory mechanics in mechanical ventilation

Respiratory mechanics can be measured in sedated mechanically ventilated patients by recording airflow and pressure at the airway opening (P_{ao}). The driving pressure required to overcome the elastic and resistive loads (E_{rs} and R_{rs}, respectively) of the respiratory system is

$$P_{ao} = R_{rs} \cdot V' + E_{rs} \cdot V$$

where V is volume. R_{rs} and E_{rs} can be computed by least squares fitting of this equation to P_{ao}, V' and V recordings.

In patients ventilated with a constant flow waveform, R_{rs} and E_{rs} can also be measured by performing a post-inspiratory pause. Flow interruption results in a sharp drop in pressure from the peak value at end inspiration (P_{max}) to P_1, followed by a slow decay to a plateau (P_2). The sudden decrease in P_{ao} is associated with the resistive load of the airways. Therefore, R_{aw} is estimated as

$$R_{aw} = (P_{max} - P_1)/V'$$

A higher value of resistance due to the contribution of tissue viscoelasticity and gas redistribution within the lungs is computed from the pressure drop to the plateau ($P_{max} - P_2$).

The additional performance of a post-expiratory pause allows E_{rs} to be computed as the ratio of pressure and volume changes at the end of the post-inspiratory and post-expiratory pauses.

Respiratory muscle strength

Since direct measurements of muscular pressure are not clinically available, respiratory muscle performance is commonly assessed by measuring maximal pressures generated at the mouth during maximal inspiratory and expiratory efforts against an occluded airway (or occluded except for a small leak). Maximum expiratory pressure ($P_{E,max}$) is measured at total lung capacity (TLC). Maximum inspiratory pressure measurements ($P_{I,max}$) are taken at either FRC or residual volume (RV). Alternatively, inspiratory muscle strength can be assessed during sniffing with one nostril occluded with a plug. Maximum pressure (sniff P_{di}) is recorded into the occluded nostril during a rapid forceful inspiratory sniff performed at FRC.

The clinical testing of maximal respiratory pressures is quick and simple but measurement is dependent on effort. The test is useful for excluding significant respiratory muscle weakness.

References

- ATS/ERS Statement on Respiratory Muscle Testing. *Am J Respir Crit Care Med* 2002; 166: 518-624.

- Beydon N, et al. An official American Thoracic Society/European Respiratory Society statement: pulmonary function testing in preschool children. *Am J Respir Crit Care Med* 2007; 175: 1304-1345.
- Farre R, et al. Noninvasive monitoring of respiratory mechanics during sleep. *Eur Respir J* 2004; 24: 1052-1060.
- Gibson GJ. Clinical tests of respiratory function. 3rd Edn. London, Hodder Arnold, 2009; pp. 3-52.
- Hyatt RE, et al. Interpretation of pulmonary function tests. A practical guide. 3rd Edn. Philadelphia, Lippincott Williams & Wilkins, 2008; pp. 75-86.
- Lucangelo U, et al. Lung mechanics at the bedside: make it simple. *Curr Opin Crit Care* 2007; 13: 64-72.
- Oostveen E, et al. The forced oscillation technique in clinical practice: methodology, recommendations and future developments. ERS task force. *Eur Respir J* 2003; 22: 1026-1041.
- Pride NB. Airflow resistance. *In*: Hughes JMB, Pride NB, eds. Lung function tests: Physiological principles and clinical applications. London, W.B. Saunders, 1999; pp. 27-44.

GAS TRANSFER ($T_{L,CO}$)

J.M.B. Hughes
National Heart and Lung Institute, Imperial College, London, UK
E-mail: mike.hughes@imperial.ac.uk

Apart from spirometry, the transfer factor of the lung for carbon monoxide ($T_{L,CO}$) is the most frequently performed pulmonary function test. It focuses on the integrity of the alveolar (gas exchanging) part of the lung. The $T_{L,CO}$ can detect abnormalities limited to the pulmonary microcirculation, the only routine test which can do so. It helps to think of the $T_{L,CO}$ as a measure of the anatomy of the alveolar region, whereas blood gas measurements (arterial oxygen (P_{a,O_2}) and carbon dioxide (P_{a,CO_2}) tension) measure a physiological efficiency, which involves airways and larger blood vessels, as well as alveolar structures. For example, the $T_{L,CO}$ is normal in asthma (alveoli are uninvolved), but the P_{a,O_2} may be considerably reduced.

Definition

The transfer factor (called the diffusing capacity of the lung for carbon monoxide ($D_{L,CO}$) in the USA) measures the surface area available for gas exchange. It is closely related to the oxygen diffusing capacity (D_{L,O_2}). $T_{L,CO}$ is the quantity of inhaled CO absorbed, per unit time and per unit CO partial pressure. The pressure gradient is the alveolar–plasma carbon monoxide tension (P_{CO}) difference. CO is chosen for alveolar–capillary exchange because, after diffusing into capillary blood, CO binds to haemoglobin (Hb) as carboxy-Hb, but at an extremely low partial pressure (P_{CO}). Plasma P_{CO} is so low that it is not usually measured, but it may reach significant levels in current smokers. CO uptake is independent of blood flow, but it is dependent on the number of Hb–binding sites, *i.e.* on capillary volume. "Transfer" is the better term, because chemical reaction as well as "diffusion" is involved.

Technique

Nearly all clinical laboratories use the single breath (sb) technique of Ogilvie *et al.* The $T_{L,CO}$ is measured during a 10-s breath-hold at maximal inspiration (volume = total lung capacity (TLC)).

Breath-holding at TLC optimises the distribution of the inhaled marker gases (He and CO), and makes $T_{L,CO}$ independent of ventilation. The breathing manoeuvre is shown in fig. 1. The subject is asked to: 1) exhale slowly to residual volume; 2) make a signal; 3) inspire *rapidly* to full inflation; and 4) breath-hold. The breath-hold is assisted by automatic closure of the inspiratory and expiratory valves for a pre-set time (9-11 s), after which exhalation occurs rapidly (there is no need for a forced expiration) and an alveolar sample taken, from which water vapour and CO_2 are absorbed before He and CO concentrations are analysed.

Calculation of the $T_{L,CO}$

The key point is that the $T_{L,CO}$ is the product of *two* measurements, the alveolar volume (V_A) and the rate of alveolar uptake of CO, given by the transfer coefficient of the lung for CO (K_{CO}). During the breath-hold at

> **Key points**
>
> - $T_{L,CO}$ measures alveolar function.
> - $T_{L,CO}$ is the product of K_{CO} and V_A.
> - K_{CO} (or T_L/V_A) is the more specific index of alveolar integrity.
> - K_{CO} is low in emphysema and fibrosis.
> - K_{CO} is high in extrapulmonary restriction.

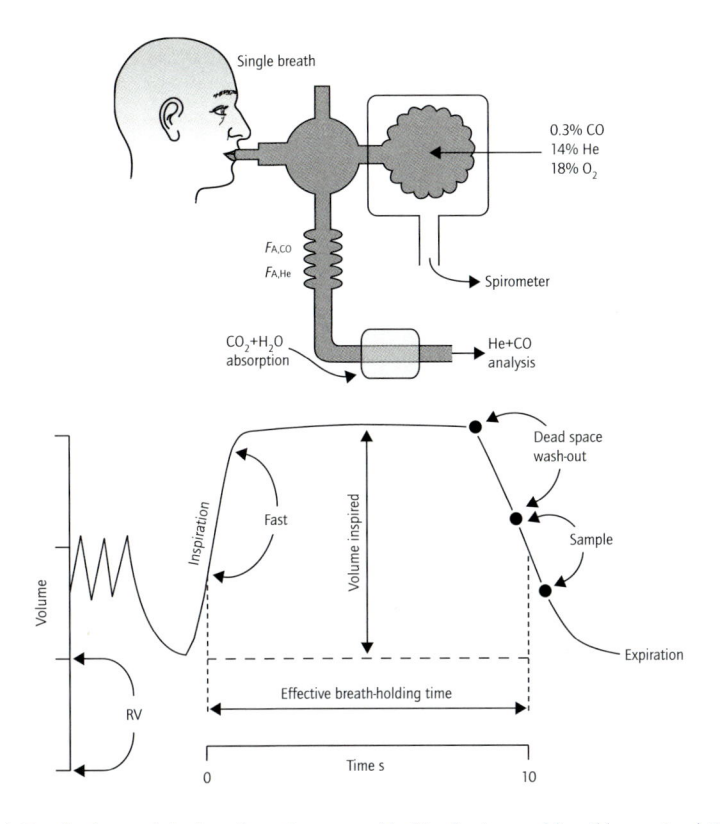

Figure 1. Transfer factor of the lung for carbon monoxide ($T_{L,CO}$) set-up and breathing protocol. The breath-hold time is set automatically, and is calculated from 0.33 × inspired time to 1 L expiratory time. $F_{A,CO}$: alveolar carbon monoxide fraction; $F_{A,He}$: alveolar helium fraction; RV: residual volume.

maximal inspiration, V_A should equal TLC minus anatomical dead space (97–98% TLC). In practice, V_A in normal subjects = 94% TLC with a lower confidence limit (-1.64 SD) of 83%. The 10-s breath-hold is insufficient time for complete gas mixing; in airflow obstruction, the measured V_A may be much less than 80% of the actual TLC (measured by multi-breath gas dilution or plethysmography).

The k_{CO} is the rate of alveolar uptake of CO during the breath-hold (the slope in fig. 2). It is a rate constant with units of s^{-1} or min^{-1}. When normalised to barometric pressure (minus water vapour pressure) (P_b^*), k_{CO}/P_b^* = K_{CO} ($min^{-1} \cdot kPa^{-1}$). The final step in the calculation of $T_{L,CO}$ is the multiplication of K_{CO} by V_A (in mmol: 1 mmol = 22.4 mL standard temperature, pressure and dry).

$$K_{CO} \times V_A = T_{L,CO} \; (mmol \cdot min^{-1} \cdot kPa^{-1})$$

$$T_{L,CO}/V_A = K_{CO} \; (mmol \cdot min^{-1} \cdot kPa^{-1} \cdot L^{-1})$$

but the units are equivalent to ($min^{-1} \cdot kPa^{-1}$).

If V_A remains constant, $T_{L,CO}$ and K_{CO} will change equally (as % predicted). There are formulae to correct $T_{L,CO}$ for anaemia, so the Hb level should always be known. Oxygen breathing with an increase in P_{A,O_2} reduces $T_{L,CO}$ and K_{CO} by competitive antagonism between O_2 and CO; it is the basis of the Roughton–Forster equation which partitions $1/T_{L,CO}$ (transfer resistance) into $1/D_M$ (alveolar–capillary membrane resistance) and $1/\theta V_c$ (transfer resistance of red cells).

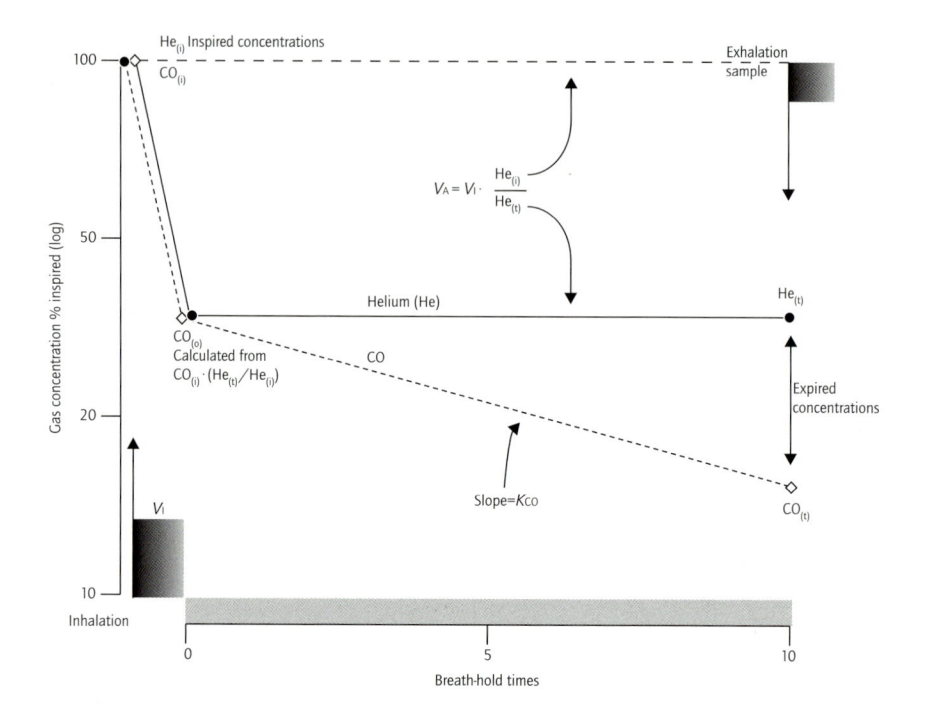

Figure 2. Transfer factor of the lung for carbon monoxide ($T_{L,CO}$): CO and He analysis. CO and He concentrations *versus* breath-hold time to illustrate the origin and calculation of the two components (slope of the transfer coefficient of the lung for CO (K_{CO}) and alveolar volume (V_A)) from which $T_{L,CO}$ is derived. CO(i) and CO(t) are CO concentrations inspired (i) and after exhalation (with dead space discard) at time t after breath-hold (the same for He(i) and He(t)). CO(0) is the calculated alveolar concentration at breath-hold start before alveolar uptake has begun. V_I: inspired volume.

When V_A is reduced, $T_{L,CO}$ and K_{CO} may change in opposite directions (table 1) if the cause is a) reduced alveolar expansion, *e.g.* extrapulmonary restriction, or b) a reduction in aerated alveolar units, *e.g.* pneumonectomy or consolidation or atelectasis. Other causes of a reduced V_A are c) diffuse alveolar damage (emphysema or fibrosis) ($T_{L,CO}$ and K_{CO} both reduced) and d) airflow obstruction (V_A low due to poor gas mixing). In d), $T_{L,CO}$ and K_{CO} are variable, being low in emphysema and normal or high in asthma.

Causes of a low K_{CO} (and $T_{L,CO}$):

- diffuse alveolar damage (fibrosis, emphysema)
- pulmonary vascular diseases
- chronic heart failure
- anaemia

Causes of a high K_{CO}:

- extrapulmonary restriction
- loss of aerated units
- increased pulmonary blood flow
- acute alveolar haemorrhage
- polycythaemia

Implications of $K_{CO} \times V_A = T_{L,CO}$

1. Transfer factor of the lung (T_L)/V_A does not correct $T_{L,CO}$ for a low V_A because a) T_L/V_A may rise when V_A falls, and b) $T_L/V_A = K_{CO} =$ the rate constant for alveolar uptake of CO.

2. The same $T_{L,CO}$ (say 60% predicted) can arise from different combinations of K_{CO} and

Table 1. Physiological influences on the transfer factor of the lung for carbon monoxide ($T_{L,CO}$) and the transfer coefficient of the lung for CO (K_{CO})

	$T_{L,CO}$	K_{CO}
Anaemia	↓	↓
Cardiac output increase	↑	↑
P_{A,O_2} increase	↓	↓
V_A ↓ (reduced alveolar expansion)	↓	↑ ↑
V_A ↓ (reduction in no. of aerated units)	↓	↑

P_{A,O_2}: alveolar oxygen tension; V_A: alveolar volume.

V_A, such as a) high K_{CO} and low V_A (extrapulmonary restriction), b) low K_{CO} and normal V_A (pulmonary vasculopathy), or c) low-ish K_{CO} and low-ish V_A (fibrosis).

References

- Hughes JMB, Pride NB. In defence of the carbon monoxide transfer coefficient K_{CO} (T_L/V_A). *Eur Respir J* 2001; 17: 168-174.
- Jones RS, Meade F. A theoretical and experimental analysis of anomalies in the estimation of pulmonary diffusing capacity by the single breath method. *Q J Exp Physiol* 1961; 46: 131-143.
- Ogilvie CM, et al. A standardized breath holding technique for the clinical measurement of the diffusing capacity of the lung for carbon monoxide. *J Clin Invest* 1957; 36: 1-17.
- Roberts CM, et al. Multi-breath and helium single breath dilution lung volumes as a test of airway obstruction. *Eur Respir J* 1990; 3: 515-520.

CONTROL OF VENTILATION

B.J. Whipp
Human Bio-Energetics Research Centre, Crickhowell, UK
E-mail: bjwhipp@dsl.pipex.com

Key points

- The slope of the $V'E$–P_{ET,CO_2} relationship ($\Delta V'E/\Delta P_{ET,CO_2}$) is driven by central "chemoreceptor" CO_2 responsiveness and, if P_{a,O_2} is not excessive, also that of peripheral chemoreceptors.

- The hyperoxic rebreathing method appreciably reduces the time demands of the steady-state, constant-concentration inspirate approach for measuring $\Delta V'E/\Delta P_{ET,CO_2}$, although $\Delta V'E/\Delta P_{ET,CO_2}$ obtained by this method reflects only the activity of the central chemoreflex.

- The isocapnic $V'E$–P_{ET,CO_2} response is curvilinear, and reflects solely the activity of the carotid chemoreceptors. It can be determined by steady-state, constant-concentration inspirates or by rebreathing.

- Expressing the $V'E$ response as a function of S_{a,O_2} yields a linear profile of hypoxic responsiveness; the actual $V'E$ stimulus, however, is P_{a,O_2} not S_{a,O_2}.

- The "Dejours" hypoxia-withdrawal test is a further means of estimating hypoxic $V'E$ responsiveness. Abruptly administering 100% O_2 from a prior hypoxic background will acutely suppress carotid body hypoxic responsiveness and cause $V'E$ to fall transiently and rapidly; the maximum decrease in $V'E$ as a fraction of the total hypoxic $V'E$ provides the hypoxic index.

The ventilatory control system is highly complex, involving the transmission of primary humoral stimuli from their sites of generation to the sensing elements; the integration of chemoreceptor afferent activity within brainstem "respiratory centres"; the generation of respiratory motor-discharge patterns; neuromuscular transmission at the respiratory muscles; and, finally, the generation of appropriate pulmonary pressure gradients to generate the required airflow and ventilation. Consequently, while the inhalation of hypercapnic or hypoxic gas mixtures, either singly or in combination, is widely utilised to assess the normalcy of ventilatory "chemoreflex" sensitivity, interpretation of the response should be made in the context of the entire "input–output" relationship. Subjects with increased airways resistance or impaired respiratory muscle function, for example, may have an abnormally low overall ventilatory CO_2 or hypoxic response despite normal chemoreceptor responsiveness.

Ventilatory response to inhaled CO_2

The relationship between minute ventilation ($V'E$) and arterial (a) or alveolar (A; typically end-tidal (ET)) carbon dioxide tension (P_{CO_2}), with the subject sequentially inhaling a series of progressively greater hypercapnic inspirates (e.g. 3–6%), each for sufficiently long to establish a steady state, is used to estimate overall ventilatory CO_2 responsiveness. The resulting $V'E$–P_{ET,CO_2} relationship is typically linear in healthy, normoxic individuals, with a slope ($\Delta V'E/\Delta P_{ET,CO_2}$) averaging ~2–3 $L \cdot min^{-1} \cdot mmHg^{-1}$. This slope reflects the CO_2 responsiveness of both the central "chemoreceptors", located predominantly on the ventral medullary surfaces, and also, if arterial oxygen tension (P_{a,O_2}) is not excessive, the peripheral chemoreceptors (predominantly, if not exclusively, the carotid bodies in humans). At P_{a,O_2} levels of ~90 mmHg, the central component accounts for 70–75% of the response with the peripheral component accounting for the remainder. However, as the "peripheral" component of CO_2 responsiveness increases with reductions of P_{a,O_2} below normal, $\Delta V'E/\Delta P_{ET,CO_2}$ increases with greater (but constant) degrees of hypoxaemia and decreases with greater (but constant) degrees of hyperoxia. This results in a "fan" of hypoxia-dependent CO_2 response slopes reflecting altered response "sensitivity" (also termed "potentiation"), with little-or-no change in the extrapolated zero $V'E$ intercept on the P_{CO_2} axis (fig. 1). By contrast, sustained metabolic acidaemia or alkalaemia results in a parallel shift in the CO_2 response relationship (i.e. no change in CO_2 "sensitivity") with a reduced or increased zero $V'E$ intercept, respectively.

The increasing $V'E/P_{ET,CO_2}$ slope with greater levels of simultaneous hypoxia reflects a progressively greater carotid body response component; it is crucial, therefore, to maintain P_{a,O_2} constant (iso-oxia) during the test. Above a P_{a,O_2} of ~200 mmHg, the carotid body component is effectively inactivated and hence the sufficiently hyperoxic CO_2 response entirely reflects that of the "central" component. Interpreting the result depends on the relationships between the typically measured P_{ET,CO_2} (or, less typically, the P_{a,CO_2}) and the P_{CO_2} (and local [H^+]) at each set of chemoreceptors; these relationships depend on factors such as the local-tissue perfusion, CO_2 production, CO_2 capacitance, H^+ buffering capacity and metabolic rate. The equilibrium process is rapid at the carotid body chemoreceptors, but is considerably delayed at the sites of central chemoreception.

It has been has proposed that three or more levels of inspired (I) P_{CO_2} should be used for the slope characterisation. Each level is maintained for ~8 min, with the average $V'E$ and P_{ET,CO_2} over the final 3 min providing the steady-state value. Consequently, the demands of the test are time consuming, although transiently "overshooting" P_{I,CO_2} beyond the required level can reduce the time required to attain the new $V'E$ steady-state level.

This concern is obviated, to a considerable extent, by the rebreathing method of READ and LEIGH, which takes a small fraction of the time to perform while providing effectively the same $\Delta V'E/\Delta P_{ET,CO_2}$ values as for the steady-state method. The subject re-breathes from a 6-7 L bag initially containing ~7% CO_2 balance O_2. The high initial P_{I,CO_2} is designed to raise the P_{a,CO_2} rapidly to, or close to, the mixed-venous level such that the subsequent rebreathing provides an effectively linear increase in P_{a,CO_2}; the high inspired oxygen tension (P_{I,O_2}) maintains P_{a,O_2} above levels for which variations in carotid chemosensitivity would influence the response slope. The rebreathing relationship is shifted to the right of the steady-state relationship, as a result of both the transit delay between the lungs and the sites of chemoreception and the kinetics of the $V'E$ response. Consequently, as the test is designed to provide a constant rate of change of P_{CO_2} at the chemoreceptor sites,

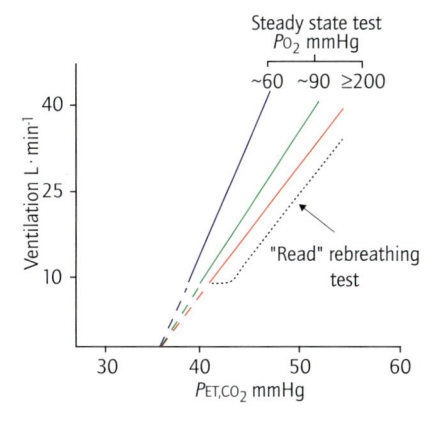

Figure 1. Steady-state ventilatory responses to inhaled carbon dioxide tension (P_{CO_2}) at constant oxygen tension (P_{O_2}; solid lines). The dotted line depicts the response to progressively increasing P_{CO_2} (hyperoxic rebreathing test). P_{ET,CO_2}: end-tidal carbon dioxide tension.

the *rate of change* of V'_E is compared with the *rate of change* of P_{ET,CO_2} ($\Delta V'_E/\Delta P_{ET,CO_2}$). This is currently the more common means of assessing CO_2 responsiveness. It is important to recognise, however, that the CO_2 responsiveness obtained by this hyperoxic method reflects only the activity of the central chemoreflex.

One must be careful, however, not to assume that hypoxia does not influence central chemoreceptor responsiveness; it does *indirectly* by increasing cerebral blood flow. This tends to "wash out" CO_2 from the region, narrowing the difference between the local tissue P_{CO_2} and P_{a,CO_2}.

Beginning at a value below the spontaneous control condition, CO_2 responsiveness is not characterised by the extrapolated dashed lines in fig. 1. Rather, there is a region of virtual insensitivity to increasing P_{CO_2}, if previously lowered by, for example, acute hyperventilation or sufficient hypoxia. The transition from the "insensitive" to the "sensitive" region is considered to reflect a ventilatory recruitment threshold. The difference between this threshold and the lower P_{ET,CO_2} at which apnoea ensues is thought to be important in conditions such as sleep apnoea. Also, as this threshold is lower in hypoxia than in hyperoxia, it can be used to further understand the interaction between peripheral and central chemoreceptor mediation. As a practical expedient, the difference in P_{ET,CO_2} between these conditions at resting ventilation can be used as an index of the threshold change (DUFFIN has suggested P_{ET,O_2} values of 150 and 50 mmHg for this assessment).

Estimation of ventilatory response to hypoxia

The ventilatory response to hypoxia, if defined under isocapnic conditions, is considered solely to reflect the activity of the carotid chemoreceptors. Both constant-concentration inspirates and rebreathing techniques have been successfully utilised for the characterisation.

The pattern of the ventilatory response to a step decrease of P_{I,O_2} is not monotonic, even with P_{ET,CO_2} being maintained constant by controlling the inspired level (*i.e.* isocapnic hypoxia): there is an initial increase to a peak, usually well within 5 min, followed by a slow reduction (termed "hypoxic ventilatory decline") to a final steady-state value (fig. 2a). The initial increase is considered to be the carotid body component and the subsequent decline is thought to result from the hypoxia-mediated increase in cerebral blood flow. This reduces the degree of central chemoreceptor stimulation as a result of cerebral CO_2 wash-out, although an involvement of altered neurotransmission has also been proposed. If the hypoxic step is limited to the initial, or primary, response phase, then the resulting V'_E–P_{a,O_2} relationship over a range of increasingly hypoxic inspirates is curvilinear, with the V'_E rate of change approaching infinity at a P_{a,O_2} of ~30 mmHg. Naturally, at higher isocapnic P_{CO_2} levels the curvature constant of the response is increased as a result of greater hypoxic–hypercapnic interaction at the carotid bodies. It is recommended that the subject be switched to air or even a mildly hyperoxic mixture between successive hypoxic steady states to avoid possible depression of brainstem respiratory neurones. If, instead of isocapnia being maintained in this test, P_{a,CO_2} is allowed to decrease spontaneously as ventilation increases (poikilocapnia), then both the peak initial response and the final level achieved after the hypoxic ventilatory decline are reduced.

A rebreathing test, notionally similar to the "Read–Leigh" test of CO_2 sensitivity, yields considerably greater data density in a significantly shorter period, although the requirement for isocapnia throughout the test does demand a degree of sophistication in obviating, by means of a CO_2-absorbing system, the otherwise progressive hypercapnia. The resulting curvilinear response to the progressive isocapnic hypoxia is shown in fig. 2b for two subjects differing markedly in hypoxic sensitivity. There is little, from a physiological standpoint, to choose

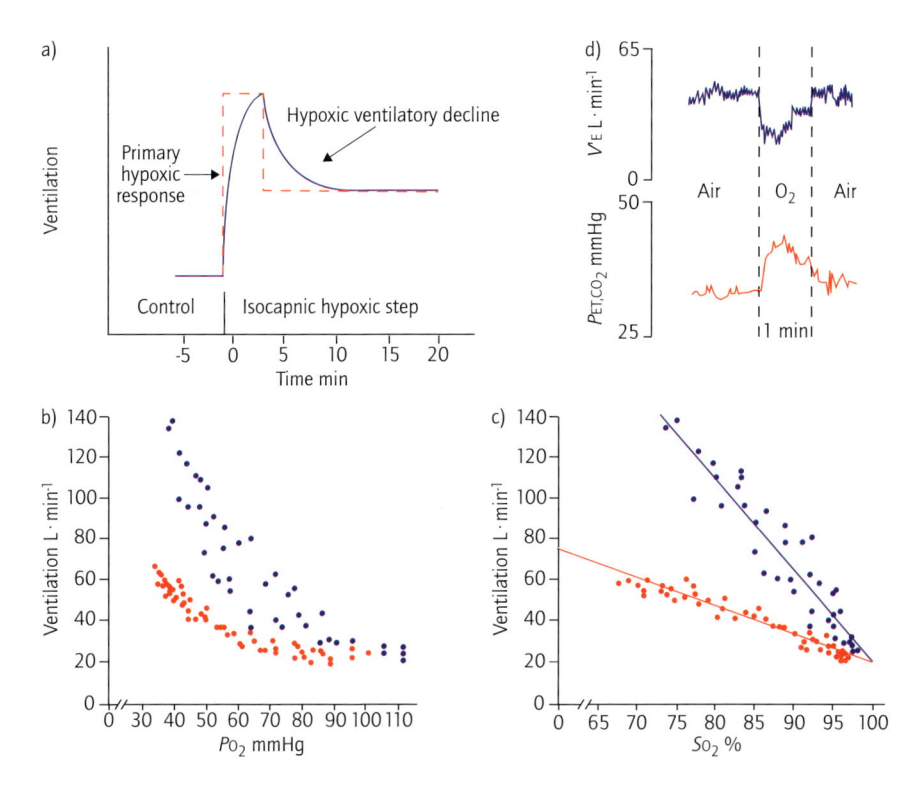

Figure 2. Ventilatory time-course to prolonged isocapnic step-decrease in end-tidal oxgen tension (P_{ET,O_2}; a). Ventilatory response to progressive isocapnic hypoxia (in two subjects) as a function of P_{ET,O_2} (b) and oxygen saturation (S_{O_2}; c; figure reproduced from REBUCK and SLUTSKY (1981), with permission from the publisher). Ventilatory time-course to an hyperoxic step-increase in an exercising hypoxic subject with alveolar proteinosis (d; figure reproduced from WASSERMAN et al. (1989), with permission from the publisher). P_{ET,CO_2}: end-tidal carbon dioxide tension; V'_E: minute ventilation; P_{O_2}: oxygen tension.

between an exponential and a hyperbolic characterisation of the response. The conflicting issues regarding the most appropriate index for hypoxic response characterisation appear to be obviated (on empirical grounds) by the demonstration that the curvilinear V'_E-P_{a,O_2} relationship can be transformed into a linear relationship by substituting arterial O_2 saturation (S_{a,O_2}) for P_{a,O_2} (fig. 2c):

$$V'_E = G \cdot S_{a,O_2} + V'_{E(0)}$$

where $V'_{E(0)}$ is the control V'_E and the slope parameter G is the hypoxic responsiveness quantifier. G has been shown to average ~1.5 ± 1.0 (average ± SD) $L \cdot min^{-1} \cdot \%$ decrease of S_{a,O_2}^{-1} in normal subjects. At higher isocapnic levels, G is increased as a result of the potentiating effect of CO_2 on carotid sensitivity, which sums with the further central CO_2-H^+ stimulation.

In addition to the ease of measuring S_{a,O_2} noninvasively by pulse oximetry, and averting any assumption regarding the difference between P_{ET,O_2} and P_{a,O_2}, the linearity of the V'_E response makes this rebreathing method a very practical means of assessing hypoxic ventilatory responsiveness. It is important to recognise, however, that the ventilatory stimulus is P_{a,O_2}; S_{a,O_2} is merely a practical expedient, with uncertainties regarding the influence of conditions altering the haemoglobin affinity for O_2.

The current degree of a subject's hypoxic ventilatory drive may be estimated by the hypoxia-withdrawal test of DEJOURS. If a particular level of Pa,O_2 is established by inhalation of a hypoxic gas mixture, or noting the spontaneous Pa,O_2 if the subject is already hypoxaemic (as in fig. 2d for an exercising subject with alveolar proteinosis), then the abrupt administration of 100% O_2 will acutely suppress carotid body hypoxic responsiveness and cause $V'E$ to fall transiently and rapidly. The maximum decrease in $V'E$ as a fraction of the total hypoxic $V'E$ provides the hypoxic index. In addition to the assumption (probably justified in humans) that the consequently high level of PO_2 actually "silences" the carotid bodies, the validity of the Dejours' test depends upon the $V'E$-decrement reaching its nadir prior to the subsequently increased Pa,CO_2 (caused by the reduced $V'E$) influencing central sites of CO_2 responsiveness. As the nadir of the response commonly occurs ~20–25 s after the hypoxic–hyperoxic transition, there is some uncertainty regarding this latter point. Although this test is quite easy to perform and provides a useful qualitative estimate of hypoxic responsiveness, it remains to be precisely standardised and quantified.

The peripheral-chemosensory potentiation of the CO_2 response by hypoxia may also be used to provide an index of hypoxic ventilatory responsiveness, as follows: 1) from the linear difference between the hyperoxic and the hypoxic CO_2 response, and 2) the increase in $V'E$ between the hyperoxic (peripheral chemoreceptors "silenced") and the hypoxic (40 mmHg Pa,O_2) CO_2 response relationship, measured at a standard target level of 40 mmHg Pa,CO_2 (ΔV_{40}).

Conclusions

While these approaches provide indices of acute ventilatory responsiveness, laboratory-based tests of more chronic blood–gas and acid–base regulatory challenges are less well standardised.

References

- Cunningham DJC, et al. Integration of respiratory responses to changes in alveolar partial pressures of CO_2 and O_2 and in arterial pH. In: Widdicombe JG, Cherniack N, eds. Handbook of Physiology, Respiration, Vol II, Control of Breathing, Part 2. Washington DC, American Physiological Society, 1986; pp. 475–528.
- Dejours P. Chemoreflexes in breathing. *Physiol Rev* 1962; 42: 335–358.
- Dempsey JA, et al. The ventilatory responsiveness to CO_2 below eupnoea as a determinant of ventilatory stability in sleep. *J Physiol* 2004; 560: 1–11.
- Edelman NH, et al. Effects of CNS hypoxia on breathing. *In:* Crystal RG, et al. The Lung: Scientific Foundations. 2nd Edn. New York, Raven Press, 1997; pp. 1757–1765.
- Duffin J. Measuring the ventilatory response to hypoxia. *J Physiol* 2007; 584: 285–293.
- Read DJC, Leigh J. Blood-brain tissue PCO_2 relationships and ventilation during rebreathing. *J Appl Physiol* 1967; 23: 53–70.
- Rebuck AS, Slutsky AS. Measurement of ventilatory responses to hypercapnia and hypoxia. *In:* Hornbein T, ed. The Regulation of Breathing. New York, Dekker, 1981; pp. 745–772.
- Severinghaus JW. Proposed standard determination of ventilatory responses to hypoxia and hypercapnia in man. *Chest* 1976; 70: Suppl. 1, 129–131.
- Wasserman K, et al. Respiratory control during exercise. *In:* Widdicombe JG, ed. International Review of Physiology, Respiratory Physiology III. Baltimore, Univ Park Press, 1981; pp. 149–211.

ARTERIAL BLOOD GAS ASSESSMENT

P. Palange[1], A.H. Ferrazza[1] and J. Roca[2]
[1] Dept of Clinical Medicine, Sapienza University of Rome, Rome, Italy
[2] Hospital Clinic IDIBAPS, CIBERES, University of Barcelona, Barcelona, Spain
E-mail: paolo.palange@uniroma1.it

The fundamental function of the lung is to contribute to the homeostasis of the system by ensuring that pulmonary uptake of oxygen (V_{O_2}) and clearance of carbon dioxide (V_{CO_2}) match with whole-body bioenergetic requirements. We must look at pulmonary function as the first step of the oxygen transport chain from the atmosphere to mitochondria.

Arterial blood gas (ABG) analysis provides direct measurements of partial pressures of oxygen (P_{a,O_2}) and carbon dioxide (P_{a,CO_2}) and pH in arterial blood. In clinical practice,

> **Key points**
>
> - ABG is mandatory for the diagnosis of respiratory failure and of A–B disorders.
> - Pulmonary gas exchange status is best evaluated by the integrated reading of P_{a,O_2} and P_{a,CO_2}.
> - A–B status is best evaluated by the integrated reading of P_{a,CO_2} and pH, with concomitant measurement of serum electrolytes.
> - Mixed A–B disorders are very common in clinical practice.
> - The correct interpolation of ABG represents a fundamental step for the diagnosis and treatment of A–B disorders.

ABG analysis is needed to assess the severity and causes of pulmonary gas exchange impairment and acid–base (A–B) disequilibrium. ABG analysis is one of the most useful diagnostic tests, not only in the critical care setting, but also in general clinical practice, to assess patients with respiratory diseases and those with other disorders with potential impact on pulmonary gas exchange and A–B disturbances (diabetes, heart failure, renal failure). Moreover, ABG analysis is mandatory to establish the diagnosis of respiratory failure.

Modern equipment to perform ABG assessment uses electrodes to measure P_{a,O_2}, P_{a,CO_2} and pH. Other variables, such as bicarbonates (actual HCO_3^- and standard HCO_3^-), base excess (BE) and oxyhaemoglobin saturation (S_{a,O_2}) are computed using well-defined equations.

A simple and practical two-step approach for ABG interpretation in the clinical setting is illustrated in figure 1. The first step aims at the analysis of pulmonary gas exchange status based primarily on P_{a,O_2} and P_{a,CO_2}, while the second step addresses the assessment of A–B status using P_{a,CO_2}, pH and, eventually, HCO_3^- (or BE).

Step 1: Evaluation of lung gas exchange

Healthy subjects at sea level breathing room air (inspired oxygen fraction (F_{I,O_2}) 0.21) show P_{a,O_2} values close to 90–95 mmHg. P_{a,O_2} values <80 mmHg are considered arterial hypoxaemia and P_{a,O_2} <60 mmHg indicates

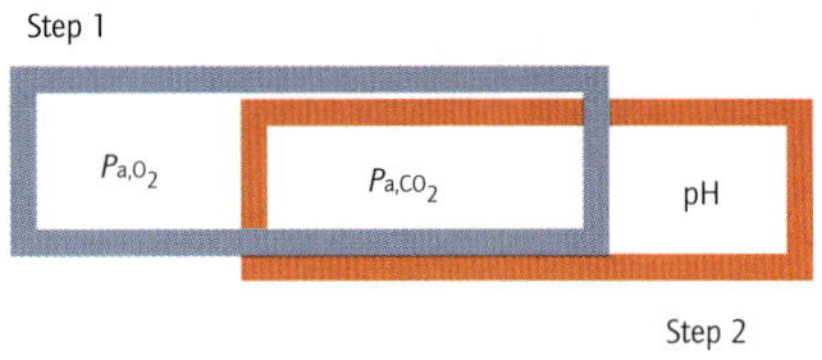

Step 1

Step 2

Figure 1. "Two-step" approach for arterial blood gas interpretation. Pa,O_2: arterial oxygen tension; Pa,CO_2: arterial carbon dioxide tension.

hypoxaemic respiratory failure. Because of the characteristics of the oxyhaemoglobin dissociation curve, a Pa,O_2 of 60 mmHg corresponds to a Sa,O_2 of ~90% and is located at the upper end of the steepest portion of the curve. Pa,O_2 values <60 mmHg will have a substantial impact, reducing arterial O_2 content and compromising tissue oxygenation. The accepted reference interval for Pa,CO_2 is 35–45 mmHg. By convention, hypercapnic respiratory failure is established at Pa,CO_2 >50 mmHg.

Abnormal levels of respiratory gases in arterial blood are generally due to impaired pulmonary gas exchange. Intrapulmonary factors that may cause arterial hypoxaemia are listed in table 1. Pulmonary ventilation–perfusion (V/Q) inequality is the most frequent determinant of hypoxaemia and hypercapnia in the clinical scenario. However, the identification of pulmonary shunt (perfusion of unventilated pulmonary units, V/Q=0) as the main cause of hypoxaemia in a patient with severe pneumonia has relevant therapeutic implications. It is of note, however, that alterations of extrapulmonary factors such as cardiac output, FI,O_2, VO_2 and minute ventilation are also determinants of Pa,O_2 and Pa,CO_2.

When Pa,CO_2 values are close to 40 mmHg, Pa,O_2 is an excellent indicator of the efficacy of the lung as an oxygen exchanger, but patients with abnormal Pa,CO_2 values (hypercapnia or hypocapnia) may benefit from the integrated reading of Pa,O_2 and Pa,CO_2 values indicated in table 1. Such an integrated view can be numerically obtained by computing the alveolar–arterial oxygen gradient ($PA\text{-}a,O_2$) using the following simplified formula:

$$PA\text{-}a,O_2 = [(PB - PH_2O) \times FI,O_2 - Pa,CO_2/R] - Pa,O_2$$

where PB is barometric pressure, PH_2O is airway water vapour partial pressure and R is respiratory quotient (the ratio VCO_2 and VO_2, ~0.8 at rest).

At sea-level, the normal expected $PA\text{-}a,O_2$ value is <15 mmHg in young subjects and <20 mmHg in the elderly. Table 1 shows the contribution of $PA\text{-}a,O_2$ in the identification of the mechanisms of alteration of ABG.

To further understand the cause of arterial hypoxaemia, the effect of supplemental oxygen breathing on Pa,O_2 should be examined, keeping in mind that in the normal lung $PA\text{-}a,O_2$ widens when breathing additional oxygen. While hypoxaemia due to pulmonary V/Q inequalities and diffusion defects is usually corrected by increasing inspired oxygen concentrations, this does not correct respiratory failure due to shunt.

A simple, but less accurate, way to compute $PA\text{-}a,O_2$ is to use the rule of "130". It is assumed that in a healthy subject, at sea-level (FI,O_2 0.21), the sum of Pa,O_2 and Pa,CO_2 should be ~130 mmHg. Consequently, the difference between 130 and the sum of Pa,O_2 + Pa,CO_2 is a surrogate of ($PA\text{-}a,O_2$). The

Table 1. Arterial-alveolar oxygen gradient ($PA\text{-}a,O_2$) in the evaluation of the causes of arterial hypoxaemia.

Cause	Pa,O_2	Pa,CO_2	$PA\text{-}a,O_2$
Hypoventilation	↓	↑	↔
V/Q mismatch	↓	↔ ↓ ↑	↑
O_2 diffusion limitation	↓	↔ ↓	↑
Shunt	↓ ↓	↔ ↓ ↑	↑ ↑

Table 2. Respiratory failure

Hypoxaemic respiratory failure
Pa,O_2 <60 mmHg, Pa,CO_2 normal or low, at sea-level (FI,O_2 0.21)

Hypoxaemia due to pulmonary V/Q mismatching (Pa,O_2 rises with FI,O_2)
Chronic respiratory diseases (only pulmonary fibrosis shows oxygen diffusion limitation with V/Q mismatch)

Hypoxaemia due to intrapulmonary shunt (lung units with V/Q = 0) ($Pa,O_2/FI,O_2$ ≤200 mmHg)

Hypercapnic respiratory failure
Pa,CO_2 >50 mmHg and Pa,O_2 low, at sea-level (FI,O_2 0.21)

"Normal" lung (PA-a,O_2 gradient preserved)
Reduced alveolar ventilation due to extrapulmonary factors

Advanced chronic respiratory disease or severe exacerbation
Hypoxaemia due to pulmonary V/Q mismatch

following examples illustrate the use of the rule. A patient with Pa,O_2 70 mmHg and Pa,CO_2 60 mmHg (130 - (Pa,O_2 70 + Pa,CO_2 60) = 10 mmHg) is hypoventilating a lung that is functionally "normal", with a PA-a,O_2 within the reference interval. On the other hand, a patient with hypoxaemic respiratory failure and hypocapnia (130 - (Pa,O_2 50 + Pa,CO_2 20) = 60 mmHg) shows worse pulmonary oxygen exchange (higher PA-a,O_2)

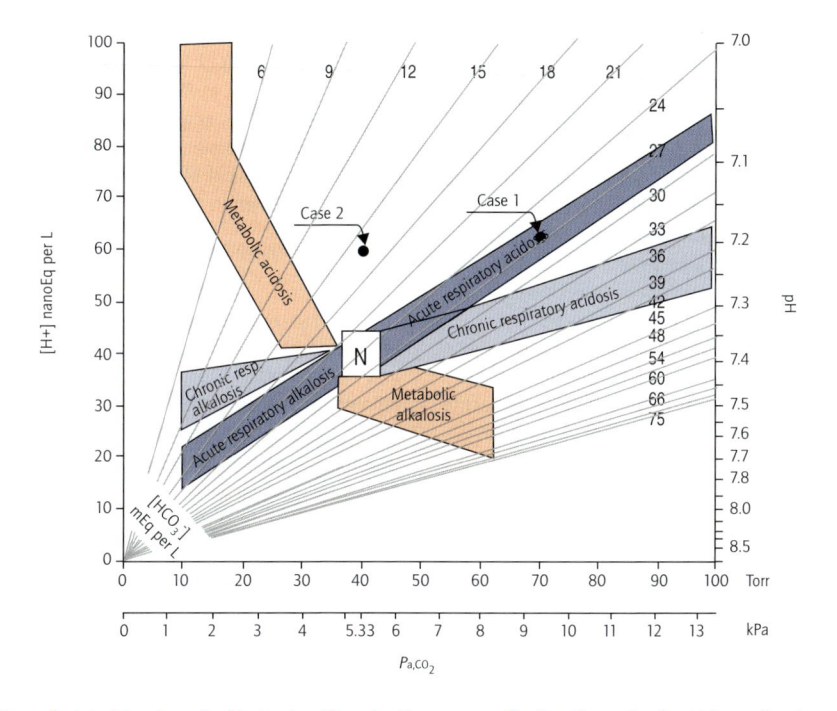

Figure 2. Arterial carbon dioxide tension (Pa,CO_2)-pH nomogram for the diagnosis of acid–base disorders. Pa,CO_2-pH values that fall into acute or chronic, respiratory and nonrespiratory (or metabolic) "bands" should be considered as "simple" disorders (Case 1: Pa,CO_2 70 mmHg, pH 7.19, acute respiratory acidosis). Pa,CO_2-pH values that fall between respiratory and metabolic "bands" should be considered as "mixed" disorders (Case 2: Pa,CO_2 40 mmHg, pH 7.20, acute respiratory and metabolic acidosis). N: normal.

Table 3. Examples of simple acid-base disorders

	pH	P_{a,CO_2}	[HCO_3^-]
Respiratory acidosis	↓	↑	↔
Respiratory alkalosis	↑	↓	↔
Metabolic acidosis	↓	↓	↓
Metabolic alkalosis	↑	↑	↑

P_{a,CO_2}: arterial carbon dioxide tension; [HCO_3^-]: bicarbonate concentration.

than a patient with respiratory failure and hypercapnia (130 - (P_{a,O_2} 50 + P_{a,CO_2} 50) = 30 mmHg). The computation P_{A-a,O_2} (and the use of the rule of 130) is not useful clinically when F_{I,O_2} increases. Calculating the $P_{a,O_2}/F_{I,O_2}$ ratio is recommended to assess the efficacy of the lung as an oxygen exchanger in critical care when comparing ABG measurements taken at different F_{I,O_2} levels. Lung injury is defined as $P_{a,O_2}/F_{I,O_2}$ <300 while acute respiratory distress syndrome (ARDS) is associated with a $P_{a,O_2}/F_{I,O_2}$ ratio <200 (table 2).

Step 2: Diagnosis of A–B disorders

Arterial pH is highly regulated to be maintained between 7.38–7.42. In the clinical assessment of A–B equilibrium, two main determinants of arterial pH must be taken into account, namely: the respiratory component (P_{a,CO_2}) and the metabolic component. Hypercapnia (high P_{a,CO_2}) generates respiratory acidosis (low pH) whereas hypocapnia (low P_{a,CO_2}) is associated to respiratory alkalosis (high pH). In simple acute respiratory disorders, for each 10 mmHg variation in P_{a,CO_2}, the expected change in pH is 0.07 for acidosis and 0.08 for alkalosis, while in simple chronic respiratory disorders it is 0.03 for both acidosis and alkalosis.

The metabolic component refers to the impact of nonvolatile molecules generating acidosis or alkalosis. The variable most often used to assess the metabolic component is bicarbonate [HCO_3^-], computed through the Henderson–Hasselbalch equation:

$$pH = 6.1 + \log([HCO_3^-] / (0.03 \times P_{a,CO_2}))$$

In the past, the role of simple rules associating changes in P_{a,CO_2} with changes in pH (and HCO_3^-) was emphasised as useful for the diagnosis of simple and mixed A–B disorders. A graphical illustration of this approach is shown in figure 2.

Table 3 displays some examples of simple A–B disorders.

The first two rows in table 3 indicate simple, uncompensated, A–B disorders. The first row may correspond to a chronic obstructive pulmonary disease patient with an episode of severe exacerbation showing acute hypercapnia leading to respiratory acidosis.

Table 4. Respiratory disorders

Respiratory acidosis
  Central nervous system depression, neuromuscolar disorders
  Chest wall abnormalities
  Lung diseases

Respiratory alkalosis
  Anxiety, central nervous system disorders
  Hormones/drugs (catecholamine, progesterone, hyperthyroidism, salicylate)
  Fever
  Hypoxia
  Liver diseases

Table 5. Metabolic disorders

Metabolic acidosis
Normochloraemic acidosis (or high anion gap acidosis)
Ketoacidosis
Lactic acidosis
Renal failure
Toxins
Hyperchloraemic acidosis (or normal anion gap acidosis)
Extra-renal loss of Na^+
Renal tubular acidosis

Metabolic alkalosis
Chloride-responsive type
Gastric fluid loss
Volume contraction
Chloride-resistant type
Mineral corticoid disorders
Milk-alkali and Bartter syndromes
Hypoalbumin

The second example fits with any situation leading to hyperventilation and low P_{a,CO_2} that generates respiratory alkalosis (*e.g.* interstitial oedema in heart failure). The third row indicates an example of acidosis due to a metabolic disturbance (*e.g.* exercise-related increase in blood lactate, ketoacidosis, renal failure). Finally, the fourth example of A–B disequilibrium corresponds to a metabolic alkalosis that may be seen in patients with liquid depletion and low intracellular and serum potassium concentrations (*e.g.* excessive diuretic therapy).

Common causes of A–B disorders are illustrated in tables 4 and 5. It is of note that although they may begin as simple disorders (respiratory or metabolic), they often evolve to become mixed A–B abnormalities.

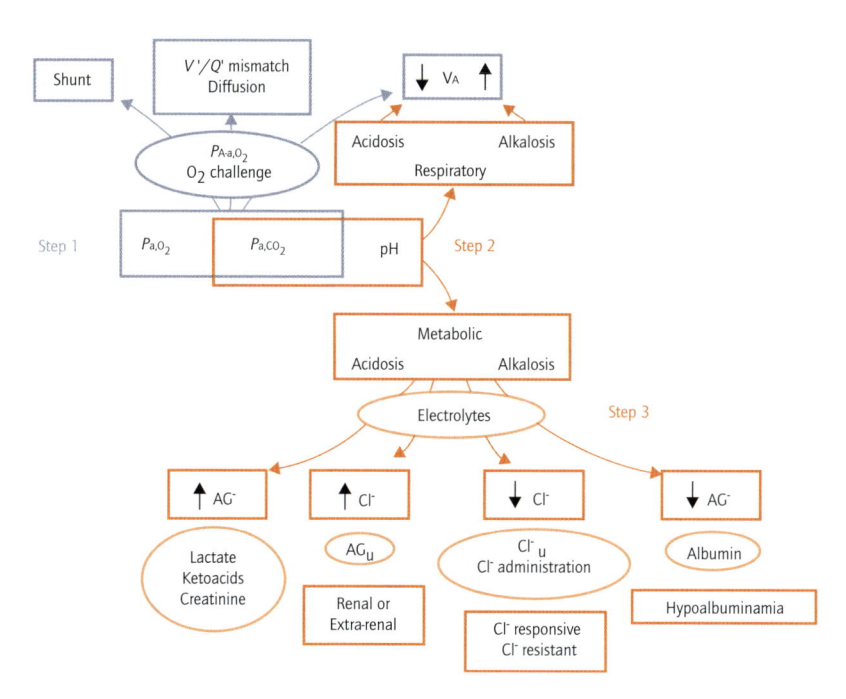

Figure 3. Comprehensive approach to interpreting arterial blood gases. *V/Q*: ventilation/perfusion; V_A: alveolar ventilation; P_{A-a,O_2}: alveolar–arterial oxygen gradient; P_{a,O_2}: arterial oxygen tension; P_{a,CO_2}: arterial carbon dioxide tension; AG: anion gap; Cl⁻: chloride; U: urinary.

Conclusion

In clinical practice, the correct interpretation of ABG provides unique information on the characteristics and severity of lung gas exchange impairment and on A–B abnormalities. It represents a fundamental step towards an appropriate diagnosis of the patient and the adoption of the treatment strategy. Figure 3 summarises the interpretative "integrative" approach to be used in the evaluation of ABG. As a first step (Step 1), the combined reading of Pa,O_2 and Pa,CO_2 values, on room air and during supplemental oxygen breathing, should be used to identify the causes and the severity of arterial hypoxaemia (blue squares and blue circles). As a second step (Step 2), the combined reading of Pa,CO_2 and pH is needed for the correct diagnosis of A–B disorders (red squares). Furthermore, the study of serum electrolytes, and in particular serum chloride, may be of great help in the identification of the causes of metabolic disorders (red squares; further step, Step 3).

References

- Astrup P. A simple electrometric technique for the determination of carbon dioxide tension in blood and plasma, total content of carbon dioxide in plasma and bicarbonate content in 'separated' plasma at fixed carbon dioxide tension. *Scand J Clin Lab Invest* 1956; 8: 33.
- Brackett NC Jr, *et al.* Carbon dioxide titration curve of normal man. Effect of increasing degrees of acute hypercapnia on acid–base equilibrium. *N Engl J Med* 1965; 272: 6–12.
- Hughes JMB. Pulmonary gas exchange. *In*: Hughes JMB, Pride NB, eds. Lung Function Tests: Physical Principles and Clinical Applications. London, WB Saunders, 1999; pp. 75–92.
- Kassirer JP, Bleich HL. Rapid estimation of plasma carbon dioxide tension from pH and total carbon dioxide content. *N Engl J Med* 1965; 272: 1067–1068.
- Kellum JA. Clinical review: reunification of acid-base physiology. *Crit Care* 2005; 9: 500–506.
- Kellum JA. Disorders of acid–base balance. *Crit Care Med* 2007; 35: 2630–2636.
- Narins RG, Emmett M. Simple and mixed acid-base disorders: a practical approach. *Medicine* 1980; 59: 161–187.
- Roca J, Wagner PD. Principles and information content of the multiple inert gas elimination technique. *Thorax* 1994; 49: 815–824.
- Riley RL, Cournand A. "Ideal" alveolar air and the analysis of ventilation-perfusion relationships in the lungs. *J Appl Physiol* 1949; 1: 825–847.
- Riley RL, Cournand A. Analysis of factors affecting partial pressures of oxygen and carbon dioxide in gas and blood of lungs: theory. *J Appl Physiol* 1951; 4: 77–101.
- Severinghaus JW, Bradley AF. Electrodes of blood PO_2 and PCO_2 determination. *J Appl Physiol* 1958; 13: 515–520.
- Stewart PA. Modern quantitative acid-base chemistry. *Can J Physiol Pharmacol* 1983; 61: 1444–1461.
- Wagner PD, The biology of oxygen. *Eur Respir J* 2008; 31: 887–890.
- West JB. Causes of carbon dioxide retention in lung disease. *N Engl J Med* 1971; 284: 1232–1236.

EXERCISE TESTING

P. Palange
Dept of Clinical Medicine, Sapienza University of Rome, Rome, Italy
E-mail: paolo.palange@uniroma1.it

The ability to exercise largely depends on the integrated physiological responses of the respiratory, cardiovascular and skeletal muscle systems. In healthy individuals exercise tolerance is influenced by age, sex and level of fitness. In patients with lung diseases, exercise tolerance is typically reduced and limited by symptoms, such as dyspnoea and leg fatigue.

Cardiopulmonary exercise testing (CPET), *i.e.* the study of ventilatory and pulmonary gas exchange variables during symptom-limited incremental exercise, is considered the "gold standard" for evaluating the degree and the causes of exercise intolerance in disease states. Moreover, CPET has been extensively utilised in patients with chronic obstructive lung disease (COPD), cystic fibrosis (CF), interstitial lung diseases (ILD) and pulmonary vascular disorders (PVD). In COPD and CF, exercise tolerance is mainly limited by pulmonary mechanic abnormalities (*e.g.* reduction in ventilatory capacity, dynamic hyperinflation); in ILD exercise tolerance is limited by ventilatory constraints and pulmonary gas exchange abnormalities (*e.g.* arterial oxygen desaturation); in PVD, both circulatory (*e.g.* reduced adaptation in cardiac output) and pulmonary gas exchange abnormalities contribute to exercise intolerance.

Some causes of exercise intolerance in lung diseases:

- ventilatory limitation to exercise,
- dynamic hyperinflation,
- increased work of breathing,
- pulmonary gas exchange abnormalities,
- excessive perception of symptoms,
- impaired cardiovascular response to exercise,
- reduced oxygen delivery, and
- peripheral muscle weakness/dysfunction.

Exercise protocols

The symptom-limited *maximal incremental exercise* protocol is recommended as a first step in the evaluation of exercise tolerance. Minute ventilation ($V'E$), cardiac frequency (fC), oxygen uptake ($V'O_2$), CO_2 output ($V'CO_2$) and the end-tidal O_2 and CO_2 are the primary variables measured, typically on a breath-by-breath basis using computerised systems. Additional required measurements include: ECG, blood pressure, dyspnoea and leg discomfort, exercise-related arterial O_2 desaturation and dynamic hyperinflation. Careful selection of patients minimises the likelihood of serious complications during maximal incremental exercise testing. Myocardial infarction (within 3–5 days), unstable angina, severe arrhythmias, pulmonary embolism, dissecting aneurysm,

---

Key points

CPET is considered the gold standard for:

- an objective measure of exercise capacity
- identifying the mechanisms limiting exercise tolerance
- establishing indices of the patient's prognosis
- evaluating the effects of therapeutic interventions

and severe aortic stenosis represent absolute contraindication to CPET. Resting lung function measurement and ECG are usually obtained before CPET. Cycle and treadmill exercise have been utilised interchangeably, although the former is largely utilised as the work rate for incremental and endurance tests is easier to quantify. As the exercise period should last 10-12 min, the work rate increment should be selected carefully. In patients with lung diseases the usual rate of workload increase is 10 Watt·min^{-1}, although slower or faster rates are possible in the very sick and in fitter patients, respectively. The maximal incremental exercise test is also utilised to determine the appropriate work rate to be used in an endurance protocol.

Constant work rate (CWR) tests, on either a cycle ergometer or a treadmill, are utilised for the measurement of exercise "endurance" tolerance and ventilatory and pulmonary gas exchange kinetics. CWR exercise results in steady-state responses when work rate is of moderate intensity (*i.e.* below the lactate threshold, θ_L); conversely, high intensity CWR exercise (*i.e.* above the θ_L) results in steady states either being delayed or not attained at all.

Walking tests, such as the 6-min walking test (6-MWT) have been increasingly utilised for the assessment of exercise tolerance in chronic lung diseases. The object of this test is to walk as far as possible for 6 min. The test should be performed indoors along a 30-m flat, straight corridor; encouragement significantly increases the distance walked. Measurements of arterial O_2 saturation by pulse oximetry (S_{p,O_2}), f_C and exertional symptoms are recommended during the 6-MWT.

Indications to CPET

In patients with lung diseases, exercise testing is mainly utilised for functional and prognostic purposes. Other indications include detection of exercise-induced bronchoconstriction, selection of candidates for surgery including lung transplant, and evaluation of the effects of therapeutic intervention including pulmonary rehabilitation.

Exercise variables and indexes

Peak oxygen uptake ($V'O_2,peak$) The classical criterion for defining exercise intolerance and classifying degrees of impairment is the $V'O_2,peak$. With good subject effort on an incremental test, $V'O_2,peak$ reflects a subject's maximal aerobic capacity ("maximum" $V'O_2$). This index is taken to reflect the attainment of a limitation in the O_2 conductance pathway from the lungs to the mitochondria. Values <80% predicted are considered abnormal while values <40% of the predicted indicate severe impairment.

Lactate threshold (θ_L) The θ_L is the highest $V'O_2$ at which arterial lactate is not systematically increased, and is estimated using an incremental test. It is considered an important functional demarcator of exercise intensity. Sub-θ_L work rates can normally be sustained for prolonged periods. θ_L is dependent on age, sex, body mass and fitness. Noninvasive estimation of θ_L requires the demonstration of an augmented $V'CO_2$ in excess of that produced by aerobic metabolism, and its associated ventilatory sequelae.

O_2 pulse The O_2 pulse is the product of the stroke volume and difference between the arterio-mixed venous O_2 content ($C_{a,O_2}-C_{v,O_2}$). Given the Fick equation ($V'O_2$ = cardiac output $\times$ ($C_{a,O_2}-C_{v,O_2}$), the O_2 pulse can be calculated as follows:

O_2 pulse = $V'O_2/f_C$

In patients with ILD, the O_2 pulse at peak exercise is lower and its rate of increase with increasing work rate is usually reduced because of the reductions in stroke volume and C_{a,O_2}. In PVD, the O_2 pulse is characteristically low at peak exercise and may not increase during incremental exercise, reflecting the abnormal CO adaptation.

Heart rate reserve (HRR) The peak cardiac frequency ($f_{C,peak}$) achieved on a symptom-limited exercise test decreases with age. The most commonly used equation to predicted peak cardiac frequency ($f_{C,peak\ pred}$)

is 220-age. HRR is defined as the difference between $f_{C,peak\ pred}$ and $f_{C,peak}$. In healthy individuals, HHR is virtually zero; a high HRR is usually observed in patients with COPD, CF and ILD.

$V'E/V'CO_2$ slope and ventilatory equivalent for CO_2 It is conventional to express the ventilatory response to exercise relative to $V'CO_2$. It can be measured as the slope of the $V'E$-$V'CO_2$ relationship ($\Delta V'E/\Delta V'CO_2$) over its linear region, i.e. typically extending from "unloaded pedalling" to the respiratory compensation point. In normal individuals, $\Delta V'E/\Delta V'CO_2$ values of ~23-25 have been reported.

The adequacy of the ventilatory response to exercise is also expressed by the ratio $V'E/V'CO_2$ that represents the litres of ventilation necessary to clear 1 L of CO_2. Up to the respiratory compensation point, $V'E/V'CO_2$ declines curvilinearly as the work rate increases. It is common practice to record the value at θL ($V'E/V'CO_2@\theta L$) or the minimum value ($V'E/V'CO_2,min$). These have each been proposed to provide noninvasive indices of ventilatory inefficiency. In normal individuals, $V'E/V'CO_2@\theta L$ values of 25-28 have been reported. Several factors may increase $\Delta V'E/\Delta V'CO_2$ and $V'E/V'CO_2@\theta L$, e.g. hypoxaemia, acidosis, increased levels of wasted ventilation and pulmonary hypertension.

Breathing reserve (BR) BR provides an index of the proximity of the ventilation at the limit of tolerance ($V'E,max$) to the maximal achievable ventilation (MVV, estimated from the subject's resting forced expiratory volume in 1 s × 40). BR can be defined as $V'E,max$ as a percentage of MVV (i.e. 1-$V'E,max$/MVV). In COPD, CF and ILD, BR is usually reduced or absent at peak CPET exercise (fig. 1). Analysis of the flow-volume loops is also emerging as an important tool to assess the degree of airflow and ventilatory limitation during exercise in patients with COPD.

Dynamic hyperinflation In normal subjects, end-expiratory lung volume (EELV)

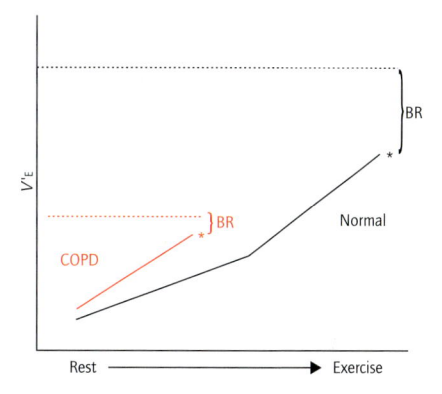

Figure 1. Ventilatory limitation to exercise. Ventilatory limitation to exercise is typically observed in patients with chronic obstructive pulmonary disease (COPD; red lines) compared with normal subjects (black lines). In COPD, but also in CF and ILD, breathing reserve (BR) is reduced at peak exercise. See text for further comments.

decreases with increasing work rate by as much as 0.5-1.0 L below functional residual capacity. Changes in EELV during exercise can be estimated by asking the subject to perform an inspiratory capacity manoeuvre at a selected point in the exercise test. In COPD, particularly in the advanced phases of the disease, EELV increases during exercise (i.e. dynamic hyperinflation) in spite of expiratory muscle activity.

Arterial O_2 desaturation During exercise, S_{p,O_2} is normally maintained in the region of ~97-98%. However, arterial oxygen desaturation can be observed in patients with moderate-to-severe ILD and in patients with primary pulmonary hypertension.

Tolerable limit of exercise (T_{lim}) and "isotime" measurements T_{lim} is expressed as a function of time measured during CWR protocols. In clinical practice, high-intensity (~70-80% Watt max) CWR protocols are utilised for the evaluation of interventions. In addition to T_{lim}, measurement of pertinent physiological variables (e.g. $V'E$, inspiratory capacity, dyspnoea) at standardised time ("isotime") are obtained.

Table 1. Cardiopulmonary exercise testing prognostic indices

	COPD	ILD	CF	PVD
↓ $V'O_2,peak$	+	+	+	+
↑ $V'E / V'CO_2$		+		
Arterial O_2 desaturation		++	+	+

COPD: chronic obstructive pulmonary disease; ILD: interstitial lung disease; CF: cystic fibrosis; PVD: pulmonary vascular disorders; ↓: decreased; $V'O_2,peak$: peak oxygen uptake; ↑: increased; $V'E$: minute ventilation; $V'CO_2$: CO_2 output.

CPET response patterns

Ventilatory response The ventilatory response to exercise in patients with lung disorders is abnormal. Conventionally, the ratio of $V'E$ at peak exercise to the estimated MVV represents the assessment of the ventilatory limitation or of the prevailing ventilatory constraints. Ventilatory limitation is commonly judged to occur when $V'E$/MVV exceeds 85%. In lung diseases, the increase in $V'E$/MVV may reflect the reduction in MVV but also the increase in $V'E$. The ventilatory response during exercise is influenced by metabolic rate ($V'CO_2$), the arterial carbon dioxide tension (Pa,CO_2) and the physiological dead space fraction of the tidal volume (VD/VT). The relationship existing among these variables is described by the following equation:

$$V'E = 863 \times V'CO_2/Pa,CO_2 \times (1-VD/VT)$$

(where 863 is a constant, Pa,CO_2 is the arterial carbon dioxide partial pressure in Torr and VD/VT is the dead space (VD) expressed as a fraction of the tidal volume (VT)). In lung diseases, for a given $V'CO_2$ and Pa,CO_2, $V'E$ is usually increased because of a higher VD/VT. $\Delta V'E/\Delta V'CO_2$ or $V'E/V'CO_2@\theta L$ are often utilised in the functional assessment of patients with lung diseases (e.g. COPD, ILD, PVD). $V'E/V'CO_2$ is usually increased, particularly in patients with PVD.

Pulmonary gas exchange The efficiency of pulmonary gas exchange can be assessed by studying the magnitude of alveolar-arterial O_2 partial pressure difference ($PA-a,O_2$), at rest and during exercise. Normally, arterial O_2 partial pressure (Pa,O_2) does not decrease during exercise, and $PA-a,O_2$ at peak exercise usually remains below 20-30 Torr. In most patients with ILD and PVD, pulmonary gas exchange efficiency is impaired, as indicated by an abnormally large $PA-a,O_2$ (>30 Torr) at peak exercise accompanied by arterial O_2 desaturation. These changes reflect regional ventilation-perfusion ratio ($V'A/Q'$) dispersion and alterations in pulmonary capillary transit time resulting from the recruited pulmonary-capillary volume becoming inadequate for the high levels of pulmonary blood flow.

Cardiovascular response CPET has proved very useful in the detection and quantification of cardiovascular abnormalities during exercise. The characteristic findings are a reduced $V'O_2,peak$, reduced θL, steeper $fC-V'O_2$ relationship (with a reduced HRR at peak exercise), and a shallower profile (or even flattening) of the O_2 pulse increase with increasing $V'O_2$. An abnormal cardiovascular response to exercise is observed in PVD and in particular in patients with idiopathic pulmonary arterial hypertension.

Exercise testing in prognostic evaluation Exercise tolerance is well recognised as a valuable predictor of mortality in healthy subjects. This also appears to be the case in chronic pulmonary diseases. Exercise testing has become an essential component in the prognostic evaluation of patients with lung diseases.

Several studies have confirmed that $V'O_2,peak$ is superior to other indexes in the risk stratification of patients with end-stage lung diseases; many centres, however, utilise field tests for prognostic purposes.

Evaluating the effects of therapeutic interventions

High-intensity endurance CWR protocols, performed on a cycle ergometer or on a treadmill, to the Tlim have been successfully utilised in COPD patients for the evaluation of the effects of therapeutic interventions (*e.g.* bronchodilators, oxygen, heliox, rehabilitation).

References

- Wasserman K, *et al*. Principles of Exercise Testing and Interpretation, 4th Edn. Philadelphia, Lippincott, Williams & Wilkins 2005.
- ERS Task Force on Standardization of Clinical Exercise Testing. Clinical exercise testing with reference to lung diseases: indications, standardization and interpretation strategies. *Eur Respir J* 1997; 10: 2662-2689.
- Johnson B, *et al*. ATS/ACCP Statement on Cardiopulmonary Exercise Testing. IV. Conceptual and physiologic basis of cardiopulmonary exercise testing measurements. *Am J Respir Crit Care Med* 2003; 167: 228-238.
- ERS Task Force, Palange P, *et al.*, Recommendations on the use of exercise testing in clinical practice. *Eur Respir J* 2007; 27: 529-541.
- Ward SA, Palange P, eds. Clinical Exercise Testing. *Eur Respir Mon* 2007, vol. 40.
- ATS statement: guidelines for the six-minute walking test. *Am J Respir Crit Care Med* 2002; 166: 111-117.
- O'Donnell DE, *et al*. Dynamic hyperinflation and exercise intolerance in chronic obstructive pulmonary disease. *Am J Respir Crit Care Med* 2001; 164: 770-777.

BRONCHIAL PROVOCATION TESTING

K-H. Carlsen
Oslo University Hospital, Rikshospitalet, Voksentoppen, Dept of Paediatrics, University of Oslo, Norwegian School of Sport Science, Oslo, Norway
E-mail: k.h.carlsen@medisin.uio.no

"En dernier lieu entre en jeu l'hyperexcitabilité de l'appareil bronchovasomoteur. Ce processus essentiel est le substratum pathologique de l'asthma. Pas l'intervention d'un méchanisme à seul, le degré de l'excitabilité bronchomotorice régit la quantité de mediateurs necessaire (quantum critique) pour l'effet ventilatoire asthmogene assurer."

Tiffenau R. Reseche quantitatives sur les médiateurs bronchoconstrictifs produits par inhalation continue d'allergènes. Pathol Biol 1959; 21: 2293-2310.

Bronchial provocation testing (BPT) may be done with several different aims in mind, as part of research and in the clinical setting, and with several different chemical substances. It may be done to test specific bronchial responsiveness (BR) to an allergen using the allergen bronchial provocation test, or to test nonspecific BR using a bronchial provocation test to histamine (a mediator substance) or metacholine (a transmitter substance), as well as several other different substances (table 1).

Methods of BPT

Testing BR has been divided into direct and indirect methods. Metacholine BPT and histamine BPT represent direct methods, using a transmitter substance (metacholine) or a mediator (histamine) as test agents. Indirect methods include exercise testing (which may also be regarded as a bronchial provocation test, but which otherwise is regarded to fall outside the present topic), inhaled AMP, mannitol and eucapnic voluntary hyperventilation tests. The indirect tests commonly act by causing mediator or transmitter release and their effect on inflammatory cells and nerves.

Previously, BPT was done qualitatively by inhaling the test substance at a 10-fold increase in concentration; however, during the last 25 yrs a quantitative assessment by doubling the concentration/dose of the test substance has been done.

Key points

- BPT with metacholine/histamine is a sensitive measure of asthma, but not so specific when compared with other chronic lung diseases.

- BPT with indirect measures (exercise, adenosine monophosphate, hypertonic saline, mannitol, eucapnic voluntary hyperpnoea) are specific, but not sensitive.

- Indirect measures of BR (exercise, *etc.*) respond rapidly (over 1-4 weeks) to inhaled steroids.

- Direct measures of BR (metacholine, histamine) respond slowly (over 3 months or more).

- Direct measures of BR (metacholine, histamine) are presently the most exact monitoring tool for asthma.

Table 1. Different types of bronchial responsiveness, assessed by different types of bronchial provocation tests

Bronchial responsiveness	Test method	Bronchial provocation test substance
Specific		Allergen bronchial provocation test
Nonspecific	Direct	Metacholine
	Direct	Histamine
	Indirect	Exercise test
	Indirect	Inhaled AMP
	Indirect	Inhaled mannitol
	Indirect	Eucapnic voluntary hyperventilation

AMP: adenosine monophosphate.

Taking bronchial provocation with metacholine as an example, fig. 1 shows the reduction in forced expiratory volume in 1 s (FEV1) caused by inhaling doubling doses of metacholine, with interpolation on the x-axis to determine the concentration of metacholine to cause a 20% decrease in FEV1 (PC20). Later, a simplification of the test was introduced by inhaling single doubling doses of metacholine, determining PD20 (the dose of the test agent causing a reduction in FEV1 of 20%). As it is easier and quicker to determine PD20 as compared with PC20, PD20 may be recommended for clinical routine use.

The test is performed under standardised conditions, with specified nebulisation rates for the tidal breathing method (PC20), inhaling the test agent for 2 min, then measuring FEV1, and then inhaling the doubling concentration. The test is stopped when FEV1 is reduced by ≥20%, and the PC20/PD20 determined by interpolating on the semi-logarithmic dose–response curve (fig. 1).

When determining BR by measuring PD20, the cumulative inhaled dose is determined. This is done by inhaling doubling doses of the test substance. The delivering device most often used at present as is an inspiration-triggered nebuliser, such as the Spira nebuliser (Spira Respiratory Care Centre, Hämeenlinna, Finland) or the Aerosol Provocation System (APS) (Jaeger, Würzburg, Germany). Alternatively a hand-held DeVilbiss nebuliser (DeVilbiss Healthcare, Somerset, PA, USA) may be used.

Determination of PC20 or PD20 are used both for BPT with metacholine and histamine as well as with AMP, and may be used for allergen BPT. A BPT with mannitol was recently developed and launched commercially by inhaling cumulative doses of mannitol through a powder inhaler. Here a 15% reduction in FEV1 (PD15) is used as the cut-off point.

Eucapnic voluntary hyperventilation (EVH) may also be seen as a bronchial provocation test. In this test, the subject inhales dry air with 5% CO_2 for 6 min at a preferred ventilation rate of 85% of maximum voluntary ventilation (MVV), often calculated

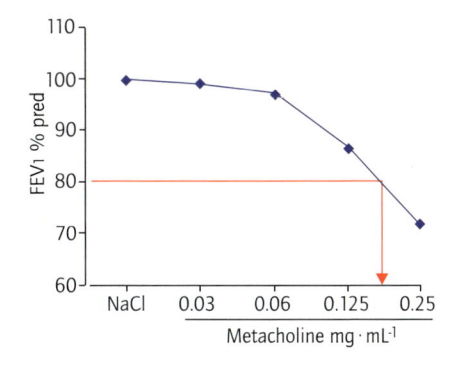

Figure 1. Determination of the concentration of metacholine to cause a 20% decrease in forced expiratory volume in 1 s (FEV1; PC20) by interpolation on the logarithmic x-axis.

Bronchial provocation testing

as FEV1 × 30, but tolerating a ventilation rate down to 65% of MVV (FEV1 × 22). A reduction in FEV1 ⩾10% is taken as a positive test. EVH test has been shown to be particularly sensitive for asthmatic athletes, in particular endurance athletes.

Clinical relevance of BPT

Previously, allergen BPT was often used qualitatively to diagnose asthma, and to demonstrate the reaction of the airways to the allergen. This has changed during recent years through fear of worsening the asthma after such a bronchial provocation test. A long-lasting worsening of nonspecific bronchial hyperresponsiveness was demonstrated after performing an allergen bronchial provocation test, thus the allergen bronchial provocation test is now mostly a tool in research projects, and is not used in clinical practice.

Conversely, the different measures of nonspecific bronchial hyperreactivity are often used, both in a research context, but also in a clinical setting. With the diagnosis of asthma in mind, the direct measures of bronchial hyperreactivity are seen as most sensitive for bronchial asthma, whereas indirect measures are considered to be more specific and less sensitive. In asthma patients from an outpatient clinic compared with healthy subjects, histamine BR was found to be more sensitive but less specific in discriminating asthmatics from healthy subjects. Compared with exercise testing, metacholine bronchial provocation tests were more sensitive, but were markedly less specific for discriminating between asthma and other chronic lung diseases; when adding cold air inhalation to exercise, a sensitivity comparable with metacholine was reached, while maintaining the sensitivity. In a general population of university students, a PC_{20} >8 mg·mL^{-1} ruled out current asthma, whereas a value <1 mg·mL^{-1} was diagnostic of current asthma symptoms.

Other differences are also found between direct and indirect BR. Indirect BR is rapidly influenced by treatment with inhaled steroids, with the first effects already appearing after 1 week, whereas metacholine BR needed several months of inhaled steroids treatment to show an effect.

Results of BPT may be used to monitor the effect of treatment in asthma. It has been shown that metacholine BPT is superior to clinical assessment and lung function measurements in the follow-up of asthma patients. By monitoring the effect of treatment of asthma with inhaled steroids by follow-up using metacholine BPT as compared with follow-up based upon clinical symptoms and lung function measurements, it was shown that follow-up by metacholine BPT improved asthma control and had a positive effect upon airways remodelling, as assessed by bronchial biopsies.

Thus, BPT with various substances and performed in a standaridsed measure is probably, at the present time, the best tool for the continuing follow-up of asthma patients.

References

- Brannan JD, *et al*. The safety and efficacy of inhaled dry powder mannitol as a bronchial provocation test for airway hyperresponsiveness: a phase 3 comparison study with hypertonic (4.5%) saline. *Respir Res* 2005; 6: 144.
- Carlsen KH, *et al*. Cold air inhalation and exercise-induced bronchoconstriction in relationship to metacholine bronchial responsiveness: different patterns in asthmatic children and children with other chronic lung diseases. *Respir Med* 1998; 92: 308-315.
- Cockcroft DW, *et al*. Allergen-induced increase in non-allergic bronchial reactivity. *Clin Allergy* 1977; 7: 503-513.
- Cockcroft DW, *et al*. Bronchial reactivity to inhaled histamine: a method and clinical survey. *Clin Allergy* 1977; 7: 235-243.
- Dickinson JW, *et al*. Screening elite winter athletes for exercise induced asthma: a comparison of three challenge methods. *Br J Sports Med* 2006; 40: 179-182.
- Essen-Zandvliet EE, *et al*. Effects of 22 months of treatment with inhaled corticosteroids and/or beta-2-agonists on lung function, airway responsiveness, and symptoms in children with asthma. The Dutch Chronic Non-specific Lung Disease Study Group. *Am Rev Respir Dis* 1992; 146: 547-554.

- Henriksen JM, Dahl R. Effects of inhaled budesonide alone and in combination with low-dose terbutaline in children with exercise-induced asthma. *Am Rev Respir Dis* 1983; 128: 993-997.
- Nieminen MM, *et al*. Methacholine bronchial challenge using a dosimeter with controlled tidal breathing. *Thorax* 1988; 43: 896-900.
- Pauwels R, *et al*. Bronchial hyperresponsiveness is not bronchial hyperresponsiveness is not bronchial asthma. *Clin Allergy* 1988; 18: 317-321.
- Sont JK, *et al*. Clinical control and histopathologic outcome of asthma when using airway hyperresponsiveness as an additional guide to long-term treatment. The AMPUL Study Group. *Am J Respir Crit Care Med* 1999; 159: 1043-1051.
- Yan K, *et al*. Rapid method for measurement of bronchial responsiveness. *Thorax* 1983; 38: 760-765.

SPUTUM AND EXHALED BREATH ANALYSIS

O. Toungoussova[1], S. Dragonieri[1], A. Zanini[2] and A. Spanevello[1,3]
[1] Fondazione Salvatore Maugeri, IRCCS, Cassano delle Murge and
[2] Tradate
[3] Department of Clinical Medicine, University of Insubria, Varese, Italy
E-mail: antonio.spanevello@fsm.it

Recently, noninvasive techniques such as induced sputum and exhaled breath analysis have been successfully established to reveal an inflammatory status and to find oxidative stress indicators in the airways involved in the pathogenesis of lung diseases. These techniques allow longitudinal sampling of various lung biomarkers of inflammation in the same individual, providing a possibility to monitor the lung damage process and evaluate treatment strategies in patients with respiratory diseases, including children.

Induced sputum

Induced sputum is one of the most referenced methods used to determine airway inflammation in asthma, chronic obstructive pulmonary disease (COPD) and chronic cough both in research and in clinical practice. The induced sputum technique is a relatively noninvasive method allowing sampling of low airway secretions from patients who are not able to produce sputum spontaneously.

Procedure Sputum induction consists of inhalation of nebulised saline solution (isotonic or hypertonic) over different time periods and subsequent expectoration of secretions into a Petri dish.

The subject is asked to inhale 200 mg of salbutamol before induction, and forced expiratory volume in 1 s (FEV_1) is monitored before and after each inhalation to either prevent or detect possible bronchoconstriction.

Key points

- Sputum and exhaled breath analysis are useful noninvasive tools to appraise airway inflammation, particularly in a longitudinal sense.
- Healthy sputum is rich in macrophages and neutrophils but poor in eosinophils, lymphocytes and epithelial cells.
- Many inflammatory mediators can be measured in the fluid phase of sputum.
- Although further validation of many assays is needed, exhaled breath analysis can reveal markers of both asthma and COPD.

After collection, sputum sample is processed according to a standardised method and centrifugation is required to separate sputum cells from the fluid phase.

Safety issues Sputum induction is a simple, safe and well-tolerated procedure even in patients with severe lung diseases and exacerbations. It is recommended to use experienced personnel and to apply standard operating procedures taking into consideration the degree of airway obstruction, to use a modified protocol for subjects with severe airway obstruction, and to assess lung function and symptoms during the procedure. Sputum induction is considered to be safe if the fall in FEV1 is within 5% of baseline after waiting 15 min. Excessive airway constriction may occur in asthmatics and patients with COPD if they show a fall in FEV1 of > 20%. This adverse effect can affect 11% of asthmatics and patients with COPD.

Cell counts in different diseases
A sputum sample from a healthy subject is rich in macrophages and neutrophils and poor in eosinophils, lymphocytes and epithelial cells. These reference parameters can be used for comparison with cell counts obtained from patients with airway inflammation pathology.

Asthma is characterised by sputum eosinophilia, which predicts a favourable response to corticosteroids. However, non-eosinopilic asthma accounts for 25–55% of steroid-naive asthmatics and it is associated with a poor response to corticosteroids.

In COPD, neutrophils are usually increased and they are associated with reduced FEV1, suggesting that neutrophilic airway inflammation is functionally relevant. Up to 40% of subjects with COPD have a high eosinophil count, which appears to predict a response to corticosteroid therapy.

In up to 40% of subjects with chronic cough, a sputum eosinophil count >3% is shown. These subjects with cough and sputum eosinophilia have an objective response to corticosteroid treatment. Conversely, patients without sputum eosinophils do not respond.

Many inflammatory mediators can be measured in the fluid phase of sputum. These mediators belong to the class of granulocyte proteins, leakage markers, cytokines and chemokines, eicosanoids and proteases. Table 1 summarises cellular and fluid phase markers of airway inflammation in different pulmonary diseases.

Reproducibility and validity
The method of induced sputum induction is reproducible, sensitive and valid. The reproducibility is documented within sample, between samples and between examiners for all types of cells. A standardised methodology of sputum induction and processing was issued in 2002

Table 1 Biomarkers in induced sputum

Parameters	Asthma	COPD	Cystic fibrosis	Sarcoidosis
Cellular phase				
TCC			↑	
Eosinophils	↑			
Neutrophils		↑	↑	
CD8+		↑		↑
Fluid phase	ECP, MPO, albumin, fibrinogen, nonkinase plasminogen activator, plasmonogen activator inhibitor, neurokinin A, IL-8, IL-13, Cys-LTs, 8-isoprostane, MMP-9/TIMP ratio	IL-8, IL-6, TNF-α, IL-10, leptin, MPO, HNL, NE, ECP, EPO, LTB-4, GRO-α, MCP-1, GM-CSF, MMP-1, -8, -9, -12, hyaluronan	IL-8, NE	

↑: increased level; COPD: chronic obstructive pulmonary disease; TCC: total cell count; ECP: eosinophil cationic protein; MPO: myeloperoxidase; IL: interleukin; Cys-LTs: cysteinyl leukotrienes; MMP-9: matrix metalloproteinasis-9; TIMP: tissue inhibitor of metalloproteinases; TNF: tumour necrosis factor; HNL: human neutrophil lipocalin; NE: neutrophil elastase; EPO: eosinophil peoxidase; LTB-4: leukotriene B-4; GRO-α: growth related oncogen-α; MCP-1: monocyte chemotactic protein-1; GM-CSF: granulocyte-macrophage colony-stimulating factor; MMP: metalloproteinases.

by the European Respiratory Society Task Force in order to provide guidance for the reproducibility of the results obtained.

Examination of samples obtained from patients with different respiratory diseases demonstrated significant differences in cell counts, confirming the validity of the technique. Reference values and the distribution of cell counts in induced sputum were established on a large number of samples from healthy subjects.

Exhaled breath

Measuring biomarkers in breath is important in monitoring airways inflammation and oxidative stress. Exhaled breath analysis can be defined as analysis of exhaled gases and/or exhaled breath condensate (EBC).

Variable-sized particles or droplets that are aerosolised from the airway lining fluid, distilled water that condenses from gas phase out of the nearly water-saturated exhalate, and water-soluble volatiles that are exhaled and absorbed into the condensing breath are the main components of EBC.

Sample collection and analysis The method of exhaled breath analysis is completely noninvasive, and it is suitable for longitudinal studies and for monitoring the response to pharmacological therapy.

Sample collection is noninvasive, simple and easy to perform in patients of any age. Home-made and commercially manufactured condensers are available.

Breath analysis consists of direct (on line) and indirect (off line) reading methods. Breath analysis is immediately available in the on-line method. The use of indirect methods generally involves collecting and trapping the breath sample and subsequently transferring it to an analytical instrument for analysis.

Various kinds of breath samples include mixed expired air and end expired air. End-exhaled-

Table 2 Biomarkers in exhaled breath condensate

Biomarker	Clinical significance in asthma	Clinical significance in COPD
F2-isoprostanes	Increased reflecting the severity of the disease and the degree of inflammation	Increased reflecting the severity of the disease and the degree of inflammation
Leukotrienes	Elevated in both adults and children	
Prostanoids		Elevated in steroid-naive and steroid-treated patients and correlate with the degree of airway inflammation
pH	Decreased and normalises with glucocorticoid therapy	
Hydrogen peroxide	Increased in both adults and children	Increased in patients with exacerbations
Nitrite/nitrate, nitrosothiol, nitrotyrosine	Increased and correlate with eosinophilic inflammation, reduced by corticosteroid therapy	Increased in early stages of exacerbations
F_{eNO}	Increased and falls after treatment with corticosteroids	Increased during exacerbations and falls after inhaled steroids in stable COPD

COPD: chronic obstructive pulmonary disease; F_{eNO}: exhaled nitric oxide fraction.

air represents the alveolar air concentration and mixed-exhaled-air represents the gas mixture coming from the dead space of the bronchial tree and the alveolar gas-exchange space.

The analysis of sample and measurement of different biomarkers are usually performed by immunoassays mass spectrometry, high-performance liquid chromatography, nuclear magnetic resonance spectra, luminometry, spectophotometry and pH-meter.

Biomarkers Several biomolecules can be detected in exhaled air of healthy subjects and patients with different inflammatory lung diseases (table 2).

Validity Immunoassays for many biomarkers still need to be validated by reference analytical techniques. Concentrations of markers are often close to the detection limit of the assays making analytical data less reliable. Dilution of airway lining fluid may influence the results of biomarker analysis in EBC. A confident dilution marker for EBC has not been standardised yet. However, dilution markers can be avoided by: 1) testing for multiple biomarkers and calculating ratios among them; and 2) identification of a substance that serves as an on-off indicator of an abnormality.

Standardisation and validation of exhaled breath analysis is important, and special attention should be given to technical issues of flow dependence, time dependence, influence of respiratory patterns, origin of markers in EBC, and possible nasal, saliva and sputum contamination.

The latest achievements in standardisation and validation of exhaled breath analysis have been presented in ATS/ERS recommendations.

Conclusions

Noninvasive methods such as induced sputum and exhaled breath analysis have been successfully introduced in clinical practice and research to study airway inflammation involved in the pathogenesis of respiratory diseases.

References

- ATS/ERS recommendations for F_{ENO} procedure. *Am J Respir Crit Care Med* 2005; 171: 912-930.
- Barnes PJ, et al. Pulmonary biomarkers in chronic obstructive pulmonary disease. *Am J Respir Crit Care Med* 2006; 174: 6-14.
- Brightling CE. Clinical applications of induced sputum. *Chest* 2006; 129; 1344-1348.
- Corradi M, Mutti A. Exhaled breath analysis: from occupational to respiratory medicine. *Acta Biomed* 2005; 76: 20-29.
- European Respiratory Society Task Force, Standardised methodology of sputum induction and processing. *Eur Respir J* 2002; 20: Suppl. 37, 1s-55s.
- Hunt J. Exhaled breath condensate: an overview. *Immunol Allergy Clin North Am* 2007; 27: 587-596.
- Montuschi P. Analysis of exhaled breath condensate in respiratory medicine: methodological aspects and potential clinical applications. *Ther Adv Respir Dis* 2007; 1: 5-23.
- Pizzichini E, et al. Indices of airway inflammation in induced sputum: reproducibility and validity of cell and fluid-phase measurements. *Am J Respir Crit Care Med* 1996; 154: 308-317.
- Spanevello A, et al. Induced sputum cellularity. Reference values and distribution in normal volunteers. *Am J Respir Crit Care Med* 2000; 62: 1172-1174.
- Spanevello A, et al. Induced sputum to assess airway inflammation: a study of reproducibility. *Clin Exp Allergy* 1997; 27: 1138-1144.

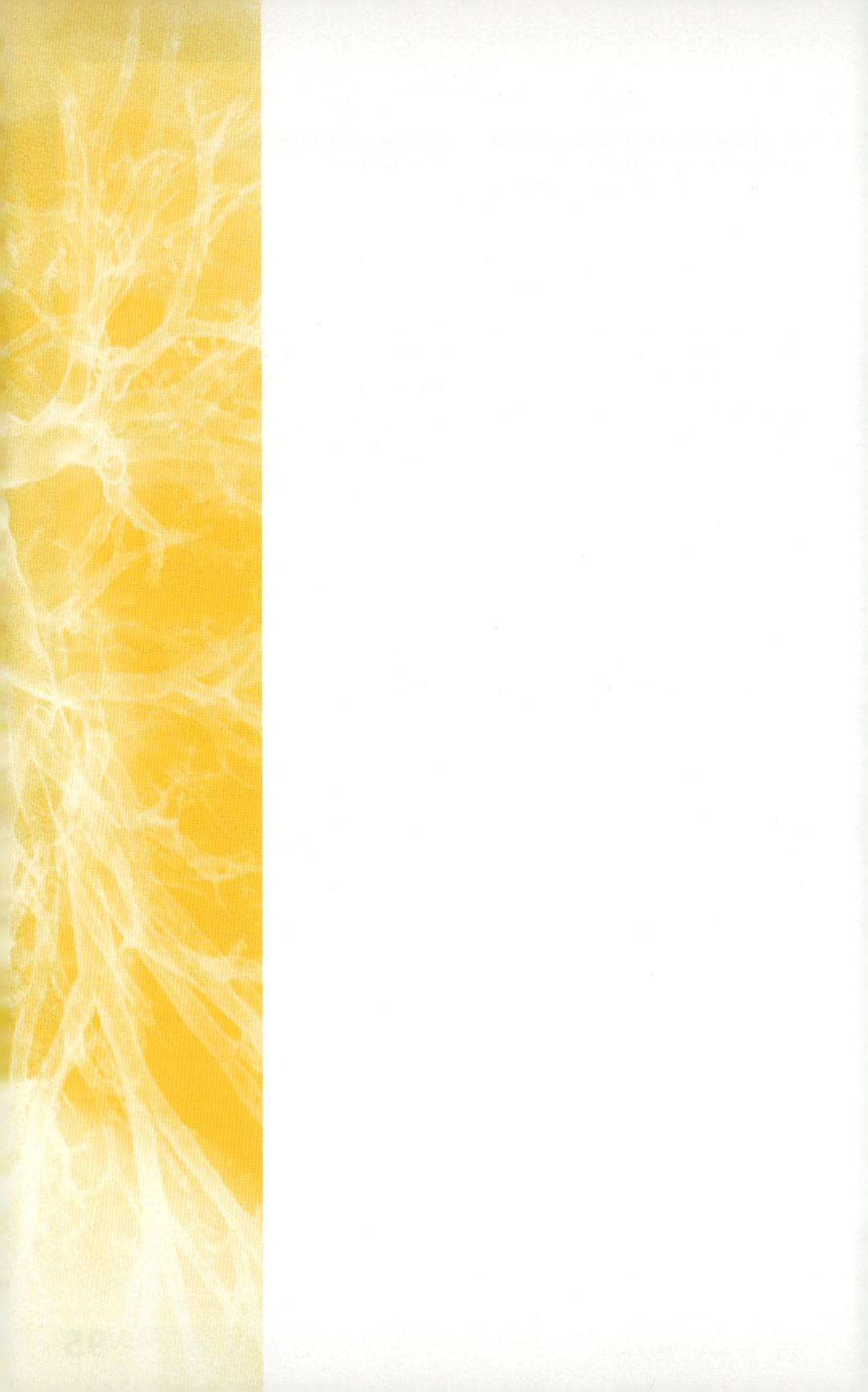

CHAPTER 4:

OTHER DIAGNOSTIC TESTS

BRONCHOSCOPY P.L. Shah	**98**
BRONCHOALVEOLAR LAVAGE P.L. Haslam	**103**
FINE-NEEDLE BIOPSY S. Gasparini	**110**
MEDICAL THORACOSCOPY/PLEUROSCOPY R. Loddenkemper	**112**
THORACENTESIS E. Canalis and M.C. Gilavert	**115**
INTERVENTIONAL PULMONOLOGY M. Noppen	**118**

BRONCHOSCOPY

P.L. Shah
Royal Brompton Hospital, London, UK
E-mail: pallav.shah@ic.ac.uk

Bronchoscopy is an essential tool for the pulmonologist that allows inspection and sampling of the airways. The procedure is usually performed with or without conscious sedation.

Equipment

The flexible bronchoscope has evolved from a fibreoptic instrument to videobronchoscopes, which are now almost universally used in most centres (fig. 1). The videobronchoscope consists of a video chip at the distal end, an instrument channel and optical fibres that illuminate the airways. The images obtained are then transmitted to a monitor. The distal end of the bronchoscope can be angled through to 180°. This, in combination with manual rotation movements, allows the bronchoscope to be manipulated in the airways.

Indications

Bronchoscopy provides diagnostic information in patients with suspected lung cancer, diffuse lung disease and in patients with persistent infection or local pulmonary infiltrates.

Key points

- Bronchoscopy provides diagnostic information in suspected lung cancer and diffuse lung disease and in patients with persistent infection or local pulmonary infiltrates.
- Bronchoscopy also has therapeutic uses in tumour treatment, as well as asthma and emphysema.

Investigation of symptoms

- Haemoptysis
- Persistent cough
- Recurrent infection

Investigation of suspected neoplasia

- Unexplained paralysis of vocal cords or hemi-diaphragm
- Stridor
- Localised monophonic wheeze
- Suspicious sputum cytology
- Unexplained pleural effusions
- Mediastinal tissue diagnosis and staging
- Assess suitability for surgery
- Staging of lung cancer

Assessment of persistent or recurrent infection

- Identification of organisms
- Evaluate airways if recurrent or persistent infection

Assessment of diffuse lung disease

Therapeutic bronchoscopy was traditionally performed for malignant disease. However, there are now a number of therapeutic procedures for emphysema and asthma:

- Clearance of airway secretions
- Removal of foreign body
- Palliation of endobronchial airway obstruction by tumour ablation or insertion of stents

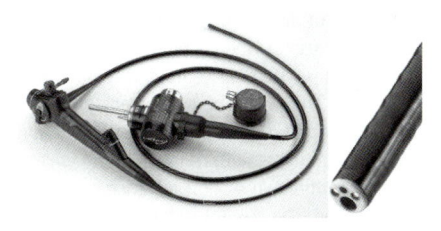

Figure 1. The flexible videobronchoscope.

- Bronchoscopic lung volume reduction for emphysema
- Bronchial thermoplasty for asthma

Patient preparation

Patients should be given a full explanation of the procedure accompanied by written information. Below is a simple pre-procedure check list:

- Patient information – verbal and written
- Informed consent
- Full blood count and clotting – before transbronchial lung biopsy
- Electrocardiogram (ECG) if history of cardiac disease
- Ensure patients do not eat or drink for at least 4–6 h before the procedure
- Ensure patients have someone to take them home following the procedure if they receive sedation
- Patients are advised not to drive or operate machinery for at least 24 h after any sedation

Patients are monitored by continuous oximetry throughout the procedure. Those with pre-existing cardiac disease or hypoxia that is not fully corrected by oxygen therapy should undergo continuous ECG monitoring.

Procedure

The oro-pharynx is anaesthetised with 4% xylocaine and the nasal passage with 2% lidocaine gel. Venous access should always be secured before the procedure, and oxygen administered *via* a single nasal cannula. Bronchoscopy can be performed with or without light sedation (fig. 2).

In the nasal approach, the bronchoscope is lubricated with 2% lidocaine gel and passed through the nares under direct vision. It is then inserted into the nasopharynx until the epiglottis is visualised.

In the oral approach, the patient is asked to bite gently onto a mouth-guard; the bronchoscope is then inserted through this mouth-guard into the posterior pharynx, to the level of the epiglottis.

The movement of the vocal cords is assessed, and they are then anaesthetised using 2-mL aliquots of 2% lidocaine. When the coughing has subsided, the bronchoscope is advanced through the widest part of the glottis, taking care not to touch the vocal cords. The subglottic area of the trachea is very sensitive, and patients initially feel as though they are choking. Further 2-mL aliquots of 2% lidocaine are administered in the trachea, carina, and right and left main bronchi. The airways are carefully inspected down to the subsegmental level for the presence of endobronchial lesions and mucosal abnormalities (fig. 3). Narrowing of the bronchial tree as a result of external compression from large lymph nodes or masses is also noted.

Bronchoscopic sampling

Bronchoscopy also provides an opportunity to obtain a variety of samples which may aid diagnosis.

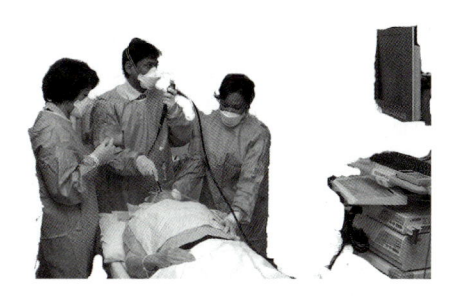

Figure 2. Performance of the bronchoscopy.

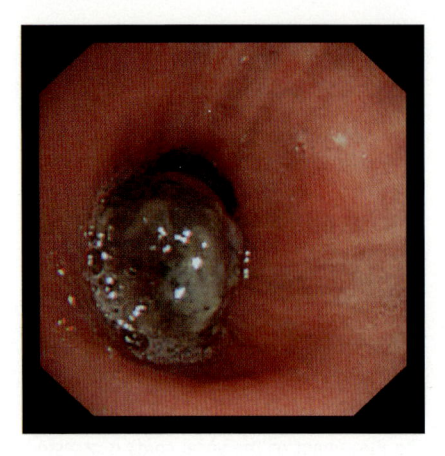

Figure 3. Image obtained through the videobronchoscope.

Bronchial washings The specimens are obtained by injection of 20 mL of normal saline into the affected segment of the lung, followed by aspiration.

Bronchial brushings A fine cytology brush may be used to scrape cells from the surface of any visible lesion or from segments when the lesion is not visible at bronchoscopy. The bronchial brush specimen may be smeared onto a slide and fixed before cytological analysis, or shaken into saline for cytospin preparations.

Bronchial biopsy Any endobronchial abnormalities should be biopsied. At least four samples should be obtained and placed in 10% formol saline solution. The diagnostic yield for polypoid lesions should be high (>90%), but is less for submucosal lesions.

Bronchoalveolar lavage (BAL) This is used in the assessment of diffuse lung disease. The bronchoscope is wedged into the segment of interest and 50–60-mL aliquots of warm saline are injected into the segment. The fluid is then slowly aspirated using low-pressure suction or direct hand suction. A total of 150–250 mL is instilled and aspirated.

Transbronchial lung biopsy Used to obtain parenchymal lung tissue for the evaluation of diffuse lung diseases. It is particularly useful when a broncho-centric component is visible on computed tomography (CT) scans. The closed biopsy forceps are advanced into a specific bronchial segment and advanced until met with resistance. The forceps are then withdrawn a short distance and the jaws opened. The patient is asked to take a deep breath and the open forceps are advanced further. When there is further resistance, the patient is asked to breathe out and a biopsy sample is taken during expiration. Samples are obtained from the periphery of the lung.

Transbronchial fine-needle aspiration (TBNA) mediastinal and hilar lymph nodes can be sampled by TBNA. The site of aspiration is planned on the basis of a cross-sectional CT. The needle is inserted at the desired point perpendicular to the airway wall. The needle is moved back and forth after penetration of the airway wall and suction applied with a 20-mL syringe. Samples collected can then be used to prepare slides or placed in cytolite or saline solution for cytological analysis. This is useful in the staging and diagnosis of suspected lung cancer. This should be performed prior to any other aspects of bronchoscopy so as not to carry over cells from endobronchial lesions into TBNA specimens and hence falsely upstage the patient. Needle aspiration of submucosal lesions may also improve diagnostic yield. Overall TBNA is a low risk procedure with a good yield.

Complications

The adverse effects of flexible bronchoscopy may be due to the sedation, the local anaesthesia or the procedure. The overall incidence of complications is about 2%. Mortality from the procedure is less than 0.02%.

Sedative drugs may depress respiration and have cardiovascular effects (*e.g.* hypotension). Lidocaine may very rarely cause bradycardia, seizures, bronchospasm or laryngeal spasm.

The procedure may cause bronchospasm, laryngospasm, hypoxaemia or cardiac arrhythmias, particularly in patients with pre-existing cardiac disease or hypoxia not corrected by oxygen supplementation. Infection can be introduced by the bronchoscope. Therefore, it is essential to clean and disinfect all instruments before use. Haemorrhage and pneumothorax may follow transbronchial lung biopsy. The risk is 5–7%, and this is increased with paroxysmal coughing. Hypoxia and precipitation of respiratory failure are the main complications of bronchoalveolar lavage particularly as the procedure is often performed in patients with diffuse lung disease.

Advanced diagnostic procedures

The airway is illuminated by blue light during fluorescence bronchoscopy. Normal tissue is visible as fluorescent green, whereas abnormal areas appear brown and red in colour. This absence of autofluorescence occurs in dysplasia, carcinoma *in situ* and invasive carcinoma, and may enable the earlier detection of endobronchial tumours. It is currently used as a research tool but may also be useful in routine practice. Narrow band imaging emphasises the blood vessels and increased capillary loops in the mucosa, which is associated with dysplasia and carcinoma *in situ*. Magnification of images and presentation at high definition further enhances the ability of the operator to detect subtle abnormalities.

Endobronchial ultrasound guided transbronchial fine needle aspiration (EBUS–TBNA) is performed with an integrated linear array ultrasound bronchoscope. It provides excellent ultrasound images of the mediastinum and tissue adjacent to the airways and allows ultrasound-guided sampling of mediastinal lymph nodes or peri-bronchial tumour masses. The sensitivity of this technique is high. Its use is rapidly expanding and is establishing an important role in the diagnosis and staging of lung cancer. A radial or mini probe system can be used for localising peripheral pulmonary masses. These probes are passed through the instrument channel of a flexible bronchoscope into the desired segment with a guide sheath.

The probe is manipulated in the airways with or without radiological guidance. Once the abnormal area is identified the sheath is maintained in position, the radial ultrasound probe is removed and washings, brushings and biopsies obtained *via* the guide sheath.

Therapeutic procedures

The therapeutic role of bronchoscopy is rapidly increasing. It is well established in the treatment of endobronchial tumour obstruction. A variety of techniques such as cryotherapy, electrocautery or laser can be utilised by flexible bronchoscopy to rapidly debulk tumours, which are obstructing the main airways. Several clinical series have demonstrated that these techniques are very effective in palliating symptoms and improving the quality of life for patients with endobronchial tumour occlusion. They also reduce the risk of post-obstructive pneumonia. Where the airway wall structure has been extensively damaged or there is extrinsic compression from the tumour, endobronchial stents can be used to support the airways. Metal self-expanding stents can be inserted *via* a flexible bronchoscopy and are available in both uncovered and covered formats.

Brachytherapy is localised radiotherapy administered to an area of tumour infiltration. A blind-ending catheter is inserted through the instrument channel of the bronchoscope into the desired airway. The bronchoscope is then removed whilst maintaining the catheter in the appropriate position. The catheter can then subsequently be loaded with a remote device which is used to insert radiotherapy beads and hence deliver local radiotherapy. This technique can also be used to treat endobronchial obstruction. However, there is a risk of acute localised oedema following the procedure and treatment carries a significant risk of severe haemorrhage.

More recently a number of innovations have been developed for the bronchoscopic treatment of patients with severe emphysema with significant hyperinflation. Endobronchial valves, such as zephyr valves and intra-bronchial valves, can be used for bronchoscopic volume reduction. Other developments include biological polymers, endobronchial coils and airway stents. A novel treatment for patients with moderate to severe asthma is also delivered bronchoscopically. A special catheter is used to apply radiofrequency energy to the airways in order to destroy airway smooth muscle.

Weblinks

- www.bronchoscopy.org.
- www.interventionalbronchoscopy.co.uk.

BRONCHOALVEOLAR LAVAGE

P.L. Haslam
National Heart and Lung Institute, Imperial College, and Royal Brompton Hospital, London, UK
E-mail: p.haslam@ic.ac.uk

What it is and when to use it

Bronchoalveolar lavage (BAL) involves using a fibreoptic bronchoscope to wash a subsegment of the lungs with sterile physiological saline to sample components from the peripheral air spaces in health and disease. These include immune and inflammatory cells, other pathological cells or features, cytokines, enzymes, lipids or other secreted products, inhaled environmental or occupational agents, and infections. Since the 1960s, BAL has been used extensively in research and to assist in the diagnosis of peripheral lung diseases, notably diffuse interstitial lung diseases (ILDs), occupational lung diseases, rare lung diseases, thoracic malignancies and lower respiratory tract infections (table 1). Numerous publications, including guidelines from the European Respiratory Society (ERS), confirm that BAL cytological or microbiological findings can often increase diagnostic confidence. However, BAL itself is rarely specifically diagnostic and must be interpreted together with clinical, physiological, radiological and other multidisciplinary investigations.

Prior to 2000, BAL was routinely included in the diagnostic work-up of parenchymal lung diseases. Currently, for ILDs, specialists consider that high-resolution computerised tomography (HRCT) patterns are often sufficiently diagnostic to avoid the need for BAL or lung biopsy. A recent American Thoracic Society/ERS consensus terminology for the idiopathic interstitial pneumonias (IIPs) has also changed the way specialists diagnose and manage this subgroup of ILDs. However, BAL is still indicated whenever the preliminary clinical investigations plus HRCT fail to establish a confident diagnosis, or where additional information is needed to confirm, strengthen or to exclude a diagnosis.

How to obtain a sample

This chapter will only describe the BAL procedure recommended in Europe for routine cytological investigation of adults with lung diseases where infection is not suspected. A modified procedure to minimise contamination with irrelevant microorganisms and target sites of maximal involvement is used for the specialist diagnosis of lower respiratory tract infections.

A standardised procedure must be followed in order to minimise variability due to the unknown dilution factor during lavage and many other potential sources of variability. There is still no globally agreed standard for the general conduct of BAL in adults for cytological and other purposes, but the ERS

Key points

- BAL is used to sample components from peripheral air spaces in health and disease.
- BAL is mainly used in the diagnosis of interstitial lung diseases or lower respiratory tract infections.
- BAL must be interpreted in conjunction with results from clinical, pathological and radiological investigations.
- A standardised procedure must be followed.

Table 1. A guide to main types of bronchoalveolar lavage (BAL) inflammatory cells and other cytological features in lower respiratory diseases

	Predominant BAL inflammatory cell types increased compared with normal range[#]	Other characteristic cytological features
Lower respiratory tract infections		
Community-acquired pneumonia; nosocomial pneumonia	Neutrophils very high in bacterial pneumonias	Intracellular bacteria active pneumonia. Identify by special stains, cultures *etc.*
Opportunistic infections in AIDS; organ transplant recipients; on chemotherapy	Neutrophils often moderately increased	*Pneumocystis carinii*, Cytomegalovirus, fungal infections, others by special stains, cultures, *etc.*
Thoracic malignancies		
Adenocarcinoma or bronchoalveolar cell carcinoma	Not of diagnostic value	Tumour cells readily detectable
Metastatic or lymphangitic spread from non-pulmonary tumours	Not of diagnostic value	Tumour cells readily detectable
B-cell lymphomas; Hodgkin's lymphoma	Lymphocytes often strikingly increased	Abnormal lymphocytes consistent with lymphoma; Reed-Sternberg cells
Rare lung diseases		
Alveolar lipoproteinosis	Not of diagnostic value	Globules of lipoprotein plus acellular debris. Original BAL fluid 'milky'
Pulmonary haemosiderosis	Mainly macrophages containing particles similar to smoking but orange-brown	Majority of macrophages heavily laden with haemosiderin: Perl stain positive
Pulmonary Langerhans cell histiocytosis	Mainly macrophages containing smoking-related particles	>5% of the cells shown to be Langerhans cells by CD1a staining or electron microscopy
Fibrosing mineral dust diseases		
Asbestosis	Moderate increases in neutrophils ± eosinophils or lymphocytes	Asbestos bodies indicating exposure
Talc pneumoconiosis	Insufficient information	Talc bodies indicating exposure
Hard metal lung disease/giant cell interstitial pneumonia	Mild increases in neutrophils ± eosinophils or lymphocytes	Refractile particles of hard metal in macrophages plus giant cells if also giant cell interstitial pneumonia

Table 1. Continued

Drug-induced lung diseases		
Amiodarone-induced pneumonitis	Lymphocytes increased	Large phospholipid inclusions in macrophages
Acute alveolar haemorrhage	Not of diagnostic value	Numerous erythrocytes & 'bloody' fluid
Drug-induced eosinophilic pneumonia	Eosinophils very high	
Other pulmonary eosinophilias		
Idiopathic eosinophilic pneumonia	Eosinophils very high	
Allergic diseases: asthma; Churg–Strauss syndrome; bronchopulmonary aspergillosis	Mild to moderate increases in eosinophils plus lymphocytes	
Parasitic infections: schistosomiasis; stronguloides	Eosinophils often high	
Acute respiratory distress syndrome	Neutrophils very high	
Idiopathic interstitial pneumonias		
Idiopathic pulmonary fibrosis	Moderate increases in neutrophils ± eosinophils	
Nonspecific interstitial pneumonitis	Mild increases in lymphocytes plus neutrophils ± eosinophils	
Cryptogenic organising pneumonia	Moderate increases in lymphocytes plus neutrophils	
Lymphoid interstitial pneumonia	Increases in lymphocytes	
Respiratory bronchiolitis associated interstitial lung disease	Mainly macrophages containing smoking-particles plus a few neutrophils	
Desquamative interstitial pneumonia	Macrophages containing smoking particles plus moderate increases in neutrophils ± eosinophils or lymphocytes	
Acute interstitial pneumonia	Neutrophils very high	

Table 1. Continued

Systemic connective tissue diseases	
Systemic sclerosis	Moderate increases in neutrophils ± eosinophils or lymphocytes
Sjorgren's syndrome	Moderate increases in neutrophils ± lymphocytes
Granulomatous lung diseases[¶]	
Sarcoidosis	Moderate increases in lymphocytes ± mild neutrophils. CD4:CD8 ratios increased in about half
Hypersensitivity pneumonitis/ extrinsic allergic alveolitis	Lymphocytes very high. Neutrophils and mast cells also increased after recent exposure. CD4:CD8 ratios frequently decreased
Chronic beryllium disease	Moderate to high increases in lymphocytes. CD4:CD8 ratios increased in nearly all. Lymphocytes proliferate to beryllium salts

#: using differential percentage BAL cell counts (see text for full explanation); ¶: excluding infections.

has long promoted BAL standardisation in a series of European guidelines. The earliest on technical aspects and clinical applications contain useful information but need some updating. However, updated guidelines for a standardised BAL procedure in adults were published in 1999. A protocol using this European standard procedure is as follows.

1) Perform BAL under local anaesthesia using fibreoptic bronchoscopy as part of pre-treatment assessment. 2) Proceed initially as for routine fibreoptic bronchoscopy: generally semi-supine patient positioning; pre-medication with a sedating compound; local anaesthesia with lidocaine removing any excess prior to lavage. 3) For lavage, gently wedge the tip of the bronchoscope into an appropriate subsegmental bronchus. The recommended standard site is right middle lobe in diffuse lung diseases and healthy controls, but the area of greatest radiographic abnormality in localised lung diseases. 4) Sequentially introduce then aspirate standard aliquots (4 × 60 mL) of sterile physiological saline pre-warmed to body temperature through the application tube of the bronchoscope. Do not exceed total introduction volume of 240 mL. 5) Aspirate each aliquot, keeping dwell time to the minimum, using very low suction pressure (3.33–13.3 kPa/25–100 mmHg) to avoid airway collapse. 6) Collect the recovered fluid into a container to which cells are poorly adherent, e.g. siliconised glass or a non-cell adherent plastic designed for suspension tissue cultures. 7) Record the lavage site, total BAL fluid introduction volume and number of aliquots and the total recovery volume. 8) Immediately send the BAL sample to the laboratory to enable processing to commence within 1 h because BAL cells deteriorate rapidly in saline. 9) Also send a patient protocol with age, sex, provisional diagnosis and other factors that influence BAL findings including smoking history (current, ex- or nonsmoker), current medications and associated diseases. 10) If biopsies are needed, perform these after BAL to avoid contamination of BAL with blood or bronchial tissue debris.

BAL is safe and side-effects are low and as for fibreoptic bronchoscopy alone, except for an increased risk of minor post-lavage pyrexia, which can be minimised by keeping total BAL introduction volumes to <300 mL.

Processing of samples for cytology

BAL cells deteriorate rapidly in saline and laboratory processing should commence within a maximum of 1 h after BAL sample collection. To delay deterioration, BAL cells should be transferred into serum-free minimum essential medium containing 25 mM HEPES buffer (MEM-HEPES), which maintains pH7 in an open system.

Non-cell adherent containers and pipettes must be used for all laboratory procedures. The processing procedure is as follows. 1) Measure the total volume of the BAL sample. 2) Record any abnormality in the gross appearance of the fluid, *e.g.* milky appearance suggestive of alveolar lipoproteinosis, very bloody suggestive of acute haemorrhagic conditions. 3) Mix sample to ensure even suspension then divide into measured aliquots for different departments if required (*e.g.* ≥20 mL for BAL cytology and flow cytometry, 10 mL for microbiology, 20 mL for electron microscopy). 4) For BAL cytology, the fluid aliquot should be mixed and a cell viability test conducted, *e.g.* trypan blue. Then make a total count of nucleated cells (per mL) using an improved Neubauer counting chamber and white cell counting stain, *e.g.* Kimura stain. If the original BAL sample is too dilute for an accurate cell count, the count should be performed after separating the cells by centrifugation and resuspending them in higher concentration. 5) Centrifuge the BAL sample at low speed ($300 \times g$ at 4°C for 10 min) to separate the cells and other insoluble components from the supernatant fluid. Aspirate the supernatant and aliquot it for storage at -70°C. Then wash the BAL cell pellet in MEM-HEPES and resuspend in a small volume (1–2 mL) to achieve a more concentrated suspension. Perform a total cell count/mL and calculate the number/mL and total in the original BAL fluid. 6) Adjust the volume of the cell suspension to a standard 1.5×10^6 cells·mL to make cytocentrifuge slide preparations. Use 100-µL aliquots (1.5×10^5 cells) per slide (spin at $90 \times g$ for 4 min). Prepare at least six slides per patient. After air drying, fix two slides in methanol (not formalin which impairs staining of mast cells). Stain with May-Grünwald–Giemsa for differential cell counting. Use other slides for special stains, *e.g.* Gomori–Grocott silver stain for fungi and *Pneumocystis carinii*, and Perl stain for haemosiderin-laden macrophages.

Mucus contamination of BAL samples, if very excessive, can cause serious technical problems in processing. When there is such heavy contamination from the upper airways, BAL results must be interpreted with caution. Mucus can be removed by filtering the lavage through cotton gauze or nylon mesh, but this can cause loss of adherent cells, dust fibres and other components. An alternative to avoid such loss is to remove mucus by treating the BAL cell pellet with the mucolytic dithiothreitol.

Some workers consider that when BAL cells are in tissue culture medium, processing can be delayed for 24 h to enable long distance transport to centralised processing centres. However, this is not advisable because granulocytes are short lived and apoptotic changes start within 9 h. Therefore, it is advisable to transfer BAL cells into tissue culture medium within 1 h and make cytocentrifuge preparations within 1–4 h. Staining of air-dried preparations can be delayed for ≥24 h if necessary. It is essential that BAL is conducted by clinical and laboratory personnel who are highly trained in the procedure, applications and interpretation.

Differential cell counting and other cytological appearances

The standard approach to counting BAL cells in cytocentrifuge preparations is to express the count of each type as a percentage of the total BAL cells (differential percentage cell count). This proportionate approach is not affected by the unknown BAL dilution factor.

Differential cell counts are performed and other cytological features identified by examining May–Grünwald–Giemsa stained cytocentifuge slide preparations by light microscopy. First, low-power magnification ($\times 10$ and $\times 25$ objectives) is used to search the entire preparation and semi-quantitatively grade (0–5) any mucus and erythrocytes, and identify any unusual cytological features, such as inorganic dust particles or fibres, globules of lipoprotein, giant cells, malignant cells or microorganisms. Secondly, higher-power magnification ($\times 40$ or $\times 60$ objectives) is used to count all the immune and inflammatory cells and any other type of nucleated cells employing random-field counting methodology until a total of $\geqslant 400$ cells have been counted. The count for each cell type is then expressed as a percentage of the total cells counted (differential percentage BAL cell count). For diagnostic purposes, all nucleated cells, not only inflammatory cells, must be included in the count to ensure that important information is not omitted (*e.g.* malignant cells, giant cells and epithelial cells). The presence of >5% of bronchial epithelial cells indicates excessive contamination from the upper airways, and such samples are inadequate as a reliable indicator of alveolar events.

Abnormal cell appearances must also be reported, including proportions of foamy macrophages, multinucleate macrophages, giant cells, macrophages containing smoking-related particles, macrophages containing refractile or bi-refringent particles indicative of inorganic dusts, or macrophages heavily laden with haemosiderin confirmed by Perl staining, indicating possible pulmonary haemosiderosis.

When neutrophil counts are very high it is important to check for intracellular bacteria, which can indicate active bacterial pneumonia.

Fungal spores or hyphae may also be seen, and their presence should be confirmed using Gomori–Grocott silver stain, which can also detect *Pneumocystis carinii*.

Normal cell counts and the effect of smoking

BAL cells from healthy nonsmokers are mainly macrophages and a few lymphocytes, but proportions of other cell types are very low. Smoking causes increases in BAL macrophages up to four-fold higher (total and per mL) in healthy smokers compared with nonsmokers; smokers also have slight increases in neutrophils. Thus, smoking must be taken into account when defining normal ranges and interpreting any BAL studies. Published normal ranges show considerable variability when cell counts are expressed per mL or absolute total numbers. However, results are very similar when expressed as differential percentage counts, consistent with these not being influenced by dilution.

The following normal ranges can be employed for differential BAL cell counts: macrophages $\geqslant 80\%$ in nonsmokers and $\geqslant 90\%$ in smokers; lymphocytes $\leqslant 20\%$ in nonsmokers and $\leqslant 10\%$ in smokers; neutrophils $\leqslant 3\%$ in nonsmokers and $\leqslant 4\%$ in smokers; eosinophils $\leqslant 0.5\%$ in nonsmokers and $\leqslant 3\%$ in smokers; mast cells $\leqslant 0.5\%$ in nonsmokers and smokers; plasma cells 0%; and ciliated or squamous epithelial cells $\leqslant 5\%$. Smoking-related inclusions are frequent in macrophages from smokers.

Main applications in the diagnostic work-up of peripheral lung diseases

Although this chapter describes BAL procedures, it would be incomplete not to include a summary indicating how BAL is used in routine clinical investigation to increase confidence in the diagnosis of many parenchymal lung diseases. A quick guide showing the main types of increased BAL inflammatory cells and other cytological features in a wide range of lower respiratory diseases is given in table 1.

References

- American Thoracic Society/European Respiratory Society International Multidisciplinary Consensus Classification of Idiopathic Interstitial

- Pneumonias. *Am J Respir Crit Care Med* 2002; 165: 277-304.
- Bradley B, Branley HM, *et al.* Interstitial lung disease guideline: the British Thoracic Society in collaboration with the Thoracic Society of Australia and New Zealand and the Irish Thoracic Society. *Thorax* 2008; 63: Suppl. 5, v1-v58.
- Bronchoalveolar lavage constituents in healthy individuals, idiopathic pulmonary fibrosis, and selected comparison groups. The BAL Cooperative Steering Group Committee. *Am Rev Respir Dis* 1990; 141: Suppl. 5, S169-S202.
- Costabel U. Ask the expert – diffuse interstitial lung disease. *Breathe* 2007; 4: 165-172.
- Dhillon DP, Haslam PL, *et al.* Bronchoalveolar lavage in patients with interstitial lung diseases: side effects and factors affecting fluid recovery. *Eur J Respir Dis* 1986; 68: 342-350.
- Haslam PL, Baughman RP, eds, Guidelines for measurement of acellular components and recommendations for standardization of bronchoalveolar lavage (BAL). Report of European Respiratory Society (ERS) Task Force. *Eur Respir Rev* 1999; 9: 66, 25-157.
- Haslam PL, Baughman RP. Report of ERS Task Force: guidelines for measurement of acellular components and standardization of BAL. *Eur Respir J* 1999; 14: 245-248.
- Haslam PL. Bronchoalveolar lavage. *Semin Respir Med* 1984; 6: 55-70.
- Klech H, Hutter C, eds. Clinical guidelines and indications for bronchoalveolar lavage (BAL): report of the European Respiratory Society of Pneumology Task Group on BAL. *Eur Respir J* 1990; 3: 937-974.
- Klech H, Hutter C, Costabel U, eds. Clinical guidelines and indications for bronchoalveolar lavage (BAL): report of the European Society of Pneumology Task Group on BAL. *Eur Respir Rev* 1992; 2: 8, 47-127.
- Klech H, Pohl W, eds. Technical recommendations and guidelines for bronchoalveolar lavage (BAL): report of the European Respiratory Society of Pneumology Task Group on BAL.: *Eur Respir J* 1989; 2: 561-585.
- Ohshimo S, Bonella F, *et al.* Significance of bronchoalveolar lavage for the diagnosis of idiopathic pulmonary fibrosis. *Am J Respir Crit Care Med* 2009; 179: 1043-1047.
- Reynolds HY, Newball HH. Analysis of proteins and respiratory cells obtained from human lungs by bronchial lavage. *J Lab Clin Med* 1974; 84: 559-573.
- Woodhead M, Blasi F, *et al.* Guidelines for the management of adult lower respiratory tract infections: report of ERS Task Force in collaboration with ESCMID. *Eur Respir J* 2005; 26. 1138-1180.

FINE-NEEDLE BIOPSY

S. Gasparini
Pulmonary Diseases Unit, Dept of Internal Medicine, Immunoallergic and Respiratory Diseases, Azienda Ospedaliero-Universitaria "Ospedali Riuniti", Ancona, Italy
E-mail: s.gasparini@fastnet.it

Percutaneous (or transthoracic) fine-needle biopsy (PFNB) is a technique that allows cytohistological diagnosis of thoracic lesions. While the first reports on the use of transthoracic needle biopsy date back to the end of the 19th century, the modern era of PFNB did not begin until the mid-1960s when NORDENSTROM (1965) introduced the use of fine needles (diameter <20 Gauge).

Indications

PFNB is indicated when a cytohistological diagnosis is required of peripheral lung lesions (nodules, mass or infiltrates) following a negative bronchoscopy. PFNB is also indicated for expansive lesions of the chest wall or for diagnosis of mediastinal masses, especially those located in the anterior mediastinum.

Contraindications

Absolute contraindications are: contralateral pneumonectomy, bleeding disorders, uncooperative patient, uncontrollable cough, and suspected arteriovenous malformation or hydatid cyst. Relative contraindications that may increase the risk of complications are: respiratory failure, severe chronic obstructive pulmonary diseases, pulmonary arterial hypertension and unstable ischaemic heart disease.

Technique

Guidance systems Biplane fluoroscopy is the traditional guidance system for PFNB. Its main advantage is the real-time visualisation of the needle during the whole procedure. In recent years, computed tomography (CT) has become the most common means of guidance. Although performing a CT scan is more time-consuming, it has several advantages: 1) it helps determine the safest needle trajectory avoiding vascular structures, fissures, bullae and necrotic areas of the tumour; 2) it allows an approach to lesions not visible on fluoroscopy; and 3) it avoid radiation exposure to the operators. However, there are no studies that demonstrate a better sensitivity of CT compared with fluoroscopy. Ultrasound can also be used as guidance system when the lesion is in contact with the thoracic wall.

Type of needle Commercially available needles are either: 1) aspiration needles that yield material satisfactory for cytological evaluation (Chiba, Franseen, Westcott, Nordenstrom); or 2) histology needles that yield a tissue core (Trucut, Menghini, Silverman). Needle diameter should be <20 Gauge and generally 20-22 Gauge needles are utilised. The use of an histology needle is recommended when either a benign

---

Key points

- PFNB is indicated when a cytohistological diagnosis of peripheral lung lesion is required.

- The most common guidance system for PFNB is CT scan. Biplane fluoroscopy and ultrasound can also be used.

- The sensitivity of PFNB for lung cancer is 85-95%.

- The most frequently reported complication is minor pneumothorax (25%).

lesion or a malignancy other than cancer (*i.e.* lymphoma) is suspected.

Results

The reported sensitivity of PFNB ranges from 60-97%. In patients with lung cancer, a diagnosis by PFNB is generally established in 85-95% of cases. Lower sensitivities are reported for benign lesions (4-14%). Sensitivity may be affected by the size and location of the lesion, number of needle passes, size of the needle, availability of immediate cytological assessment and experience of the operator. False-positive results are rare and the specificity of the technique is extremely high. However, it is important to emphasise that a nondiagnostic PFNB does not rule out the possibility of malignancy.

Complications

The most frequently reported complication is minor pneumothorax, with an incidence of ~25%. Major pneumothorax, requiring chest tube drainage, occurs in 5% of cases. Haemoptysis occurs in 5-10% of cases and is generally mild and self-limited. Rare complications include air embolism (0.07%), haemothorax, empyema, tumour implantation along the needle tract and haemopericardium.

References

- Gasparini S, *et al*. Integration of transbronchial and percutaneous approach in the diagnosis of peripheral pulmonary nodules or masses. *Chest* 1995; 108: 131-137.
- Gould MK, *et al*. Evaluation of patients with pulmonary nodules: when is it lung cancer. *Chest* 2007; 132: Suppl. 3, 108s-130s.
- Nordenstrom B. A new technique for transthoracic biopsy of lung cancer. *Br J Radiol* 1965; 38: 550-553.
- Shaham D. Percutaneous transthoracic needle biopsy. *Radiol Clin North Am* 2000; 38: 525-534.

MEDICAL THORACOSCOPY/ PLEUROSCOPY

R. Loddenkemper
Former Chief, Dept of Pneumology II, Lungenklinik Heckeshorn, HELIOS
Klinikum Emil von Behring, Berlin, Germany
E-mail: rloddenkemper@dzk-tuberkulose.de

Key points

- MT/P has the advantage compared with VATS that it can be performed under local anaesthesia or conscious sedation, in an endoscopy suite using nondisposable rigid (or semi-rigid) instruments. Thus, it is considerably less expensive.

- The leading indications for MT/P are pleural effusions, both for diagnosis – mainly in exudates of unknown aetiology – or for staging in diffuse malignant mesothelioma, lung cancer, and for talc poudrage, the best conservative method today for pleurodesis.

- MT/P can also be used efficiently in the management of early empyema and pneumothorax.

- In the above indications, MT/P can replace most surgical interventions, which are more invasive and more expensive.

- MT/P is a safe procedure, even easier to learn than flexible bronchoscopy, provided sufficient experience with chest-tube placement has been gained.

- MT/P as part of the new field of interventional pulmonology should be included in the training programme of chest physicians.

Thoracoscopy was first used 100 yrs ago, primarily as a diagnostic procedure, but soon also as a therapeutic technique for lysis of pleural adhesions by means of thoracocautery ('Jacobaeus operation') to facilitate pneumothorax treatment of tuberculosis. At the end of the last century, the addition of the term 'medical' was necessary in order to distinguish this procedure from 'surgical' thoracoscopy, which is much more invasive, using general anaesthesia, a double-lumen endotracheal tube and multiple points of entry. Surgical thoracoscopy is better described as video-assisted thoracic surgery (VATS), whereas medical thoracoscopy can be performed under local anaesthetic or conscious sedation in an endoscopy suite using nondisposable rigid or semi-rigid (semi-flexible) instruments. It is therefore considerably less invasive and less expensive.

Medical thoracoscopy/pleuroscopy (MT/P) are invasive techniques that would be used only when other more simple methods fail. Today, it is considered to be one of the main areas of interventional pulmonology. As with all technical procedures, there is certainly a learning curve before full competence is achieved. Therefore, appropriate training is mandatory. Actually, the technique is very similar to chest-tube insertion by means of a trocar, the difference being that, in addition, the pleural cavity can be visualised (fig. 1) and biopsies can be taken from all areas of the pleural cavity including the chest wall, diaphragm, mediastinum and lung.

There are two different techniques of diagnostic and therapeutic thoracoscopy, as

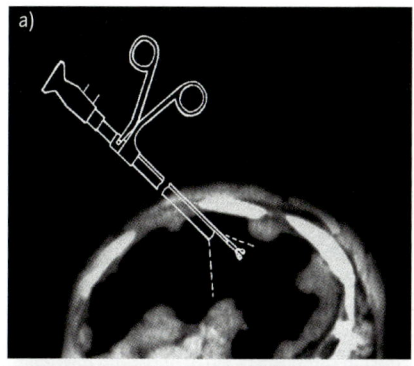

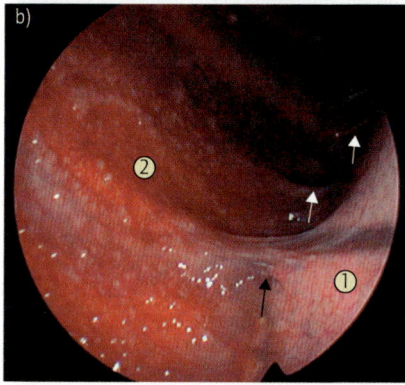

Figure 1. a) Diagram of a computed tomography scan showing several malignant lesions of the parietal pleura for which biopsies can be taken under visual control through the thoracoscope. b) Tuberculous pleural effusion. After drainage of 800-mL serous effusion, typical sago-like nodules on the reddened inflamed posterior chest wall, firm adhesions between right lower lobe (1) and chest wall (2). Reproduced from LODDENKEMPER *et al.* (2010), with permission from the publisher.

performed by the pneumologist. The one, very similar to the technique first described by Jacobaeus for diagnostic purposes, uses a single entry with a rigid 9-mm thoracoscope with a working channel for accessory instruments and an optical biopsy forceps under local anaesthesia. This single-entry technique has now been modified by the introduction of an autoclavable semi-flexible pleuroscope (Olympus), which has the advantage that handling is very simple, similar to a flexible bronchovideoscope.

The other technique uses two entries, one with a 7-mm trocar for the rigid examination telescope and the other with a 5-mm trocar for accessory instruments, including the biopsy forceps. For this technique, neuroleptic or general anaesthesia is preferred.

For cauterisation of adhesions and blebs, or in case of bleeding after biopsy, electrocoagulation should be available. For pleurodesis of effusions, 4–6 g of a sterile, dry, asbestos-free talc is insufflated through a rigid or flexible suction catheter with a pneumatic atomiser. In pneumothorax patients, 2–3 g of talc is sufficient. After thoracoscopy, a chest tube is introduced through which immediate suction is started carefully.

MT/P is a safe examination if the contraindications are observed and if certain standard criteria are fulfilled. An obliterated pleural space is an absolute contraindication. Relative contraindications include bleeding disorders, hypoxaemia and an unstable cardiovascular status, and persistent uncontrollable cough. The most serious, but fortunately least frequent, complication is severe haemorrhage due to blood-vessel injury during the procedure. However, this and also pulmonary perforations, can be avoided by using safe points of entry and a cautious biopsy technique. Reported mortality rates (<0.001) are very low. The most frequent complication is nonspecific, transient fever.

Pleural effusions are by far the leading indication for MT/P, both for diagnosis, mainly in exudates of unknown aetiology, and for staging in diffuse malignant mesothelioma or lung cancer, and for treatment by talc pleurodesis in malignant or other recurrent effusions, or in cases of empyema. Spontaneous pneumothorax for staging and for local treatment is also an excellent indication. For those who are familiar with the technique, other (mainly diagnostic) indications are biopsies from the diaphragm, the lung, *e.g.* in interstitial lung diseases, the mediastinum and the pericardium. In addition, MT/P offers a remarkable tool for research as a 'gold standard' in the study of pleural effusions.

```
Needle          Effusion         Medical
biopsy         (cytology)      thoracoscopy
  |                |                |
  44              62               95
   \              / \              /
    \            /   \            /
     74                  96
       \                /
        \              /
              97
```

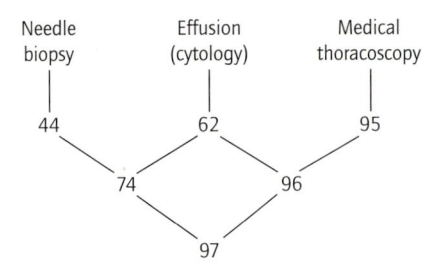

Figure 2. The different biopsy techniques used in the diagnosis of malignant pleural effusions and their sensitivity expressed in percentages (cytological and histological results combined). Prospective intrapatient comparison (n=208). Reproduced from LODDENKEMPER (1998).

Malignant pleural effusions represent the leading diagnostic and therapeutic indication for MT/P. MT/P has a much higher diagnostic sensitivity and specificity in malignant pleural effusions than closed needle biopsy and pleural fluid cytology (fig. 1). Biopsies can be taken under direct visual control not only of the costal pleura, but also of the visceral and diaphragmatic pleura. An additional advantage is that the diagnostic procedure can easily be combined with the therapeutic procedure of talc poudrage for pleurodesis. MT/P is helpful in the staging of lung cancer, diffuse malignant mesothelioma and metastatic cancers. In lung cancer patients, thoracoscopy can determine whether the tumour spread to the pleura is secondary to venous or lymphatic obstruction or is parapneumonic. As a result, it may be possible to avoid exploratory thoracotomy or

```
Needle          Effusion         Medical
biopsy          (culture)      thoracoscopy
  |                |                |
  51              28               99
   \              / \              /
    \            /   \            /
     61                 100
```

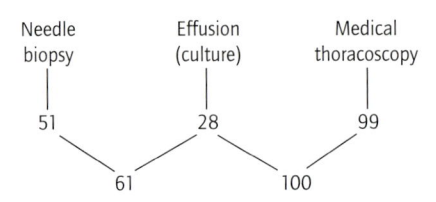

Figure 3. The different biopsy techniques used in the diagnosis of tuberculous pleural effusions and their sensitivity expressed in percentages (cytological and histological results combined). Prospective intrapatient comparison (n=100). Reproduced from LODDENKEMPER (1998).

to determine operability. In diffuse malignant mesothelioma, MT/P provides an earlier diagnosis and a better histological classification due to larger and consequently more representative biopsies, as well as a more precise staging.

In tuberculous pleural effusion, MT/P has a high diagnostic sensitivity of almost 100% (fig. 2). It provides much more often a bacteriological confirmation of the diagnosis of TB and thus the possibility to perform susceptibility tests. In parapneumonic pleural effusion (empyema), MT/P offers the possibility to remove fibrinopurulent membranes and break up loculations, thus creating one single pleural cavity for successful local treatment.

In other pleural effusions, when the origin remains indeterminate, the main diagnostic value of MT/P lies in its ability to exclude, with high probability, malignant or tuberculous disease. In pneumothorax patients, MT/P allows talc poudrage for pleurodesis, which is highly effective in recurrence prevention.

References

- Diacon AH, *et al*. Diagnostic tools in tuberculous pleurisy: a direct comparative study. *Eur Respir J* 2003; 22: 589–591.
- Loddenkemper R, *et al*. Medical Thoracoscopy/Pleuroscopy: Manual and Atlas. New York, Thieme, 2011.
- Loddenkemper R. Thoracoscopy – state of the art. *Eur Respir J* 1998; 11: 213–221.
- Loddenkemper R, *et al*. Treatment of parapneumonic pleural effusion and empyema – conservative view. *Eur Respir Mon* 2004; 29: 199–207.
- Noppen M. Pleural biopsy and thoracoscopy. *Eur Respir Mon* 2010; 48: 119–132.
- Rodriguez-Panadero F, *et al*. Thoracoscopy: general overview and place in the diagnosis and management of pleural effusion. *Eur Respir J* 2006; 28: 409–422.
- Tassi GF, *et al*. Advanced techniques in medical thoracoscopy. *Eur Respir J* 2006; 28: 1051–1059.
- Tschopp JM, *et al*. Management of spontaneous pneumothorax: state of the art. *Eur Respir J* 2006; 28: 637–650.
- Vansteenkiste J, *et al*. Medical thoracoscopic lung biopsy in interstitial lung disease: a prospective study of biopsy quality. *Eur Respir J* 1999; 14: 585–590.

THORACENTESIS

E. Canalis[1] and M.C. Gilavert[2]
[1] Thoracic Surgery Service
[2] Intensive Care Unit, Hospital Universitari Joan XXIII, IISPV, URV, Tarragona, Spain
E-mail: emilio.canalis@urv.cat

Thoracentesis (pleural tap; fig. 1) is a frequently performed procedure that is used to remove and analyse pleural fluid. Its goals may be diagnostic and/or therapeutic.

Diagnostic thoracentesis should be performed on almost all patients with a pleural effusion of unknown origin. Its main purpose is to differentiate between transudate and exudate. The number of diagnoses established by pleural fluid analysis varies with the population being evaluated. Careful history and physical examination, radiological evaluation, and ancillary blood tests are crucial in establishing a pre-test diagnosis.

The main purpose of therapeutic thoracentesis is to relieve dyspnoea and respiratory insufficiency caused by pleural effusion.

Patient position

A sitting position is preferred in conscious patients, as this will help the fluid to settle in the posterior and basal regions of the lung (usually the 7th to 8th intercostal spaces, although clinical examination may reveal different locations of the fluid).

Once a comfortable position for operating on the patient is achieved, the site for the puncture must be selected. This is decided according to the results of the physical examination and the radiological findings, which will indicate characteristics such as the size and localisation of the main effusion and whether it is free-organised, free-floating or encapsulated. Ultrasound examination is valuable to assess fluid presence accurately.

The puncture should be guided by ultrasound or attempted one intercostal space further down from where dullness on percussion starts. At least in pleural effusions of smaller size, ultrasound guidance is strongly recommended.

The thoracentesis set

The thoracentesis set is detailed in table 1.

Procedure

1. Under sterile conditions, the selected region of puncture is disinfected with povidone iodine or alcohol, and a sterile draping, preferably with a centre hole, is taped to the patient's back.

2. Local anaesthesia is injected stepwise, at first with an intradermal injection producing a small wheal, then infiltrated subcutaneously and into the intercostal muscle down to the parietal pleura at the upper rim of the lower rib in order to avoid the intercostal nerve and vessels. During the injection, alternating aspiration is performed until the parietal pleura is penetrated and pleural fluid is

> **Key points**
>
> - Thoracentesis may be diagnostic or therapeutic in patients with a pleural effusion.
> - Ultrasound examination is valuable in guiding the procedure.
> - There are no absolute contraindications, and complications are rare, but the possibility should be taken into account.

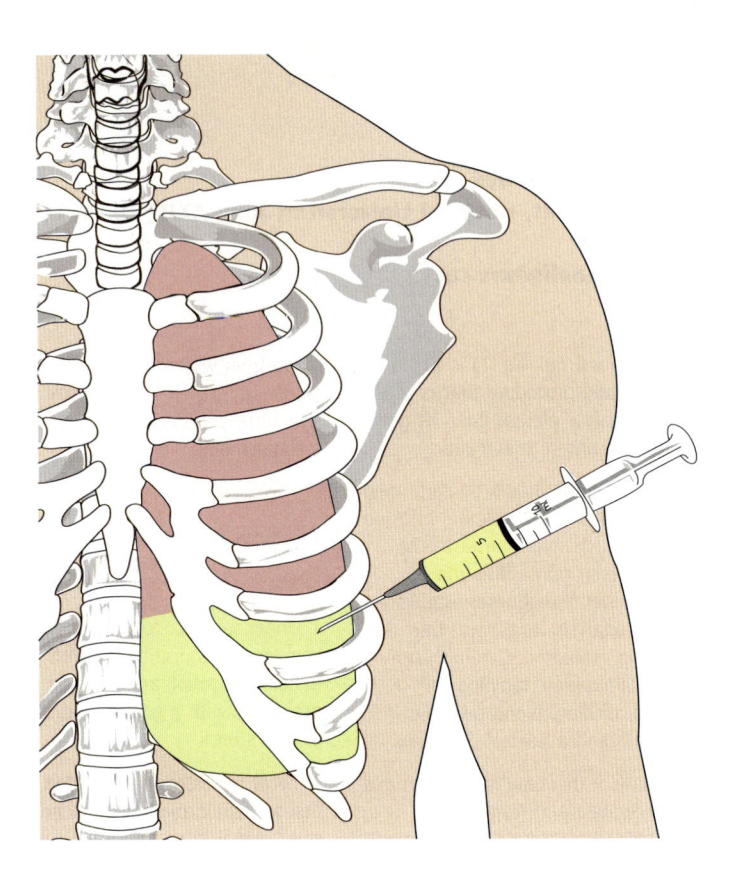

Figure 1. Thoracentesis needle through the intercostal space.

aspirated. Then 20–60 mL of pleural fluid should be aspirated for fluid analysis.

Diagnostic thoracentesis can occasionally be carried out without local anaesthesia if the adult patient is calm, the puncture is anticipated to be easy, the subject is not obese and the operator is experienced.

3. For therapeutic thoracentesis, a catheter should be used, which is immediately connected to a closed three-way stop-cock. This allows aspiration syringes to be changed or facilitates connection to a suction device.

4. As soon as the procedure is finished, the needle or the catheter is removed and pressure is applied to the wound for a few minutes, followed by a sterile dressing.

5. Chest radiography should be carried out to exclude the development of a pneumothorax, unless the procedure has been performed under ultrasound guidance without any problems.

Contraindications

Diagnostic thoracentesis has no absolute contraindications provided that it is done with caution by experienced persons. The following are relative contraindications.

- Altered coagulation. A decision must be taken as to whether thoracentesis is really needed. If so, it may be necessary to reverse anticoagulation or to administer fresh frozen plasma or platelets.

Table 1. Thoracentesis set

Povidone iodine solution or alcohol
Sterile drapes, gloves and gauzes
Abbocath-type needle catheters
Local anaesthesia
Syringes
Three-way stopcock
Aspiration set (if therapeutic)
Adhesive strips
Instrumentation table

- Mechanical ventilation with positive pressure at the end of expiration. Whenever possible, mechanical ventilation is suspended briefly. If this is not possible, thoracentesis must be carried out with caution using ultrasound guidance.
- Local skin infections such as cellulitis or *Herpes zoster*.
- Small effusions (this should be done under ultrasound control).

Complications

As with any invasive investigation, complications may occur, but these are rare. Patients have to be informed about possible complications when asked to give their informed consent. The most important are:

- Pneumothorax. This is usually only small if caused by entrance of air into the pleural cavity through the needle or the aspiration system. It can become larger if the lung is injured by the needle.
- Hypotension. This may be induced by a vaso-vagal reaction when the parietal pleura is punctured. It can be avoided by careful local anaesthesia and prevented by administering atropine (not routinely necessary).
- Bleeding. This can be prevented by avoiding the lower rim of the upper rib and by excluding coagulopathies.
- Haemopneumothorax. This is rare when the above-described technique is observed and the patient has no bleeding disorder.
- Re-expansion pulmonary oedema. This can be prevented by removing <1–1.5 L of pleural fluid.

Additional recommendations

1. The region from the mid-clavicular line to the sternum should be avoided, as here the vessels are located in the centre of the intercostal space.

2. Sterile conditions are mandatory during the whole procedure to prevent infection which may lead to empyema.

3. For diagnostic purposes, 20 mL of pleural fluid is usually sufficient to assess the appearance of the fluid and for chemical, cytological, and bacteriological analysis. Recent work recommends ~60 mL for cytology in case of suspected malignancy.

References

- Abouzgheib W, *et al*. A prospective study of the volume of pleural fluid required for accurate diagnosis of malignant pleural effusion. *Chest* 2009; 135: 999–1001.
- Alcaide MJ, *et al*. Toracocentesis y drenaje pleural. *In*: De Mendoza D, *et al*. Medicina Intensiva Respiratoria. Tarragona, Silva ed., 2008.
- Chest Trauma. *In*: Advanced Trauma Life Support (ATLS) Course Manual. 7th Edn. Chicago, American College of Surgeons, 2004; pp. 107–121.
- Capizzi SA, Prakash UB. Chest roentgenography after outpatient thoracentesis. *Mayo Clin Proc* 1988; 73: 948–950.
- Dev SP, Nascimento B Jr. Videos in clinical medicine. *N Engl J Med* 2007; 357: l5.
- Duncan DR, *et al*. Reducing iatrogenic risk in thoracentesis: establishing best practice *via* experiential training in a zero-risk environment. *Chest* 2009; 135: 1315–1320.
- Feller-Kopman D, *et al*. Assessment of pleural pressure in the evaluation of pleural effusions. *Chest* 2009; 135: 201–209.
- Gaba DM, Dunn WF. Procedural risks in thoracentesis: process, progress, and proficiency. *Chest* 2009; 135: 1120–1123.
- Sahn SA. Diagnostic value of pleural fluid analysis. *Clin Chest Med* 1995; 16: 269–278.
- Swiderek J, *et al*. Prospective study to determine the volume of pleural fluid required to diagnose malignancy. *Chest* 2010; 137: 68–73.

INTERVENTIONAL PULMONOLOGY

M. Noppen
University Hospital UZ Brussel, Brussels, Belgium
E-mail: Marc.Noppen@uzbrussel.be

Interventional pulmonology encompasses both diagnostic and therapeutic bronchoscopic, thoracoscopic and other techniques that go beyond everyday "simple" procedures performed by pulmonary clinicians. In the context of pulmonary function testing and interventional pulmonology, this chapter will be limited towards the effects on interventional bronchoscopy of pulmonary function tests.

Interventional bronchoscopy here is limited to all (rigid and flexible) bronchoscopic procedures designed to reopen obstructed central airways (including laser, electrocautery, cryotherapy, brachytherapy and photodynamic therapy) or to establish airway patency (airway stenting).

The literature on interventional bronchoscopy has, during the past few decades, mainly focused on the "technicality" of the various procedures; data pertaining to the functional assessment and evaluation are relatively scarce. Certainly in the "pioneer era" of interventional pulmonology, patients were referred in a (very) late stage of disease, with severe dyspnoea and/or stridor or signs of post-obstructive disease, requiring prompt intervention without additional testing. In stable and nonlife-threatened patients with or without symptoms, however, additional testing before proceeding an intervention may be helpful in patient selection, and post-procedure testing may focus the usefulness and efficacy of an intervention. Thus, as more centres successfully perform various interventional bronchoscopic techniques, the need is increasing for a critical evaluation and selection of patients in order to understand the physiological effects of these interventions and gain an evidence-based, algorithmic integration of these techniques in the overall care of these patients. Alternatively, abnormalities observed during pulmonary function testing may prompt the clinician to suspect an upper (or central) airway stenosis (UAS).

In patients suffering from malignant airway stenosis, which is not candidate for, or unresponsive to, "classical" oncological treatments, the main interest of interventional pulmonological treatment should lie in the improvement of quality of life and the avoidance of death by suffocation.

Pulmonary function tests in UAS

Inspection of the maximal inspiratory and expiratory flow–volume loop is currently the most widely used method to detect/suspect

> **Key points**
>
> - Symptoms of central airway stenosis occur late, after at least 50% (on exercise) or 80% (at rest) of the tracheal lumen is obstructed.
> - The diagnostic accuracy of spirometric indices and visual flow–volume loop criteria in detecting central airway stenosis is relatively poor.
> - Interventional bronchoscopic techniques have been shown to significantly improve objective pulmonary function and quality of life.

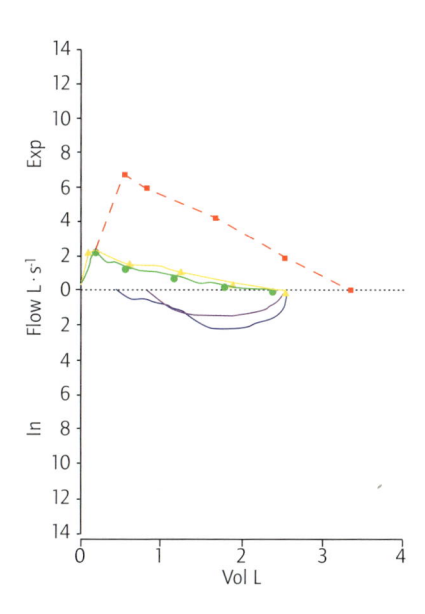

Figure 1. A typical flattened "coffin" flow–volume loop curve in a patient with severe fixed tracheal obstruction due to an inoperable intrathoracic goitre. ●: pre; ▲: post.

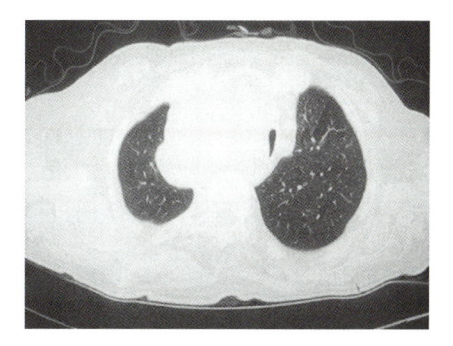

Figure 2. Computed tomography image of the patient in fig. 1.

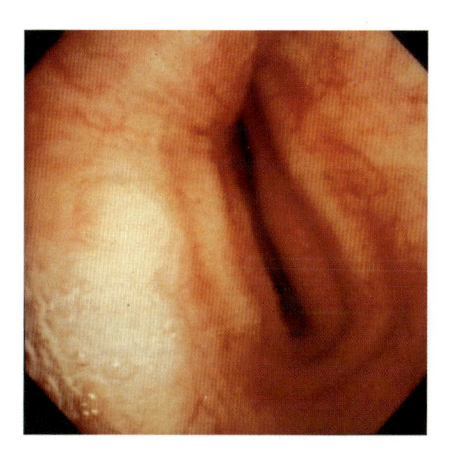

Figure 3. Bronchoscopic image of the patient in figs 1 and 2.

the presence of UAS (figs 1–3). However, significant changes in spirometry appear relatively late in the course of the stenosing process. The airway cross-sectional area indeed has to be reduced by ⩾50% in order to cause breathing impairment, a clinical observation that recently has been corroborated by a fluid dynamics study of tracheal stenosis. There is also a very poor or even absent correlation between the severity of the UAS as determined by the flow loop analysis and its spirometrically derived indices, and breathing symptoms or radiological assessment of UAS. UAS becomes more easily symptomatic during exercise (from a tracheal diameter ⩽8 mm), whereas at rest the diameter has to be ⩽5 mm before symptoms occur. All of this may explain why the diagnostic accuracy of the various individual spirometric indices and visual flow-volume loop criteria in detecting UAS is relatively poor (receiver-operating-curve analysis <0.52).

Typical flow–volume appearances, however, may be helpful: a typical "coffin" or "box" appearance of the flow–volume curve is suspicious for a fixed UAS due to severe tracheal obstruction; an isolated plateau during expiration is suspicious for an intrathoracic airway stenosis; an isolated plateau of the inspiratory loop suggests extrathoracic obstruction. Obstructive lesions at multiple airway sites and associated abnormalities such as severe chronic obstructive pulmonary disease may cause atypical flow–volume loop characteristics.

Interventional pulmonology

UAS may lead to typical flow–volume loop abnormalities and spirometric derived indices, but

- the diagnostic accuracy in detecting UAS of these tests is (very) low;
- symptoms of UAS occur relatively late in the UAS process; and
- symptoms of UAS occur earlier during exercise.

The most commonly used quantitative criteria to detect UAS include maximal expiratory flow at 50% of forced vital capacity (FVC; MEF50%)/maximal inspiratory flow at 50% of FVC (MIF50%) (<0.30 for intrathoracic, and >1 for extrathoracic stenosis), forced expiratory volume in 1 s (FEV1)/maximum expiratory flow (>10 mL·L^{-1}·min^{-1}), MIF50% (<100 L·min^{-1}), and FEV1/FEV0.5 (>1.5). The visual criteria are the presence of a plateau, biphasic shape, or oscillations in the inspiratory or expiratory curves.

Impact of interventional bronchoscopy on pulmonary function

In most patients, but not all, pulmonary function significantly improves after restoration of central airway patency. EISNER *et al.* (1999) demonstrated mean improvements of 388 mL for FVC, 1,288 mL for peak expiratory flow, and 550 mL for FEV1 after stenting in nine patients. GELB *et al.* (1992) showed increases in FVC from 64% to 73% predicted, and in FEV1 from 49% to 72% predicted after stenting in 17 patients. VERGNON *et al.* (1995) showed mean improvements in FEV1 (440 mL), peak expiratory flow (920 mL·s^{-1}), maximum expiratory flow 25–75% (470 mL·s^{-1}), and forced inspiratory volume in 1 s (310 mL) after stenting in a total of 24 patients. Improvements were more outspoken in intra- and extrathoracic tracheal stenosis as compared with bronchial stenosis. NOPPEN *et al.* (2004) showed improvements after tracheal stenting for inoperable benign thyroid disease (FEV1 +470 mL, FVC +620 mL, peak expiratory flow +79 L·min^{-1}) and after tracheal laser debulking and/or stenting for inoperable malignant thyroid disease (FEV1 +540 mL, FVC +730 mL, peak expiratory flow +96 L·min^{-1}) (figs 4 and 5).

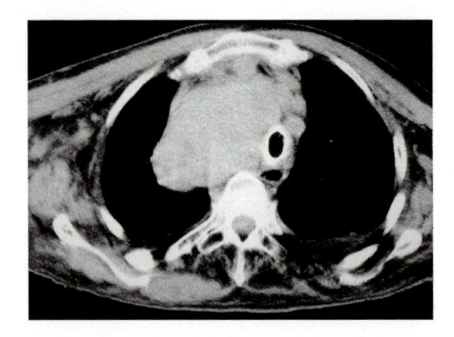

Figure 4. Computed tomography image of the same patient after stenting.

ERNST *et al.* (2007) showed improvements in some but not all patients stented for severe tracheomalacia, in respiratory symptoms, quality of life, and in functional status assessed by exercise testing and FEV1. Overall, these retrospective and prospective observational case series, in selected patients, show significant but not homogeneous improvements in a number of functional parameters. Data on physiological effects of repermeabilisation techniques without additional stenting are even more scarce: objective improvements in pulmonary function was seen in 58% of patients after cryotherapeutic debulking of central airways,

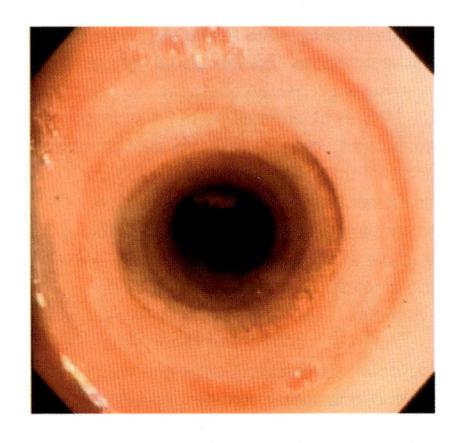

Figure 5. The same patient, 1 yr after stent insertion.

and a trial of 19 patients with major airway obstruction due to lung cancer showed significant improvements in a variety of parameters including FEV1, FVC and ratio of forced expiratory/forced inspiratory flow rate at 50% of vital capacity, after endobronchial radiotherapy.

A breakthrough article by MIYAZAWA et al. (2004) shed more light on the underlying physiological phenomena occurring after airway stenting, including the heterogeneity of response. A total of 64 patients with extrinsic airway stenoses due to advanced malignancy were studied; patients were classified by location of the stenosis (tracheal, carinal, bronchial or multi-site). Pulmonary function tests and CT were performed before and after stenting. Prior to stent insertion, patients underwent endobronchial ultrasound to evaluate the airway walls and ultrathin bronchoscopy to evaluate airway patency distal to the obstruction. Stents were placed at the visualised flow-limiting segments (choke points). Distinctive flow–volume loop patterns were found for each of the four types of stenosis. Most patients showed symptomatic improvement after stenting, and most flow–volume loops returned to normal. All 10 patients with multi-site, extensive stenosis, however, showed persistent choke points, associated with only minor improvements in symptoms and spirometry. Repeat endoscopy in these patients showed upstream displacement of choke points (distally from the inserted stents), and ultrasound showed destructed cartilage at these sites. Additional stenting at these sites then improved symptoms and pulmonary function to levels comparable with the other groups. This additional physiological and imaging information excluded all therapeutic failures.

Conclusions

When patients with UAS present with dyspnoea at exertion, and certainly with dyspnoea at rest, severe central airway stenosis is already present. In these patients, flow–volume loop analysis and spirometry will most probably show aberrations typical for UAS. However, as a screening tool in a general population, these abberations show a poor accuracy in predicting UAS. In extremely symptomatic, almost suffocating patients, immediate intervention with repermeabilisation/stenting is warranted. In nonlife-threatening cases, pre-intervention pulmonary function testing may yield useful information on the type, site and extent of the stenosis, whereas post-procedure testing may be used to focus the response and can be used as a basis for post-procedure follow-up. In the case of a multi-site, extensive airway stenosis, its relatively typical flow–volume loop pattern may be predictive of therapeutic failure of single-site stenting and may predict the necessity of additional stenting at upstream choke points. Interventional bronchoscopic procedures offer immediate (and often longstanding) palliation of respiratory symptoms, improvements in quality of life (and frequently length of life as well), and objective improvements in pulmonary function in the majority of patients. When used judiciously, they have become an invaluable tool in the armamentarium of modern pulmonology.

References

- Amjadi K, et al. Impact of interventional bronchoscopy on quality of life in malignant airway obstruction. *Respiration* 2008; 76: 421–442.
- Brouns M, et al. Tracheal stenosis: a flow dynamics study. *J Appl Physiol* 2007; 102: 1178–1184.
- Eisner MD, et al. Pulmonary function improves after expandable metal stent placement for benign airway obstruction. *Chest* 1999; 115: 1006–1011.
- Empay DW. Assessment of upper airways obstruction. *BMJ 1972* 5825; 3: 503–505.
- Ernst A, et al. Airway stabilization with silicone stents for treating adult tracheobronchomalacia: a prospective observational study. *Chest* 2007; 132: 609–616.
- Ernst A, et al. Central airway obstruction. *Am J Respir Crit Care Med* 2004; 169: 1278–1297.
- Gelb AF, et al. Physiologic studies of tracheobronchial stents in airway obstruction. *Am Rev Respir Dis* 1992; 146: 1088–1090.
- Gittoes NJ, et al. Upper airways obstruction in 153 consecutive patients presenting with thyroid enlargement. *BMJ* 1996; 312: 484.

- Goldman JM, et al. Physiological effect of endobronchial radiotherapy in patients with major airway occlusion by carcinoma. Thorax 1993; 48: 110-114.
- Lund ME, et al. Airway stenting: applications and practice management considerations. Chest 2007; 131: 579-587.
- Melissant CF, et al. Lung function, CT-scan and X-ray in upper airway obstruction due to thyroid goitre. Eur Respir J 1994; 7: 1782-1787.
- Miller RD, Hyatt RE. Evaluation of obstructing lesions of the trachea and larynx by flow-volume loops. Am Rev Respir Dis 1973; 108: 475-481.
- Miyazawa T, et al. Stenting at the flow-limiting segment in tracheobronchial stenosis due to lung cancer. Am J Respir Crit Care Med 2004; 169: 1096-1102.
- Modrykamien AM, et al. Detection of upper airway obstruction with spirometry results and the flow-volume loop: a comparison of quantitative and visual inspection criteria. Respir Care 2009; 54: 474-479.
- Noppen M, et al. Interventional bronchoscopy for treatment of tracheal obstruction secondary to benign or malignant thyroid disease. Chest 2004; 125: 723-730.
- Rotman HH, et al. Diagnosis of upper airway obstruction by pulmonary function testing. Chest 1975; 68: 796-799.
- Vincken W, et al. Flow oscillations on the flow-volume loop: a nonspecific indicator of upper airway dysfunction. Bull Eur Physiopathol Respir 1985; 21: 559-567.
- Vergnon JF, et al. Efficacy of tracheal and bronchial stent placement on respiratory functional tests. Chest 1995; 107: 741-746.
- Walsh DA, et al. Bronchoscopic cryotherapy for advanced bronchial carcinoma. Thorax 1990; 45: 509-513.

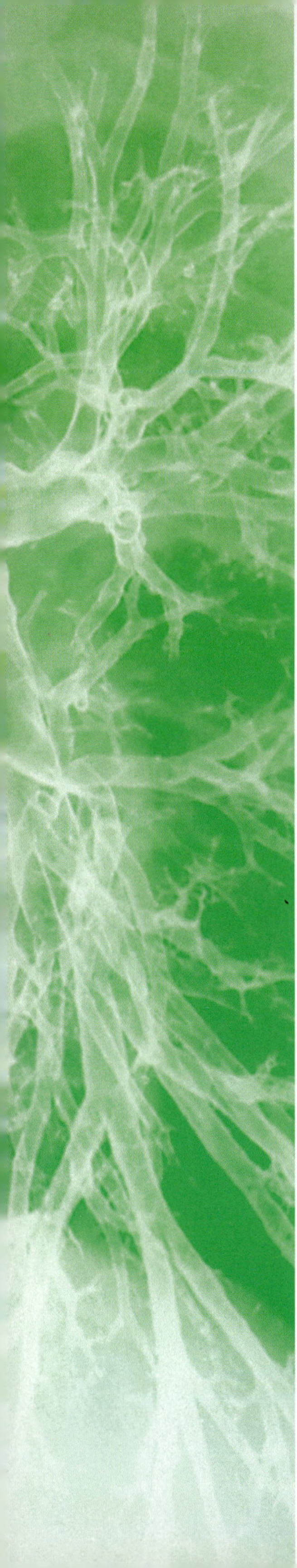

CHAPTER 5:

LUNG IMAGING

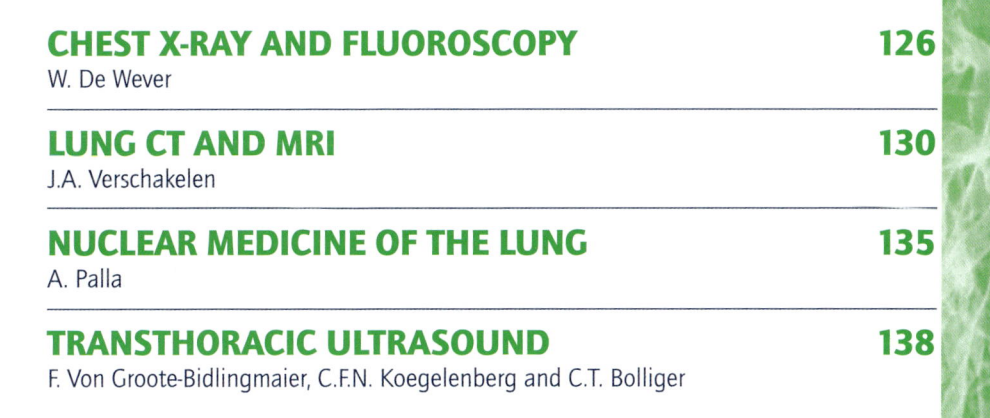

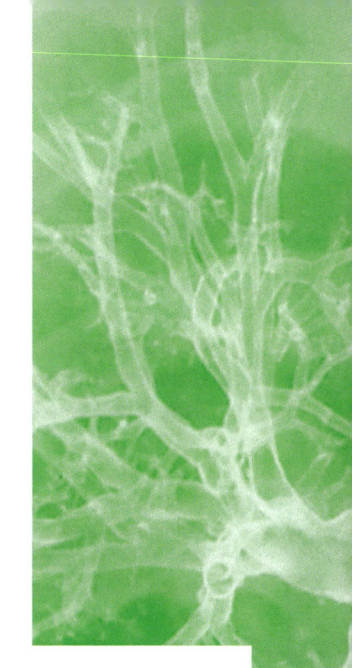

CHEST X-RAY AND FLUOROSCOPY — 126
W. De Wever

LUNG CT AND MRI — 130
J.A. Verschakelen

NUCLEAR MEDICINE OF THE LUNG — 135
A. Palla

TRANSTHORACIC ULTRASOUND — 138
F. Von Groote-Bidlingmaier, C.F.N. Koegelenberg and C.T. Bolliger

CHEST X-RAY AND FLUOROSCOPY

W. De Wever
University Hospitals Leuven, Leuven, Belgium
E-mail: walter.dewever@uz.kuleuven.be

Chest radiography is the most frequently used radiological chest imaging technique and also one of the most challenging. The technical aspects of this imaging modality are studied extensively. New approaches to image acquisition and display have been introduced in the past decade. As a general rule, establishing the presence of a lung disease process on the radiograph should constitute the first step in radiological diagnosis of chest disease.

Basic radiographic techniques

Diagnostic accuracy in chest disease is partly related to the quality of the radiographic images themselves. Several variables such as patient position, patient respiration and film exposure factors must be taken into account to ensure image quality (table 1). Positioning of the patient must be such that the X-ray beam is properly centred, the patient's body not rotated and the scapulas rotated so that they are projected away from the lungs. Patient respiration must be fully suspended, preferably at total lung capacity. Film exposure factors should be such that faint visualisation of the thoracic spine and the intervertebral disks on the postero–anterior (PA) radiograph is possible and that lung markings behind the heart are clearly visible. Exposure should be as short as possible, consistent with the production of adequate contrast. A high-kilo voltage technique appropriate to the film speed should be used.

Projections

PA and lateral projection The most satisfactory routine radiographic views for evaluating the chest are the PA and lateral projections with the patient standing (fig. 1). The combination of these two projections provides very good three-dimensional information. In patients who are too ill to stand up, antero–posterior (AP) upright or supine projections offer alternative but considerably less satisfactory views. The AP projection is of inferior quality because of the shorter focal-film distance, the greater magnification of the heart, and often the restricted ability of these patients to suspend respiration or achieve full inspiration. Based on a review of the literature and recommendations of the American College of Radiology and the American Thoracic Society, recommendations on the use of chest radiographs are summarised in table 2.

Lateral decubitus projection For the lateral decubitus projection, the patient lies on one side and the X-ray beam is oriented

> **Key points**
>
> - Chest radiography is the first step in radiological diagnosis of chest diseases.
> - Although it is a common technique, achieving high image quality is challenging and depends on getting several factors right.
> - The move from film to digital imaging offers exciting opportunities to improve image consistency and data management.

Table 1. Key points to obtaining a good chest radiograph

Radiographic appearance
Frontal view (PA view)
- Area from the lower cervical spine to below the costophrenic angles
- Sterno-clavicular joints symmetrical about the midline
- Shadows of the scapulae away from the lung field

Lateral view
- Soft tissues of the axillae should be included

Respiration
End of normal inspiration

Positioning of the patient
Erect position
- Very ill patients: horizontal or semi-erect
Postero-anterior (PA) position

Film exposure factors
High kilo voltage
Focus-film distance
- Must be kept constant for any particular department
- 150–180 cm

horizontally. This technique is particularly helpful for the identification of small pleural effusions. <100 mL of fluid may be identified on well-exposed radiographs in this position. Radiography in the lateral decubitus position is also useful to demonstrate a change in position of an air–fluid level in a cavity or a freely moving intracavitary loose body (e.g. fungus ball in aspergilloma).

Lordotic projection The lordotic projection can be made in AP or PA projection. For this projection, the patient stands erect and the X-ray tube is angled 15° cephalad. The main advantage of this modification is its reproducibility. The lordotic projection can be used: 1) for improving visibility of the lung apices, superior mediastinum and thoracic inlet, and 2) for identifying the minor fissure in suspected cases of atelectasis of the right middle lobe.

Oblique projection Oblique studies are sometimes useful in locating a pleural or chest wall disease process (e.g. pleural plaque); however, in most situations, computed tomography is preferred.

Inspiratory–expiratory radiography

Comparison of radiographs exposed in full inspiration and maximal expiration may supply useful information in two specific situations. The first indication is the evaluation of air trapping, either focal or general. With air trapping, diaphragmatic excursion is reduced symmetrically and lung density changes little between expiratory and inspiratory radiographs. The second indication is when a pneumothorax is suspected and when the visceral pleural line is not visible on the standard inspiratory radiograph or the findings are equivocal. In these situations, a film taken in full expiration may show the line more clearly.

Bedside radiography

Chest radiography, performed at the bedside with portable apparatus, is one of the most frequently performed radiological examinations; however, this technique is also the examination with the most variation in image quality. The amount of diagnostic information provided by chest examinations done with portable apparatus is high, and many abnormalities are detected. These examinations are useful 76–94% of the time. However, poor image quality and day-to-day variations in film density interfere with the detection of interval changes in patients with pulmonary diseases. The need to improve the image quality of this examination has long been recognised, but it is a difficult problem to solve.

Digital chest radiography

There have been many remarkable advances in conventional thoracic imaging over the past decade. Perhaps the most remarkable is the rapid conversion from film-based to digital radiographic systems. Digital radiography (DR) is the common name for different technologies that are characterised by a direct readout matrix that covers the whole exposure

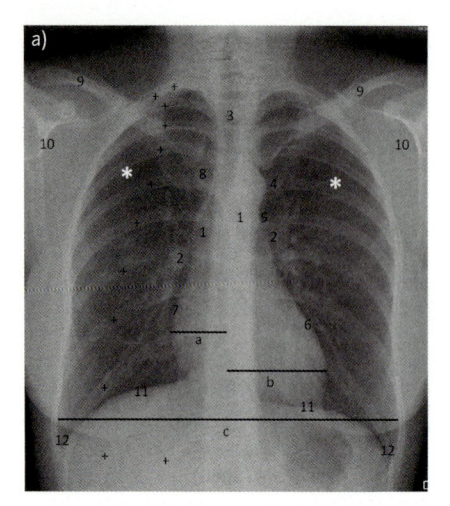

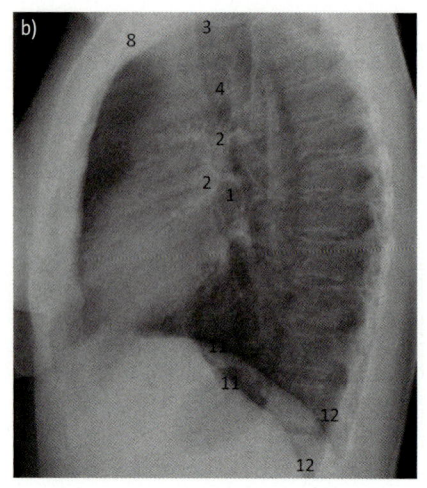

Figure 1. Posteo-anterior chest radiograph. Normal lungs are visible as black fields (air) (*) with superposition of multiple white linear structures (vessels and walls of airways). The lunghili consist of bronchi (main stem (1) and lobar bronchi) and vascular structures (pulmonary arteries (2) and pulmonary veins). A normal pleura is not visible on a chest radiograph. In the mediastinum we can visualise the trachea (3) as a translucent tube on the midline, the aortic arch (4), the pulmonary trunk (5), the left border or the heart formed by the left ventricle (6) and the right border of the heart formed by right atrium (7). A normal heart has a normal cardiothoracic index: (a+b)/maximal diameter of the chest (c) must be less than 0.5. The bony components of the chest visible on the frontal view are: the ribs (+), the manubrium sternum (8), the claviculae (9), the scapulae (10) and the vertebral bodies on the midline. The diaphragm (11) is sharply delineated and also the costophrenic angles (12) must be sharp and free. b) Lateral chest radiograph. The lateral chest film can be used to localise better the findings on the frontal view. Numbers and symbols are as for a).

Table 2. Recommendations for the use of chest radiography

Indications
Signs and symptoms related to the respiratory and cardiovascular system
Follow-up of previously diagnosed thoracic disease for evaluation of improvement resolution, or progression
Staging of intrathoracic and extrathoracic tumours
Pre-operative assessment of patients scheduled for intrathoracic surgery
Pre-operative evaluation of patients who have cardiac or respiratory symptoms or patients who have a significant potential for thoracic pathology that may lead to increased peri-operative morbidity or mortality
Monitoring of patients who have life support devices and patients who have undergone cardiac or thoracic surgery or other interventional procedures
No indications
Routine screening of unselected populations
Routine pre-natal chest radiographs for the detection of unsuspected disease
Routine radiographs solely because of hospital admission
Mandated radiographs for employment
Repeated radiograph examinations after admission to a long-term facility

area. Conversion of X-ray intensity into electrical signals can either be direct (selenium-based systems) or indirect (scintillator/photodiode systems). Advantages of DR systems are a high image quality and the potential for dose reduction. This technique is now the preferred imaging modality for bedside chest imaging because of its more consistent image quality. DR is rapidly replacing film-based chest units for in-department PA and lateral examinations. The final aim is to realise a completely integrated digital radiology department throughout the hospital connected to a large digital image archiving system. This concept, referred to as picture archiving and communication systems (PACS), represents the logical culmination of the extensive research that is continuing in this area.

Chest fluoroscopy

Chest fluoroscopy was a popular procedure a generation ago. Patients were examined fluoroscopically in various projections, and multiple spot radiographs were obtained with barium in the oesophagus. Examinations to evaluate pericardial effusion also were frequent. Overall diminution in cardiac pulsation and greater pulsation of the posterior cardiac wall in the lateral projection were thought to be signs of effusion. Other indications for fluoroscopy included the investigation of foreign bodies determined by air trapping and appropriate mediastinal shift and the evaluation of diaphragmatic paralysis. This evaluation of diaphragmatic paralysis is still an indication for fluoroscopy today.

References

- American College of Radiology. ACR Standard for the Performance of Pediatric and Adult Chest Radiography. Reston, American College of Radiology, 1997; p. 27.
- American Thoracic Society, Chest x-ray screening statements. *Am Thoracic News* 1984; 10: 14.
- MacMahon H, Doi K. Digital chest radiography. *Clin Chest Med* 1991; 12: 19-32.
- Rigler LG. Roentgen diagnosis of small pleural effusions: a new roentgenographic position. *JAMA* 1931; 96: 104-108.
- Schaefer-Prokop C, et al. Digital radiography of the chest: detector techniques and performance parameters. *J Thorac Imaging* 2003; 18: 124-137.
- Wandtke JC. Bedside chest radiography. *Radiology* 1994; 190: 1-10.
- Zinn B, Monroe J. The lordotic position in fluoroscopy and roentgenography of the chest. *Am J Roentgenol Radium Ther Nucl Med* 1956; 75: 682-700.

LUNG CT AND MRI

J.A. Verschakelen
University Hospitals Leuven, Belgium
E-mail: johny.verschakelen@uz.kuleuven.ac.be

Computed tomography (CT) is the second most important imaging modality of the chest and is, together with chest radiography, one of the two basic imaging techniques for visualising the lungs. Although there are indications to perform a CT of the chest in patients with normal chest radiography, this examination usually succeeds a chest X-ray on which a lesion is seen or suspected.

Magnetic resonance imaging (MRI) of the chest is, except for visualisation of the heart and great vessels, used less frequently in daily clinical practice. In selected cases, this imaging technique can sometimes add information to what is seen on CT. Since its introduction CT has undergone several technical changes and improvements. The first scanners were "incremental" CT scanners. In order to complete one cross-sectional image, the patient needed to suspend respiration for a few seconds. After that, the table was moved and the next scan was performed. This was repeated about 25 times in order to image the entire thorax.

Spiral scanning (also known as helical or continuous-volume scanning) has radically altered CT scanning protocols (table 1). In this technique, there is continuous patient movement with simultaneous scanning by a constantly rotating X-ray tube and detector system. While the first spiral CT scanners had only one row of detectors, today's scanners have multiple rows (multislice, multirow or multidetector-row CT). This allows for simultaneous acquisition of multiple images in the scan plane with one rotation of the X-ray tube around the patient. It also offers flexible image reconstruction options such as reconstructing images at various image

Key points

- CT is the second most important imaging modality of the chest.
- CT diagnosis of lung diseases is based on the study of their appearance and distribution patterns together with a careful analysis of patient data.
- CT interpretation of diffuse and interstitial lung diseases requires a formal multidisciplinary approach.
- MRI is second to CT when it comes to visualising pulmonary structure and pathology.

thickness and two-dimensional and three-dimensional reconstructions.

Thin-section or high-resolution CT (HRCT) is a special type of acquisition technique that uses 0.5–1-mm slice thickness and high-frequency reconstruction algorithms to produce high-detail images. It is used when detailed information about the lung parenchyma is needed. These thin slices can be obtained with the "incremental" acquisition technique in which 1-mm slices are produced with an image interval of 10–20 mm. However, with multislice spiral CT, it has become possible to produce a continuous set of thin slices of the entire chest. Although the quality of the individual images may be somewhat lower when the multislice acquisition is used, the overall information obtained is usually larger. Indeed, instead of a small number of axial slices with an image gap between, a continuous dataset is obtained that allows the

Table 1. Advantages of spiral computed tomography scanning

Sectional imaging without superposition of structures
Rapid acquisition within one breath-hold
Very good blood vessel opacification in vascular studies using limited amount of contrast
No respiratory misregistration between scans improving nodule detection
Fast and high-quality multiplanar and three-dimensional reconstructions

production of additional slices in different imaging planes. For this reason multislice is replacing the "incremental" technique in most institutions especially when it is the initial CT examination in a patient with a suspected lung problem. An inportant drawback, however, may be the increased radiation dose. On the other hand, the lung parenchyma is very suitable for reduction of the radiation dose without important quality loss and first reports on the use of low-dose CT in demonstrating lung disease are indeed promising.

As mentioned earlier, CT of the chest is usually performed when the chest radiography is abnormal or suspicious for the presence of pathology, although there are certainly indications for doing this examination even when the chest radiograph does not show any (obvious) abnormalities. Table 2 lists the most frequent indications for a CT of the chest.

Generally the diagnosis of lung disease on a chest CT is based on three elements:

- Recognition of the appearance pattern of the disease, *i.e.* classifying the abnormalities in a category that is based on their appearance.

- Determination of location and distribution of the abnormalities in the lung: the distribution pattern.

- Careful analysis of the patient data that are available at the time the CT scan is performed.

Although in some cases a diagnosis or a narrow differential diagnosis list can be proposed purely based on the study of the appearance and the distribution pattern of the disease on CT, the abnormalities seen in the lung should be carefully correlated with observations made on other radiological examinations and with all the clinical data available at the time of the CT examination. In particular diffuse and interstitial lung diseases are often very difficult to diagnose

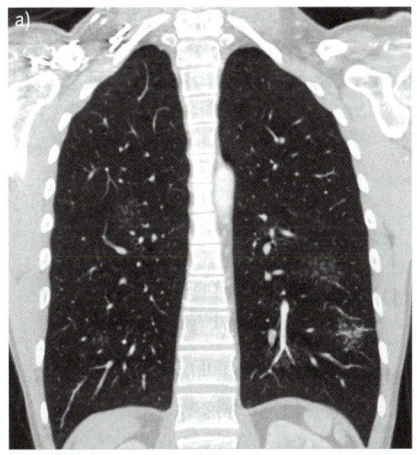

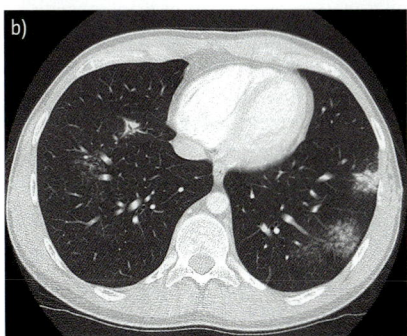

Figure 1. Thin-slice computed tomography of the lung obtained with the multislice spiral acquisition technique in a patient with sarcoidosis. The combination of axial (a) and coronal (b) views allows a better study of the appearance and distribution pattern of the lung lesions.

Table 2. Indications for computed tomography of the chest

Abnormal chest radiography
  Further evaluation of a chest wall, pleural, mediastinal or lung abnormality seen on a chest radiograph
  Rule out or confirm a lesion seen on a chest radiograph
  Lung cancer staging and follow-up
  Assessment of thoracic vascular lesion

Normal chest radiography
  Detection of diffuse lung disease
  Detection of pulmonary metastases from a known extrathoracic tumour
  Demonstration of pulmonary embolism
  Investigation of a patient with haemoptysis
  Investigation of patients with clinical evidence of a disease that might be related to the presence of chest abnormalities (*e.g.* pulmonary infection in an immunocompromised patient with fever)

when the interpretation is based only on the CT presentation. Ideally, cooperation should be established between the clinician responsible for the patient, the radiologist and, when pathological information is present or probably required, the pathologist.

Continuous efforts are being made to improve the image quality and the diagnostic performance of CT imaging of the lung. A further increase in the number of detector rows is feasible and may reduce acquisition time and hence improve image quality. Automated and semi-automated software packages will help to interpret the CT images. Dual-energy CT scanning may become helpful to study pulmonary perfusion in patients with pulmonary embolism.

Magnetic resonance imaging

Like CT, MRI produces multiplanar cross-sectional images, but it allows for a greater tissue characterisation because it has a better contrast resolution than CT. It also has the benefit of not using ionising radiation.

Tissue protons are exposed to a strong external magnetic field and realign along the plane of the magnetic gradient. From this position they are deflected momentarily by applying a so-called radio frequency (RF) pulse. As they return to their original alignment, the protons emit a faint electromagnetic signal which is detected by a receiving RF coil. When in addition a suitable gradient is set up along the magnetic field, signal detection can be confined to a pre-selected body plane. Processing of the data then yields a sectional image of the plane of interest.

MRI has an established role in the imaging of the heart and the great thoracic vessels. Concerning the chest wall, the diaphragm, the mediastinum and the lung, MRI was for many years considered a useful problem-solving technique for specific instances when used in addition to CT. These instances include the identification of tumour invasion in the chest wall and the mediastinal structures, differentiation between solid and vascular hilar masses, assessment of diaphragmatic abnormalities and the study and follow-up of mediastinal lymphoma during treatment. As mentioned earlier, however, most centres now use multidetector spiral CT for thoracic imaging, including the areas thought earlier to be the domain of "problem-solving" MRI.

Although it has become clear that MRI will always be second to CT when it comes to visualising pulmonary structure, disease and patterns with high spatial resolution, the many research and development efforts that have been made in recent years have resulted in new and valuable applications that are very promising and that may be implemented in clinical practice. There has been much interest in the role of MRI in the diagnosis of pulmonary embolism as a radiation-free

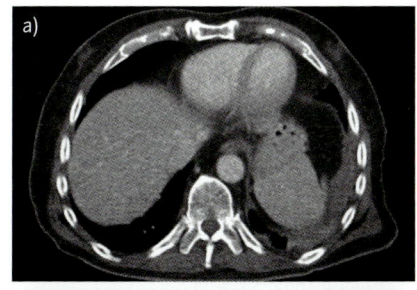

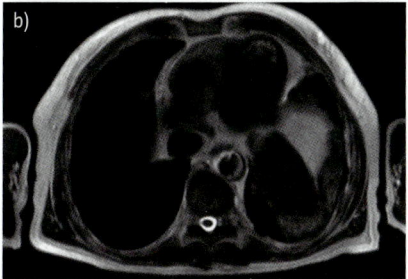

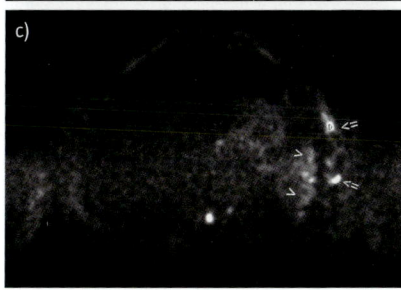

Figure 2. Patient with left-sided malignant mesothelioma. Both CT (a) and MRI (b) show irregular and nodular pleural thickening. There is suspicion of invasion in the diaphragm and spleen. Diffusion-weighted MRI (c) shows increased signal in the spleen (arrowheads) indicating tumour invasion in this structure. In addition an increased signal is seen in the chest wall (arrows) suggesting chest-wall invasion.

alternative to CT. Studies have shown that direct visualisation of the thrombus in the pulmonary artery is possible, while others have concentrated on the study of lung perfusion, looking for decreased-signal areas in the lung that represent underperfused lung tissue on gadolinium-enhanced MRI. Imaging of pulmonary ventilation by MRI has also become possible. Hyperpolarised ^{3}He gas has been used to demonstrate perfusion changes in patients with asthma, chronic obstructive pulmonary disease and cystic fibrosis. Hyperpolarized xenon-129, fluorine and oxygen-enhanced lung MRI are methods of gas imaging that have opened up the field of imaging pulmonary ventilation by MRI. Diffusion-weighted (DW) MRI is another interesting application. This technique provides a measurement that reflects the random Brownian motion of water protons in tissue. This motion causes signal loss that can be measured with the use of diffusion-sensitive sequences and that can be quantified by calculating the apparent diffusion coefficient. In the chest, it has been used successfully to differentiate between malignant and benign lesions.

Most of these techniques remain in the experimental domain, but it can be expected that some of them will reach daily clinical practice.

References

- Amundsen T, et al. Pulmonary embolism: detection with MR perfusion imaging of lung-a feasibility study. *Radiology* 1997; 203: 181-185.
- Bergin CJ, et al. Magnetic resonance imaging of lung parenchyma. *J Thorac Imaging* 1993; 8: 12-17.
- Bergin CJ, et al. MR evaluation of chest wall involvement in malignant lymphoma. *J Comput Assist Tomogr* 1990; 14: 928-932.
- Brown LR, Aughenbaugh GL. Masses of the anterior mediastinum: CT and MR imaging. *AJR Am J Roentgenol* 1991; 157: 1171-1180.
- Dawn SK, et al. Multidetector-row spiral computed tomography in the diagnosis of thoracic diseases. *Respir Care* 2001; 46: 912-921.
- de Hoop B, et al. A comparison of six software packages for evaluation of solid lung nodules using semi-automated volumetry: What is the minimum increase in size to detect growth in repeated CT examinations. *Eur Radiol* 2009; 19: 800-808.
- Gruden JF. Thoracic CT performance and interpretation in the multi-detector era. *J Thorac Imaging* 2005; 20: 253-264.
- Gupta A, et al. Acute pulmonary embolism: diagnosis with MR angiography. *Radiology* 1999; 210: 353-359.
- Heelan RT, et al. Superior sulcus tumors: CT and MR imaging. *Radiology* 1989; 170: 637-641.

- Kalender WA, et al. Spiral volumetric CT with single-breath-hold technique, continuous transport, and continuous scanner rotation. *Radiology* 1990; 176: 181-183.
- Kauczor HU, et al. Normal and abnormal pulmonary ventilation: visualization at hyperpolarized He-3 MR imaging. *Radiology* 1996; 201: 564-568.
- Klingenbeck-Regn K, et al. Subsecond multi-slice computed tomography: basics and applications. *Eur J Radiol* 1999; 31: 110-124.
- MacFall JR, et al. Human lung air spaces: potential for MR imaging with hyperpolarized He-3. *Radiology* 1996; 200: 553-558.
- Matoba M, et al. Lung carcinoma: diffusion-weighted mr imaging–preliminary evaluation with apparent diffusion coefficient. *Radiology* 2007; 243: 570-577.
- Mirvis SE, et al. MR imaging of traumatic diaphragmatic rupture. *J Comput Assist Tomogr* 1988; 12: 147-149.
- Muller NL Computed tomography, magnetic resonance imaging, past, present and future. *Eur Respir J* 2002; 35: Suppl. 35, 3s-12s.
- Muller NL, et al. Value of MR imaging in the evaluation of chronic infiltrative lung diseases: comparison with CT. *AJR Am J Roentgenol* 1992; 158: 1205-1209.
- Oudkerk M, et al. Comparison of contrast-enhanced magnetic resonance angiography and conventional pulmonary angiography for the diagnosis of pulmonary embolism: a prospective study. *Lancet* 2002; 359: 1643-1647.
- Padhani AR. Spiral CT: thoracic applications. *Eur J Radiol* 1998; 28: 2-17.
- Padovani B, et al. Chest wall invasion by bronchogenic carcinoma: evaluation with MR imaging. *Radiology* 1993; 187: 33-38.
- Thieme SF, et al. Dual energy CT for the assessment of lung perfusion–correlation to scintigraphy. *Eur J Radiol* 2008; 68: 369-374.
- Silverman PM, et al. Common terminology for single and multislice helical CT. *AJR Am J Roentgenol* 2001; 176: 1135-1136.
- Webb WR. Magnetic resonance imaging of the mediastinum, hila, and lungs. *J Thorac Imaging* 1985; 1: 65-73.

NUCLEAR MEDICINE OF THE LUNG

A. Palla
Cardiothoracic and Vascular Dept, University of Pisa, Pisa, Italy
E-mail: a.palla@med.unipi.it

Nuclear medicine may contribute to the diagnosis of pulmonary embolism (PE) and inflammatory diseases, and the diagnosis and staging of lung cancer. Among several techniques available, pulmonary perfusion and ventilation scintigraphy (PLS and VLS, respectively), gallium-67 scintigraphy and positron emission tomography (PET) scintigraphy are of interest in clinical practice.

Diagnosis of PE

Thanks to its noninvasiveness, safety and low cost, PLS still remains the cornerstone of the diagnosis and follow-up of PE.

Perfusion lung scintigraphy has been proven to be useful for:

- diagnosis of PE
- detection of recurrences under treatment or after its discontinuation
- differential diagnosis between thromboembolic and nonthromboembolic pulmonary hypertension

Two main scintigraphic criteria must be considered for the diagnosis: 1) identification of perfusion defects corresponding to one or more pulmonary segments and 2) diversion of pulmonary blood flow from lower and posterior lung regions. Perfusion defects typically are multiple, wedge-shaped and often bilateral. PLS has a sensitivity of 100% in that it allows exclusion with certainty when the diagnosis is negative. The specificity varies in different reported series, but on average does not reach acceptable values; to increase the specificity, VLS has been introduced, but is cumbersome, time-consuming and poorly available. Nowadays, VLS is only indicated in some individual patients with PE, since similar results can be obtained by using chest radiography. A few years ago, a new classification of perfusion defects was published in order to optimise its diagnostic usefulness in conjunction with chest radiography; such a method has made it possible to obtain a diagnostic accuracy similar to that shown by angio-computed tomography (CT). PLS also plays a leading role in the follow-up of patients with PE, as it helps to monitor the efficacy of treatment in the first days, it allows promptly detection of early and late recurrences and evolution towards pulmonary hypertension, and it may

Key points

- Nuclear medicine of the lung has a role in the diagnosis of pulmonary embolism and inflammatory diseases, and in the diagnosis and staging of lung cancer.
- Perfusion scintigraphy is key in the diagnosis and follow-up of pulmonary embolism as it is safe, cheap and noninvasive.
- Gallium-67 scintigraphy is useful in identifying and localising intrathoracic inflammation and infection.
- FDG PET and PET/CT are used in diagnosis, treatment targeting and treatment in lung cancer.

differentiate between thromboembolic pulmonary hypertension and other types of pulmonary hypertension.

Diagnosis of inflammatory diseases

Gallium-67 citrate is the most widely employed positive tracer in order to identify and localise intrathoracic inflammations and infections. To acquire images, a scintillation gamma-camera with a low energy collimator is required. Gallium scintigraphy may help in evaluating the activity of granulomatous disorders and the efficacy of steroid treatment. In patients with sarcoidosis, it shows a high diagnostic sensitivity; in some cases, the presence of highly specific signs, such as *panda* or *lambda* signs, allows avoidance of invasive diagnostic tests. Moreover, this tracer may differentiate between sarcoidosis and non-Hodgkin's lymphoma, and detect multiple extrapulmonary sites of sarcoidosis. Also, gallium scintigraphy is indicated in investigating metabolic activity in pulmonary infections and the efficacy of proper therapy. In the diagnosis of pulmonary tuberculosis, gallium scintigraphy may indicate the necessity of a bronchoalveolar lavage and the site where it should be performed. This occurs mostly in cases of suspected re-infection of areas of pleuroparenchymal fibrosis, in cases of suspicion where sputum is repeatedly negative, and in immunocompromised patients. Finally, gallium scintigraphy may be of value in the evaluation of efficacy of chemotherapy in lymphomatous diseases and may help differentiate post-attinic fibrosis from residual tumour foci when a lung density persists after radiotherapy.

Diagnosis of lung cancer

PET is a nuclear medicine technique that produces a three-dimensional imaging of functional and biochemical processes within the body. Recently, PET has been combined with CT (PET/CT) (fig. 1); such fusion generally improves diagnostic accuracy by upgrading specificity when compared with PET alone. The most frequently used tracer is 2-[^{18}F]-fluoro-2-deoxy-D-glucose (FDG), a glucose analogue, whose tissue concentration is directly related to the glucose metabolism. The uptake of FDG may be evaluated by a semiquantitative measurement, the "standardised uptake value" (SUV), *i.e.* the ratio between the amount of tracer in a specific area and the same amount potentially present if the tracer had been evenly distributed in the body.

FDG PET is proven useful in:

- diagnosing and staging lung cancer
- monitoring the efficacy of treatment
- defining the biological target volume for radiation treatment planning

An indication of increasing clinical relevance of FDG PET and PET/CT is the differentiation of benign from malignant solitary pulmonary nodules by replacing invasive modalities of investigation. A SUV of 2.5 has been reported as a guideline for the cut-off between benign (SUV <2.5) and malignant (SUV >2.5) lesions. A meta-analysis from 40 studies showed a sensitivity of 97% but a lower specificity (78%) due to FDG uptake within inflammatory/granulomatous lesions. However, a high rate of false-negative FDG results can occur when nodules are <1 cm (sensitivity of 69% for nodules of 5–8 mm). Moreover, some histotypes, such as bronchoalveolar carcinomas and well-differentiated neuroendocrine tumours, usually present a low glucose metabolic activity and cannot be correctly depicted by FDG imaging.

FDG PET is also a standard modality for staging nonsmall cell lung cancer. Several studies have demonstrated that PET is more accurate than CT in the staging of mediastinum (N state). Due to its high negative predicted value, invasive staging procedures (mediastinoscopy) can be omitted in patients with a negative FDG PET for mediastinal lymph node involvement. On the contrary, a positive finding should not preclude mediastinoscopy. Moreover, the addition of FDG PET to the standard work-up can prevent useless thoracotomies and

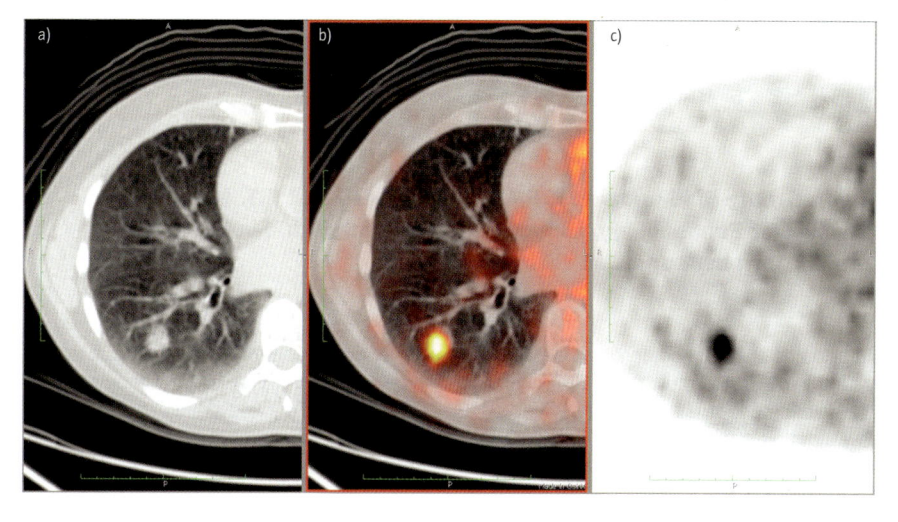

Figure 1. Solitary pulmonary nodule as it appears on a) chest computed tomography (CT), c) 2-fluoro-2-deoxy-D-glucose positron emission tomography (PET), and b) a combination of CT and PET.

change therapeutic approach in a significant percentage of patients. PET is useful in disclosing distant metastases (M state) with a high sensitivity and specificity. However, PET cannot replace CT or magnetic resonance imaging for detecting brain metastases. Moreover, the measurement of FDG SUV within the tumour correlates negatively with patient prognosis; early changes of FDG SUV during radiotherapy and chemotherapy can predict therapy efficacy; and PET is more accurate than contrast-enhanced CT for detecting residual tumour after radiotherapy and chemotherapy.

A recent indication of PET/CT is the definition of the "biological target volume" for radiation treatment planning. This approach has the goal of increasing the dose to the tumour and focusing the treatment planning to the biological target, which reveals an elevated glucose metabolism.

Thanks to D. Volterrani, Nuclear Medicine, University of Pisa, Pisa, Italy, for active assistance.

References

- Bryant AS, Cerfolio RJ. The maximum standardized uptake values on integrated FDG-PET/CT is useful in differentiating benign from malignant pulmonary nodules. *Ann Thorac Surg* 2006; 82: 1016-1020.
- De Geus-Oei LF, et al. Predictive and prognostic value of FDG-PET in nonsmall-cell lung cancer: a systematic review. *Cancer* 2007; 110: 1654-1664.
- Kita T, et al. Clinical significance of the serum IL-2R level and Ga-67 scan findings in making a differential diagnosis between sarcoidosis and non-Hodgkin's lymphoma. *Ann Nucl Med* 2007; 21: 499-503.
- Liu SF, et al. Monitoring treatment responses in patients with pulmonary TB using serial lung gallium-67 scintigraphy. *Am J Roentgenol* 2007; 188: 403-408.
- Miniati M, et al. Perfusion lung scintigraphy for the diagnosis of pulmonary embolism: a reappraisal and review of the prospective investigative study of pulmonary embolism diagnosis methods. *Semin Nucl Med* 2008; 38: 450-461.
- Sostman HD, et al. Sensitivity and specificity of perfusion scintigraphy combined with chest radiography for acute pulmonary embolism in PIOPED II. *J Nucl Med* 2008; 49: 1741-1748.
- Stein PD, et al. Multidetector computed tomography for acute pulmonary embolism. *N Engl J Med* 2006; 354: 2317-2327.
- Van Tinteren H, et al. Effectiveness of positron emission tomography in the preoperative assessment of patients with suspected non-small-cell lung cancer: the PLUS multicentre randomised trial. *Lancet* 2002; 359: 1388-1393.

TRANSTHORACIC ULTRASOUND

F. von Groote-Bidlingmaier, C.F.N. Koegelenberg and C.T. Bolliger
Division of Pulmonology, University of Stellenbosch, South Africa
E-mail: florianv@sun.ac.za

Transthoracic ultrasonography can be performed with the most basic ultrasound (US) equipment. It is used for the investigation of chest wall abnormalities, pleural thickening and pleural tumours, and the qualitative and quantitative description of pleural effusions. Lung tumours, pulmonary consolidations and other parenchymal pulmonary processes abutting the pleura can also be visualised. Furthermore, US is ideal to guide thoracentesis, drainage of effusions and other thoracic interventions. US is particularly useful in intensive care units where radiographic equipment is unavailable.

Advantages of thoracic US include its mobility, dynamic properties, lack of radiation and low cost.

The ultrasonographic appearance of the normal thorax and the most common pathologies are reviewed in this chapter.

General technical aspects and appearance of the normal thorax

A low-frequency probe (*e.g.* 3.5 MHz) is routinely used for screening purposes, while detailed assessment of an abnormal chest wall or pleura can be performed with a high-frequency probe (*e.g.* 8 MHz).

Superficial muscles and fascia planes appear as a series of echogenic layers during the initial surveillance of a normal chest. Curvilinear structures on transverse scans, associated with posterior acoustic shadowing represent the ribs.

The visceral and parietal pleura normally appear as one highly echogenic line.

Movement of the lung with the respiratory cycle in relation to the chest wall on real-time US is called the "lung sliding" sign. Its presence is strong evidence against a pneumothorax.

US cannot visualise normal aerated lung tissue. The large change in acoustic impedance at the pleura–lung interface, however, causes horizontal artefacts that are seen as a series of echogenic parallel lines equidistant from one another below the pleura. These bright but formless lines are known as reverberation artefacts (fig. 1).

Chest wall pathology

Soft-tissue masses, such as abscesses, lipomas and a variety of other lesions, can be detected by US. These lesions are mostly benign, but variable echogenicity and nonspecific US findings make differentiation between various aetiologies difficult. Supraclavicular and axillary lymph nodes are usually accessible, and US may even help to distinguish benign from malignant lymph nodes. Hypoechoic masses disrupting the normal structure of a

---

Key points

- Transthoracic US can be used to investigate chest wall abnormalities, pleural thickening and pleural tumours, and to describe pleural effusions.
- Advantages of the technique include its mobility, dynamic properties, lack of radiation and low cost.

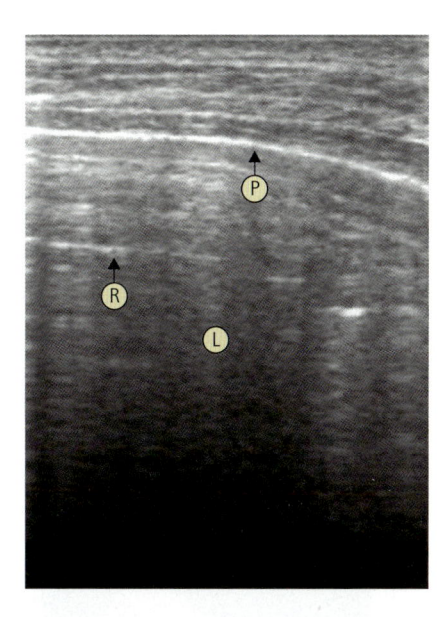

Figure 1. The typical appearance of a normal chest on ultrasound (US). A transverse view through the intercostal space is shown. The chest wall is visualised as multiple layers of echogenicity representing muscles and fascia. The visceral and parietal pleura appear as an echogenic bright line (two distinct lines sliding during respiration are visible on real-time US). Reverberation artefacts beneath the pleural lines imply an underlying air-filled lung. P: pleura; L: lung; R: reverberation artefact.

rib may represent bony metastases and can be seen on US.

Pleural pathology

Transthoracic US is most commonly used to investigate pleural effusions, and is more sensitive than decubitus radiographs at demonstrating minimal or loculated effusions. The US appearance of a pleural effusion depends on its nature and chronicity. Four appearances based on the internal echogenicity are recognised: anechoic; complex but nonseptated; complex and septated; and homogenously echogenic. Transudates are invariably anechoic, unseptated and free flowing, whereas complex, septated or echogenic effusions are usually exudates. Malignant effusions are

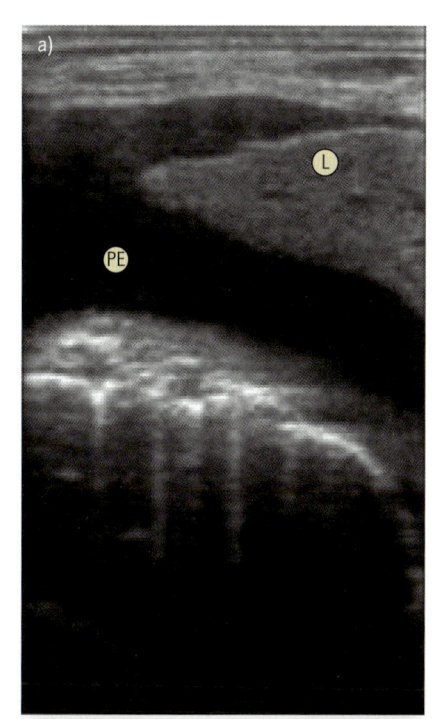

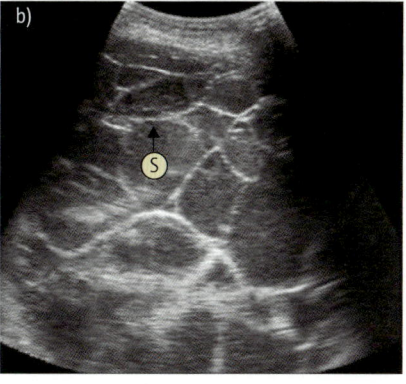

Figure 2. Example of an anechoic pleural effusion is shown in a). It presents as an echo-free space between the visceral and parietal pleura. Compressive atelectasis of the lung may be seen as a tongue-like structure in a large effusion. Note the difference to the effusion on b), which is classified as complex septated. Multiple septa form many compartments in the same effusion. PE: pleural effusion; L: lung; S: septum.

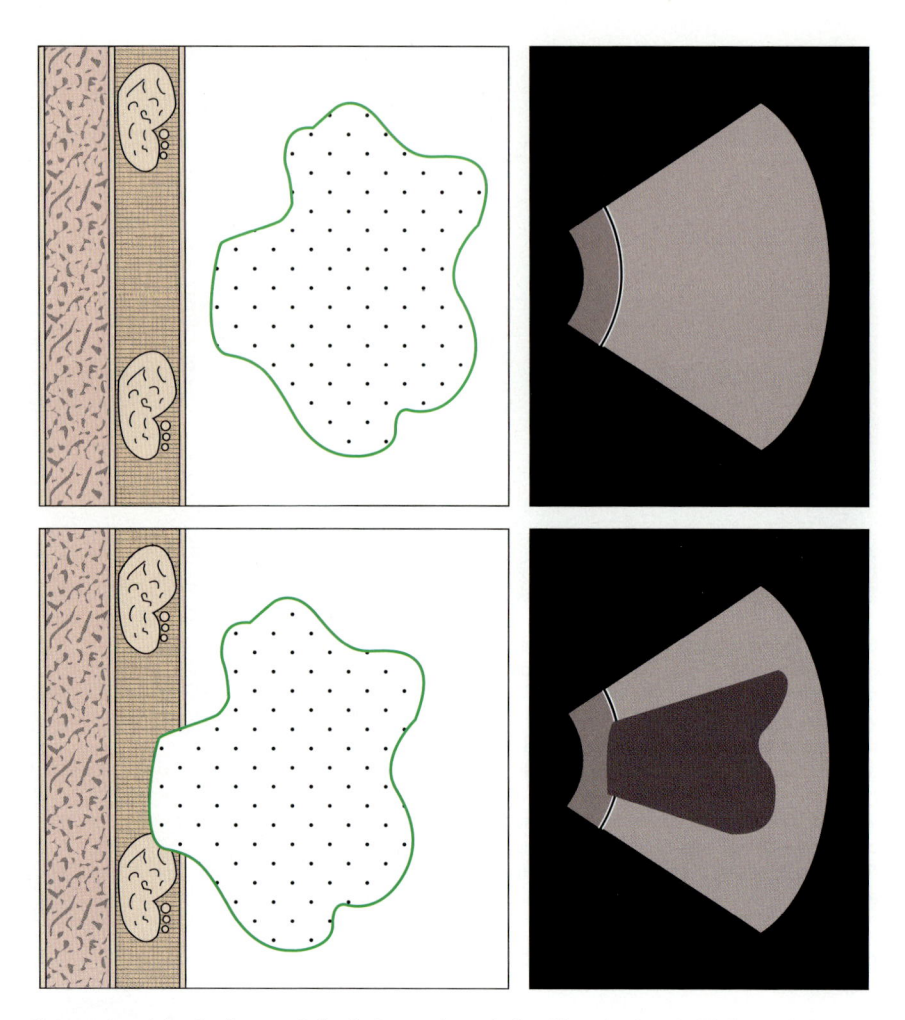

Figure 3. A peripheral pulmonary lesion is shown schematically without (top) and with (bottom) pleural contact. Only the lesion with pleural contact is visible on ultrasound. Reproduced from DIACON *et al.* (2005), with permission from the publisher.

frequently anechoic. The atelectatic lung inside a large effusion may appear as a tongue-like structure within the effusion. Inflammatory effusions are often associated with strands of echogenic material and septations that show more or less mobility with respiration and the cardiac cycle (fig. 2).

The volume of a pleural effusion can be estimated using the following classification: minimal, if the echo-free space is confined to the costophrenic angle; small, if the space is greater than the costophrenic angle but still within the range of the area covered with a 3.5 MHz curvilinear probe; moderate, if the space is greater than a one-probe range but within a two-probe range; and large, if the space is bigger than a two-probe range.

Both small effusions and pleural thickening may appear as hypoechoic on US, so differentiation might be difficult. An important sign in favour of an effusion is mobility on real-time US.

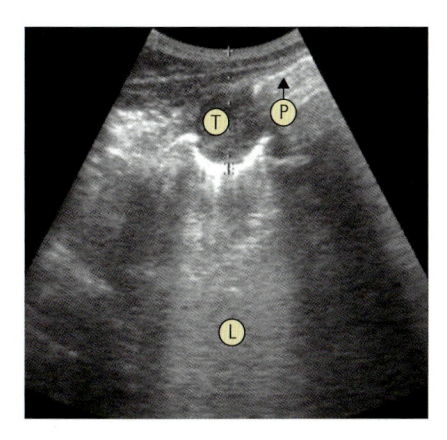

Figure 4. A sonographic image showing a solid lung lesion with posterior echo enhancement. Note that the tumour is abutting the pleura and is therefore visible on ultrasound. P: pleura; L: lung; T: tumour.

Metastatic pleural tumours and malignant mesothelioma can be visualised as polypoid pleural nodules or irregular sheet like pleural thickening. They are often associated with large pleural effusions. Benign pleural tumours are rare.

QURESHI et al. found that pleural thickening >1 cm, pleural nodularity and diaphragmatic thickening >7 mm were highly suggestive of malignant disease. In their study, US correctly identified 73% of malignant effusions.

The absence of normal lung sliding, the loss of comet-tail artefacts and exaggerated horizontal reverberation artefacts are reliable signs for the presence of a pneumothorax.

Pulmonary pathology

A lung tumour abutting the pleura will be detectable by US (fig. 3). In most cases these tumours present as a hypoechoic mass with posterior acoustic enhancement (fig. 4).

Visceral pleura or chest wall involvement is important for staging of malignant lung tumours. Loss of movement of a visualised tumour with respiration suggests infiltration beyond the parietal pleura.

US can detect pneumonic consolidations provided they have contact with the pleura. Non-infective causes of consolidations with similar appearance on US include pulmonary infarction, haemorrhage and bronchoalveolar carcinoma.

A hypoechoic lesion with a well-defined or irregular wall abutting the pleura might represent a lung abscess. The centre of the abscess is most often anechoic, but may reveal septations and internal echoes.

Conclusion

The value of US for chest physicians is firmly established. Basic thoracic ultrasonography is an elegant and inexpensive investigation that extends the physicians' diagnostic and interventional potential at the bedside in peripheral lung, pleural, and chest wall disease.

References

- Diacon AH, et al. Transthoracic ultrasound for the pulmonologist. *Curr Opin Pulm Med* 2005; 11: 307-312.
- Evans AL, Gleeson FV. Radiology in pleural disease: state of the art. *Respirology* 2004; 9: 300-312.
- Gorg C, et al. Sonography of malignant pleural effusion. *Eur Radiol* 1997; 7: 1195-1198.
- Herth FJ, et al. Diagnosis of pneumothorax by means of transthoracic ultrasound: a prospective trial. *Eur Respir J* 2004; 24: S491.
- Hirsch JH, et al. Real-time sonography of pleural opacities. *Am J Roentgenol* 1981; 136: 297-301.
- Kocijancic I, et al. Imaging of pleural fluid in healthy individuals: *Clin Radiol* 2004; 59: 826-829.
- Koegelenberg CF, et al. Pleural Ultrasound. *In*: Light RW, Lee YC, eds. Textbook of Pleural Disease, 2nd Edn. London, Hodder & Stoughton, 2008; pp. 271-28.
- Koh DM, et al. Transthoracic US of the chest: clinical uses and applications. *Radiographics* 2002; 22: e1.
- Lichtenstein DA, Menu Y. A bedside ultrasound sign ruling out pneumothorax in the critically ill. *Chest* 1995; 108: 1345-1348.
- Mathis G. Thoraxsonography – part I: chest wall and pleura. *Ultrasound Med Biol* 1997; 23: 1131-1139.
- Mayo PH, Doelken P. Pleural ultrasonography. *Clin Chest Med* 2006; 27: 215-217.

- Qureshi NR, et al. Thoracic ultrasound in the diagnosis of malignant pleural effusion. *Thorax* 2009; 64: 139–143.
- Tsai TH, Yang PC. Ultrasound in the diagnosis and management of pleural disease. *Curr Opin Pulm Med* 2003; 9: 282–290.
- Yang PC, et al. Value of sonography in determining the nature of pleural effusion: analysis of 320 cases. *Am J Roentgenol* 1992; 159: 29–33.
- Yang PC. Ultrasound-guided transthoracic biopsy of peripheral lung, pleural, and chest wall lesions. *J Thorac Imaging* 1997; 12: 272–284.

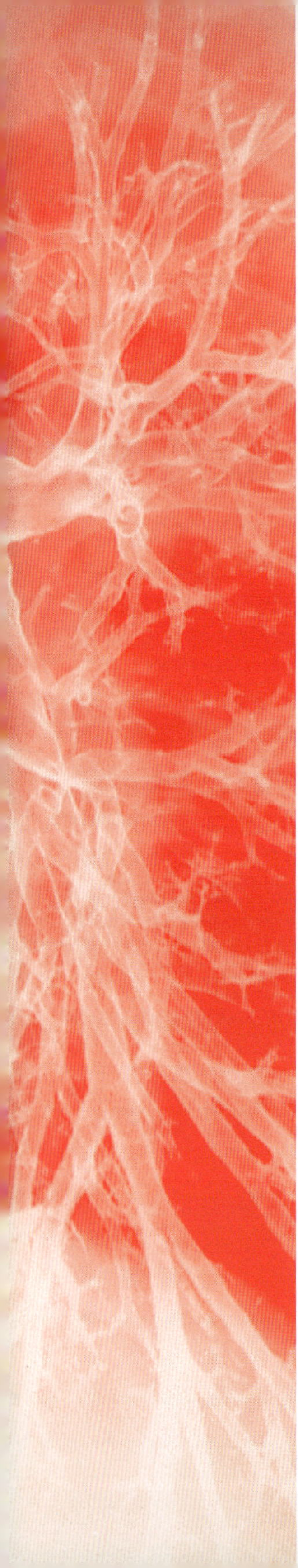

CHAPTER 6:

LUNG INJURY AND RESPIRATORY FAILURE

LUNG INJURY   146
B. Schönhofer

RESPIRATORY FAILURE   148
N. Ambrosino and F. Guarracino

OXYGEN THERAPY AND VENTILATORY SUPPORT   151
A.K. Simonds

INTENSIVE CARE AND HIGH-DEPENDENCY UNIT   154
S. Nava and P. Navalesi

ASSESSMENT FOR ANAESTHESIA/SURGERY   156
M.M. Schuurmans, C.T. Bolliger and A. Boehler

LUNG INJURY

B. Schönhofer
Abteilung für Pneumologie und Internistische Intensivmedizin, Krankenhaus Oststadt-Heidehaus, Klinikum Region Hannover, Hanover, Germany
E-mail: Bernd.Schoenhofer@t-online.de

Acute lung injury (ALI) and its most severe manifestation, the acute respiratory distress syndrome (ARDS), are defined by physiological (*i.e.* ratio of arterial oxyen tension (P_{a,O_2}) to inspiratory oxygen fraction (F_{I,O_2}) $\leqslant 300$ mmHg for ALI and $\leqslant 200$ mmHg for ARDS, independent of positive end-expiratory pressure) and bilateral pulmonary infiltrates as radiological criteria.

Cardiac failure must be excluded based either on pulmonary artery wedge pressure (<18 mmHg) or on clinical evaluation of left ventricular function if the invasive measurement is unavailable.

These criteria should be re-evaluated after 24 h, since their persistence is essential for the correct diagnosis of ALI/ARDS. Furthermore, timing may be of influence on the development of ALI/ARDS.

Lung oedema may evaluated by computed tomography or other established methods.

ALI/ARDS may be caused by various aetiologies: direct lung injury, *e.g.* pneumonia, aspiration, toxic inhalation, near drowning or lung contusion; or indirect lung injury *e.g.* sepsis, burn, pancreatitis or massive blood transfusion. The two aetiologies may coexist.

The exact incidence of ALI/ARDS is not known; its annual mortality rate has been estimated to be $>30,000$ patients per year in the USA. Despite recent advances in the understanding of the pathophysiology of ARDS, improvements in supportive care, and multiple therapeutic efforts directed at modifying the course of the condition, mortality rates are persistently 35–40%.

The pathophysiology of ALI/ARDS is related to altered pulmonary capillary permeability and increased intrapulmonary shunt, which is associated with impaired gas exchange. ARDS has been divided into three stages in which an initial inflammatory phase (exudative) is followed by fibro-proliferation, which can lead to established interstitial and intra-alveolar fibrosis, the final phase.

Mechanical ventilation itself can seriously damage lung parenchyma (ventilator-induced lung injury). ALI/ARDS often has systematic

Key points

- ALI and its most severe manifestation ARDS are defined as $P_{a,O_2}/F_{i,O_2}$ $\leqslant 300$ mmHg and $\leqslant 200$ mmHg, respectively, in addition to bilateral infiltrates as radiological criteria.

- Principles of protective ventilator settings for patients with ALI/ARDS are low tidal volume (*i.e.* $V_T = 6$ mL·kg^{-1} ideal body weight, plateau pressure <30 cmH$_2$O and peak pressure <35 cm H$_2$O.

- Permissive hypercapnia may be helpful to realise protective mechanical ventilation.

- Protection of the lungs may also be provided by the pump-driven veno-venous extracorporeal membrane oxygenation (ECMO) or pumpless extra corporeal lung assist (ILA).

manifestations, triggering systemic inflammatory response syndrome (SIRS), or *in extremis* multiple organ dysfunction syndrome (MODS).

In general the spectrum of treatment ALI/ARDS includes supportive care, ventilator support and pharmacological treatment. The first principle of treatment is to identify potential underlying causes of ALI/ARDS. Furthermore, secondary lung injury has to be avoided, such as aspiration, barotraumas, nosocomial infections and oxygen toxicity. The main aims of supportive care are maintaining oxygen delivery to end organs by avoiding anaemia and optimising cardiovascular function and body fluid balance; additionally catabolism and nutritional support have to be balanced.

With regard to mechanical ventilation, the main goal is to improve oxygenation without increasing the iatrogenic effects caused by mechanical ventilation; there are different methods available. Among the methods related to the ventilatory setting, those found really effective are to reduce tidal volume and pressures and to apply positive end-expiratory pressure (PEEP) to reduce the amount of nonaerated atelectatic lung.

Principles of protective ventilator settings for patients with ALI/ARDS are:

- Tidal volume 6 mL·kg^{-1} ideal body weight.
- Plateau pressure, <30 cmH$_2$O, peak pressure <35 cmH$_2$O.
- This strategy of protective mechanical ventilation may be associated with permissive hypercapnia.

The "optimal" setting of PEEP is not clear, since several methods have been proposed without any clear advantages over each other.

Higher PEEP (>15 cmH$_2$O) might be recommended in more severe ARDS patients. Prone position might be recommended in more severe ARDS patients, according to the expertise of the clinicians. Alternative methods of ventilation include include high-frequency ventilation and airway pressure release ventilation.

Protection of the lungs may also be provided by pump-driven veno-venous extracorporeal membrane oxygenation, which improves both oxygenation and carbon dioxide removal, either by leaving the lungs "at rest" (apnoeic oxygenation) or by using low-tidal-volume low-frequency ventilation. Recently, a pumpless extracorporeal lung assist was developed using arterio-venous bypass, in which a gas exchange membrane is integrated ("interventional lung assist" (ILA)). ILA provides effective carbon dioxide elimination and a moderate improvement in oxygenation.

Concerning pharmacological treatments of ALI/ARDS, inhaled nitric oxide has not been found to be really effective and there is no clear convincing data suggesting the widespread use of corticosteroids in both early and late phases of ALI/ARDS.

Finally, based on experimental models a series of molecular mechanisms offer innovative opportunities for cell or gene therapy. These need to be elaborated in human studies, however.

References

- Dreyfuss D, Saumon G. Ventilator-induced lung injury. Lessons from experimental studies. *Am J Respir Crit Care Med* 1998; 157: 294-323.
- Gattinoni L, Pesenti A. The concept of 'baby lung'. *Intensive Care Med* 2005; 31: 776-784.
- International consensus conference in intensive care medicine: ventilator-associated lung injury in ARDS. *Am J Respir Crit Care* 1999; 160: 2118-2124.
- Marini JJ, Gattinoni L. Ventilatory management of acute respiratory distress syndrome - a consensus of two. *Crit Care Med*, 2004; 32: 250-255.
- Matthay MA, Zimmerman GA. Acute lung injury and the acute respiratory distress syndrome: four decades of inquiry into pathogenesis and rational management. *Am J Respir Cell Mol Biol* 2005; 33: 319-327.
- The Acute Respiratory Distress Syndrome Network. Ventilation with lower tidal volumes as compared with traditional tidal volumes for acute lung injury and the acute respiratory distress sydrome. *N Engl J Med* 2000; 342: 1301-1308.

RESPIRATORY FAILURE

N. Ambrosino and F. Guarracino
Cardio-Thoracic Dept, University Hospital, Pisa, Italy
E-mail: n.ambrosino@ao-pisa.toscana.it

The respiratory system consists of two parts. The lung performs gas exchange, and the pump ventilates the lung. The pump consists of the chest wall, including the respiratory muscles, the respiratory controllers in the central nervous system (CNS) linked to respiratory muscles through spinal and peripheral nerves.

When respiratory failure (RF) ensues, the respiratory system fails in one or both of its gas exchange functions, *i.e.* oxygenation of mixed venous blood and/or elimination of carbon dioxide (CO_2) (fig. 1).

The diagnosis of RF is not clinical but based on arterial gas assessment: RF is defined by an arterial oxygen tension (P_{a,O_2}) <60 mmHg and/or arterial CO_2 tension (P_{a,CO_2}) >45 mmHg. These values are not rigid; they must serve as a general guide in combination with the history and clinical evaluation. RF may be acute, chronic, or acute on chronic, with clinical presentation quite different between the types.

Acute respiratory failure (ARF) may be life-threatening in clinical presentation, arterial blood gases and acid–base status; chronic respiratory failure (CRF) is clinically indolent to unapparent, due to mechanisms of compensation of respiratory acidosis.

RF due to lung diseases (*e.g.* pneumonia, acute lung injury, adult respiratory distress syndrome (ARDS), emphysema, interstitial lung disease) leads to hypoxaemia with normocapnia or even hypocapnia (type I RF).

Four pathophysiological mechanisms are responsible for hypoxaemic RF:

- ventilation/perfusion (V'/Q') ratio inequalities
- shunt
- diffusion impairment
- hypoventilation

Hypoxaemia with hypoventilation is characterised by normal alveolar–arterial oxygen difference, whereas disorders due to any of the other three mechanisms are characterised by a widening of the alveolar–arterial gradient.

Abnormal desaturation of systemic venous blood in the face of extensive lung disease is an important mechanism of hypoxaemia.

Several non-chronic obstructive pulmonary disease (COPD) diseases may lead to hypoxaemic ARF, which is defined as a P_{a,O_2} to oxygen inspiratory fraction (F_{I,O_2}) ratio ⩽300 (table 1).

Hypoxaemia is treated with an increase in F_{I,O_2} (the lower the V'/Q', the less the effect), and by recruiting airspaces with assisted ventilation. Airspace derecruitment occurs when the transpulmonary pressure falls below the airspace collapsing or closing pressure, and when the transpulmonary pressure applied during inspiration fails to exceed airspace opening pressure. Accordingly, airspace opening can be facilitated by increasing the

Key points

- Respiratory failure is failure of one or both of the respiratory system's gas exchange functions.
- It is diagnosed by arterial blood gas assessment.
- The clinical presentations of acute, chronic, and acute on chronic respiratory failure can differ greatly.

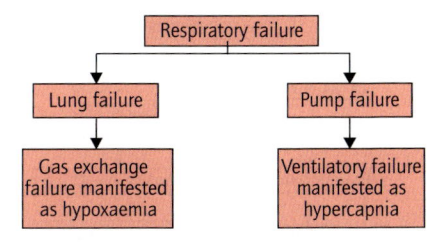

Figure 1. Types of respiratory failure. The respiratory system can be considered as consisting of two parts: the lung and the pump. Reproduced from Roussos and Koutsoukou (2003).

transpulmonary pressure applied at end expiration (continuous positive airway pressure (CPAP) or positive end-expiratory pressure (PEEP)) and at end inspiration (*i.e.* inspiratory positive airway pressure).

Failure of the pump (*e.g.* neuromuscular diseases, opiate overdose) results in alveolar hypoventilation and hypercapnia with parallel hypoxaemia (type II RF).

In some diseases (*e.g.* COPD, cardiogenic pulmonary oedema), both conditions may coexist, hypoxaemia usually appearing first.

Hypercapnic RF may be the result of CNS depression, functional or mechanical defect of the chest wall, imbalance of energy demands and supplies of the respiratory muscles, and/or adaptation of central controllers in order to prevent respiratory muscle injury and avoid or postpone fatigue (table 2). Hypercapnic RF may occur either acutely, insidiously, or acutely upon a chronic CO_2 retention. In all of these conditions, the pathophysiological, common mechanism is reduced alveolar ventilation for a given CO_2 production.

Table 1. Most common causes of acute hypoxaemic respiratory failure

Cardiogenic pulmonary oedema
Acute respiratory distress syndrome and acute lung injury
Alveolar haemorrhage
Lobar pneumonia
Atelectasis

Acute exacerbations of COPD (AECOPD) are periods of acute worsening which greatly affect the health status of patients with an increase in hospital admission and mortality. Estimates of in-patient mortality range 4–30%, but patients admitted due to ARF experience a higher rate, in particular elderly patients with comorbidities (up to 50%) and those requiring intensive care unit admission (11–26%).

Many causes may potentially be involved in determining ARF during AECOPD, such as bronchial infections, bronchospasm, left ventricular failure, pneumonia, pneumothorax and thromboembolism. Acute on chronic RF due to AECOPD is characterised by the worsening of hypoxaemia and a variable degree of hypercapnia and respiratory acidosis. The capacity of the patient to maintain acceptable indices of gas exchange during an AECOPD or the development of ARF depends both on the severity of the precipitating cause and on the degree of physiological dysfunction during the stable state and the subsequent physiological reserve. Worsening in V'/Q' mismatching is probably the leading mechanism in the occurrence of the hypoxaemia by the enlargement of physiological dead space and the rise of wasted ventilation. The increase in airway resistance and the need for a higher minute ventilation may result in expiratory flow limitation, dynamic hyperinflation and related intrinsic PEEP (PEEPi) with subsequent increased inspiratory threshold load and dysfunction of the respiratory muscles, which may lead to their fatigue. A rapid shallow breathing pattern may ensue in attempting to maintain adequate alveolar ventilation (V_A) when these additional resistive, elastic and inspiratory threshold loads are imposed on weakened respiratory muscles. Nevertheless, despite increased stimulation of the respiratory centres, and large negative intrathoracic pressure swings, CO_2 retention and acidaemia may occur. Dyspnoea, right ventricular failure, and encephalopathy characterise severe AECOPD complicated by ARF. Arterial pH reflects the acute worsening of V_A and, regardless of the chronic Pa,CO_2

Table 2. Causes of acute hypercapnia

Decreased central drive
 Drugs
 CNS diseases

Altered neural and neuromuscular transmission
 Spinal cord trauma
 Myelitis
 Tetanus
 Amyotrophic lateral sclerosis
 Poliomyelitis
 Guillan-Barrè
 Myasthenia gravis
 Organophosphate poisoning
 Botulism

Muscle abnormalities
 Muscular dystrophies
 Disuse atrophy
 Prematurity

Chest wall and pleural abnormalities
 Acute hyperinflation
 Chest wall trauma

Lung and airway diseases
 Acute asthma
 Acute exacerbation of COPD
 Cardiogenic and noncardiogenic pulmonary oedema
 Pneumonia
 Upper airway obstruction
 Bronchiectasis

Other causes
 Sepsis
 Circulatory shock

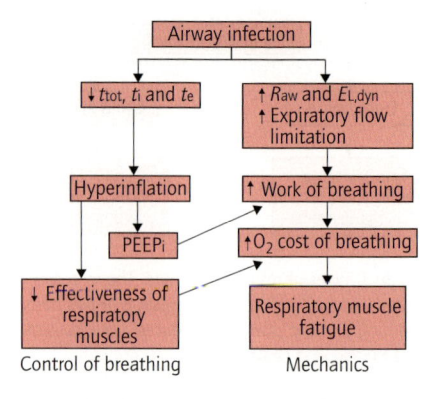

Figure 2. Schematic representation of the sequence of responsible mechanisms that lead to acute-on-chronic respiratory failure in chronic obstructive pulmonary disease patients. t_{tot}: total respiratory cycle; t_I: inspiratory time; t_e: expiratory time; R_{aw}: airway resistance; $E_{L,dyn}$: dynamic elastance of the lung; PEEPi: intrinsic positive end-expiratory pressure; ↓: decrease; ↑: increase. Reproduced from ROUSSOS and KOUTSOUKOU (2003).

level, it represents the best marker of the ARF severity. Figure 2 shows a schematic representation of the sequence of responsible mechanisms that lead to acute-on-chronic respiratory failure in COPD patients.

Besides medical treatment of the underlying disease, oxygen supplementation and eventually ventilator assistance is appropriate therapy for acute on chronic respiratory failure. The goals of assisted ventilation (either invasive or noninvasive) during AECOPD, is to unload the respiratory muscles and to reduce CO_2 by increasing V_A, thereby stabilising arterial pH until the underlying problem can be reversed.

References

- Ambrosino N, et al. Advanced chronic obstructive pulmonary disease. *Monaldi Arch Chest Dis* 1997; 52: 574–578.
- Ambrosino N, Vagheggini G. Noninvasive positive pressure ventilation in the acute care setting: where are we? *Eur Respir J* 2008; 31: 874–886.
- Calverley PMA. Respiratory failure in chronic obstructive pulmonary disease. *Eur Respir J* 2003; 22: Suppl. 47, 26s–30s.
- Donaldson GC, Wedzicha JA. COPD exacerbations – 1: epidemiology. *Thorax* 2006; 61: 164–168.
- Koutsoukou A, Roussos C. Acute and chronic respiratory failure: pathophysiology and mechanics. *In*: Fein AM, Kamholz S, Ost D, eds. Respiratory Emergencies. London, Hodder Arnold, 2006; pp. 17–30.
- Patil SP, et al. In-hospital mortality following acute exacerbations of chronic obstructive pulmonary disease. *Arch Intern Med* 2003; 163: 1180–1186.
- Plant PK, Elliott MW. Chronic obstructive pulmonary disease – 9: management of ventilatory failure in COPD. *Thorax* 2003; 58: 537–542.
- Rossi A, et al. Intrinsic positive end-expiratory pressure (PEEPi). *Intensive Care Med* 1995; 21: 522–536.
- Roussos C, Koutsoukou A. Respiratory failure. *Eur Respir J* 2003; 22: Suppl. 47, 3s–14s.

OXYGEN THERAPY AND VENTILATORY SUPPORT

A.K. Simonds
Royal Brompton Hospital, London, UK
E-mail: A.Simonds@rbht.nhs.uk

Acute oxygen therapy

Oxygen therapy is prescribed to correct hypoxaemia, rather than to reduce breathlessness, and so should always be titrated to arterial saturation (S_a,O_2) or blood gas measurements. In acutely ill patients, high-concentration oxygen therapy should be delivered to correct S_a,O_2 to 94–98%. In those with hypercapnic respiratory failure or at risk of ventilatory decompensation (*e.g.* severe chronic obstructive pulmonary disease (COPD), neuromuscular disease, obesity hypoventilation syndrome, chest wall disorder), a target S_a,O_2 of 88–92% should be the aim. If this cannot be achieved without progressive acidosis and hypercapnia, ventilatory support should be added. In emergency situations, oxygen therapy can be delivered by a high concentration reservoir mask at a flow rate of 15 L·min^{-1}. In hypercapnic patients, 28% and 24% Venturi masks can be used. All acute patients require regular or continuous assessment by oximetry to ensure hypoxaemia has been corrected and dose is still appropriate. Blood gas measurements are indicated if there is deterioration in S_a,O_2, features of CO_2 retention, such as drowsiness or flap, metabolic conditions or low cardiac output state.

Long-term oxygen therapy (LTOT)

Chronic hypoxaemia occurs either due to ventilation–perfusion mismatch, alveolar hypoventilation or diffusion problems in chronic lung disease, and in some conditions, *e.g.* COPD, all factors may be present. LTOT is used to correct hypoxaemia diurnally and nocturnally in the majority of patients. It has an additional use to palliate symptoms in those with end-stage or terminal conditions. In COPD, LTOT increases survival, reduces polycythaemia and, in some patients, may improve sleep quality and/or neuropsychiatric symptoms. LTOT is prescribed for >15 h a day, *e.g. via* concentrator, to correct S_a,O_2 to ≥90% in those listed in table 1.

Ambulatory O_2 therapy is added to correct hypoxaemia on exercise. In sedentary patients using LTOT, ambulatory O_2 is usually prescribed at the same flow rate as daytime use. In active and mobile LTOT recipients and patients who desaturate on exertion but do not fulfil criteria for LTOT, optimum flow rates can be derived from a standard 6-min or shuttle walk, again aiming to correct S_a,O_2 to

---

Key points

- Oxygen therapy is prescribed to correct hypoxaemia and should thus be titrated to arterial oxygen saturation.

- Long-term oxygen therapy can also palliate symptoms in patients with end-stage or terminal disease.

- NIV is the gold standard in treating acute hypercapnic COPD exacerbations, but is not useful in all acute respiratory situations.

- Long-term NIV home care can be more useful than oxygen therapy in chest wall and neuromuscular conditions.

Table 1. Criteria for long-term oxygen therapy

Chronic arterial oxygen tension (P_{a,O_2}) ⩽7.3 kPa
P_{a,O_2} 7.3–8.0 kPa if additional pulmonary hypertension, secondary polycythaemia, right heart failure or nocturnal desaturation

>90%. There is no evidence to support the use of short-burst O_2 therapy.

Acute ventilatory support

The term respiratory support embraces invasive ventilation (*via* endotracheal tube or tracheostomy), noninvasive positive pressure ventilation (delivered through oronasal, nasal, oral or helmet interfaces), noninvasive negative pressure ventilation using an iron lung or cuirass-type device and continuous positive airway pressure (CPAP). CPAP does not augment minute ventilation greatly, and is therefore insufficient to control arterial carbon dioxide tension (P_{a,CO_2}) in markedly hypercapnic patients.

On respiratory and high-dependency wards, noninvasive positive pressure ventilation (NIV) is now gold standard therapy in managing acute hypercapnic exacerbations of COPD as it has been shown to reduce mortality by about half and to decrease the need for intubation and invasive ventilation, thereby reducing pressure on intensive care unit (ICU) beds. NIV can also facilitate weaning and reduce the need for re-intubation. However, in patients with acute lung injury, more than two system failures, and moderate or severe bulbar problems, NIV is unlikely to be successful. In those with poor cough efficiency, *e.g.* due to neuromuscular disease, NIV can be combined with cough-assist devices such as the cough in–exsufflator.

There is no evidence that one type of noninvasive ventilator is superior, but bilevel pressure support models are most commonly used, often starting at initial settings of inspiratory positive airway pressure 10–12 cmH$_2$O and expiratory positive airway pressure 4 cmH$_2$O, increasing according to comfort and arterial blood gas control. A close-fitting, comfortable mask/interface with minimal deadspace is also important to success rates.

Home ventilatory support

The evidence supporting long-term home NIV is not as secure as acute NIV use in COPD exacerbations but does have a longer track record in restrictive disorders. Long-term NIV is more effective than LTOT in patients with chest wall disease, and is the treatment of choice in neuromuscular patients, *e.g.* those with amyotrophic lateral sclerosis (ALS)/motor neurone disease with mild-to-moderate bulbar involvement and Duchenne muscular dystrophy, where NIV use extends life expectancy. O_2 use in neuromuscular disease may exacerbate hypercapnia and should not be used without close monitoring. Nocturnal NIV should be initiated in patients with symptomatic nocturnal hypoventilation, or daytime hypercapnia.

Home ventilation in COPD patients is more controversial. Several randomised studies of LTOT *versus* LTOT plus NIV have been performed but few had the power to examine survival and, in some, quality of life impact seems variable. There is some evidence that NIV in severe COPD may reduce ICU admissions and hospital admissions in COPD patients with recurrent hospitalisations for hypercapnic exacerbations, although larger studies are required.

Tracheostomy ventilation is required in patients with severe bulbar weakness, aspiration and in those in whom ventilatory failure cannot be controlled with NIV.

References

- British Thoracic Society, Guideline for emergency oxygen use in adult patients. *Thorax* 2008; 63: Suppl. 6, vi1–vi68.
- Domiciliary oxygen therapy services: Royal College of Physicians Report. London, Royal College of Physicians, 1999.
- Elliott MW. Non-invasive ventilation in acute exacerbations of chronic obstructive lung disease. *In:* Simonds AK, ed. Non-Invasive Respiratory Support: A Practical Handbook. London, Hodder Arnold, 2007; pp. 39–56.
- Medical Research Council Working Party Report. Long term domiciliary oxygen therapy in chronic

hypoxic cor pulmonale complicating chronic bronchitis and emphysema. *Lancet* 1981; i: 681–685.
- Nocturnal Oxygen Therapy Trial Group. Continuous or nocturnal oxygen therapy in hypoxaemic chronic obstructive lung disease, a clinical trial. *Ann Intern Med* 1980; 93: 391–398.

Weblinks

- Emergency O_2: http://www.brit-thoracic.org.uk/ClinicalInformation/EmergencyOxygen/tabid/219/Default.aspx.
- Non-invasive ventilation: http://www.rcplondon.ac.uk/pubs/brochure.aspx?e=258.

INTENSIVE CARE AND HIGH-DEPENDENCY UNIT

S. Nava[1] and P. Navalesi[2]
[1] Respiratory Intensive Care Unit, Fondazione S. Maugeri, Istituto Scientifico di Pavia, Pavia
[2] Intensive Care Unit SCDU Anestesia, Terapia Intensiva e Rianimazione Generale Eastern Piedmont University "A. Avogadro" University Hospital, Maggiore della Carità, Novara, Italy
E-mail: snava@fsm.it

The respiratory intensive care unit (RICU), sometimes referred to as the "high dependency unit", is intended for patients with respiratory failure who do not require full ICU care but are considered to need more care than can usually be offered in a general ward.

The main reasons for admission to RICU are: 1) acute respiratory failure requiring noninvasive mechanical ventilation (NIV); 2) weaning of patients considered ventilator-dependent, and eventually their discharge home with a long-term ventilatory programme;

Key points

- The main reasons for admission to RICU are use of "acute" NIV, weaning from mechanical ventilation and requirement of intensive monitoring.

- RICUs have three levels of care: 1) RICU, 2) respiratory intermediate care unit, and 3) respiratory monitoring unit.

- The approach to the patients admitted to a RICU is usually multidisciplinary.

- All the diagnostic (*e.g.*, CT scans, NMR imaging) and therapeutic (*e.g.* major surgery) options should be readily available.

- RICUs should provide a fair amount of physical and pulmonary rehabilitation.

and 3) requirement of intensive monitoring (preferably noninvasive).

The main expectations from a RICU are the possibility to relieve congestion of ICU beds, to guarantee a high level of nursing assistance, to adequately respond to potential sudden changes in a patient's clinical condition and, under certain conditions, to provide a multidisciplinary rehabilitative approach to patients of high complexity.

The European Respiratory Society Task Force on RICU has defined three levels of care: 1) RICU, capable of applying both NIV and invasive ventilation, with a high nurse–patient ratio ($>$1:3) and an attending physician 24 $h \cdot day^{-1}$, 7 $days \cdot week^{-1}$; 2) respiratory intermediate care unit, capable of applying both NIV and invasive ventilation, with a nurse–patient ratio of 1:3–1:4 and the availability of a physician 24 $h \cdot day^{-1}$, 7 $days \cdot week^{-1}$; and 3) respiratory monitoring unit with a nurse–patient ratio $<$1:4, a physician on call within the hospital and the possibility of applying NIV.

These facilities may be located inside or outside a so-called "acute care hospital". It should be borne in mind, however, that access to these different environments may differ internationally or even regionally within the same country.

Concerning the admission criteria, these are pretty well established for those patients who require "acute" application of NIV. As opposed to NIV application in the ward, the closely monitored setting permits safe application of NIV also in tenuous patients. Noninvasive management of such patients, including those with severe acute respiratory acidosis (*i.e.* pH <7.30) secondary to exacerbation of chronic obstructive pulmonary disease and those with hypoxaemia (*i.e.* arterial oxygen tension to inspiratory oxygen fraction ratio <200) requires a skilled, experienced staff and preparedness to promptly intubate the patient who deteriorates despite NIV. Delays in intubation and application of invasive ventilation may harm the patient. Theoretically, the worse the derangement in arterial blood gases, the higher the level of care should be (*i.e.* RICU *versus* respiratory monitoring unit).

There is still disagreement about the definition of a ventilator-dependent patient, in whom the transfer from the ICU to RICU may be useful in an attempt to ameliorate the chances of weaning. Various authors have used times limits as short as 48–72 h and as long as 30 days. Realistically, ~20% of patients in an ICU require mechanical ventilation for more than a week, and about half are successfully weaned over the following few days. Therefore, a limit of 2 weeks has been chosen by most authors to define the threshold for "ventilator-dependency".

A definition, however, based only on time does not consider that for a particular patient to be regarded as ventilator-dependent (and, therefore, eligible for transfer to a RICU), the precipitating cause of the respiratory failure must have been reversed.

Some patients affected by an acute respiratory disorder may not fit the criteria of enrolment for mechanical ventilation when admitted to the hospital. However, their fragility and, very often, the high number of comorbidities do not allow the clinicians to make any firm statement about the immediate prognosis and risk of progression towards overt respiratory failure. These patients are likely to benefit from closer monitoring in a specialised environment, to avoid a delay in applying the appropriate treatment in case of worsening. Furthermore, in a subset of patients discharged from the ICU without the need for mechanical ventilation, but still having a tracheotomic tube in place, an associated increased mortality has been shown. An "intermediate step" in a protected environment after ICU discharge may be useful in these patients, primarily to allow better management of artificial airways.

The approach to the patients admitted to a RICU is usually multidisciplinary, in all cases involving physicians, respiratory therapists and nurses, and, in some cases, also involving dieticians, psychologists, physical and speech therapists, and social workers, as needed.

All the diagnostic (*e.g.* computed tomography (CT) scans, nuclear magneic resonance (NMR) imaging) and therapeutic (*e.g.* major surgery) options should be readily available. Because most of the units are located within an acute care hospital, this is a problem in most cases. Furthermore, these units should be able to allow a reasonable level of privacy, to favour rest and permit, compared with ICUs, longer visiting hours for relatives and friends. Last but not least, these units should provide a fair amount of physical and pulmonary rehabilitation, which has been shown to help in freeing patients from mechanical ventilation and restoring them to an acceptable level of autonomy.

References

- European Respiratory Task Force on epidemiology of respiratory intermediate care in Europe, Respiratory intermediate care units: a European survey. *Eur Respir J* 2002; 20: 1343–1350.
- Ambrosino N, Vagheggini G. Noninvasive positive pressure ventilation in the acute care setting: where are we? *Eur Respir J* 2008; 31: 874–886.
- Engoren M, *et al.* Hospital and long-term outcome after tracheostomy for respiratory failure. *Chest* 2004; 125: 220–227.
- Gosselink R, *et al.* Physiotherapy for adult patients with critical illness: recommendations of the European Respiratory Society and European Society of Intensive Care Medicine Task Force on Physiotherapy for Critically Ill Patients. *Intensive Care Med* 2008; 34: 1188–1199.
- Nava S, *et al.* Time of non-invasive ventilation. *Intensive Care Med* 2006; 32: 361–370.

ASSESSMENT FOR ANAESTHESIA/SURGERY

M.M. Schuurmans[1], C.T. Bolliger[2] and A. Boehler[1]
[1] University Hospital, Zurich, Switzerland
[2] Tygerberg Academic Hospital, Cape Town, South Africa
E-mail: capybara@compuserve.com

Pre-operative assessment of pulmonary risk is important in order to identify patients at risk for peri-operative morbidity and mortality, to determine possible pre-operative interventions that are beneficial for the outcome and to identify patients where surgery may be prohibitive.

Pre-operative evaluation for lung resection evaluates to which extent lung tissue can be resected without unacceptably increasing post-operative morbidity and mortality.

A careful history and physical examination are the most important tools for assessment of risk for post-operative pulmonary complications. Symptoms suggesting occult underlying lung disease (exercise intolerance, unexplained dyspnoea and cough) and the following risk factors for increased post-operative pulmonary complications need to be assessed.

Surgery-specific risk factors include: upper abdominal procedures; aortic, thoracic, and head and neck surgery, including neurosurgery; surgery lasting >3 h; and emergency procedures.

Definite risk factors include: chronic obstructive pulmonary disease (COPD); congestive heart failure; diminished general health status (American Society of Anesthesiologists (ASA) class >2 (table 1); malnutrition (serum albumin <35 mg·L^{-1}); and use of pancuronium as a neuromuscular blocker.

Probable risk factors include: obstructive sleep apnoea; general anaesthesia (when

> **Key points**
>
> - A careful history and physical examination is necessary to assess the risk of post-operative pulmonary complications.
>
> - Pulmonary function testing is not routine except in the case of evaluation for lung resection.
>
> - A number of strategies are available to reduce the risk of complications.

compared with spinal or epidural anaesthesia); abnormal chest radiograph; cigarette use within previous 8 weeks; and current upper respiratory tract infection.

It is noteworthy that pulmonary function tests are not part of routine pre-operative assessment unless patients are being evaluated for lung resection (see "Pulmonary resection") or have unexplained dyspnoea or exercise intolerance. Clinical evaluation cannot determine whether airflow obstruction has been optimally reduced in patients with previously diagnosed COPD or asthma. Well-controlled asthma (free of wheezing, peak flows >80% predicted, or personal best) has been shown not to carry any added risk. Age and blood gases have no definitive role in the risk assessment when confounding issues such as comorbidities have been considered.

Patients with high risk (surgery-specific risk factor + one or more definite risk factors) will

Table 1. American Society of Anesthesiologists (ASA) classification of pre-operative risk

ASA class	Systemic disturbance	PPC %	Mortality %
1	Healthy patient with no disease outside of the surgical process	1.2	<0.03
2	Mild-to-moderate systemic disease caused by the surgical condition or by other pathological processes, medically well-controlled	5.4	0.2
3	Severe disease process that limits activity but is not incapacitating	11.4	1.2
4	Severe incapacitating disease process that is constant threat to life	10.9	8
5	Moribund patient not expected to survive 24 h with or without an operation	NA	34
E	Suffix to indicate emergency surgery for any class	Increased	Increased

PPC: post-operative pulmonary complications; NA: not applicable.

benefit from strategies to reduce pulmonary complications.

Pre-operative interventions: smoking cessation for 8 weeks; inhaled ipratropium or tiotropium for patients with clinically significant COPD; inhaled β-agonists for symptomatic COPD and asthma patients; pre-operative systemic glucocorticoids for COPD and asthma patients who are not optimised on inhalative treatment; delay elective surgery if respiratory infection present; antibiotics for patients with purulent sputum or change in sputum character; and inspiratory muscle training.

Intraoperative interventions: choose alternative procedure lasting <3 h when possible (video-assisted thoracoscopic and laparoscopic procedures have ~1/10th the pulmonary complication rates of open procedures); minimise duration of anaesthesia; regional anaesthesia (nerve block) in very high-risk patients; and avoid pancuronium.

Post-operative interventions: deep-breathing exercises or incentive spirometry; and epidural analgesia instead of parenteral opioids.

Cardiac evaluation: history, physical examination and resting ECG are frequently required for the initial estimate of the peri-operative cardiac risk. The definitive assessment of cardiac risk should respect current guidelines for cardiologists.

Pulmonary resection

Pulmonary resection is a high-risk procedure with a mortality of 2–3% for lobectomy and 4–6% for pneumonectomy in experienced centres. The clinical evaluation should focus on respiratory and cardiovascular pathology. Air flow limitation should be optimised before further evaluation and cardiac disease identified and managed either medically or surgically. Initial pulmonary function evaluation should include at least forced expiratory volume in 1 s (FEV1), forced vital capacity (FVC) and transfer capacity of the lung for carbon monoxide ($T_{L,CO}$). Values >80% pred for FEV1 and $T_{L,CO}$ are associated with an uncomplicated surgical course for resection up to a pneumonectomy. All other candidates should undergo a formal exercise test. Patients with a peak oxygen uptake (V'_{O_2}) >20 mL·kg^{-1}·min^{-1} (or >75% pred) tolerate pulmonary resection up to a pneumonectomy, and values >15 mL·kg^{-1}·min^{-1} are sufficient for lobectomy. Values <10 mL·kg^{-1}·min^{-1} are predictive of major post-operative complications and disability. Further evaluation according to a validated algorithm (fig. 1) necessitates the estimation of the relative contribution of the tissue earmarked for resection by means of the predicted post-operative (ppo) values for FEV1, $T_{L,CO}$ and $V'O_2$ ("split function"). The ppo values of these parameters are equal to their pre-operative values × (1 – fractional contribution of the tissue earmarked for resection). There are three acceptable ways of estimating the relative functional contribution or split lung function: anatomical calculation; quantitative computed tomography (CT) scanning; or split perfusion scanning. Anatomical calculations are by far the simplest: the number of patent (or functional) segments that are due for resection is subtracted from the total number of segments (19) and this value is divided by 19 to give a fraction. The FEV1-ppo is estimated to be equal to the pre-operative FEV1 × ((19 – patent segments removed)/19). Anatomical calculations have been shown to overestimate the functional loss so that patients who are deemed operable by anatomical calculations will generally not require radiological calculations.

Calculated ppo values on the basis of lung perfusion scans (with technetium 99m-labelled macroaggregates) have been shown to correlate best with actual post-operative values. Densitometric calculations on the basis of CT scans are marginally less accurate than perfusion scans. The advantage of this method is the availability of the information since most lung resection candidates invariably have a pre-operative chest CT scan and modern software simplifies the three-dimensional reconstruction for the calculation of the relative volume of lung to be resected.

The recent revival of simple stair climbing as a low-cost alternative to assess exercise capacity and operative risk is still under investigation. One large study showed a significant correlation between the ability to climb to a 20.6-m elevation and an uncomplicated surgical course.

Lung volume reduction surgery for end-stage emphysema has partly redefined the limits of lung resection. Many patients with pre-operative FEV1 and $T_{L,CO}$ between 20–40% pred have benefited from targeted removal of the most emphysematous lung regions.

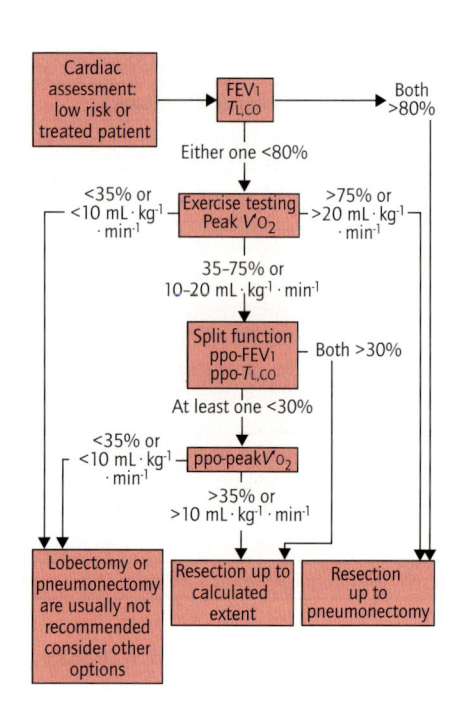

Figure 1. Algorithm for assessment of cardiopulmonary reserve before lung resection in lung cancer patients. FEV1: forced expiratory volume in 1 s; $D_{L,CO}$: diffusing capacity of the lung for carbon monoxide; $V'O_2$: oxygen uptake; ppo: predicted post-operative. Modified from BRUNELLI et al. (2009).

References

- Bolliger CT, et al. Prediction of functional reserves after lung resection: comparison between quantitative computed tomography, scintigraphy, and anatomy. *Respiration* 2002; 69: 482–489.
- Brunelli A, et al. ERS/ESTS clinical guidelines on fitness or radical therapy in lung cancer patients (surgery and chemoradiotherapy). *Eur Respir J* 2009; 34: 17–41.

- Brunelli A, et al. Stair climbing test predicts cardiopulmonary complications after lung resection. *Chest* 2002; 121: 1106-1110.
- Eagle KA, et al. ACC/AHA guideline update for perioperative cardiovascular evaluation for noncardiac surgery - executive summary: a report of the American College of Cardiology/American Heart Association Task Force on Practice Guidelines (Committee to Update the 1996 Guidelines on Perioperative Cardiovascular Evaluation for Noncardiac Surgery). *J Am Coll Cardiol* 2002; 39: 542.
- Koegelenberg CFN, et al. Preoperative pulmonary evaluation. *In:* Albert RK, et al. eds. Clinical Respiratory Medicine, 3rd Edn. Amsterdam, Elsevier, 2008; pp. 275-283.
- Schuurmans MM, et al. Functional evaluation before lung resection. *Clin Chest Med* 2002; 23: 159-172.

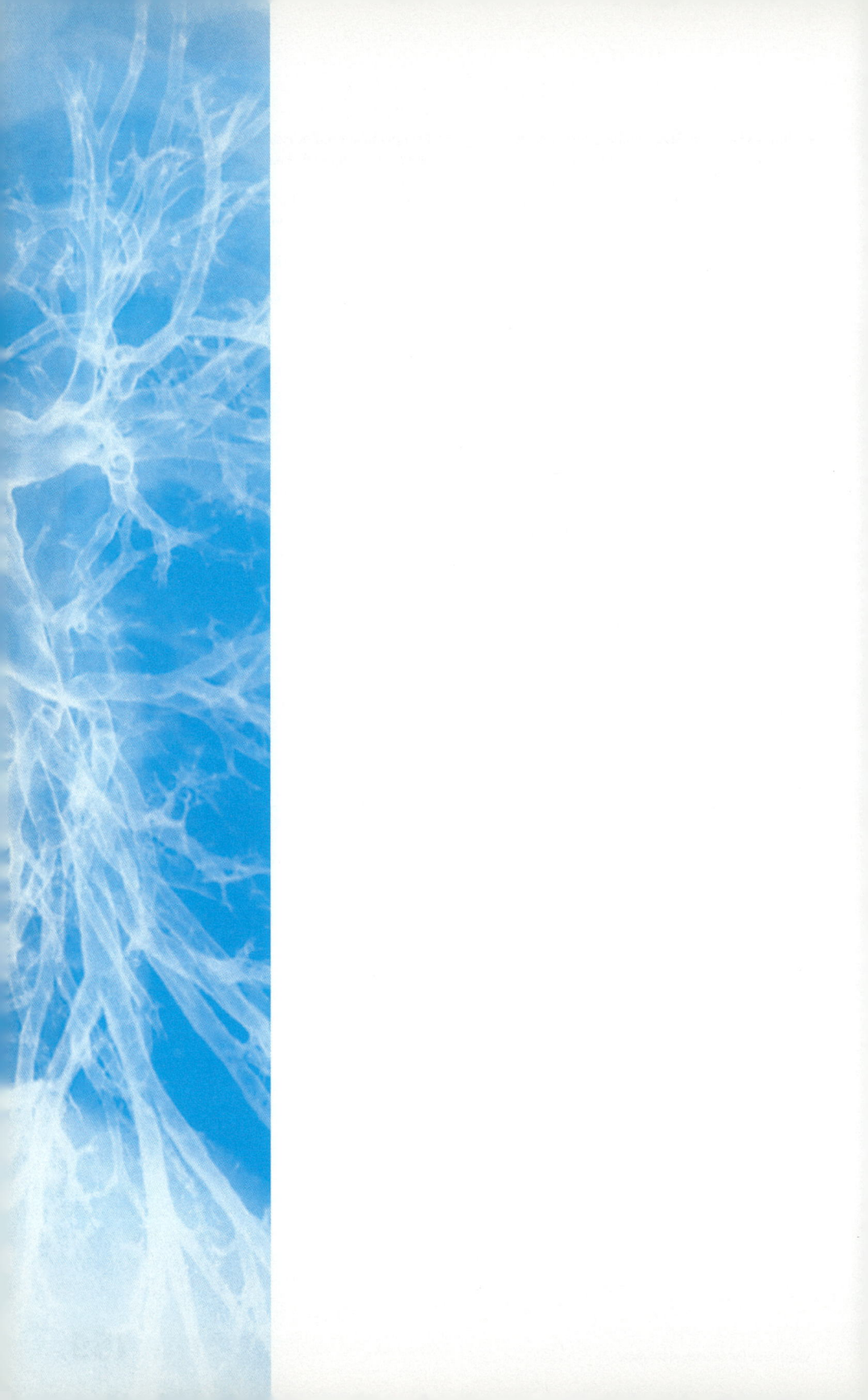

CHAPTER 7:

RESPIRATORY INFECTIONS

MICROBIOLOGY TESTING AND INTERPRETATION M. Ieven	162
UPPER RESPIRATORY TRACT INFECTIONS G. Rohde	168
INFECTIVE EXACERBATIONS OF COPD M. Miravitlles	172
PNEUMONIA M. Woodhead	176
HOSPITAL-ACQUIRED PNEUMONIA F. Blasi	180
PNEUMONIA IN THE IMMUNOCOMPROMISED HOST S. Ewig	183
PLEURAL INFECTION AND LUNG ABSCESS C. Hooper and N. Maskell	186
INFLUENZA, PANDEMICS AND SARS W.S. Lim	191

MICROBIOLOGY TESTING AND INTERPRETATION

M. Ieven
Laboratory for Microbiology, Vaccine and Infectious Disease Institute, University of Antwerp, Wilrijk, Antwerp, Belgium
E-mail: Greet.Ieven@uza.be

In primary care, microbiological work-up in respiratory infections is primarily meant as an epidemiological investigation in order to guide future empiric antimicrobial policies. Hardly any study has shown that initial microbiological studies in primary care affect the outcome of respiratory infections. Nevertheless an aetiologic diagnosis, of both bacteria and viruses and mixtures of these in community-acquired pneumonia (CAP) or lower respiratory tract infections (LRTI) may be helpful in guiding treatment, particularly in the more severely ill patients. Diagnostic testing should not lead to delays in initiation of therapy, however. Even with extensive diagnostic testing, a specific aetiology is usually identified in only half of all patients, generally at least 1–2 days after the clinical diagnosis is made. With the advent of recently developed rapid techniques such as immunochromatographic tests, urinary antigen tests and particularly nucleic acid amplification tests (NAATs) that produce results within 30 min or 4–5 h, microbiological information is becoming clinically useful (table 1).

Key points

For the aetiologic diagnosis of lower respiratory tract infections (LRTIs):

- Gram stain and culture of a good quality sputum can be valuable for the microbiological diagnosis of LRTI caused by *Streptococcus pneumoniae* or *Haemophilus influenzae*.

- Urinary antigen detection is a very helpful and rapid test for the diagnosis of pneumococcal or *Legionella* infections.

- Serology is rarely helpful in the management of the individual patient with LRTI.

- Molecular tests for the detection of respiratory viruses and atypical pathogens in specific patient populations are desirable.

Conventional culture techniques

Blood culture For the diagnosis of pneumonia, blood cultures have a very high specificity but are positive in only about 10–20% of untreated cases. In some studies, a direct correlation has been found between the severity (based on the Fine Severity Index) of pneumonia and blood culture positivity rate. Two blood cultures should be obtained as early as possible in the disease and before any antibiotic treatment is started. Blood cultures are more sensitive for the detection of *Streptococcus pneumoniae* than for the detection of *Haemophilus influenzae*. Despite their low sensitivity, blood cultures in CAP are considered the gold standard because the organisms are recovered from a normally sterile source. Results may be available after 24–48 h.

Sputum Gram stain and culture The most frequently submitted specimen in cases of

Table 1. Diagnostic approach for the most common specific agents in lower respiratory tract infections

Pathogen	Specimen	Rapid tests	Conventional tests	Comments
S. pneumoniae	Blood		Blood culture	Positive in 10–20% of cases when collected within 4 days
	Sputum	Gram stain	Culture	Only purulent samples acceptable. Obtained in 35–40% of patients; informative if >90% Gram-positive, diplococci most relevant if Gram stain informative
	Pleural exudates	Gram stain	Culture	Specific, only considered if less invasive methods nondiagnostic
	Urine	Antigen test		Sensitivity 50–80% of bacteraemic cases, lacks specificity in children, more evaluation necessary
H. influenzae	Blood		Blood culture	Less frequently positive than for S. pneumoniae
	Respiratory specimens	Gram stain	Culture	
Legionella spp.	Urine	Antigen test		Sensitivity 66–95%
	Respiratory specimens	NAAT	Culture	Culture: on appropriate media, late results, less sensitive than NAAT
	Serum		IgM and IgG serology	Acute and convalescent specimens. Retrospective diagnosis
C. pneumoniae M. pneumoniae	Respiratory specimens	NAAT	Culture	Culture: on appropriate medium; low sensitivity compared to NAAT
	Serum		IgM and IgG serology	Acute and convalescent specimens. Lack of sensitivity, specificity, not appropriate for individual patient management. Retrospective results
Respiratory viruses	Respiratory specimens	Direct antigen tests, NAAT	Virus isolation	Requirement for appropriate infrastructure. Isolation less sensitive than NAAT

S. pneumoniae: Streptococcus pneumoniae; H. influenzae: Haemophilus influenzae; C. pneumoniae: Chlamydophila pneumoniae; M. pneumoniae: Mycoplasma pneumoniae; BAL: bronchoalveolar lavage; PSB: protected specimen brush; NAAT: nucleic acid amplification test; Ig: immunoglobulin

LRTI and more specifically in pneumonia is sputum. To be of value for microbial diagnosis and early guidance to therapy, sputum specimens must be representative of lower respiratory secretions, and must be interpreted according to strict criteria by an experienced observer. The most widely used method to assess acceptability in this regard is based on cytological criteria. The specimen should therefore be screened by microscopic examination for the relative number of polymorphonuclear cells and squamous epithelial cells in a lower power (10×) field. Invalid specimens ($\geqslant 10$ squamous epithelial cells and $\leqslant 25$ polymorphonuclear cells/field) should not be examined further. It may be difficult to obtain good-quality, purulent sputum. Many LRTI or pneumonia patients, particularly older ones, do not produce sputum. Satisfactory sputum specimens can be obtained in 32–55% of patients.

Large studies on the diagnostic value of Gram staining in primary care patients are lacking, but some hospital-based studies show that in good-quality Gram-stained sputum, the presence of a single or a preponderant morphotype of bacteria ($\pm$90%) may be diagnostic. This is based on correspondence with the organisms recovered from blood cultures obtained in parallel, and which are the gold standard. The sensitivity and specificity for the detection of *S. pneumoniae* are ~35–79% and 96%, respectively, and 42% and 99% respectively for *H. influenzae*. Sputum with a mixed flora in the Gram stain has no diagnostic value. The sputum Gram stain is therefore valuable in guiding the processing and interpretation of sputum cultures.

The sensitivity and specificity of sputum cultures are reduced by contamination with flora colonising the upper respiratory tract. The value of sputum cultures in establishing a bacterial cause of LRTI depends on how the specimens are collected and processed. The reported yield of sputum cultures has varied widely, from <20% for outpatients to >90% for hospitalised patients. The sputum Gram stain is valuable in guiding the processing and interpretation of sputum cultures. Sputum culture results are most convincing when the organism(s) isolated in culture are compatible with the morphology of the organisms present in the Gram stain. In the absence of an informative Gram stain, the predictive value of sputum culture is very low.

Rapid antigen tests

Urinary antigen tests The *S. pneumoniae* urinary antigen test in adult CAP has been shown to have a sensitivity of 65–100% and a specificity of >90%; however, weak positive results should be interpreted with caution. There is a relation between the degree of *S. pneumoniae* urinary antigen test positivity and the pneumonia severity index. Therefore, the test could be reserved for high-risk patients for whom demonstrative results of a sputum Gram stain are unavailable.

The urinary antigen test may also be applied on pleural fluid with a high sensitivity and specificity, and on serum samples with a sensitivity of 50% in bacteraemic patients and 40% in nonbacteraemic patients. Vaccination does not result in a positive urinary antigen test. The immunochromatographic urinary antigen test for *S. pneumoniae* is therefore useful for the aetiologic diagnosis of severe CAP, especially for patients without demonstrative results of a sputum Gram stain.

Urinary antigen detection is currently the most helpful rapid test for the diagnosis of a *Legionella* infection. Several test formats have been developed, the enzyme immunoassay (EIA) format being more suited to test a larger number of specimens and taking a few hours to complete. The immunochromatographic format is better suited for single specimens, and produces a result within minutes. These tests are particularly useful since culture of *Legionella* spp. is slow and takes 3–4 days. *Legionella* urinary antigen detection is frequently the first positive laboratory test in this infection. The sensitivity of the tests varies between 65–70% in unconcentrated urine and increases significantly after concentration of the specimen. In *Legionella* infection, there is also a relationship between the degree of positivity of the urinary antigen test and the severity of disease: for patients with mild Legionnaires' disease, test sensitivities range from only 40–50%, whereas for patients with severe Legionnaires' disease who need immediate special medical care, sensitivities reach 88–100%.

Antigen tests on pharyngeal specimens A variety of antigen tests have been evaluated on respiratory specimens. For respiratory infections due to viruses, the optimal specimen is the nasopharyngeal aspirate. During recent years, a considerable number of previously unknown respiratory viral agents have been discovered whose *in* vitro culture is very slow or even unrealised: the human metapneumovirus, the novel coronaviruses NL 63, HKU1 and human bocavirus. Antigens of the many common respiratory viruses, influenza virus, respiratory syncytial virus (RSV), adenovirus and parainfluenza viruses, can be detected by direct immunofluorescence (DIF) or by commercially available EIAs. The sensitivities of these tests vary from 50->90% depending on the virus and the patient population studied. For the detection of influenza virus infections, the sensitivity of immunofluorescence can be increased by inoculation of the clinical sample on appropriate cells, followed by immunofluorescence after 48 h. Several common respiratory viruses can be detected simultaneously by the use of pooled monoclonal antibodies. The sensitivity of the DIF test is lower in adults and older people than in children. Rapid methods for the detection of influenza virus are of particular interest because of the availability of antiviral agents that must be given within 48 h after onset of symptoms.

Serology

Efforts have been made to diagnose infections caused by slowly growing or difficult to grow organisms by serology. This holds particularly for *Mycoplasma pneumoniae, Chlamydophila pneumoniae, Legionella* infections and respiratory viruses. It should be remembered that the most reliable serologic evidence of an ongoing infection is based on a fourfold increase in titre of immunoglobulin (Ig)G (or IgG+IgM) antibodies during the evolution of the disease episode based on two serum samples collected at an interval of 14-21 days or longer, and/or the appearance of IgM antibodies during the evolution of the disease. IgM tests are usually less sensitive and specific than fourfold changes in antibody titres between paired specimens separated by several weeks. Solitary high IgG titers have no diagnostic meaning for an acute infection since the moment of the seroconversion is unknown and necessarily took place some time before the illness under observation started.

The sensitivity and specificity of serologic tests are related to the antigen used. For *M. pneumoniae* and *C. pneumoniae*, a great number of antigen preparations have been proposed: whole organisms, protein fractions, glycoprotein fractions and recombinant antigens. Several studies illustrate a lack of standardisation of antigens of *M. pneumoniae*.

For a number of respiratory agents, a variety of tests are available commercially. Some assays lack both sensitivity and specificity, emphasising the need for more validation and quality control.

IgM antibodies against *M. pneumoniae* require up to 1 week to reach diagnostic titres, and sometimes much longer. Anti-*M. pneumoniae* IgM antibodies can be detected in 7-25% (depending on the test applied) of acute sera and IgG antibodies in 41-63% of convalescent sera depending on the timing of the second sample illustrating the low incidence of IgM antibodies in the acute-phase serum specimens and importance of the delay between the two serum samples. *Legionella* antibody tests also have a sensitivity of only 61-64% depending on the assay applied and also do not substantially improve the diagnosis of legionellosis. The acute antibody test for *Legionella* in Legionnaires' disease is usually negative or demonstrates very low titres. As for other aetiologies, high titres of IgG and/or IgM, above a certain threshold, present early during the disease, have been interpreted as diagnostic but at least one study showed that this titre had a very low positive predictive value.

For respiratory viral infections such as for influenza and RSV, a significant or fourfold IgG antibody increase is detected by EIA in ~80-90%% of patients at only 20-30 days after the onset of disease.

The serologic measurement of specific antibody responses can mostly not offer an early diagnosis and therefore has limited application for an aetiologic diagnosis and for the routine management of the individual patient with LRTI. Consequently, it is rather an epidemiological than a diagnostic tool.

Nucleic acid amplification tests

The newest approach in the diagnosis of respiratory tract infections is the detection of microbial nucleic acids by NAATs. Culture procedures for viruses and fastidious bacteria, *M. pneumoniae, C. pneumoniae, Legionella pneumophila, Bordetella pertussis*, which normally do not colonise the human respiratory tract, are too insensitive and too slow to be therapeutically relevant and these pathogens therefore should be detected using NAATs, whose sensitivity is almost always superior to that of the traditional procedures.

A multitude of reports has appeared on the epidemiology of LRTIs but most are restricted to a few viruses (influenza, sometimes together with RSV, to rhino-, metapneumo- or coronaviruses) and/or to some population groups, *e.g.* children, adults or the elderly. Great variations occur in function of time, place and the age-groups studied. Although the role of some new viruses is becoming more clear in specific patient populations, more studies are needed to identify the clinical relevance of some others, such as the bocavirus. All these studies were done with the traditional NAATs that require at least 1–2 days, producing *a posteriori* results that were unavailable to the clinician in time to have an impact on patient management. Real-time multiplex NAATs offer the solution. To cover the wide spectrum of aetiologic respiratory agents, a number of uni- and/or multiplex reactions are performed simultaneously. Both in-house and commercially available multiplex NAATs for the simultaneousl detection of two, three or up to 22 different respiratory pathogens, including the "atypical" *M. pneumoniae, C. pneumoniae* and *L. pneumophila,* and respiratory viruses, with a mixture of primers have been developed.

The combined use of single target assays or of multiplex assays has increased the diagnostic yield in respiratory infections by 30–50%: combined with traditional bacteriological techniques to diagnose *S. pneumoniae* infections, >50% – and in some studies of CAP up to 70% – of aetiologic agents can be detected.

The wider application of multiplex reactions during recent years has resulted in the detection of numerous simultaneous viral infections with widely varying incidences: from 3% to even 23% or 35%, depending on whether bacterial agents are also included. The divergent incidences may result from the variety of diagnostic panels applied. Combined viral and viral–bacterial infections are diagnosed but no preferential combinations have been found. The clinical significance of combined infections remains to be further clarified. Respiratory viruses have also been increasingly recognised as causes of severe LRTIs in immunocompromised hosts. Respiratory infections are more common in solid organ recipients, particularly in lung transplant recipients. Infections are especially dangerous prior to engraftment and during 3 months after transplantation, in the setting of graft *versus* host disease. The origin of the infections is community-acquired as well as nosocomial.

As more epidemiological information on the role of a panel of respiratory viral pathogens becomes available, it is clear that screening for these viruses in specific patient populations such as transplant patients, very young children or the elderly is desirable and preventive and therapeutic recommendations may take this information into account.

NAATs are, however, not required for every purpose. For cohorting RSV-infected paediatric patients, the DIF tests can be as sensitive as an RT-PCR with results available within 60 min (and at lower cost than with NAATs). Very rapid chromatographic tests are also available for RSV, which can be done in the laboratory outside virology laboratory operating hours. These tests lack sensitivity, however, when applied to respiratory samples of adult patients.

Conclusion

In recent years significant progress has been made in the microbiological diagnosis of respiratory infections. A straightforward interpretation of a good-quality, Gram-stained sputum sample has been established, and has been shown to be important for rapid diagnosis of pneumonia and the interpretation of culture results in severely ill patients.

The number of possible aetiologic agents, viruses and fastidious bacteria has been extended and their epidemiology has been clarified. Sensitive and rapid methods for their detection have been developed and are increasingly validated in clinical settings.

Amplification techniques are at present more expensive than conventional approaches. However, improvements in standardisation and automation for sample preparation and technical advances will lead to increased use of amplification methods and cost reductions to rates competitive with conventional methods. Several studies have tended to show cost efficiency of rapid diagnosis of acute respiratory infections resulting from reduced antibiotic use and complementary laboratory investigations but most significantly from shorter hospitalisation and reduced isolation periods. Serologic diagnosis of those cases that remain undetected by the NAATs is of no clinical use since it is available only after many days or even weeks.

References

- Beersma MF, *et al*. Evaluation of 12 commercial tests and the complement fixation test for *Mycoplasma pneumoniae*-specific immunoglobulin G (IgG) and IgM antibodies, with PCR used as the "gold standard". *J Clin Microbiol* 2005; 43: 2277-2285.
- Genne D, *et al.* Enhancing the etiologic diagnosis of community-acquired pneumonia in adults using the urinary antigen assay (Binax NOW). *Int J Infect Dis* 2006; 10: 124-128.
- Ieven M. Currently used nucleic acid amplification tests for the detection of viruses and atypicals in acute respiratory infections. *J Clin Virol* 2007; 40: 259-276.
- Ieven M.: Diagnosis of community acquired pneumonia. *In:* Torres A, ed. Community Acquired Pneumonia. Chichester, John Wiley and Sons Ltd, 2007; pp. 43-61.
- Loens K, *et al.* Minireview: Optimal sampling sites and methods for detection of pathogens possibly causing community-acquired lower respiratory tract infections. *J Clin Microbiol* 2009; 47: 21-31.
- Loens K, *et al.* Molecular diagnosis of *Mycoplasma pneumoniae* in respiratory tract infections. *J Clin Microbiol* 2003; 41: 4915-23.
- Mahony JB. Detection of respiratory viruses by molecular methods. *Clin Microbiol Reviews* 2008; 21: 716-741.
- Templeton KE, *et al.* Improved diagnosis of the etiology of community-acquired pneumonia with real-time polymerase chain reaction. *Clin Infect Dis* 2005; 41: 345-351.
- Woodhead M, *et al.* Guidelines for the management of adult lower respiratory tract infections. *Eur Respir J* 2005; 26: 1138-1180.

UPPER RESPIRATORY TRACT INFECTIONS

G. Rohde
Dept of Respiratory Medicine, Maastrict University Medical Centre, Netherlands
E-mail: gernot.rohde@mumc.nl

Upper respiratory tract infections (URTIs) are the most common infectious illness in the general population. They are the leading cause for people missing work or school.

Prevalence

URTIs usually occur during the cold months, mainly due to overcrowding inside buildings. The mean frequency is 2–4 episodes annually for adults. In children it is higher. Antigenic variation of 100s of respiratory viruses allows repeated circulation in the community.

Spectrum

The upper respiratory tract consists of the nose, paranasal sinuses, pharynx, larynx, trachea and bronchi. The most prevalent illness is the common cold (rhino-sinusitis), followed by sinusitis, pharyngitis/tonsillitis, laryngitis and sometimes tracheobronchitis (table 1).

Onset of symptoms usually begins after 1–3 days after exposure to a microbial pathogen. The duration of the symptoms is typically 7–10 days but may persist longer.

Transmission and predisposition

Transmission of pathogens happens by aerosol, droplet, or direct hand-to-hand contact. The pathogens invade the respiratory epithelium of the corresponding area. Sinusitis and acute bronchitis are often preceded by a common cold. There are predisposing conditions as allergic rhinoconjunctivitis, nasal septum deviation, immundeficiency, or cocaine abuse. Smoking or exposure to second-hand smoke and travel are additional risk factors.

Key points

- URTIs are the most common infectious illness in the general population, and are the leading cause of missed work and school.

- Most URTIs are viral in origin, and typical agents are rhinoviruses, coronaviruses, adenoviruses, coxsackieviruses, influenza- and parainfluenzaviruses, human metapneumovirus, and respiratory syncytial virus.

- URTIs rarely cause permanent sequelae or death, but can progress to otitis media, bronchitis, bronchiolitis, pneumonia, sepsis, meningitis, intracranial abscess, and other infections.

- Diagnosis is usually purely clinical; diagnostic investigations should only be performed in special circumstances, such as influenza, group A streptococcal pharyngitis, infectious mononucleosis and pneumonia.

- Infection will often be self-limiting, with no specific treatment necessary; the only indications for antibiotic treatment are group A streptococcal pharyngitis, bacterial sinusitis and pertussis.

Table 1. Signs and symptoms

Upper respiratory tract infection	Symptoms	Signs
Common cold	Nasal congestion, mucopurulent nasal discharge, sneezing, sore throat, halitosis	Low-grade fever, nasal vocal tone, inflamed nasal mucosa
Sinusitis	Unilateral facial pain, maxillary toothache, headache, purulent nasal discharge	Swelling, redness, tenderness to palpation or percussion overlying the affected sinuses, abnormal transillumination
Pharyngitis	Sore throat, odynophagia, or dysphagia, fever, absence of cough, halitosis	Pharyngeal erythema and exudate, palatal petechiae (doughnut lesions), tender anterior cervical lympadenopathy, scalartiniform rash, pharyngeal or palatal vesicles and ulcers (herpangina), tonsillar hypertrophy
Laryngitis	Hoarseness, voicelessness, dry cough, odynophagia, or dysphagia, halitosis	Low-grade fever, cervical lymphadenopathy, inspiratory stridor, tachypnoea
Tracheo-bronchitis	Dry or productive cough, dyspnoea	Low-grade fever, anterior cervical lymphadenopathy, tachypnoea, rhonchi

Pathogens

Most URTIs are viral in origin. More than 200 different viruses are known to cause the common cold. Typical viral agents that cause URTIs are rhinoviruses, coronaviruses, adenoviruses, coxsackieviruses, influenza- and parainfluenzaviruses, human metapneumovirus, respiratory syncytial virus and others.

Group A, but also group C and G *Streptococci* can cause pharyngitis (10–20% of cases), as well as other bacteria like *Neisseria gonorrhoeae*, *Corynebacterium diphtheriae* and atypical bacteria (*Chlamydia*, *Mycoplasma*). *Streptococcus pneumoniae*, *Haemophilus influenzae* and *Moraxella catarrhalis* can be the bacterial cause of rhinosinusitis or tracheobronchitis. *Bordetella pertussis* or *Bordetella parapertussis* are the cause of whooping cough associated with laryngotracheitis.

Complications

URTIs rarely cause permanent sequelae or death. However they can progress to otitis media, bronchitis, bronchiolitis, pneumonia, sepsis, meningitis, intracranial abscess, and other infections. Specific complications can occur with untreated group A streptococcal pharyngitis resulting in acute rheumatic fever (ARF), acute glomerulonephritis, peritonsillar abscess, and toxic shock syndrome. Sinusitis can extend into surrounding deep tissue leading to orbital cellulitis, subperiosteal abscess, orbital abscess, frontal and maxillary osteomyelitis, subdural abscess, meningitis, and brain abscess. Epiglottitis, a presentation of laryngitis caused by *H. influenzae* type B, poses a risk of death due to sudden airway obstruction and other complications, including septic arthritis, meningitis, empyema and mediastinitis.

Diagnosis

In most cases, the diagnosis is purely clinical. History, inspection, palpation, percussion and auscultation (see table 1) are sufficient. Additional diagnostic investigations should only be performed in special circumstances. These include suspicion of:

- Influenza (perform pharyngeal swab for PCR).
- Group A streptococcal pharyngitis (perform pharyngeal swab for rapid antigen detection test).
- Infectious mononucleosis (there are usually additional symptoms such as hepatosplenomegaly and lymphocytosis; perform mononucleosis spot test in blood).
- Pneumonia (perform C-reactive protein and chest radiography).

Differential diagnosis

Influenza viruses can cause mild URTIs but also systemic disease. The definition of influenza-like illness is fever $>38.5°C$) and one of the following: cough, sore throat, headache and muscle ache.

Allergic rhinoconjunctivitis is characterised by oedema of the conjunctiva, itching and increased lacrimation additional to symptoms of rhinitis. Is shows seasonal variation related to allergen exposure.

Acute thyroiditis can present as sore throat, a common symptom in URTIs. Investigation of thyroid hormones, thyroid-specific autoantibodies, ultrasound and radioactive iodine uptake can help with diagnosis.

Gastro-oesophageal reflux disease (GORD) can clinically present as laryngopharyngitis and/or tracheobronchitis. History and oesophagogastroduodenoscopy in more severe cases should be performed.

Wegener's granulomatosis should be considered in patients with sinusitis not responding to therapy. Classic antineutrophil cytoplasmic antibodies and biopsy are key to diagnosis.

Asthma should be considered in patients with a nonresolving cough for >3 weeks.

Treatment

The vast majority of URTIs are viral in origin. In most cases the infection will be self-limiting and no specific treatment is necessary. Sufficient fluid intake should be advocated. The effect of zinc and vitamin C is still debated. Echinacea seems to be effective in prevention and treatment of the common cold. Nonsteroidal anti-inflammatory drugs relieve fever, headache and malaise. In general, there is no role for antibiotic therapy in the management of common cold or any mild URTI. The only indications for antibiotic treatment are group A streptococcal pharyngitis (oral penicillin or macrolide), bacterial sinusitis (aminopenicilline + β-lactamase inhibitor, cephalosporin 2nd/3rd generation) and pertussis (erythromycin or trimethoprim-sulfamethoxazole). Nasal decongestants decrease symptoms in rhinitis and sinusitis, topical nasal steroids improve sinusitis. Confirmed cases of influenza can be considered for a therapy with neuraminidase inhibitors according to Centers for Disease Control and Prevention guidelines (www.cdc.gov/flu). New treatment options for the most prevalent respiratory pathogens, human rhinoviruses, are under development.

Prevention

Direct hand-to-hand contact is an important mechanism of pathogen transmission. Hence, frequent hand washing or disinfection in healthcare can limit spread of infection significantly. Influenza vaccination has been shown to be very beneficial and has to be advocated. In children, the routine administration of *H. influenzae* type B (Hib) vaccination has practically eradicated Hib as a cause of URTI. A herd effect could be demonstrated, as the introduction of the pneumococcal vaccine in children with significant reduction in invasive pneumococcal disease in adults.

References

- Arroll B, *et al.* Antibiotics for the common cold and acute purulent rhinitis. *Cochrane Database Syst Rev* 2005; CD000247.
- Choby BA. Diagnosis and treatment of streptococcal pharyngitis. *Am Fam Physician* 2009; 79: 383–390.
- Lund VJ. Therapeutic targets in rhinosinusitis: infection or inflammation? *Medscape J Med* 2008; 10: 105.

- Musher DM. How contagious are common respiratory tract infections? *N Engl J Med* 2003; 348: 1256-1266.
- Poole MD, Portugal LG. Treatment of rhinosinusitis in the outpatient setting. *Am J Med* 2005; 118: Suppl. 7A, 45S-50S.
- Rohde G. Drug targets in rhinoviral infections. *Infect Disord Drug Targets* 2009; 9: 126-132.
- Rohde G. Therapeutic targets in respiratory viral infections. *Curr Med Chem* 2007; 14: 2776-2782.
- Shah SA, et al. Evaluation of echinacea for the prevention and treatment of the common cold: a meta-analysis. *Lancet Infect Dis* 2007; 7: 473-480.
- Tiwari T, *et al.* Recommended antimicrobial agents for the treatment and postexposure prophylaxis of pertussis: 2005 CDC Guidelines. *MMWR Recomm Rep* 2005; 54: 1-16.

Weblinks

- http://emedicine.medscape.com/article/302460-overview.
- www.clevelandclinicmeded.com/medicalpubs/diseasemanagement/infectious-disease/upper-respiratory-tract-infection/.
- www.cdc.gov/flu.

INFECTIVE EXACERBATIONS OF COPD

M. Miravitlles
Fundació Clínic, Institut d'Investigacions Biomèdiques August Pi i Sunyer (IDIBAPS), Hospital Clínic, Barcelona, Spain
E-mail: marcm@separ.es

A recent American Thoracic Society (ATS)/European Respiratory Society (ERS) task force has defined the exacerbation of chronic obstructive pulmonary disease (COPD) as: "an increase in respiratory symptoms over baseline that usually requires medical intervention". In fact, the chronic and progressive course of COPD is often aggravated by short periods of increasing symptoms, particularly increasing cough, dyspnoea and production of sputum, which can become purulent. Patients with moderate-to-severe COPD present a mean of between one and two of these episodes or exacerbations per year, but this number is dependent on the degree of functional impairment at baseline. Patients with more advanced disease may suffer from an increasing number of exacerbations.

Outcomes of exacerbations: risk factors for failure

The failure rate of ambulatory treatment of exacerbations of COPD ranges 12–26%, and failure may lead to hospital admission. The mortality of patients admitted to hospital with COPD exacerbation is ~10–14% and the mortality of those admitted to an intensive care unit (ICU) may be as high as 24%. Hospitalisation has an important impact on COPD patients, and after the first admission to hospital the mean survival time has been estimated to be 5.7 yrs. Frequent exacerbations have been demonstrated to have a negative impact on health-related quality of life in patients with COPD and survival is significantly related to the frequency and severity of exacerbations.

Identification of risk factors for failure of ambulatory treatment may allow the implementation of more aggressive broad-spectrum treatment and closer follow-up (table 1).

Aetiology of exacerbations

A variety of causes may deteriorate the clinical stability of patients with COPD: cold temperature, air pollution, lack of compliance with respiratory medication, worsening of comorbidities, and pulmonary embolism, among others. However, up to three-quarters of exacerbations can be infectious in origin, with bacteria being responsible for three quarters of these exacerbations. In addition, co-infection with respiratory viruses may be frequent in patients with severe COPD. The most frequent microorganisms causing exacerbations are presented in table 2.

Key points

- Up to 75% of COPD exacerbations are of infective aetiology.
- *Haemophilus influenzae* is the most frequent pathogen causing exacerbations.
- The relapse rate may be as high as 20%.
- Risk factors and bacterial resistance to antibiotics are the criteria used for the selection of antibiotics.

Table 1. Risk factors for failure after ambulatory treatment of exacerbations of COPD

Coexisting cardiopulmonary disease
Increasing number of visits to the GP for respiratory problems ($>3\cdot yr^{-1}$)
Increasing number of previous exacerbations ($>3\cdot yr^{-1}$)
Increasing baseline dyspnoea
Severity of FEV1 impairment (FEV1 <35% predicted)
Use of home oxygen
Inadequate antibiotic therapy

GP: general practitioner; FEV1: forced expiratory volume in 1 s.

The role of bacteria in exacerbations has been a matter of controversy since the respiratory secretions of some patients with stable COPD carry significant concentrations of bacteria. Therefore, the isolation of such microorganisms during exacerbations should not always be interpreted as a definite demonstration of their pathogenic role. However, studies performed with specific invasive techniques have shown that both the number of patients with pathogenic bacteria in respiratory secretions and their concentrations in bronchial secretions increase during exacerbations. The change in the colonising strain of bacteria is an important mechanism originating exacerbations. The host does not have protective specific antibodies against the new strain of bacteria and the microorganism can thereby proliferate and cause the exacerbation.

Diagnosis of infective exacerbations

The combination of symptoms described by ANTHONISEN *et al.*, *i.e.* increased dyspnoea and increased production or purulence of sputum, have been widely used to identify exacerbations that require treatment with antibiotics. However, new studies have demonstrated that the presence of green (purulent) sputum as opposed to white (mucoid) is one of the best and easiest methods to predict the bacterial aetiology and the need for antibiotic therapy.

Unfortunately, no signs or symptoms can help the clinician to differentiate bacterial from viral exacerbations. Both viral and bacterial agents may co-infect a patient with COPD, and mixed infection is associated with higher inflammation, more severe symptoms and prolonged recovery time.

The degree of airflow impairment in COPD patients indicates the presence of different microorganisms during the course of exacerbations. Individuals with severe pulmonary function impairment, manifested by FEV1 <50% predicted, are at a six-fold

Table 2. Aetiology of exacerbations of COPD

Infectious exacerbations (~60-80% of all exacerbations)	

Frequent (70–85% of infectious exacerbations)
  Haemophilus influenzae
  Streptoccocus pneumoniae
  Moraxella catarrhalis
  Viruses (influenza/parainfluenza, rhinoviruses, coronaviruses)
	Infrequent (15-30% of infectious exacerbations)
	  Pseudomonas aeruginosa
	  Opportunistic Gram-negative
	  Staphyloccocus aureus
	  Chlamydia pneumoniae
	  Mycoplasma pneumoniae

Noninfectious exacerbations (20–40% of all exacerbations) Heart failure Pulmonary embolism Nonpulmonary infections Pneumothorax	

higher risk of developing acute exacerbations caused by *Haemophilus influenzae* or *Pseudomonas aeruginosa* than patients presenting FEV1 >50% pred. Those with FEV1 <30% pred have an even higher risk for *P. aeruginosa*.

However, the clinical presentation of exacerbation is not characteristic of any particular microorganism and no microbiological diagnostic test is available for differential diagnosis in primary care. The use of biomarkers such as procalcitonin to identify bacterial exacerbations is promising, but more studies are required.

Antibiotic treatment of exacerbations

Antibiotics have been shown to be superior to placebo in the treatment of exacerbations when all of the Anthonisen criteria are present; *i.e.* increased dyspnoea, increased production and purulence of sputum. The purulence of sputum has recently been demonstrated to be very sensitive and specific for the diagnosis of bacterial exacerbation and indicates the need for antibiotic therapy. Therefore, most guidelines also recommend antibiotic therapy in patients with two of the three aforementioned criteria if one of them is increased in purulence of sputum.

The antibiotic of choice may vary from country to country based on the prevalence of different bacteria and, more importantly, the differences in susceptibility of the causative bacteria to antibiotics. As an example, in 2000, the prevalence of macrolide-resistant *Streptoccocus pneumoniae* in the UK was 12.2%, but in France it was 58.1%, while the production of β-lactamase by *H. influenzae* was 13.9% in the UK and 33.1% in France.

Guidelines recommend the use of so-called first-line antibiotics, such as amoxicyllin or tetracyclin, in low-risk patients in countries with a low prevalence of antibiotic resistance, such as the Netherlands, UK and other North European countries. However, in countries with a high percentage of resistant strains or in patients with risk factors for treatment failure, the choice of an antibiotic must consider amoxycillin/clavulanate, the new fluorquinolones (moxifloxacin, levofloxacin) or cephalosporins (cefditoren, cefuroxime). Table 3 describes the antibiotic alternatives according to the severity of COPD.

Nonantibiotic treatment of exacerbations

Acute exacerbations of COPD present with increasing dyspnoea in most cases. Both infectious and noninfectious exacerbations are the result of an ongoing inflammatory reaction in the bronchial mucosa making anti-inflammatory and bronchodilator therapy mandatory.

A short course of oral corticosteroids has been demonstrated to accelerate recovery from exacerbations and reduce the rate of relapse in patients with moderate-to-severe COPD. Patients can be treated with 0.5 mg·kg^{-1}·day^{-1} of methylprednisolone or equivalent in a single morning dose for 7–14 days. Treatment for >14 days has not been demonstrated to be more beneficial and increases the likelihood of adverse side-effects. Inhaled bronchodilators, particularly short-acting inhaled $β_2$-agonists, must be given at increased doses during exacerbations. The short-acting bronchodilators may be prescribed with a chamber of inhalation or by nebulisation. In acute phase, repeated doses every 30–60 min can be administered with close monitoring of clinical signs and arterial gas exchange with a pulse oximeter. If a prompt response to these drugs does not occur, the addition of an anticholinergic is recommended.

Oxygen therapy should be provided in cases of hypoxaemia. Adequate levels of oxygenation are arterial oxygen tension >8.0 kPa or 60 mmHg, or arterial oxygen saturation >90%. These levels are easy to achieve in uncomplicated exacerbations. When oxygen is started, arterial blood gases should be checked 30–60 min later to ensure satisfactory oxygenation without CO_2 retention or acidosis.

The clinical and gasometric evolution of the patients will guide the decision to step down the treatment and discharge the patient from

Table 3. Risk classification and suggested antimicrobial therapy

	FEV1 % pred	Most frequent microorganisms	Suggested treatment
Mild-to-moderate COPD without risk factors	>50	Haemophilus influenzae Moraxella catarrhalis Streptoccocus pneumoniae Chlamydophilia pneumoniae Mycoplasma pneumoniae	Amoxycillin, tetracycline In areas of high incidence of resistance: amoxycillin-clavulanate Cefditoren, cefuroxime
Mild-to-moderate COPD with risk factors[#]	>50	H. influenzae M. catarrhalis PRSP	Amoxycillin-clavulanate Moxifloxacin/levofloxacin Cefditoren, cefuroxime
Severe COPD	30-50	H. influenzae M. catarrhalis PRSP Enteric Gram-negative	Amoxycillin-clavulanate Moxifloxacin/levofloxacin
Very severe COPD	<30	H. influenzae PRSP Enteric Gram-negative Pseudomonas aeruginosa	Moxifloxacin/levofloxacin Ciprofloxacin if *Pseudomonas* is suspected Amoxicillin-clavulanate (if allergy to quinolones)[¶]

FEV1: forced expiratory volume in 1 s; PRSP: penicillin-resistant *S. pneumoniae*. [#]: risk factors are explained in table 1. [¶]: in the case of intravenous therapy, other antibiotics can be used, such as piperacillin-tazobactam, imipenem or cefepime.

the emergency department or hospital. Family and home support is crucial in the first days after discharge.

In mild and moderate ambulatory exacerbations, clinical evaluation is required 48–72 h after initiation of therapy. In mild cases, this evaluation can be performed by telephone contact.

References

- Anthonisen NR, *et al.* Antibiotic therapy in exacerbations of chronic obstructive pulmonary disease. *Ann Intern Med* 1987; 106: 196–204.
- Balter MS, *et al.* Canadian guidelines for the management of acute exacerbations of chronic bronchitis. *Can Respir J* 2003; 10: Suppl. B, 3B–32B.
- Miravitlles M, *et al.* Antimicrobial treatment of exacerbation in chronic obstructive pulmonary disease: 2007 consensus statement. *Arch Bronconeumol* 2008; 44: 100–108.
- Niewoehner DE, *et al.* Effect of systemic glucocorticoids on exacerbations of chronic obstructive pulmonary disease. *N Engl J Med* 1999; 340: 1941–1947.
- Papi A, *et al.* Infections and airway inflammation in chronic obstructive pulmonary disease severe exacerbations. *Am J Respir Crit Care Med* 2006; 173: 1114–1121.
- Seemungal T, *et al.* Respiratory viruses, symptoms, and inflammatory markers in acute exacerbations and stable chronic obstructive pulmonary disease. *Am J Respir Crit Care Med* 2001; 164: 1618–1623.
- Sethi S, *et al.* New strains of bacteria and exacerbations of chronic obstructive pulmonary disease. *N Engl J Med* 2002; 347: 465–471.
- Soler-Cataluña JJ, *et al.* Severe acute exacerbations and mortality in patients with chronic obstructive pulmonary disease. *Thorax* 2005; 60: 925–931.
- Stockley RA, *et al.* Relationship of sputum color to nature and outpatient management of acute exacerbations of COPD. *Chest* 2000; 117: 1638–1645.
- Woodhead M, *et al.* Guidelines for the management of adult lower respiratory tract infections. *Eur Respir J* 2005; 26: 1138–1180.

PNEUMONIA

M. Woodhead
Dept of Respiratory Medicine, Manchester Royal Infirmary, Manchester, UK
E-mail: mark.woodhead@cmft.nhs.uk

Background and definitions

Pneumonia is a condition caused by microbial infection within the lung parenchyma. This infection, together with the associated host inflammatory response, impairs normal alveolar function (*i.e.* gas exchange), which, together with the systemic effects of the infection, causes the clinical features of pneumonia. The gold standard for recognition of pneumonia is the presence of new lung shadowing on the chest radiograph in the setting of a compatible clinical illness.

Pneumonia is classified according to the origin of the infection as community-acquired (CAP) or hospital-acquired (nosocomial (NP)). Additional pneumonia types are in the immunocompromised and aspiration pneumonia. In each group, the causative pathogens and hence the management are different.

Key points

- Pneumonia is very common and has a significant mortality.
- Severity assessment, aided by a severity assessment score, is a key management step.
- A variety of different pathogens can cause pneumonia.
- Antibiotic management is initially empirical and based on guidelines and knowledge of local microbial patterns and resistance rates.

CAP is that which occurs in the absence of immunocompromise or prior hospital admission within the previous 7 days.

Epidemiology

CAP occurs in between one and 10 per 1,000 of the adult population each year. It is more common in children aged <5 yrs and becomes progressively more common from age 40 yrs onwards with a peak in the very elderly. It is more common in those with comorbidity, *e.g.* chronic obstructive pulmonary disease (COPD), bronchiectasis, chronic cardiac and renal disease. It occurs throughout the year with a peak during the winter months.

NP can occur in anyone resident in hospital for $\geqslant$7 days. It is especially common on the intensive care unit after endotracheal intubation (ventilator-associated pneumonia (VAP)) with risk being proportional to duration of intubation.

Two types of immune dysfunction predispose to pneumonia: humoral immune dysfunction, *e.g.* immunoglobulin deficiencies; and cell-mediated immune function in *e.g.* cancer chemotherapy, solid organ transplantation and bone marrow transplantation.

Aspiration pneumonia occurs especially in those with swallowing impairment and neurological impairment.

Most cases of CAP are managed in the community with a variable, but significant, proportion requiring hospital admission. Of those admitted, 5-10% may die and of those reaching the intensive care unit, 30-50% may die. Mortality is generally higher in NP and pneumonia in the immunocompromised.

Clinical features

The duration of illness before presentation is usually short. Classically there is an abrupt onset with fever, shivers and pleuritic chest pain. A slower onset over a few days may also occur. Other common symptoms include cough, sputum production, which may be purulent or blood-stained, breathlessness, muscle aches, headaches and anorexia. Nausea and diarrhoea are less common. In elderly patients, symptoms of cerebral dysfunction, such as confusion, incontinence or falls, may be the presenting feature.

Abnormalities on clinical examination include focal signs on chest examination, most commonly crackles, but occasionally the classical features of lung consolidation – dullness to percussion, bronchial breathing and enhanced vocal resonance. In addition, raised temperature, raised heart and respiratory rates, low blood pressure and mental confusion may be found.

Clinical features are not helpful in predicting the causative organism.

Investigations including radiology

Investigations are unnecessary outside hospital but in those admitted are performed to aid precise diagnosis, assess illness severity and identify the microbial cause.

The chest radiograph is essential to confirm new lung shadowing in those admitted. Classically such shadowing conforms to a lobar pattern and is associated with air bronchograms. Shadowing may occupy less than a whole lobe and may also be patchy, multilobar and bilateral. Additional features may include pleural effusion and less commonly cavitation and pneumothorax. The lower lobes are most commonly affected.

Of routine blood tests, peripheral blood white cell count may be raised, especially in bacterial infection, but C-reactive protein and procalcitonin are probably more specific. Blood urea and creatinine are helpful in severity assessment and the assessment of renal impairment, and liver function tests may be abnormal. Measures of gas exchange such as oxygen saturation and/or arterial blood gases also aid assessment of illness severity and guide management.

In routine practice, tests to identify a microbial cause are positive in only about 15% of cases of CAP and hence seldom influence management. They are probably not indicated unless the patient is severely ill. In such cases blood culture, sputum Gram stain and culture, and urine for pneumococcal and legionella antigen are indicated. Blood antibody levels or nose/throat secretion PCR-based tests for microbe-specific nucleic acids can be used for the detection of viruses and less common bacteria such as *Legionella, Mycoplasma* and *Coxiella*.

In NP, and especially in VAP, lower respiratory secretions should be sampled either by tracheal aspirate or from bronchoscopic specimens. The latter may be of value also in the immunocompromised.

Differential diagnosis

This includes acute bronchitis, COPD exacerbation, left ventricular failure, pulmonary embolism, exacerbation of pulmonary fibrosis and rare lung disorders, *e.g.* pulmonary eosinophilia.

Microbial aetiology and resistance

Some 10 pathogens commonly cause CAP, with *Streptococcus pneumoniae* being the most common overall and the most important cause of severe illness and death. *Mycoplasma pneumoniae* is also a common cause of mild illness, especially in young adults. Severe illness is most likely to be associated with *S. pneumoniae*, legionella, staphylococcal or Gram-negative bacterial infection. *Legionella* infection may occur in outbreaks associated with a water aerosol source such as showers or decorative fountains. Staphylococcal infection is especially common following influenza virus infection. Influenza occurs in seasonal outbreaks during the winter months and occasional pandemics. It is the commonest viral cause of CAP.

Table 1. CURB65 (or CRB65) score

Score 1 for each of:	
C = mental confusion	
U = blood urea >7 mmol·L^{-1}	
R = respiratory rate ≥30·min^{-1}	
B = systolic blood pressure <90 mmHg or diastolic blood pressure ≤60 mmHg	
65 = age ≥65 yrs	
Score: mild 0–1 (mortality 1.5%), moderate 2 (9%), severe 3–5 (22%)	

Clinically significant resistance to penicillins in *S. pneumoniae* is rare, but clinically significant macrolide resistance is more common, especially in Southern Europe (see www.earss.rivm.nl). This varies in frequency between countries.

NP is most commonly caused by Gram-negative enterobacteria or *Staphylococcus aureus*. *Pseudomonas aeruginosa* and multiresistant bacteria (*e.g.* methicillin-resistant *S. aureus* (MRSA)) are important causes of VAP.

Humoral immune deficiency is associated with bacterial infection and cell-mediated immune defects with viral and fungal infections such as *Pneumocystis jirovecii*.

Anaerobic bacteria may be important in aspiration pneumonia.

Severity assessment

Severity assessment is the key to deciding place of care and should also guide diagnostic tests and antimicrobial therapy. This should be done through clinical judgement guided by objective severity scores. There are many of these, but the best validated for CAP are the CURB65 (and its derivative CRB65) and the pneumonia severity index (PSI). The latter is based on a score from 20 variables and is often not practical in routine practice. The former is simpler and based on the number of severity variables present (table 1). The Clinical Pulmonary Infection Score (CPIS) may be useful in NP.

Management

Correction of gas exchange and fluid balance abnormalities and the provision of appropriate antimicrobial therapy are the cornerstones of management. Outside hospital rest, oral fluids and an oral antibiotic may all that is required. In hospital, oxygen at a concentration to maintain arterial oxygen saturation (>92%) should be delivered. If this cannot be achieved continuous positive airway pressure may be helpful. If there is an unacceptable rise in arterial carbon dioxide tension then assisted

Table 2. European Respiratory Society antibiotic guidelines for CAP

CAP severity	Preferred	Alternative
Nonsevere	Aminopenicillin ± macrolide or co-amoxiclav ± macrolide or penicillin G ± macrolide or third-generation cephalosporin ± macrolide	Levofloxacin or moxifloxacin
Severe	Third-generation cephalosporin + macrolide	Third-generation cephalosporin + (levofloxacin or moxifloxacin)
Severe + risk factors for *Pseudomonas aeruginosa*	Autopseudomonal cephalosporin + ciprofloxacin	Piperacillin/tazobactam + (ciprofloxacin or levofloxacin) or carbapenem + (ciprofloxacin or levofloxacin)

ventilation should be considered. A place for noninvasive ventilation in pneumonia management has yet to be proven.

Initial antibiotic therapy must be empirical and directed by illness severity according to national or international guidelines (table 2). A single antibiotic for nonsevere CAP and dual therapy for severe CAP is usual. Treatment for NP should be guided by knowledge of local microbial causes and that for pneumonia in the immunocompromised by the type of immune suppression and likely pathogens. Duration of therapy is usually 7 days in the uncomplicated, but may need to be prolonged in severe illness. Failure to respond should prompt a re-evaluation of the correct diagnosis and a more detailed search for microbial cause, for example by bronchoscopy, as long as gas exchange function will allow.

Prevention

The main preventable risk for pneumonia is tobacco smoking. In those with comorbid disease and in the elderly, influenza and pneumococcal vaccination is indicated. Recent evidence suggests that conjugate pneumococcal vaccination in children not only reduces invasive pneumococcal infection in this group, but also in adults.

References

- European Respiratory Society Task Force Report, Guidelines for management of adult community-acquired lower respiratory tract infections. *Sheffield, European Respiratory Society, 2009; in press.*
- Lim WS, *et al.* Severity prediction rules in community acquired pneumonia: a validation study. *Thorax* 2000; 55: 219–223.
- Pugin J, *et al.* Diagnosis of ventilator-associated pneumonia by bacteriologic analysis of bronchoscopic and nonbronchoscopic "blind" bronchoalveolar lavage fluid. *Am Rev Respir Dis* 1991; 143: 1121–1129.
- Torres A, *et al.* Defining, treating and preventing hospital acquired pneumonia: European perspective. *Intensive Care Med* 2009; 35: 9–29.
- Torres A, *et al.* Respiratory Infections. London, Hodder Arnold, 2006.

HOSPITAL-ACQUIRED PNEUMONIA

F. Blasi
Thoracopulmonary and Cardiocirculatory Dept, Università degli Studi di Milano and IRCCS Fondazione Cà Granda Ospedale Maggiore Policlinico, Milan, Italy
E-mail: francesco.blasi@unimi.it

The currently proposed classification of hospital-acquired pneumonias includes hospital-acquired pneumonia (HAP), ventilator-associated pneumonia (VAP) and healthcare-associated pneumonia (HCAP) (table 1).

However, a recent statement issued by the European Respiratory Society/European Society of Clinical Microbiology and Infectious Diseases/European Society of Intensive Care Medicine calls for a redefinition of HCAP, particularly in terms of risk factors and microbial aetiology.

Epidemiology

The incidence of HAP is ~0.5–2.0% among all hospitalised patients and it is the second most common nosocomial infection, yet the first in terms of mortality (ranging 30->70%). The incidence in different hospitals and different wards of the same hospital varies considerably. The main risk factors are age, type of hospital and type of ward. Patients aged <35 yrs are less prone to develop HAP than elderly patients; the incidence of HAP may vary between 5–15 episodes per 1,000 discharges. In large teaching hospitals, the incidence is higher than in district hospitals, possibly relating to differences in patient complexity. HAP is quite uncommon in paediatric and obstetric wards, and clearly most common in surgical wards and intensive care units (ICUs), particularly in ventilated patients in whom the incidence may be >35 episodes per 1,000 patient-days.

Table 1. Definitions of hospital-acquired pneumonias

HAP	Pneumonia that occurs ⩾48 h after admission, which was not incubating at the time of admission
VAP	Pneumonia that arises >48–72 h after endotracheal intubation
HCAP	Pneumonia that occurs in any patient who was hospitalised in an acute care hospital for ⩾2 days within 90 days of the infection; resided in a nursing home or long-term care facility; received intravenous antibiotic therapy, chemotherapy, or wound care within the 30 days prior to the current infection; or attended hospital or haemodialysis clinic

Key points

- Incidence of hospital-acquired pneumonias is ~0.5–2%, with risk factors including age, type of hospital and type of ward.
- Mortality is high (30–70%).
- Diagnosis can be difficult, and requires a combined clinical and bacteriological approach.
- Antimicrobial therapy must be both prompt and appropriate, and should be modified as culture results become available.

Pathogenesis and risk factors

The understanding of the pathogenesis of HAPs is a fundamental step for the comprehension of risk factors involved. The main sources of HAP pathogens include healthcare devices, the environment, the transfer of microorganisms

Table 2. Main recommendations for the management of modifiable risk factors for HAP and VAP

Host related	Adequate nutrition, enteral feeding *via* orogastric tubes
	Reduction/discontinuation of immunosuppressive treatments
	Prevent unplanned extubation (restraints, sedation)
	Kinetic beds
	Incentive spirometry, deep breathing and pain control
Device/treatment related	Minimise use of sedatives and paralytics
	Avoid gastric overdistention
	Avoid intubation and reintubation
	Expeditious removal of endotracheal and nasogastric tubes
	Semirecumbent positioning
	Drain condensate from ventilator circuits
	Endotracheal tube cuff pressure (>20 cmH$_2$O prevents leakage of bacterial pathogens around the cuff into lower respiratory tract)
	Continuous aspiration of subglottic secretions
	Use of heat moisture exchangers (reduces ventilator circuit colonisation but not VAP incidence)
Environment related	Attention to infection-control procedures, *i.e.* staff education, hand washing, patient isolation
	Microbiological surveillance programme

between the patient and staff or other patients, and oropharyngeal and gastric colonisation, with subsequent aspiration of their contents into the lungs in patients with impaired mechanical, cellular and humoral defences. Risk factors for the development of HAP can be differentiated into modifiable and non-modifiable conditions (table 2).

Microbiology

Gram-negative pathogens are the main cause of HAP. *Pseudomonas aeruginosa*, *Acinetobacter baumannii*, microorganisms belonging to the family *Enterobacteriaceae* (*Klebsiella* spp., *Enterobacter* spp., *Serratia* spp., *etc.*) and, under certain conditions, microorganisms such as *Haemophilus influenzae* are involved in HAP aetiology. Among Gram-positive pathogens, *Staphylococcus aureus*, *Streptococcus* spp. and *Streptococcus pneumoniae* are the most common agents, accounting for 35–39% of all cases. Nonbacterial pathogens such as *Aspergillus* spp. and viruses (cytomegalovirus) have been described.

In general, there are significant geographical differences in the rates of resistance between some European areas and even within countries, from one hospital to another.

Taking into account the time course of pneumonia development, the expected pathogens in early-onset pneumonia (onset in ⩽4 days of hospital admission) include *S. aureus*, *S. pneumoniae* and *H. influenzae*, as well as nondrug-resistant Gram-negative enteric bacteria (GNEB), and in late-onset pneumonia (onset >4 days of hospital admission) include methicillin-resistant *S. aureus*, drug-resistant

Table 3. Major points for HAP diagnosis

Medical history and physical examination
Chest radiograph (posteroanterior and lateral)
Blood gas analysis
Blood cultures
Thoracentesis if pleural effusion
Endotracheal aspirate, bronchoalveolar lavage or protected brush sample for culture before antibiotic (negative results do not rule out viral or Legionella infections)
Extrapulmonary site of infection should be investigated

Table 4. Antimicrobial treatment of nosocomial pneumonia

	Recommended treatment options	Recommended dosages
Early-onset pneumonia without any additional risk factors[#]	Aminopenicillin plus β-lactamase-inhibitor or Second/third generation cephalosporin or Respiratory fluoroquinolone	Amoxi-clav 3×2.2 g; ampicillin–sulbactam 3×3 g Cefuroxime 3×1.5 g; cefotaxime 3×2 g; ceftriaxone 1×2 g Levofloxacin 1×750 mg; moxifloxacin 1×400 mg
Late-onset or risk factors for multidrug-resistant pathogens	Anti-*Pseudomonas* β-lactams or Carbapenems **PLUS** Fluoroquinolone Addition of coverage for MRSA if suspected	Piperacillin-tazo 3×4.5 g; ceftazidime 3×2 g Imipenem 3×1g; meropenem 3×1 g Ciprofloxacin 3×400 mg; levofloxacin 1×750 mg Vancomicin 2×1 g; linezolid 2×600 mg

MRSA: methicillin-resistant *Staphylococcus aureus*. [#]: Ertapenem has been suggested; however, its use on a regular basis would lead to a considerable risk of overtreatment.

GNEB, *P. aeruginosa* and *A. baumannii* among other potentially drug-resistant microorganisms.

Diagnostic strategy

The clinical diagnosis of HAP is often difficult to establish. The American Thoracic Society/Infectious Diseases Society of America guidelines suggest the use of a combined clinical and bacteriological strategy. Table 3 summarises the major points and recommendations of the guidelines.

In case of doubt or relevant disagreement between the clinical presentation and the radiological findings, it is recommended to perform a computed tomography scan. The presence of new chest radiographic infiltrates plus one of the three clinical variables (fever >38°C, leukocytosis or leukopenia and purulent secretions) is sufficient to start antimicrobial treatment.

Treatment

Prompt administration of appropriate antimicrobial treatment is crucial in order to achieve an optimal outcome, and inappropriate antimicrobial treatment is associated with an excess mortality from pneumonia. Antibiotic selection for empirical therapy of HAP should be based primarily on the risk of multidrug-resistant pathogen infection. Table 4 shows the proposed empirical treatment approach.

Once the results of respiratory tract and blood cultures become available, therapy should be focused or narrowed, based on the identity of specific pathogens and their susceptibility to specific antimicrobials. An 8-day antibiotic course can be appropriate provided that the patient has a good clinical response and difficult-to-treat pathogens are not involved as an aetiological agent.

References

- American Thoracic Society, Infectious Diseases Society of America, Guidelines for the management of adults with hospital-acquired, ventilator-associated, and healthcare-associated pneumonia. *Am J Respir Crit Care Med* 2005; 171: 388–416.
- Torres A, *et al*. Defining, treating and preventing hospital acquired pneumonia: European perspective. *Intensive Care Med* 2009; 35: 9–29.

PNEUMONIA IN THE IMMUNOCOMPROMISED HOST

S. Ewig
Thoraxzentrum Ruhrgebiet, Kliniken für Pneumologie und Infektiologie, Evangelisches Krankenhaus Herne und Augusta-Kranken-Anstalt Bochum, Germany
E-mail: ewig@augusta-bochum.de

In contrast to community- and hospital-acquired pneumonia, pneumonia in the immunocompromised host is not defined by the setting of pneumonia acquisition but by the immune status of the host. In this context, immune suppression is best defined as a relevant risk for so-called opportunistic pathogens such as fungi, viruses, mycobacteria and parasites.

The expected pathogen patterns differ according to the type of immune suppression (table 1). Overall, there are five main types of immunosuppression:

- iatrogenic (through steroidal and nonsteroidal agents)
- neutropenia (usually through antineoplastic chemotherapy)
- haematopoetic stem-cell transplantation (HSCT)
- solid organ transplantation
- HIV infection

Each immunosuppressive condition confers characteristic risk profiles for pulmonary infections according to the type of immune failure. Some conditions additionally show time- or extent-dependent risk profiles.

Pulmonary infections in the immunocompromised host usually consistute an emergency. Thus, immediate appropriate antimicrobial treatment is mandatory. Since the spectrum of potential pathogens is far more diverse than in immunocompetent hosts, a systematic approach to the management of these patients is required. This approach should include a comprehensive diagnostic evaluation, indications for empirical initial antimicrobial treatment, also in the absence of definite pathogen identification, and for salvage management in case of treatment failure.

The basic diagnostic evaluation should include history, physical examination and chest radiography as well as a basic microbiological work-up (sputum, blood cultures). A computed tomography (CT) scan of the lung (multi-slice scan and high-resolution (HR)CT) is usually indicated in patients in whom a straightforward diagnosis cannot be made. It can be particularly valuable in patients at risk of fungi (*Pneumocystis* and *Aspergillus*). Bronchoscopy is usually indicated in patients with bilateral infiltrates, unusual clinical and radiographical

Key points

- Different types of immunosuppression confer vulnerability to different respiratory pathogens, which may be bacterial, viral, mycobacterial or fungal.
- The approach to treatment should include comprehensive diagnostic evaluation, indications for empirical antimicrobial treatment and a plan in case of treatment failure.

Table 1. Types of immunosuppression and typical infectious complications

Type of complication	Main immune disorder	Typical Infections
Iatrogenic (steroids)	Macrophages, T-cells	Bacteria, fungi (*Aspergillus* spp.), *Mycobacterium tuberculosis*
Iatrogenic (anti-TNF-α)	TNF-α	*M. tuberculosis*
Neutropenia, stem cell transplantation	Neutrophils	
	Short duration (<10 days)	Bacteria
	Long duration (>10 days)	Additionally: fungi (*Aspergillus* spp.)
Solid organ transplantation	Early (month 1): neutrophils	Bacteria
	Intermediate (months 2-6): macrophages, T-cells	Fungi, viruses, parasites
	Late (months >6): depends on extent of immune suppression	Variable
HIV infection	T-cells (CD-4)	
	CD4 >500·μL^{-1}	No risk
	CD4 200-500·μL^{-1}	Bacteria, *M. tuberculosis*
	CD4 <200·μL^{-1}	Additionally: *Pneumocystis jirovecii*
	CD4 <50·μL^{-1}	Additionally: *Aspergillus* spp., atypical mycobacteria

TNF: tumour necrosis factor.

presentations and those with treatment failure. When performing bronchoscopy, particular care has to be taken to comply with the methodology of retrieving uncontaminated samples of the lower respiratory tract, and a comprehensive evaluation of the samples retrieved. Bronchoalveolar lavage (BAL) is the most important sample, and stains and cultures should be investigated for all relevant pathogens. Occasionally, transbronchial biopsies and/or transbronchial needle aspiration may be rewarding.

In the following, typical pneumonias in the immunosuppressed host are described in more detail.

Pneumocystis jirovecii pneumonia (PJP)

PJP in HIV-infected patients presents with at least one of the following symptoms: fever, cough and dyspnoea on exertion. Chest radiograph typically discloses bilateral interstitial infiltrates in a perihilar distribution but may also be normal in the early course. In the latter case, HRCT may reveal ground glass opacities in a patchy or geographical distribution. Atypical cystic presentations may occur. Blood gas analysis shows wide alveolar–arterial gradients. The typical laboratory finding is an elevated lactate dehydrogenase. Specific diagnosis is required and may be established by examination of induced sputum or BAL. The treatment of choice (also for prophylaxis) is trimethoprim-sulfamethazole. Second-line options include pentamidine and clindamycin/primaquin. Adjunctive steroids are indicated in patients with acute respiratory failure.

PJP in non-HIV patients differs in that it presents more frequently as an acute onset pneumonia and tends to be associated with higher mortality.

Cytomegalovirus pneumonia (CMVP)

CMVP is defined as pulmonary signs and symptoms and the detection of CMV in pulmonary samples. Nevertheless, patients may shed CMV in the absence of CMVP. Co-infections with other opportunistic pathogens are frequently encountered. After introduction of CMV prophylaxis, the incidence in allogeneic HSCT is 10–30%, with the highest risk in seropositive recipients, while it is rare in autologous HSCT (< 10%). Also, the onset is shifted to >100 days. Clinical presentation is unspecific. Radiologically, there is typically an interstitial pattern with tiny pulmonary nodules and patchy areas of consolidation. HRCT is more sensitive. Diagnosis is made by demonstration of inclusion bodies within epithelial cells of the lower respiratory tract (sensitivity 90%, specificity 98%). Culture of BAL fluid lacks specificity. The value of CMV pp65 antigen and PCR is controversial. The treatment of choice is ganciclovir and valganciclovir, combined with CMV immune globulin. Second-line agents are foscarnet and cidofovir. Antiviral prophylaxis and monitoring are the main preventive strategies.

Tuberculosis (TB)

Patients with lowered CD-4 cell counts as well as on chronic steroid and anti-tumour necrosis factor (TNF)-α treatment are at increased risk of TB. Co-infection with TB and HIV alters the natural history of both diseases. TB in HIV-infected patients presents like primary infection (patchy infiltrates, mediastinal lymph node enlargement, pleural effusion and bacteraemia). Concurrent treatment of TB and HIV is challenging due to the many complex interactions of anti-TB drugs and antiretroviral agents. Patients who are candidates for chronic steroid or anti-TNF-α treatment should be evaluated for TB infection and, in case of positive skin testing or interferon-γ release assay, receive prophylaxis.

Aspergillus pneumonia (AP)

Definite diagnosis of AP in neutropenic patients requires tissue biopsy and can only rarely be established. Therefore, probable and possible diagnosis is based on a set of clinical, microbiological and radiographic criteria. HRCT is the method of choice to detect AP early in its course. Typical, albeit not specific signs of AP include the "halo" sign, as well as nodular and peripheral patchy densities near to vessels. The "air crescent" sign, representing cavitation, is a late marker of AP. The galactomannan antigen test in serum and BAL has a sensitivity of $\sim$70% and a specificity of 90%. Bronchoscopy is usually indicated. Early initiation of treatment is crucial. The treatment of choice for definite AP is voriconazole, or alternatively liposomal amphotericin B. Second-line options include caspofungin and posaconazole. Mortality reaches $\sim$50–60%.

References

- Agusti C, Torres A.: Pulmonary Infection in the Immunocompromised Patient. Strategies for Management. Oxford, Wiley-Blackwell, 2009.
- Boersma WG, et al. Bronchoscopic diagnosis of pulmonary infiltrates in granulocytopenic patients with hematologic malignancies: BAL versus PSB and PBAL. *Respir Med* 2007; 101: 317-325.
- Chan KM, Allen SA. Infectious pulmonary complications in lung transplant recipients. *Semin Respir Infect* 2002; 17: 291-302.
- D'Avignon LC, et al. Pneumocystis pneumonia. *Semin Respir Crit Care Med* 2008; 29: 132-140.
- Davis JL, et al. Respiratory infection complicating HIV infection. *Curr Opin Infect Dis* 2008; 21: 184-190.
- Duncan MD, Wilkes DS. Transplant-related immunosuppression: a review of immunosuppression and pulmonary infections. *Proc Am Thorac Soc* 2005; 2: 449-455.
- Feller-Kopman D, Ernst A. The role of bronchoalveolar lavage in the immunocompromised host. *Semin Respir Infect* 2003; 18: 87-94.
- Rañó A, et al. Pulmonary infiltrates in non-HIV immunocompromised patients: a diagnostic approach using non-invasive and bronchoscopic procedures. *Thorax* 2001; 56: 379-387.
- Rosen MJ. Pulmonary complications of HIV infection. *Respirology* 2008; 13: 181-190.

PLEURAL INFECTION AND LUNG ABSCESS

C. Hooper and N. Maskell
North Bristol Lung Centre, University of Bristol, UK
E-mail: nick.maskell@bristol.ac.uk

Pleural infection

Pleural infection occurs when microorganisms, most commonly bacteria, enter the pleural space. It can be confirmed when pleural fluid has a positive Gram stain or culture, is frankly purulent or, in the context of sepsis, has an acidic pH. Pleural infection is a common and serious medical problem. It is associated with a mortality rate of 15–20%.

Epidemiology
- Greatest incidence in the elderly and children but can occur at any age.
- Twice as common in males.
- 20% of adults with pleural infection have diabetes mellitus.
- Other important risk factors include aspiration, immunosuppression, poor dentition, pleural procedures, thoracic surgery and penetrating chest trauma.

Pathophysiology

Pleural infection most frequently follows community-acquired pneumonia (CAP) with bacterial migration from the lung parenchyma into a parapneumonic effusion. It may also follow hospital-acquired and aspiration pneumonia with effusion, traumatic or iatrogenic pleural penetration or be a primary phenomenon. Primary pleural infection is probably the consequence of bacteraemia, the origin of which has not been fully elucidated. Microbiological data has suggested the oropharynx as one possible source.

Bacteriology

Bacteria are ultimately cultured from either pleural fluid or blood in 60–70% of cases of pleural infection. The microbiology of community-acquired pleural infection is different from that of hospital-acquired pleural infection and CAP such that these should be considered three distinct diseases requiring different empirical antibiotic regimes.

In community-acquired pleural infection, *Streptococcus* species (largely *Streptococcus milleri* and *Streptococcus pneumoniae*) account for 50% of positive cultures with *Staphylococcus* species, anaerobic and Gram-negative organisms making up the other half. Anaerobic organisms commonly co-exist with aerobes, particularly the *Streptococcus milleri* group. Atypical pneumonia organisms such as *Legionella* and *Mycoplasma* species are extremely unusual causes of pleural infection.

Key points

- Pleural infection is common and serious, with a mortality rate of 15–20%.
- Blood, in addition to pleural fluid, should always be cultured.
- Initial management is with broad spectrum antiobiotics and prompt chest drainage.
- Lung abscess has a 10% mortality rate.
- Invasive procedures are only required when lung abcess does not respond to prolonged empirical antibiotics or underlying neoplasm is suspected.

Table 1. Clinical classification of pleural infection.

	Simple parapneumonic effusion	**Complicated parapneumonic effusion**	**Empyema**
Pleural fluid appearance	Straw-coloured, bloody or turbid	Straw-coloured, bloody or turbid	Frank pus
Pleural fluid pH	>7.2	Usually ⩽7.2	Should not be measured
Pleural fluid Gram stain	Negative	May be positive	May be positive
Pleural fluid culture	Negative	May be positive	May be positive
Thoracic ultrasound appearance	Usually anechoic but septation can occur. No pleural thickening	Can be anechoic, complex septated or complex nonseptated	Homogenously echogenic. Usually evidence of pleural thickening
Immediate management	Antibiotics for pneumonia. This does not represent pleural infection	Intravenous antibiotics and chest tube drainage	Intravenous antibiotics and chest tube drainage

In nosocomial pleural infection, *Staphylococcus* species (including MRSA) and Gram-negative organisms are responsible for most positive cultures.

Investigations

- When a patient presents with sepsis and clinical and chest radiographic signs of a pleural effusion, a diagnostic pleural aspiration should always be performed to establish the presence of pleural infection.

- Pleural fluid should always be sent for culture and cytological examination. The pH of nonpurulent pleural fluid should be measured using a heparinised arterial blood gas syringe and blood gas machine, and fluid should also be sent for protein and lactate dehydrogenase.

- In the correct clinical context, a pleural fluid pH of ⩽7.2, positive pleural fluid culture or Gram stain, purulent pleural fluid and loculation on thoracic ultrasound differentiate pleural infection from simple parapneumonic effusion and indicate the need for chest tube drainage.

- Blood cultures should be sent (along with standard baseline blood tests) as they may achieve a microbiological diagnosis when there is no growth from pleural fluid.

Radiology

- Chest radiography often demonstrates a pleural effusion and consolidation. When pleural fluid has entered the organising phase there may be a lentiform pleural opacity (fig. 1).

- Ultrasound may demonstrate an anechoic, complex septated, complex nonseptated or homogenously echogenic (reflecting pus in empyema) appearance in pleural infection and is important in guiding aspiration and drain site.

- Contrast-enhanced computed tomography (CT) scans demonstrate brightly enhancing pleural thickening in the organising phase of pleural infection. CT is only required when initial drainage of fluid is incomplete for the planning of further drains or thoracic surgical intervention or if other pathology such as pulmonary abscess, neoplastic lesions or oesophageal rupture is suspected.

Management

Immediate treatment The following steps should be implemented.

- Broad-spectrum intravenous antibiotics.
- Chest tube drainage.

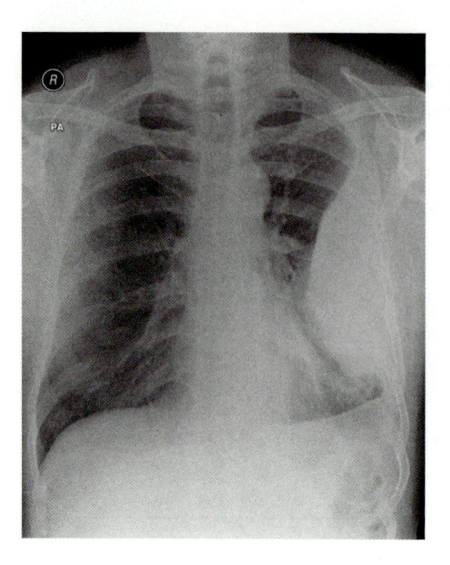

Figure 1. Chest radiograph of left empyema demonstrating a D- shaped, lentiform pleural opacity.

- Nutritional supplementation (oral or nasogastric).
- Thromboprophylaxis.
- Vigilant monitoring for evidence of worsening sepsis indicating need for early thoracic surgery.

It is not possible to reliably identify, by presenting radiological, pleural fluid or clinical features, for which patients' primary medical management will not achieve resolution of sepsis, necessitating thoracic surgery.

Antibiotics Examples of suitable empirical antibiotic regimes with broad-spectrum coverage and good penetration to the pleural space include penicillin-clavulanic acid combinations in community-acquired infection and carbopenems with vancomycin in nosocomial infection. When cultures are available, antibiotics should be modified accordingly. As anaerobes can be difficult to culture, their presence should be assumed and cover continued (unless *Streptococcus pneumoniae*, which is not known to co-exist with anaerobes, is isolated). Conventionally, $\geqslant 5$ days' *i.v.* antibiotics is followed by 2–4 weeks of oral treatment.

Chest tube drainage Small-bore (12-14 f) chest tubes are now generally preferred to large-bore tubes as they can be placed *via* a seldinger technique and are more comfortable for patients. There is no evidence that large-bore tubes acheive superior fluid drainage (although this is still the subject of significant debate). Regular saline flushes (20 mL 6-hourly) may help to maintain tube patency and larger-volume 0.9% saline irrigation of the pleural space has been adopted by some European centres with reports of improved primary treatment sucess rates (not yet supported by published evidence).

The viscosity and degree of septation of pleural fluid may impair tube drainage but routine use of intrapleural fibrinolytics has not been shown to be of benefit.

Thoracic surgery The most compelling indication for referral for surgical intervention is failure of sepsis to improve despite appropriate antibiotics and tube drainage. This assessment is usually made after 5 days' medical treatment. While surgical and anaesthetic complications are more common in the elderly and frail, the vast majority of deaths as a result of pleural infection are in patients aged >65 yrs, and this group in particular should be considered at an early stage for limited surgical drainage procedures.

Available surgical approaches include:

- video-assisted thoracoscopic surgery (VATS).
- open thoracotomy and decortication.
- rib resection and open drainage (often performed under local anaesthetic).
- mini-thoracotomy (usually VATS-assisted)

Outcome

- Patients should be followed up for $\geqslant 3$ months to allow the early detection of recurrent sepsis or persistent breathlessness.

- 20–30% of patients ultimately require surgical intervention.
- Pleural infection in the elderly and hospital-acquired disease have a particularly poor outcome.
- Mean mortality rates of 15–20% have been reported in recent series.

Lung abscess

In contrast to pleural infection, the incidence and mortality rate of lung abscess have steadily declined since the advent of penicillin.

Risk factors include:

- more common in males (2:1).
- immunocompromised states.
- aspiration of any cause.
- pneumonia (particularly *Staphylococcus aureus* and *Klebsiella pneumoniae*).
- bronchial obstruction (*e.g.* endobronchial neoplasm in 10–20% cases).
- haematogenous spread of infection.

Diagnosis

Symptoms may be acute or insidious in onset and commonly include cough, fever, chest pain, night sweats, weight loss and purulent or bloodstained sputum. There may be no specific examination findings or chest auscultation may mimic pneumonia. Anaemia is common in patients with a chronic lung abscess.

Radiology

- Plain chest radiography classically demonstrates a well circumscribed opacity within the lung field. Right-sided abscesses are twice as common as left. Dependent segments are most commonly affected when the abscess follows aspiration.
- CT is often required to distinguish a parenchymal abscess from empyema and may assist in the detection of neoplastic lesions.
- On CT, abscesses have an irregular wall and an indistinct outer margin that makes an acute angle with the chest wall. In contrast, an empyema is lenticular, well defined and causes compression of the underlying lung with vascular crowding (fig. 2).

Conditions with a similar radiological presentation to lung abscess:

- Neoplastic lesions
- Pulmonary vasculitis
- Pulmonary infarction
- Bullae and cysts
- Rheumatoid nodules
- Pneumoconiosis

Bacteriology and obtaining cultures

The microbiology of lung abscesses has changed over recent decades due to immunocompromise and immunosupression being at least as aetiologically important as aspiration.

- Polymicrobial in $\geqslant 50\%$.
- Anaerobes (*e.g. Fusobacterium*, *Prevotella* sp., *Peptostreptococcus* sp.) present in 30–50%.
- Aerobic bacteria now appear to be cultured more commonly than anaerobes (particularly *Klebsiella pneumoniae* and *Staphylococcus aureus*).
- Fungae, *Nocardia*, mycobacteria, *Amoeba*, *Actinomycosis* and *Echinococcus* are more unusual causes of a parenchymal abcess.

Most patients are treated effectively with broad-spectrum antibiotics in the absence of a microbiological diagnosis. Blood cultures should be sent and sputum cultured if available.

- Bronchoscopy should be employed when there is particular suspicion of an underlying endobronchial neoplasm or inhaled foreign body. Culture of bronchial

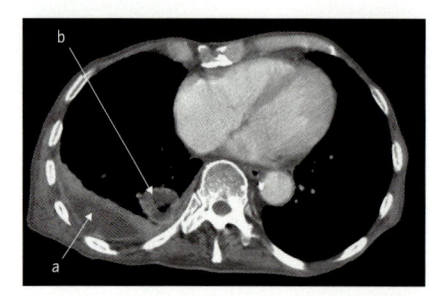

Figure 2. Computed tomography scan of a right pleural empyema (a) and cavitating pulmonary abscess (b).

washings is of relatively low accuracy and often fails to focus antibiotic selection beyond empirical choices.

- Image-guided (CT, ultrasound or fluoroscopic) percutaneous aspiration is associated with a 14% risk of pneumothorax but obtains a microbiological diagnosis in 80–90% of cases and changes antibiotic choice in up to 47%. It is usually reserved for cases that do not respond to empirical broad-spectrum antibiotics.

Management

A prolonged course (4–6 weeks depending on clinical and radiological response) of antibiotics is the foundation of treatment. β-lactam/β-lactamase-inhibitor combinations cover the majority of causative bacteria and are a good empirical choice. Local antibiotic policies differ.

Fever and infective symptoms usually settle within a week of appropriate antibiotics. Sustained resolution of sepsis is the most important marker of successful conservative management (radiological resolution can take >3 months).

The elderly, immunocompromised and patients with very large abscesses (>6 cm) or bronchial obstruction are most likely to require invasive intervention.

Drainage When appropriate antibiotic therapy fails, image guided percutaneous drainage is preferred to surgery. Successful drainage and avoidance of surgery has been reported in 84% of cases. It can be achieved with CT, ultrasound or fluoroscopic guidance. Complications, such as bronchopleural fistulae, haemothorax and empyema, are infrequent.

Percutaneous drainage should be considered if signs of systemic sepsis persist after 2 weeks of broad-spectrum antibiotic therapy.

Surgery Surgical excision can be avoided in >90% of patients. It should only be considered at an early stage when there evidence of localised obstructing malignancy or life-threatening complications such as intractible haemoptysis, bronchopleural fistula or empyema.

Perioperative mortality rates of up to 16% have been reported following surgery for lung abscess.

Prognosis Lung abcesses are associated with a 10% mortality rate.

The elderly or immunocompromised and those with large abscesses (>6 cm), underlying malignancy, malnutrition or delay in diagnosis and treatment have a particularly poor outcome.

References

- Davies CWH, et al. The British Thoracic Society Guidelines for the management of pleural infection. Thorax 2009; 58: Suppl. 2, ii18–ii28.
- Davies CW, et al. Predictors of outcome and long-term survival in patients with pleural infection. Am J Respir Crit Care Med 1999; 160: 1682–1687.
- Maskell NA, et al. The bacteriology of pleural infection by genetic and standard methods and its mortality significance. Am J Respir Crit Care Med 2006; 174: 817–823.
- Mwandumba HC, Beeching NJ. Pyogenic lung infections: factors for predicting clinical outcomeof lung abscess and thoracic empyema. Curr Opin Pulm Med 2000; 6: 234–239.
- Peña Griñan N, et al. Yield of percutaneous needle lung aspiration in lung abscess. Chest 1990; 97: 67–94.
- van Sonnenberg E, et al. Lung abscess: CT guided drainage. Radiology 1984; 151: 337–341.

INFLUENZA, PANDEMICS AND SARS

W.S. Lim
Respiratory Medicine, Nottingham University Hospitals NHS Trust, Nottingham, UK
E-mail: WeiShen.Lim@nuh.nhs.uk

Seasonal and pandemic influenza

Virology Influenza viruses are RNA orthomyxoviruses with three main types, A, B and C. Viral surface proteins include haemagglutinin (H) and neuraminidase (N) which are involved in viral attachment and release respectively. There are 16 haemagglutinin (H1 to H16) and 9 neuraminidase types (N1 to N9). Influenza viruses are described in a standardised manner according to their type/location of first isolate/laboratory strain number/year of isolate/H and N subtypes. For example: influenza A/Hong Kong/1/68/H3N2 (the cause of the 1968 "Hong Kong" pandemic).

The natural reservoir hosts of all influenza A virus subtypes are water birds. The host specificity of the various influenza A virus subtypes is partially determined by the binding affinity of hemagglutinin to sialic acid residues on the host cell.

A notable feature of influenza A viruses is their propensity to undergo antigenic variation. The appearance of a novel antigenic type demonstrating efficient human-to-human transmission is a prerequisite for a pandemic. Only influenza A viruses have been associated with pandemics.

Seasonal influenza Influenza is mostly a self-limiting viral upper respiratory tract infection that is managed in the community. In temperate climates, outbreaks of infections occur almost exclusively in winter. Attack rates are highest in young children and the elderly.

Influenza is highly transmissible. Human-to-human transmission occurs through large droplet spread and direct contact with secretions (or fomites). There is also evidence supporting aerosol transmission although the extent and importance of this is debated.

Key points

- Influenza is mostly a self-limiting viral upper respiratory tract infection that is managed in the community. Pneumonia is the most frequent serious complication of influenza.
- The neuraminidase inhibitors, oseltamivir and zanamivir, are effective in the prophylaxis and treatment of influenza A infection.
- The 2009 influenza A(H1N1) pandemic was of low severity compared to the 1918 pandemic.
- SARS coronavirus (SARS-CoV) is the causative agent of SARS. Wild mammals, such as the palm civet cat, were most likely the pre-epidemic source of SARS-CoV. Bats are most likely the natural reservoir for coronaviruses.
- The management of SARS is chiefly supportive. Basic infection control measures are the cornerstone of containment of any future outbreak.

The mean incubation period is 2–4 days with a range up to 7 days. An abrupt onset of high fever (up to 41°C) is the main presenting feature. The fever peaks within the first 24 h of illness and usually lasts for 3 days. Cough is the next commonest symptom (85%) which may be associated with sputum production in up to 40% of cases. Malaise (80%), chills (70%), headaches (65%) and myalgia (50%) may be prominent. Coryza and sore throat are reported in about half of patients. In addition, children may present with vomiting, diarrhoea and abdominal pain but these symptoms are uncommon in adults. The mean duration of symptoms is 4 days.

Two main classes of drug are active against influenza. The M2 ion channel inhibitors, amantadine and rimantadine, are effective against influenza A. However, their use is hindered by the rapid emergence of resistance to these drugs together with a high incidence of side-effects. The neuraminidase inhibitors, oseltamivir and zanamivir, are effective against influenza A and B. Fortunately, although resistance to oseltamivir has been reported, this is not widespread in seasonal influenza A(H3N2). Oseltamivir is often preferred over zanamivir because of ease of administration (oral *versus* inhaled/intravenous). Other neuraminidase inhibitors are also being developed, such as peramivir (intravenous). A Cochrane meta-analysis of randomised controlled trials of neuraminidase inhibitors in the treatment of influenza reported that the efficacy of oral oseltamivir at 75 mg daily was 61% (risk ratio 0.39, 95% CI 0.18–0.85) and of inhaled zanamivir at 10 mg daily was 62% (risk ratio 0.38, 95% CI 0.17–0.85). In clinical terms, this benefit translates to a shortening of the illness by 0.5–1 day. The review found the published evidence insufficient to answer the question whether neuraminidase inhibitors are effective in reducing the complications of lower respiratory tract infection, antibiotic use, or admissions to hospital. Oseltamivir use was associated with nausea (odds ratio 1.79, 95% CI 1.10–2.93).

Chemoprophylaxis and vaccination Both oseltamivir and zanamivir taken as prophylactic agents reduce the chance of symptomatic laboratory-confirmed influenza (risk ratio 0.38, 95% CI 0.17–0.85 for zanamivir 10 mg daily; risk ratio 0.39, 95% CI 0.18–0.85 for oseltamivir 75 mg daily). However, the effect of neuraminidase inhibitors on the prophylaxis of *influenza-like illness*, which includes infections other than influenza, is uncertain. Oseltamivir has also been demonstrated to be 58–84% efficacious as post-exposure prophylaxis.

Immunisation is the backbone of influenza prevention. The relative protective efficacy in children and young healthy adults is 70–>90%. Efficacy is lower (~40%) in the elderly.

Oseltamivir resistance In 1977, influenza A(H1N1) re-emerged and co-circulated with influenza A(H3N2), with the latter remaining the dominant seasonal human influenza virus (fig. 1). During the 2007/2008 influenza season, oseltamivir-resistant seasonal influenza A(H1N1) viruses emerged suddenly and spread globally. These viruses carried a histidine-to-tyrosine mutation at residue 275 of the neuraminidase protein (H275Y). Laboratory and limited epidemiological data indicated that the viral fitness and virulence of these oseltamivir-resistant influenza A(H1N1) viruses were no different from oseltamivir-susceptible strains.

In Europe, over the 2008/2009 influenza season, influenza A(H3N2) continued to predominate but almost all co-circulating seasonal influenza A(H1N1) viruses were oseltamivir-resistant. In contrast, in the USA, oseltamivir-resistant influenza A(H1N1) viruses predominated in the 2008/2009 season, prompting the USA to issue guidelines recommending the use of zanamivir or a combination of oseltamivir and rimantadine when seasonal influenza A(H1N1) virus infection was suspected.

H275Y mutations in 2009 pandemic influenza A(H1N1) viruses have also been identified. Fortunately, such oseltamivir-resistant isolates have been infrequent and

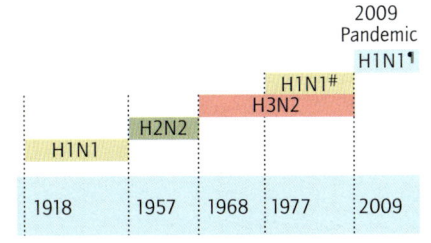

Figure 1. Influenza pandemics and subtypes, 1918-2009. #: re-emergence of H1N1, possibly from accidental laboratory release – strain closely related to 1950 strain. ¶: new reassortment of six gene segments from triple reassortant North American swine influenza virus lineages and two gene segments from Eurasian swine influenza virus lineages.

sporadic. They have been found mainly in immunosuppressed patients being treated with oseltamivir.

Complications of influenza Although influenza is mostly a self-limiting illness even without specific treatment, some patient groups experience significant morbidity and mortality. Persons at risk of complications from influenza include pregnant women, the frail elderly, those who are immunosuppressed and those with chronic medical conditions such as heart disease, chronic respiratory disease (mostly asthma and chronic obstructive pulmonary disease(COPD)), cancer, diabetes, renal disease, rheumatologic disease, dementia and stroke. Rates of hospitalisation and death are increased in all these patient groups.

Pneumonia is the most frequent serious complication of influenza. Two main clinical patterns are described: primary viral pneumonia and secondary bacterial pneumonia.

Patients with primary viral pneumonia typically become breathless within the first few days of onset of fever. This may be associated with tachypnoea, cyanosis and bilateral lung crackles on chest examination. A leukocytosis is usual. The commonest chest radiographic abnormality is of diffuse bilateral interstitial infiltrates similar to pulmonary congestion. Progression to respiratory failure is well recognised. Mortality rates of 6-40% have been reported. In severe cases, pathological findings are similar to those seen in acute respiratory distress syndrome.

Patients with secondary bacterial pneumonia complicating influenza typically experience an amelioration of the initial symptoms of viral infection. However, 4-10 days later, a recurrence of fever together with breathlessness and a productive cough ensues. Clinical features at this point are indistinguishable from community-acquired bacterial pneumonia. The three commonest pathogens implicated are *Streptococcus pneumoniae*, *Staphylococcus aureus* and *Haemophilus influenzae*.

In children, the commonest respiratory complication, though not the most serious, is otitis media.

In addition to the specific complications listed in table 1, patients with influenza may also experience a worsening of a pre-existing medical illness such as COPD or cardiac failure.

Management of the complications of influenza should follow the same principles for each specific condition regardless of influenza. In the case of influenza A primary viral pneumonia, higher doses of neuraminidase inhibitors (oseltamivir 150 mg *b.i.d.*) have been advocated based on experience with human cases of viral pneumonia resulting from avian influenza A H5N1 infection. There are no randomised trials of therapy in primary viral pneumonia.

Pandemic influenza In the 20th century, pandemics occurred in 1918 (H1N1), 1957 (H2N2) and 1968 (H3N2) (fig. 1). Each of these pandemics had a different impact and tempo. The 1918 pandemic was the most deadly, claiming the lives of an estimated 40-100 million people globally. In contrast, the subsequent two pandemics were much less severe, accounting for an estimated 1-2 million deaths each.

Table 1. Complications of influenza in adults and children.

Complication	Incidence	
	Adults	**Children**
Otitis media	Common	Very common
Secondary bacterial pneumonia	Common	Uncommon
Primary viral pneumonia	Uncommon	Uncommon
Myositis	Uncommon	Rare
Myocarditis	Rare	Rare
Encephalitis/encephalopathy	Rare	Rare
Reye's syndrome	-	Rare
Febrile convulsions	-	Common

In early April 2009, the first cases of the most recent influenza pandemic were identified in Mexico. The 2009 pandemic influenza A(H1N1) virus is a triple-reassortant virus containing genes from human, swine and avian influenza viruses. It caused an infection that was clinically similar to seasonal influenza. Gastrointestinal symptoms amongst adults were commoner than in seasonal influenza. Mainly children and young adults were affected and most illnesses were self-limiting. In persons aged >60 yrs, it is likely that pre-existing cross-reactive antibodies due to previous exposure to antigenically related influenza viruses provided protection against infection.

Compared to the 1918 pandemic, hospitalisation and mortality rates were low. In Canada, the risk of hospital admission amongst laboratory-confirmed cases was ~4.5% and the case-fatality rate was 0.3%. In the UK, the overall estimated case-fatality rate was 26 per 100,000; lowest for children aged 5-14 yrs (11 per 100,000) and highest for those aged ≥65 yrs (980 per 100,000). Hospitalisation rates varied between countries. Of those hospitalised, 9-31% required intensive care support, predominantly because of diffuse viral pneumonitis. Mortality of ICU admitted patients was 14-46%.

Patients at risk of complications from seasonal influenza were similarly at risk from 2009 H1N1 virus infection. In addition, pregnant women, especially in the third trimester and with HIV co-infection, were at higher risk of severe infection. Some non-trial data suggested that early treatment of 2009 influenza A(H1N1) virus infection with neuraminidase inhibitors reduced the duration of hospitalisation and the risk of progression to severe disease. Many critically ill patients received increased doses of antivirals for extended durations during the pandemic (*e.g.* oseltamivir 150 mg *b.i.d.* for 10 days in adults). This practice was not based on evidence from randomised controlled trials.

Severe acute respiratory syndrome (SARS)

Epidemiology The global outbreak of severe acute respiratory syndrome (SARS) in 2002/2003 affected 8,096 individuals in 26 countries, 774 of whom died. The three most severely affected regions were mainland China, Hong Kong and Taiwan with 5,327, 1,755 and 674 cases, respectively.

The first human case was identified in the city of Foshan, Guangdong Province, China on November 16, 2002 and the last known case of the initial outbreak experienced the onset of symptoms on June 16, 2003 in Taiwan.

A novel coronavirus, the SARS coronavirus (SARS-CoV), was identified as the causative agent of SARS in April 2003. Close human–animal contact associated with many of the early cases in China supported the concept of SARS as a zoonotic infection. The palm civet cat *Paguma larvata* has been identified as the likely main pre-epidemic animal source. Bats are most probably the natural reservoir for coronaviruses. Coronaviruses sharing 87–92% genome nucleotide identity with SARS-CoV have been found in horseshoe bats *Rhinolophus* sp. Accordingly, one hypothesis is that coronaviruses were transmitted from horseshoe bats to civet cats and then to humans (fig. 2).

Infections later in the course of the outbreak were due mainly to human-to-human transmission. Molecular evolutionary changes of the SARS-CoV have been described that might explain the shift in mode of transmission. Nosocomial transmission was particularly high, with attack rates amongst healthcare workers in some centres ranging from 10–60%. In contrast, community transmission rates were much lower with typically <10% of contacts infected.

The mean incubation period of SARS is estimated at 4–6 days with a maximum incubation period of 10 days. Overall, SARS may be considered to be low to moderately transmissible. A few remarkable "super-spreading events" (SSEs) were associated with SARS in which single individuals were responsible for infecting many more individuals than average. In one SSE at the Prince of Wales Hospital, Hong Kong, a single patient infected 143 people.

Clinical features The clinical presenting features of SARS infection are nonspecific. Fever (93%), chills (61%), malaise (46%), cough (41%) and rigors (38%) were the predominant symptoms recorded in the Hong Kong-wide clinical database of SARS patients. High-volume, watery, nonbloody diarrhoea is present in a sizeable minority of patients (~20%) in the early stages of disease and increases in frequency (up to 70%) by the second week of illness. It is usually self-limiting. Similarly, respiratory symptoms of cough, breathlessness and sputum production are less frequently (<50%) encountered in the first 4 days of illness, but increase to a peak (70%) by day 9–10 of illness. Typically, a dry cough is the first respiratory symptom. This is followed by breathlessness, which worsens at the start of the second week.

Radiological changes of airspace consolidation are usually unilateral and localised in the first week. The infiltrates are commoner in the lower lobes (70%) and the periphery (75%). Cavitation, lymphadenopathy and pleural effusions are not described in association with SARS infection. The extent of radiological abnormality correlates with severity of illness and prognosis.

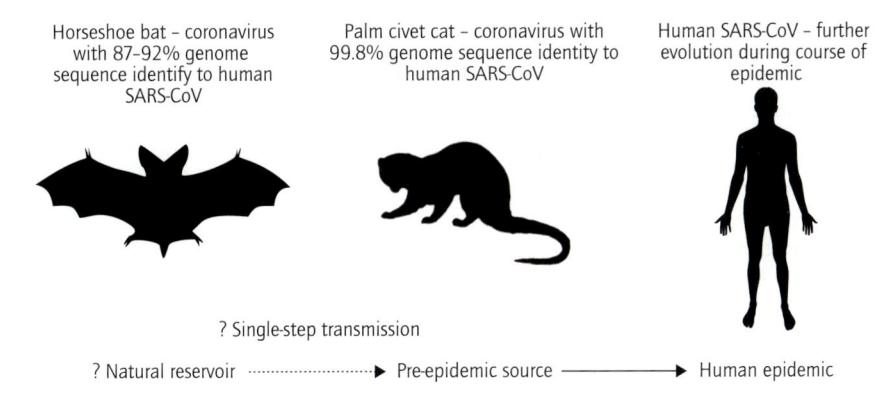

Figure 2. Possible origin of SARS, based on phylogenetic studies.

Laboratory test abnormalities include lymphopenia, neutropenia, thrombocytopenia and raised levels of lactate dehydrogenase (LDH), alanine aminotransferase, creatinine kinase, and activated partial thromboplastin time.

Respiratory failure occurs in 20–25% of patients, mainly adults. Unusually, the incidence of barotrauma (manifest as a pneumothorax or pneumomediastinum) was observed to be higher in severely ill patients with SARS than might be expected despite the use of low-volume, low-pressure mechanical ventilation strategies. The reason for this is unclear. Patients with SARS requiring critical care support have a mortality of ~25%. Features associated with a poor prognosis include advanced age, male sex, presence of comorbid illness, high serum LDH and neutrophilia at presention, and an initial radiograph with more than one zone of involvement. Overall, adults suffer a more severe disease than children.

Virology SARS-CoV is detectable by RT-PCR and by culture from respiratory tract, faecal and urine samples. Virus RNA is also detectable in serum, plasma and cerebrospinal fluid thus indicating multisystem infection. Diagnostic yields are better with nasopharyngeal aspirates and faeces compared to throat swabs. A retrospective diagnosis of SARS is possible using serological tests.

Clinical management The management of SARS is chiefly supportive. Chemical compounds that have reported activity against SARS-CoV include glycyrrhizin, baicalin, reserpine, noclosamide, ribavarin, protease inhibitors (lopinavir, nelfinavir), interferon (IFN)-α and IFN-β. A comparative study using IFN alfacon-1 (n=22), and another using a lopinavir/ritonavir combination (n=41), suggested clinical benefit. However, there are no randomised controlled trials of treatment.

Corticosteroids were used during the SARS outbreak as an immunomodulatory agent with the intention of limiting damage that might be caused by the host immune response. In reported series, there were large variations in type, dose, route and duration of corticosteroids used. Unsurprisingly, different conclusions about the efficacies of corticosteroids were drawn.

Basic infection control measures are the cornerstone of containment of any future outbreak. As subclinical infection with SARS has not been described and the peak in viral load occurs late (second week), effective infection control measures can often be instituted prior to widespread transmission.

Practice points regarding the clinical diagnosis of influenza or SARS

The early symptoms in both influenza and SARS are nonspecific, comprising primarily a fever in association with respiratory symptoms such as cough and systemic symptoms such as malaise or chills. A clinical diagnosis of influenza or SARS is therefore crucially dependent on epidemiological features. In the case of influenza, an influenza-like illness (ILI) in the setting of local or community circulation of influenza viruses (*e.g.* during an influenza season, or during a pandemic) greatly increases the likelihood that the illness is due to influenza virus infection – the positive predictive value of an ILI for laboratory-confirmed influenza can range from 20–70%. Alternative pathogens to consider in instances of an ILI include parainfluenza virus, adenovirus, rhinovirus, *Mycoplasma pneumoniae* and even *S. pneumoniae*. Similarly, a clinical diagnosis of SARS requires the establishment of an epidemiological link with another patient with SARS, or exposure to likely animal sources of SARS-CoV. Virological testing is necessary to make a definitive diagnosis in both influenza and SARS.

References

- Cleri DJ, *et al*. Severe acute respiratory syndrome (SARS). *Infect Dis Clin North Am* 2010; 24: 175–202.
- Jefferson T, *et al*. Neuraminidase inhibitors for preventing and treating influenza in healthy

- adults. *Cochrane Database Syst Rev* 2010; 2: CD001265.
- Lew TW, *et al.* Acute respiratory distress syndrome in critically ill patients with severe acute respiratory syndrome. *JAMA* 2003; 290: 374-380.
- Miller E, *et al.* Incidence of 2009 pandemic influenza A H1N1 infection in England: a cross-sectional serological study. *Lancet* 2010; 375: 1100-1108.
- Monto AS, Whitley RJ Seasonal, pandemic influenza, a 2007 update on challenges and solutions. *Clin Infect Dis* 2008; 46: 1024-1031.
- Palese P Influenza, *old and new threats. Nat Med* 2004; 10: S82-S87.
- Peiris JS, *et al.* The severe acute respiratory syndrome. *N Engl J Med* 2003; 349: 2431-2441.
- Writing Committee of the WHO Consultation on Clinical Aspects of Pandemic (H1N1) 2009 Influenza, Clinical aspects of pandemic 2009 influenza A (H1N1) virus infection. *N Engl J Med* 2010; 362: 1708-1719.
- Yip CW, *et al.* Phylogenetic perspectives on the epidemiology and origins of SARS and SARS-like coronaviruses. *Infect Genet Evol* 2009; 9: 1185-1196.

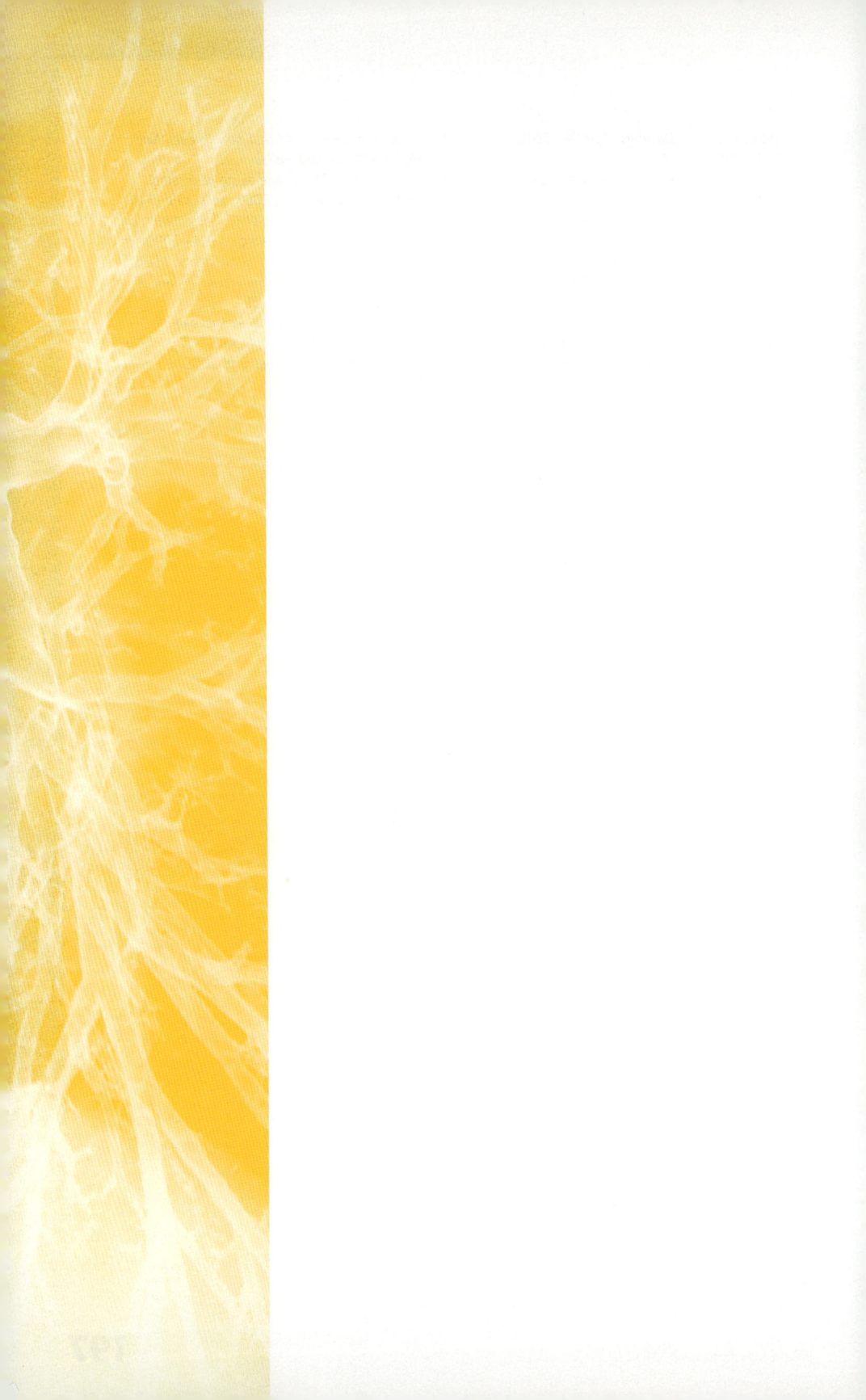

CHAPTER 8:

TUBERCULOSIS

PULMONARY TUBERCULOSIS G. Sotgiu, C. Lange and G.B. Migliori	200
EXTRAPULMONARY TUBERCULOSIS A. Bossink	209
TUBERCULOSIS IN THE IMMUNOCOMPROMISED HOST M. Sester	212
LATENT TUBERCULOSIS J-P. Zellweger	215
NONTUBERCULOUS MYCOBACTERIAL DISEASES C. Piersimoni	218

PULMONARY TUBERCULOSIS

G. Sotgiu[1], C. Lange[2] and G.B. Migliori[3]
[1] Hygiene and Preventive Medicine Institute, University of Sassari, Sassari
[2] Division of Clinical Infectious Diseases, Medical Clinic, Research Center Borstel, Borstel, Germany
[3] WHO Collaborating Centre for TB and Lung Diseases, Fondazione S. Maugeri, Care and Research Institute, Tradate, Italy
E-mail: giovannibattista.migliori@fsm.it

The World Health Organization (WHO) has declared tuberculosis (TB) a global emergency due to its burden in terms of cases and deaths. Among the factors contributing to maintenance of the TB pandemic are: the large number of patients co-infected with HIV; bacterial multidrug resistance (MDR) to anti-TB drugs (*i.e.* strains resistant to at least isoniazid and rifampicin); migration from high-incidence countries; and the social determinants of the disease (poverty, drug abuse and homelessness).

TB can affect virtually every organ, most importantly the lungs (pulmonary TB), and is typically associated with granuloma formation.

Aetiology

TB is an infectious disease caused by slightly bent, thin, aerobic, non-motile, non-spore-forming beaded rods belonging to the family *Mycobacteriaceae* and to the order *Actinomycetales*. Of the pathogenic species belonging to the *Mycobacterium tuberculosis* complex, the most frequent and important agent of human disease is *M. tuberculosis*. Mycobacteria are 2–4 μm long and 0.2–5 μm wide. They are defined as acid-fast bacilli (AFB) due to the cell wall structure, crucial to their survival and characterised by a significant content of mycolic acid attached to the underlying peptidoglycan-bound polysaccharide arabinogalactan. Another important carbohydrate structural antigen of the cell wall is lipoarabinomannan, which facilitates the survival of mycobacteria within macrophages. The peptidoglycan network, located just outside the cell membrane, confers cell wall rigidity.

This structure provides a barrier that is responsible for many of the medically challenging characteristics of TB, including resistance to antibacterial agents and to host defence mechanisms. It has been clearly demonstrated that the quality and quantity of the cell wall components affect mycobacterial virulence, pathogenicity and growth rate.

> **Key points**
>
> - With 9.27 million new cases (0.5 being multidrug-resistant tuberculosis) and 1.77 million deaths, tuberculosis is a first-class health priority.
> - Diagnosis of pulmonary tuberculosis is simple, being primarily based on bacteriology (sputum smear microscopy and culture).
> - Treatment of pan-susceptible cases of pulmonary tuberculosis is effective and cheap.
> - Management of pulmonary tuberculosis in multidrug-resistant and HIV co-infected cases is particularly complicated.

Pathogenesis

Mycobacteria are spread through air droplets expelled when those with infectious pulmonary TB cough, sneeze or speak. Close contacts (those with prolonged, frequent or intense contact with pulmonary TB sufferers) are at highest risk of becoming infected. Bacteria are carried on droplet nuclei in the air and can enter the body through the airways. The majority of the bacilli are trapped in the upper parts of the airways where the mucus-secreting goblet cells are located. The mucus catches antigens, and the cilia on the surface of the cells constantly beat the mucus and its entrapped particles upward for removal. This system provides humans with an initial physical first-line defence that prevents infection in most contacts of pulmonary TB patients.

Bacteria in small droplets that can bypass the mucociliary system and reach the alveoli are quickly surrounded and engulfed by alveolar macrophages, which are part of the innate immune system and are the most abundant phagocytic cells located in the alveolar spaces; they are readily available without requiring previous exposure. Numerous bacterial and host mechanisms are involved in the uptake of the mycobacteria, such as mycobacterial lipoarabinomannans, ligands for macrophages' receptors or the complement proteins C2a and C3b that bind to the cell wall and enhance recognition of the mycobacteria by effector macrophages. The subsequent phagocytosis starts a cascade of events that results in successful control of the infection, followed by latent TB infection (LTBI) in the majority of cases; rarely, infection progresses to active disease, called primary progressive pulmonary TB (common among children aged $\leqslant 4$ yrs). The outcome is essentially determined by the balance that occurs between host defences and the invading mycobacteria.

During the initial phase (2–12 weeks) of pulmonary TB, the bacteria continue to multiply slowly (a cell division every 25–35 h) and T-lymphocytes are attracted by cytokines released by macrophages. In the immunocompetent, the next defensive stage is formation of granuloma around mycobacteria, which limits bacterial replication and spread to other pulmonary sites. This condition establishes latency of the infection. Lesions in those with an adequate immune system generally undergo fibrosis and calcification, while in immunocompromised subjects, they progress to primary progressive pulmonary TB.

The majority of infected individuals who ultimately develop pulmonary TB do so within the first year or two after infection; dormant bacilli, however, may persist for years before being reactivated to produce secondary pulmonary TB, which is often infectious. Overall, it is estimated that lifetime risk of developing TB is 10% in those who are immunocompetent and $\leqslant 50\%$ in HIV-positive individuals. Age is an important determinant of the risk of disease after infection. Among infected subjects, the incidence is highest in childhood up to the age of 8 yrs, with a second peak during adolescence and early adulthood. The risk may increase in the elderly, possibly because of waning immunity and comorbidities (*i.e.* diabetes).

Epidemiology

WHO estimates that 9.27 million new cases of TB occurred in 2007 compared with 9.24 million in 2006. Of them, an estimated 44% or 4.1 million were infectious (new pulmonary sputum smear-positive cases). India, China, Indonesia, Nigeria and South Africa have the highest numbers of incident cases. Asia (South-East Asia and the Western Pacific region) accounts for 55% of global cases and Africa for 31%; the other three regions (the Americas, Europe and the Eastern Mediterranean region) account for small fractions of global cases. Among the 15 countries with the highest estimated TB incidence rates, 13 are in Africa, a phenomenon linked to high rates of HIV co-infection. In both the African and European regions, prevalence rates increased substantially during the 1990s.

There were an estimated 13.7 million prevalent cases of TB in 2007, a slight decrease from 13.9 million in 2006. Of these cases, an estimated 5% were HIV positive. Of the 511,000 incident cases of MDR-TB in 2007, 68% were sputum smear-positive.

Overall, 1.77 million TB deaths occurred in 2007. An estimated 456,000 were of people who were HIV-positive. Deaths from TB among HIV-positive individuals accounted for 23% of the estimated 2 million HIV deaths that occurred in 2007.

The World Health Assembly outcome targets (*i.e.* to achieve a case-detection rate of ⩾70% for new smear-positive cases and a treatment success rate of ⩾85% for such cases) provide a quantitative indication of the effectiveness of national TB programmes in finding, diagnosing and successfully treating those with TB.

The 2.6 million new smear-positive cases in 2007 represent 64% of the 4.1 million estimated cases. This is a small increase from 63% in 2006, following a slow increase from 35 to 43% between 1995 and 2001, and a more rapid increase from 43 to 60% between 2001 and 2005. Africa had the lowest case-detection rate (47%). Globally, the rate of treatment success was 85% in 2006; the target for treatment success was reached because of the high treatment success rates reported from South-East Asia and the Western Pacific region (87 and 92%, respectively).

Clinical features

Before the recognition of HIV infection, >75–80% of all TB cases were limited to the lungs. In recent decades, increases have been seen in extrapulmonary cases alone, and in pulmonary and extrapulmonary cases.

Primary pulmonary TB Pulmonary mycobacterial entry is often asymptomatic. Associated paratracheal lymphadenopathy may occur because the bacilli spread from the lungs through the lymphatic system. In the majority of cases, the lesion heals spontaneously and may later be evident as a small calcified nodule (Ghon lesion). If the primary lesion enlarges, mainly seen in children and in individuals with impaired immunity, pleural effusion is a typical finding. This effusion develops because the bacilli infiltrate the pleural space from an adjacent subpleural focus. The effusion may remain small, resolving spontaneously, or it may become large enough to induce clinical symptoms such as fever, pain and dyspnoea.

Secondary pulmonary TB Secondary pulmonary TB results from endogenous reactivation of LTBI and is frequently localised to pulmonary segments, where the high oxygen concentration favours mycobacterial replication (upper lobes).

Early signs and symptoms are often nonspecific and insidious, consisting mainly of fatigue (decreased muscle mass), general malaise, weakness, weight loss (lack of appetite and altered metabolism associated with systemic inflammatory response to mycobacteria), and a low-grade fever accompanied by chills and night sweats. Cough eventually develops in the majority of patients; it could be initially non-productive, but subsequently it may be accompanied by the production of purulent sputum often streaked with blood. Haemoptysis may be due to: the destruction of a vessel located in a pulmonary cavity; the rupture of a dilated vessel in a cavity (Rasmussen's aneurysm); or the formation of an aspergilloma in an old cavity. In some patients, the presence of inflamed subpleural parenchyma may cause pleuritic pain. Extensive disease may lead to dyspnoea or orthopnoea. Although numerous individuals with pulmonary TB have no physical characteristics, rales may be detected over involved areas during inspiration, particularly after coughing. Haematologic examinations might reveal mild or moderate anaemia, strictly related to the weakness, and leukocytosis. Chronic cough (*e.g.* cough lasting for 2–3 weeks) has to be considered the main clinical symptom.

Diagnosis

At >100 yrs old, sputum smear microscopy is still the most widely used technique for the diagnosis of pulmonary TB. Although highly specific, the lower limit for detection of microscopy is $0.5–1 \times 10^4$ organisms·mL^{-1} sputum and only about half of all culture-positive cases have sputum smear-positive results. There is evidence that sensitivity may be lower among HIV-infected subjects. AFB microscopy is simple to perform but suboptimal results are described where adequate quality-assurance programmes are absent. WHO has proposed a case definition for sputum smear-negative pulmonary TB based on three negative sputum smears, radiographic abnormalities consistent with active pulmonary TB, and no response to a course of broad-spectrum antibiotics. Although smear-negative pulmonary TB cases are not considered to be infectious, their high number is causing increasing concern in high HIV-prevalence, low-income settings.

Sputum induction with hypertonic saline is a useful technique for diagnosing pulmonary TB in individuals who are either sputum smear negative or unable to produce sputum. Repeated sputum induction increases the yield of both smear and culture. It avoids invasive procedures and provides a means of diagnosis in resource-poor settings. It is worth noting that sputum induction should be carefully conducted in a well-ventilated setting, as it is a cough-inducing procedure with a high risk of transmission.

Mycobacterial culture is considered the gold standard; however, false-positive results do occur, primarily as a consequence of laboratory contamination. Moreover, several weeks are required for the performance of culture-based methods, although the use of liquid media has decreased pulmonary TB diagnosis time. Presently, in Europe, a "definite" case of TB is a culture-positive case, while all other cases (including culture negative, sputum smear positive) are "other than definite". Drug susceptibility testing for first- and second-line drugs is also useful in order to better define the phenotype of the isolated strain in culture-confirmed cases.

Molecular techniques, based on gene amplification, offer increased sensitivity and specificity for diagnosis. The major limitation, mainly for low-income countries, is their current high cost and the risk of contamination (false-positive results).

Chest radiology (fig. 1) and computed tomography (CT) are useful tools that complement bacteriological examinations in the diagnosis of pulmonary TB. Although over- and under-reading have been described, these tools can offer important information to the clinician. Chest radiography is commonly used to screen individuals harbouring a significantly higher risk of pulmonary TB (*e.g.* prisoners, contacts of infectious cases, *etc.*) than the general population. Among the tools indirectly used to detect mycobacterial infection, the tuberculin skin test (TST) deserves to be mentioned; it must be noted, however, that it has several limitations, including poor specificity, difficult administration and the risk of anergy.

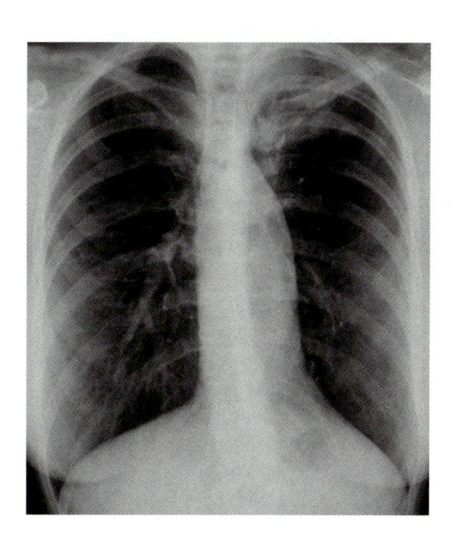

Figure 1. Pulmonary tuberculosis due to multidrug-resistant strains of *Mycobacterium tuberculosis*. A 21-yr-old female with isolated left upper lobe infiltrate.

False-negative reactions are common in immunosuppressed patients and in those with overwhelming pulmonary TB. Positive results are obtained when patients have been infected with *M. tuberculosis* but do not have active disease, and when subjects have been sensitised by nontuberculous mycobacteria or bacille Calmette-Guèrin (BCG) vaccination.

Finally, interferon (IFN)-γ release assays (IGRAs) have recently been introduced into clinical practice. Their application in specimens collected from the infected organ or tissue is still under evaluation. These techniques can increase the low specificity of TST based on the immune response (release of IFN-γ) to early-secreted antigenic target protein (ESAT)-6 and culture filtrate protein (CFP)-10, which are antigens specific to *M. tuberculosis* and are not produced by *Mycobacterium bovis* BCG.

Treatment

Due to their higher bacillary burden, individuals with active TB and positive sputum smear test results are the main source of TB transmission in the community. The highest priority in TB control programmes is the rapid identification of new cases of sputum smear-positive pulmonary TB and effective treatment. It has been estimated that case-finding and effective treatment of smear-positive individuals could decrease the number of TB cases globally by one half within a decade.

The longer the interval between doses, the easier and less expensive the task of providing treatment to large numbers of patients, particularly in high-prevalence countries. Short-course regimens are divided into an initial or bactericidal phase and a continuation or sterilising phase. Pan-susceptible TB is defined as TB susceptible to all first-line agents.

WHO recommends treatment of new cases of pulmonary TB (both sputum smear-positive cases, belonging to Category I, and sputum smear-negative cases, belonging to Category III) with a standardised regimen of four first-line anti-TB drugs, including isoniazid, rifampicin, pyrazinamide and ethambutol for 2 months, followed by isoniazid and rifampicin for 4 months (tables 1 and 2). Because of the higher probability of drug resistance, re-treatment cases (Category II) require a fifth drug during the continuation phase (streptomycin for 2 months). Both the intensive and the continuation phases of treatment (3 and 5 months, respectively) are longer in Category II than in Categories I and III (table 2).

MDR-TB is caused by mycobacteria that are resistant to at least isoniazid and rifampicin, the two most potent first-line anti-TB drugs. While MDR-TB has been documented for many years, a new term, extensively drug-resistant (XDR)-TB, appeared in the literature for the first time in March 2006. It describes a severe form of TB caused by strains of *M. tuberculosis* that are resistant to at least isoniazid and rifampicin (*i.e.* MDR-TB), as well as any fluoroquinolone and at least one of three injectable drugs used in anti-TB treatment: capreomycin, kanamycin and/or amikacin.

To achieve a regimen designed to treat the majority of patients with a minimum of four effective drugs as is recommended, it may be necessary to use five, six or more drugs to cover all the possible patterns of resistance when drug susceptibility testing (DST) results for second-line agents are not available (table 3). An injectable agent and a fluoroquinolone form the core of the preferred regimen.

The most recent WHO guidelines propose different treatment strategies for individuals suspected to harbour MDR-TB strains. Depending on specific country conditions, treatment protocols may recommend a standardised treatment regimen for all MDR-TB cases (*e.g.* in countries where DST is not widely available), or may alternatively recommend individualised treatment based on individual DST results. If standardised combinations of second-line drugs are chosen, representative national data on predominant resistance patterns to specific treatment

Table 1. Anti-tuberculosis (TB) drugs, dosages and common adverse effects

Anti-TB drugs	Recommended daily dosage	Common adverse effects (not exclusive)
Group 1: first-line oral agents		
Isoniazid	5 mg·kg^{-1} q.d. Should not exceed 300 mg per day Always consider co-administering vitamin B6	Elevated transaminases; hepatitis; peripheral neuropathy; GI intolerance; CNS toxicity
Rifampicin	10 mg·kg^{-1} q.d. >50 kg: 600 mg; <50 kg: 450 mg	Elevation of liver enzymes; hepatitis; hypersensitivity; fever; gastrointestinal disorders: anorexia, nausea, vomiting, abdominal pain; discoloration (orange or brown) of urine, tears and other body fluids; thrombopenia
Ethambutol	15-25 mg·kg^{-1} q.d. Maximum 2.0 g per day	Optic neuritis; hyperuricaemia; peripheral neuropathy (rare)
Pyrazinamide	30 mg·kg^{-1} q.d. Maximum 2.0 g per day	Arthralgia; hyperuricaemia; toxic hepatitis; gastro-intestinal discomfort
Group 2: injectables		
Streptomycin[#]	0.75-1 g q.d. <50 kg: 0.75 g per day; >50 kg: 1 g per day Maximum cumulative dose 50 g	Auditory and vestibular nerve damage (non-reversible); renal failure (usually reversible); allergies; nausea; skin rash, neuromuscular blockade
Amikacin[¶]	0.75-1 g q.d. <50 kg: 0.75 g per day; >50 kg: 1 g per day Maximum cumulative dose 50 g	Auditory and vestibular nerve damage (non-reversible); renal failure (usually reversible); allergies; nausea; skin rash, neuromuscular blockade
Capreomycin[#]	0.75-1 g q.d. <50 kg: 0.75 g per day; >50 kg: 1 g per day Maximum cumulative dose 50 g	Auditory and vestibular nerve damage (non-reversible); renal failure (usually reversible); Bartter-like syndrome; allergies; neuromuscular blockade
Kanamycin[¶]	375-500 mg b.i.d. <50 kg: 0.75 g per day; >50 kg: 1 g per day Maximum cumulative dose 50 g	Auditory and vestibular nerve damage (non-reversible); renal failure (usually reversible); allergies; nausea; skin rash, neuromuscular blockade
Group 3: fluoroquinolones		
Levofloxacin[+]	500-1,000 mg q.d.	Gastrointestinal discomfort, CNS disorders, tendon rupture (rare); hypersensitivity *Clostridium difficile* colitis
Ciprofloxacin[+]	500-750 mg b.i.d.	Gastrointestinal discomfort, CNS disorders, tendon rupture (rare); hypersensitivity *Clostridium difficile* colitis

Table 1. Continued

Moxifloxacin[+]	400 mg *q.d.*	Gastrointestinal discomfort; headache; dizziness, hallucinations; increased transaminases QT prolongation: *Clostridium difficile* colitis
Group 4: second-line oral agents		
Rifabutin	150–450 mg *q.d.* Consider to monitor drug levels	Anaemia; gastrointestinal discomfort; discoloration (orange or brown) of urine and other body fluids; uveitis; elevated liver enzymes
Ethionamid	0.75–1 g *q.d.*	Severe gastrointestinal intolerance; nausea; vomiting; hepatitis; CNS disorders
Prothionamide	0.75–1 g *q.d.*	Severe gastrointestinal intolerance; nausea; vomiting; hepatitis; CNS disorders
Cycloserine	250 mg *t.i.d.* Maximum 1,000 mg per day	CNS disorders; anxiety; confusion; dizziness; psychosis; seizures; headache
Terizidone	250 mg *t.i.d.* Maximum 1,000 mg per day	CNS disorders; anxiety; confusion; dizziness; psychosis; seizures; headache
Para-amino-salicylic acid	4 g *t.i.d.*	Gastrointestinal intolerance; nausea; diarrhoea; vomiting; hypersensitivity
Thiacetazone	50 mg *t.i.d.*	Hypersensitivity; gastrointestinal intolerance; vertigo; hepatitis
Group 5: oral reserve drugs with uncertain anti-TB activity		
Linezolid	600 mg *q.d.* (recommended for 600 mg *b.i.d.* dosage for MRSA and VRE infections)	Thrombopenia, anaemia, neuropathy
Clofazimine	100 mg *q.d.*	Ichthyosis; gastrointestinal discomfort; nausea; vomiting; discoloration of the skin
Amoxicillin-clavunate	875-125 mg *b.i.d.* or 500-250 mg *t.i.d.*	Gastrointestinal discomfort; diarrhoea; rash
Clarithromycin	500 mg *b.i.d.*	Gastrointestinal discomfort

CNS: central nervous system MRSA: methicillin-resistant *Staphylococcus aureus*; VRE: vancomycin-resistant Enterococcus. [#]: intravenous/intramuscular administration only; [¶]: intravenous administration only; [+]: also available for intravenous injection.

categories are needed. An alternative approach is to design a regimen on the basis of the individual history of previous anti-TB therapy, and eventually redesign it guided by individual DST. Relevant laboratory capacity is necessary if this option is chosen, as DST on most second-line drugs must be performed.

Although an individual patient's treatment duration should be guided by sputum smear and culture conversion, in general an injectable agent should be continued for at least the first 6 months of treatment. The entire treatment should be no less than 18 months after culture conversion.

Table 2. World Health Organization (WHO)-recommended treatment categories and regimens

Patient treatment category	Patient diagnostic category	Treatment regimens[#] Initial phase	Continuation phase
New pulmonary TB cases			
Category I	New smear-positive patients, new smear-negative patients with extensive parenchymal involvement, concomitant HIV-related diseases	Preferred: 2 HRZE Optional: 2 HRZE Optional: 2 HRZE$_3$[¶]	Preferred: 4 HR; 4 HR$_3$ Optional: 6 HE Optional: 4 HR$_3$
Category III	New smear-negative pulmonary TB (other than in Category I)	Preferred: 2 HRZE Optional: 2 HRZE Optional: 2 HRZE$_3$	Preferred: 4 HR, 4 HR$_3$ Optional: 6 HE Optional: 4 HR$_3$
Re-treatment pulmonary TB cases			
Category II	Relapses, treatment after default[+]	Preferred: 2 HRZES/1 HRZE Optional: 2 HRZES$_3$/1 HRZE$_3$	Preferred: 5 HRE Optional: 5 HRE$_3$

TB: tuberculosis; H: isoniazid; R: rifampicin; Z: pyrazinamide; E: ethambutol; S: streptomycin. [#]: Numbers preceding regimens indicate the length of treatment in months. Numbers following regimens indicate the frequency of administration per week. Where no number is given after the regimen, administration is daily. [¶]: The thrice weekly treatment was less effective than daily treatment as measured by conversion rates at 2 months, with a suggestion of less favourable outcomes overall; although the difference in outcome from the 8-month daily regimen was negligible. [+]: In settings with proven high prevalence of drug-resistant or multidrug-resistant TB cases, national programmes can design standardised regimens or can allow the use of individualised regimen, including second-line drugs to treat treatment failures of Category I.

Table 3. General principles for designing an empiric regimen to treat multidrug-resistant tuberculosis

Basic principles	Comments
Use at least four drugs of known effectiveness or that are highly likely to be effective	Effectiveness is supported by a number of factors (the more of them that are present, the more likely it is the drug will be effective): 1) susceptibility seen upon drug susceptibility testing 2) no previous history of treatment failure with drug 3) no known close contacts with resistance to drug 4) drug resistance screening indicates resistance is rare in similar patients 5) no common use of drug in the area If at least four drugs are not certain to be effective, use from five to seven drugs, depending on the specific drugs and level of uncertainty
Do not use drugs for which resistance crosses over	1) Rifamycins (rifampicin, rifabutin, rifapentin, rifalazil): have high level of cross-resistance 2) Fluoroquinolones: variable cross-resistance; *in vitro* data show some higher-generation agents remain susceptible when lower-generation agents are resistant (clinical significance of the phenomenon still unknown) 3) Aminoglycosides and polypeptides: not all cross-resist; in general, only kanamycin and amikacin fully cross-resist
Eliminate drugs likely to be unsafe for the patient	1) Known severe allergy or difficult-to-manage intolerance 2) High risk of severe adverse effects, including renal failure, deafness, hepatitis, depression and/or psychosis 3) Unknown or questionable drug quality

Table 3. Continued

Include drugs from groups 1–5 in a hierarchical order, based on potency	1) Use any group 1 (oral first-line) drugs that are likely to be effective (see the first entry in the Comments column of this table) 2) Use an effective injectable aminoglycoside or polypeptide (group 2) 3) Use a fluoroquinolone (group 3) 4) Use the remaining group 4 drugs to create a regimen consisting of at least four effective drugs. For regimens with up to four effective drugs, add second-line drugs that are likely to be effective, to give up to five to seven drugs in total, with at least four of them highly likely to be effective. The number of drugs will depend on the degree of uncertainty 5) Use group 5 drugs as needed so that at least four drugs are likely to be effective
Be prepared to prevent, monitor and manage adverse effects for each of the drugs selected	1) Ensure laboratory services for haematology, biochemistry, serology and audiometry are available 2) Establish a clinical and laboratory baseline before starting the regimen 3) Initiate treatment gradually for a difficult-to-tolerate drug, splitting daily doses of Eto/Pto, Cs and PAS 4) Ensure ancillary drugs are available to manage adverse effects 5) Organise intake supervision for all doses

Eto: ethionamide; Pto: prothionamide; Cs: cycloserine; PAS: P-amino salicylic acid.

Treatment with second-line anti-TB chemotherapy in MDR- and XDR-TB is frequently influenced by the occurrence of adverse drug events. Unfortunately, reliable indicators to individually guide the duration of anti-TB drug treatment are not available. For all the reasons previously listed, treatment of MDR- and XDR-TB cases should be managed in highly specialised reference centres, identified by national authorities.

Scaling-up of culture and DST capacities, and the expanded use of high-technology assays for rapid determination of resistance are necessary if better control of MDR- and XDR-TB is to be achieved. The majority of resistant cases can be treated successfully if well-designed regimens are used and surgical options are carefully considered. Nevertheless, the development of new (more effective and less toxic) drugs to treat patients is urgently needed. Adherence to internationally agreed standards of care and control practices is imperative.

References

- Fitzgerald D, Haas DW. *Mycobacterium tuberculosis. In*: Mandell GL, *et al.*, eds. Principles and Practice of Infectious Diseases. 6th Edn. Philadelphia, Churchill Livingstone, 2005; pp. 2852–2886.
- Frieden TR, *et al.* Tuberculosis. *Lancet* 2003; 362: 887–899.
- Hopewell PC, *et al.* International standards for tuberculosis care. *Lancet Infect Dis* 2006; 6: 710–725.
- Knechel NA. Tuberculosis: pathophysiology, clinical features and diagnosis. *Crit Care Nurse* 2009; 29: 34–43.
- Mack U, *et al.* LTBI: latent tuberculosis infection or lasting immune responses to *M. tuberculosis*? A TBNET consensus statement. *Eur Respir J* 2009; 33: 956–973.
- Raviglione MC, O'Brien RJ. Tuberculosis. *In*: Fauci AS, *et al.*, eds. Harrison's Principles of Internal Medicine. 17th Edn. New York, McGraw-Hill Medical Publishing Division Inc., 2008; pp. 1006–1020.
- Sotgiu G, *et al.* Epidemiology and clinical management of XDR-TB: a systematic review by TBNET. *Eur Respir J* 2009; 33: 871–881.
- World Health Organization. Global tuberculosis control 2009. Epidemiology, Strategy, Financing. Geneva, WHO, 2009.
- Wright A, *et al.* Epidemiology of antituberculosis drug resistance 2002-07: an updated analysis of the Global Project on Anti-Tuberculosis Drug Resistance Surveillance. *Lancet* 2009; 373: 1861–1873.

EXTRAPULMONARY TUBERCULOSIS

A. Bossink
Diakonessenhuis, Utrecht, The Netherlands
E-mail: aikbossink@mac.com

The World Health Organization (WHO) definition of extrapulmonary tuberculosis (EPTB) is: "A patient with tuberculosis of organs other than the lungs, *e.g.* pleura, lymph nodes, abdomen, genito-urinary tract, skin, joints and bones, and meninges. Diagnosis should be based on one culture-positive specimen, or histological or strong clinical evidence consistent with active extrapulmonary disease, followed by a decision by a clinician to treat with a full course of anti-tuberculosis chemotherapy".

A patient diagnosed with both pulmonary tuberculosis (PTB) and EPTB should be classified as a case of PTB.

The definition mentions neither the eyes nor the ear–nose–throat region. However, these tissues are also, but scarcely, possible localisations.

General aspects of EPTB

Only a minority of cases (<30%) suffer from EPTB. However this could be biased by the definition because in countries with a differentiated registry (PTB, EPTB, and EPTB+PTB), EPTB localisations comprise nearly 50% of all the cases.

In low-income countries, males appear to be affected by tuberculosis (TB) more often than females. However, this difference is not so clear in high-income countries; the mechanism is not clearly understood. No evidence is available to suggest that EPTB affects one of the sexes more frequently.

Immunosuppression appears to be an important cause for EPTB and is reflected by a sharp incline in reported cases of EPTB with the rise of the incidence of HIV infection. In high-income countries, and countries with a lower incidence of HIV infection, biological agents like tumour necrosis factor-α inhibitors are relatively important causes of EPTB.

"The result of tuberculous bacillaemia must be the insemination in various parts of the body of foci most of which remain latent." Therefore, EPTB can be the result of a primary infection in severely immunocompromised hosts or can be the result of reactivation of dormant bacilli in previously infected subjects.

Sites of EPTB

The two most common localisations of EPTB are the cervical lymph nodes and the pulmonary pleura. Other sites are, in declining order, bones and joints, meninges and central nervous system (CNS), abdominal lymph nodes, peritoneum and gastrointestinal tract, genito-urinary tract and pericardium.

> **Key points**
>
> - EPTB localisations appear in up to 50% of TB patients.
> - Obtaining culture confirmation is essential in the treatment of both PTB and EPTB.
> - Treatment of EPTB does not differ from PTB in the majority of EPTB localisations.

It should be noted that gastric aspirate in children with PTB often contains mycobacteria. This is, however, not an indication of EPTB but should be considered as a local spread of mycobacteria by swallowing sputum.

In immunocompromised hosts, the presentation of EPTB is often different compared with immunocompetent hosts. Dissemination of the disease is more common and clinicians should be aware of other localisations. Dissemination is more likely because ill-formed granuloma occur more frequently in immunocompromised hosts.

The term miliary TB refers to a radiological finding of the chest radiography and should not be used in this context.

Diagnosis

In countries with all possible diagnostic resources on average 70% of all the TB cases are culture confirmed. One can imagine that in EPTB samples are more difficult to obtain compared with PTB. Furthermore some of the EPTB localisations contain only few mycobacteria. Culture or PCR confirmation will thus be lower in these cases. Using the Dutch TB registry PTB is culture confirmed in nearly 80% and EPTB in about 60% of the cases.

Specific staining is in low-income countries often the only available diagnostic tool and because of the relative simplicity should always be undertaken.

Some promising reports on interferon-γ release assays in the diagnosis of EPTB (pleural and meningitis TB) have been published. However, these tests are no proof of active infection, they will not provide culture results or drug susceptibility reports and can therefore only be supportive in the search for mycobacteria. However, it remains most important to obtain materials for culture and drug susceptibility tests (DST).

Treatment

In general, treatment for EPTB does not differ from that for PTB. Depending on local or national guidelines, the treatment consists of a full course of at least four anti-TB drugs (isoniazid, rifampicin, ethambutol and pyrazinamide) in the first 2 months and than another 4-7 months of isoniazid and rifampicin in culture confirmed cases with normal drug susceptibility [D]. In countries with a high prevalence of drug resistance for one or more of these drugs, a fifth or even sixth drug should be added awaiting culture and DST.

Specific localisations

Cervical lymph nodes Involvement of the lymph nodes or lymphadenitis is the most common localisation of EPTB. Concomitant pulmonary infection occurs in 5-10% of the cases and therefore generalised symptoms are unusual. During medical treatment the lymph nodes can rapidly increase in size (paradox reaction) and to prevent fistula, fine-needle aspiration of its content may prove beneficial. In children, lymphadenitis is often caused by nontuberculous mycobacteria and this requires a different treatment approach. Confirmation of the causative organism is therefore crucial.

Other lymph nodes Other common sites of lymph node involvement are axillary, inguinal and abdominal. Culture results (*Mycobacterium tuberculosis* versus nontuberculous mycobacteria) for these localisations do not differ between children and adults.

TB of the pleura In general, the pleurisy is one sided and the majority of cases have a tendency toward spontaneous resolution. Therefore the diagnosis can be delayed for a prolonged period until a new effusion appears. Large amounts of pleural fluid are often observed with relatively low numbers of mycobacteria. An accompanying hypersensitivity reaction is held responsible for this phenomenon. Because of this low bacterial burden, the confirmation of TB can often be difficult. TB empyema is a rare condition compared with pleurisy and often requires surgical drainage and decortication combined with medical treatment.

TB of the meninges and CNS Meningitis is the most common presentation of involvement of the nervous system. The infection can cause hydrocephalus and through involvement of the cranial nerves paralysis of the nervus abducens. Classically the patient is not able to look outward with one eye and this eye is rotated towards the nose. Neurological deterioration is classified in three grades based on the performance on the Glasgow Coma Scale. Apart from antibiotic treatment, it is recommended to add steroids (0.5 mg·kg^{-1}) in stages II and III. Survival is positively influenced by this regimen, but neurological outcome is not better in the groups treated with steroids. Others recommend steroids independent of the stage. Antibiotic treatment should be at least 9 months. However, according to the British guidelines, treatment should be continued for 1 yr. The WHO recommends to replace ethambutol by streptomycin in TB meningitis

TB of the pericardium This condition is sometimes difficult to diagnose because, just like pleural effusion, the bacterial load is low. Pericardial effusion and, at a later stage, constrictive pericarditis can cause severe inflow limitation resulting in serious haemodynamic problems. Steroids are recommended to reduce the effusion and to prevent thickening of the pericardium adjuvant. No data is available on the amount and duration of steroid treatment. It appears reasonable to prescribe 0.5 mg·kg^{-1} for the first 2 months and than decrease the dose gradually to zero over a period of 4 months.

Bone and joint TB Any bone or joint can be affected, but the classical lesion is a fracture of the vertebrae resulting in a kyphotic change of the spine (Pott's disease). In general, the larger bones and joints are more often affected compared with the smaller ones. Joint involvement presents as a mono-arthritis. Diagnosis of both bone and joint involvement is generally made by biopsy. Aspiration of synovial fluid seldom yields the diagnosis. Medical treatment is the treatment of choice and should be prolonged to 9 months. Surgery is reserved for complicated cases such as neurological involvement or instability of the spine.

References

- World Health Organization. Global tuberculosis control – epidemiology, strategy, financing. Geneva, WHO, WHO/HTM/TB/2009.411.
- Wilkinson MC. Pathogenesis of non-pulmonary tuberculosis. *Br Med J* 1940; 2: 660-661.
- Thwaites GE, *et al*. Dexamethasone for the treatment of tuberculous meningitis in adolescents and adults. *N Engl J Med* 2004; 351: 1741-1751.
- Thwaites G, *et al*. British Infection Society guidelines for the diagnosis and treatment of tuberculosis of the central nervous system in adults and children. *J Infect* 2009; 59: 167-187.

Weblinks

- www.who.int/tb/publications/global_report/en/.
- ecdc.europa.eu/en/publications/Publications/1003_SUR_tuberculosis_surveillance_in_europe_2008.pd.
- www.kncvtbsurvey.nl/ziekte/index.php.
- www.who.int/tb/publications/tb_treatmentguidelines/en/index.html.

TUBERCULOSIS IN THE IMMUNOCOMPROMISED HOST

M. Sester
Dept of Transplant and Infection Immunology, Institute of Virology, University of the Saarland, Homburg, Germany
E-mail: martina.sester@uks.eu

The incidence of active tuberculosis (TB) is increased in patients with impaired cellular immunity, such as HIV-infected patients, solid-organ and stem cell transplant recipients, patients receiving tumour necrosis factor (TNF)-α antagonists and patients with end-stage renal failure. This emphasises the particular importance of the cellular arm of the adaptive immune response for efficient control of *Mycobacterium tuberculosis*. Moreover, the presence of *M. tuberculosis*-specific CD4 T-cell immunity is used as a surrogate marker for a previous contact. Consequently, a detailed knowledge of the pathomechanisms leading to increased incidence of TB in immunocompromised patients has also contributed to a better understanding of the principles of decreased test sensitivity in this vulnerable patient group.

Pathomechanisms of impaired TB control

The general incidence of TB in immunocompromised patients may vary depending on the geographical location and may range from <1% to up to 15% in low- and high-prevalence countries, respectively. The relative risk to develop TB and its underlying pathomechanisms may differ widely among the various groups due to differences in the cause and extent of immunodeficiency (table 1). The dramatic reduction in CD4 T-cell numbers in HIV-infected patients, in particular in those with AIDS, not only contributes to a severely impaired control of TB, but also to a high percentage of false-negative diagnoses by immune-based tests. Similarly, immunosuppressive drug-treatment after transplantation is associated with a decrease in T-cell function and may lead to a progressive decrease in *M. tuberculosis* specific T-cell immunity over time. This not only facilitates reactivation but also contributes to a decreased sensitivity of immune-based testing. The uraemia-associated immunodeficiency syndrome in patients with end-stage renal failure has been characterised by a defect in co-stimulatory signals to antigen-specific T-cells thereby contributing to an impaired efficiency of vaccinations and increased risk of infectious complications including TB. Finally, an increased incidence of active TB in patients receiving TNF-α antagonists is attributed to an impaired T-cell function and failure to maintain the integrity of granuloma in latently infected patients.

> **Key points**
>
> - TB has a higher incidence among people with impaired cellular immunity.
> - Diagnosis is often delayed owing to early lack of symptoms or unusual presentation.
> - Screening for latent TB infection prior to immunosuppresive treatments can be a useful preventive measure.

Table 1. Pathomechanisms and relative risk for TB in immunocompromised patients relative to persons without known risk factors (risk=1)

Risk factor	Relative risk	Pathomechanism
HIV infection (AIDS)	100–170	Low CD4 T-cell counts
HIV infection (no AIDS)	50–100	
Transplantation	20–74	Decreased T-cell function and numbers
Chronic renal failure	10–25	Co-stimulation deficiency, chronic inflammation
TNF-α antagonists	2–9	Disintegration of granuloma

Clinical presentation of active TB

Active TB in immunocompromised patients can pose a number of challenges. Due to the impaired immune response, patients may be clinically oligosymptomatic in the beginning of active disease and its diagnosis is often delayed due to atypical presentations and more frequent extrapulmonary dissemination. Active TB is further aggravated by a significantly higher morbidity due to a more fatal course in the face of a weakened immune system. In addition, treatment is frequently complicated due to complex drug interactions and altered pharmacokinetics. The treatment of TB is also more difficult to manage in HIV-infected patients, as immune restoration induced by anti-retroviral therapy may be responsible for a paradoxical worsening of TB manifestations, a phenomenon defined as immune reconstitution inflammatory syndrome.

Preventative approaches

The increased risk of active TB in immunocompromised patients may result from an immunosuppression-induced reactivation of a previously acquired latent TB infection (LTBI) or new infections. While the extent of new infections is difficult to control as it largely depends on the overall prevalence of TB, the risk of progression from LTBI to active disease may be minimised by the early identification and treatment of latently infected patients. Although risk assessment in immunocompromised patients is often hampered by a low sensitivity of commonly used immune-based tests, current guidelines recommend a regular screening for evidence of LTBI and, if possible, treatment prior to conditions of immunodeficiency, i.e. screening and treatment prior to transplantation or TNF-α antagonist therapy. Until recently, LTBI screening was exclusively carried out by the use of tuberculin skin-testing, where the cut-off of positivity is defined by the extent of immunodeficiency. At present, however, novel interferon-γ release assays (IGRA) are more widely applied that are of higher specificity as compared with skin-testing. In addition, accumulating evidence suggests that IGRA may be of higher sensitivity in immunocompromised patients although large studies, in particular in highly immunocompromised patients, are still lacking.

Conclusions

TB in immunocompromised patients is more frequent as compared with the general population, and morbidity and mortality is high. Risk assessment needs integrative approaches that should consider clinical findings, the extent of immunodeficiency and the overall prevalence of TB.

References

- Aaron L, et al. Tuberculosis in HIV-infected patients: a comprehensive review. *Clin Microbiol Infect* 2004; 10: 388–3983.
- Cooper AM. Cell-mediated immune responses in tuberculosis. *Ann Rev Immunol* 2009; 27: 393–422.
- Gardam MA, et al. Anti-tumour necrosis factor agents and tuberculosis risk: mechanisms of action and clinical management. *Lancet Infect Dis* 2003; 3: 148–155.
- Girndt M, et al. Molecular aspects of T- and B-cell function in uremia. *Kidney Int Suppl* 2001; 78: S206–S211.
- Menzies D, et al, Meta-analysis: new tests for the diagnosis of latent tuberculosis infection: areas of uncertainty and recommendations for research. *Ann Intern Med* 2007; 146: 340–354.

- Sester U, et al. Impaired detection of *Mycobacterium tuberculosis* immunity in patients using high levels of immunosuppressive drugs. *Eur Respir J* 2009; 34: 702–710.
- Singh N, Paterson DL. *Mycobacterium tuberculosis* infection in solid-organ transplant recipients: impact and implications for management. *Clin Infect Dis* 1998; 27: 1266–1277.
- Torre-Cisneros J, et al. Tuberculosis after solid-organ transplant: incidence, risk factors, and clinical characteristics in the RESITRA (Spanish Network of Infection in Transplantation) Cohort. *Clin Infect Dis* 2009; 48: 1657–1665.

LATENT TUBERCULOSIS

J-P. Zellweger
Swiss Lung Association, Berne, Switzerland
E-mail: zellwegerjp@swissonline.ch

Individuals who are in close contact with a patient with a transmissible form of tuberculosis (TB; usually smear-positive pulmonary TB) may inhale droplets containing mycobacteria, which settle in the airways and give rise to a local inflammatory reaction. The risk of infection is related to the concentration of mycobacteria in the air and the duration of contact. Some exposed individuals develop an active disease (TB) within a couple of weeks or months; others will control the incipient infection and stay for a prolonged period (up to years) in a state of equilibrium called 'latent infection' or 'latent TB'or LTBI.

LTBI and risk of TB

Individuals with latent TB have no signs or symptoms of active TB, and only immunological markers of a prior contact with mycobacteria. It is impossible to know if individuals with latent TB still harbour living mycobacteria. The only gold standard for the infection is the development of the disease, which happens in a minority of exposed individuals. Why and how the infected individuals will develop TB is unknown. Estimates are that ~10% of infected individuals may develop TB, half of them within 2 yrs after infection, and 90% will never develop the disease. Some infected individuals have a higher risk of later reactivation than others (for instance immunocompromised individuals, patients receiving immunosuppressive therapy and small children). As only a minority of contacts develop TB, there is a possibility that most contacts eradicate the mycobacteria but still retain an immunological marker of the primary contact, even in the absence of living mycobacteria.

Treatment of latent TB

As the persons in contact with a case of TB have a much higher risk of developing the disease in the future than the average population, particularly if they have a positive tuberculin reaction or a positive interferon-γ release assay (IGRA) test, the detection of latent TB among exposed contacts is important because a preventive treatment can reduce this risk. In countries or populations with a low incidence of TB, the search for latent infection among contacts and the

Key points

- The risk of latent TB infection (LTBI) depends on the intensity and duration of exposure to a source case with untreated pulmonary TB.

- Some infected contacts will develop TB at a later time-point. Timely detection of infected contacts and preventive treatment of those at highest risk of reactivation is cost-effective and reduces the pool of future cases of active TB.

- Before prescribing a preventive treatment, active TB should be excluded by a chest radiograph and, if abnormal, by a bacteriological examination of sputum.

- The tests for the detection of latent infection are the tuberculin skin test and the Interferon-Gamma Release Assays (IGRAs). The latter have the advantage of a greater specificity.

prescription of preventive treatment may contribute to the control of the disease by reducing the pool of potential future cases. The currently recommended preventive treatments are 9 months of isoniazid, 4 months of rifampicin or 3 months of an association of isoniazid and rifampicin.

As the immunological reaction after the contact with mycobacteria needs several days or weeks to be complete, the proof of a recent sensitisation is usually not present before this time (the window period). Therefore, the search for latent infection is usually performed only 4–8 weeks after the last contact. In some cases, where the progression from infection to disease may be rapid (such as immunocompromised contacts or children aged <5 yrs), a first testing with a clinical examination may be performed as soon as possible after the last contact and repeated several weeks later, if the results are negative. A test performed immediately after the last contact will usually indicate a prior sensitisation and may be observed among contacts born in a region with high prevalence of TB and in elderly people, independently of recent contacts.

Tests for detection of LTBI

The tests used for the detection of latent infection are all indirect and rely on the reaction between sensitised lymphocytes and antigens from *Mycobacterium tuberculosis*. The traditional test is the *tuberculin skin test* measuring the cutaneous reaction elicited by the intradermal injection of a mixture of antigens from *M. tuberculosis* cultures. New tests have recently been developed and introduced on the market, measuring *in vitro* the release of cytokines (interferon-γ) by lymphocytes incubated with two or three specific antigens present in *M. tuberculosis* but absent in *Mycobacterium bovis bacille-Calmette-Guerin* and in most nontuberculous mycobacteria (IGRAs). The *in vitro* tests are (at least) equally sensitive as the tuberculin test but have the advantage of a greater specificity, and therefore avoid in practice the false-positive skin reactions elicited by prior BCG vaccination or contact with nontuberculous mycobacteria.

Detection in low-prevalence countries

In low-prevalence countries, the search for infected individuals is usually performed among persons who recently had a contact with a patient with pulmonary TB (contact investigation), in healthcare workers potentially exposed to untreated cases of TB and in immunocompromised patients with a risk of reactivation higher than the general population. Infected contacts considered at risk of developing TB in the future are either followed clinically or offered a preventive treatment. All contacts with immunological signs of infection (positive tuberculin skin test or IGRA) should have at least a chest radiograph for detecting signs of past or recent TB. Before prescribing a preventive treatment in contacts with an abnormal chest radiograph, the presence of an active TB should be excluded by a bacteriological examination of sputum. The efficiency of the preventive treatment largely depends on the rate of treatment completion.

Detection in high-prevalence countries

In high-prevalence countries, formal contact investigations are usually not performed, as most of the contacts may already have immunological signs of prior infection, but it is currently recommended to search for the presence of secondary cases of TB among the close relatives and to consider the protection of small children with a preventive treatment if one of the parents has a form of transmissible TB.

Controversies and open questions

There are still controversies about the definition of infectiousness (only smear-positive cases or all cases with pulmonary TB), the extent of the contact investigation (only close and prolonged contacts or all contacts) and about the indications of preventive treatment (only infected contact with a high risk of reactivation or all contacts or individuals with a positive tuberculin or IGRA reaction). Prospective studies on the risk of reactivation among contacts with a positive immunological reaction will help to clarify these issues.

References

- American Thoracic Society, Targeted tuberculin testing and treatment of latent tuberculosis infection. Joint Statement of the American Thoracic Society (ATS) and the Centers for Disease Control and Prevention (CDC). *Am J Respir Crit Care Med* 2000; 161: S221-S247.
- Andersen P, et al. The prognosis of latent tuberculosis: can disease be predicted? *Trends Mol Med* 2007; 13: 175-182.
- Cardona PJ. New insights on the nature of latent tuberculosis infection and its treatment. *Inflamm Allergy Drug Targets* 2007; 6: 27-39.
- Diel R, et al. Cost-effectiveness of isoniazid chemoprevention in close contacts. *Eur Respir J* 2005; 26: 465-473.
- Diel R, et al. Predictive value of a whole-blood IFN-γ assay for the development of active TB disease. *Am J Respir Crit Care Med* 2008; 15: 1164-1170.
- Ferebee SH. Controlled chemoprophylaxis trials in tuberculosis A general review. *Adv Tuberc Res* 1970; 17: 28-106.
- Landry J, Menzies D. Preventive chemotherapy. Where has it got us? Where to go next? *Int J Tuberc Lung Dis* 2008; 12: 1352-1364.
- Mack U, et al. LTBI: latent tuberculosis infection or lasting immune responses to *M. tuberculosis*? A TBNET consensus statement. *Eur Respir J* 2009; 33: 956-973.
- Moran-Mendoza O, et al. Tuberculin skin test size and risk of tuberculosis development: a large population-based study in contacts. *Int J Tuberc Lung Dis* 2007; 11: 1014-1020.
- Pai M, et al. Systematic review: T-cell-based assays for the diagnosis of latent tuberculosis infection: an update. *Ann Intern Med* 2008; 149: 177-184.

NONTUBERCULOUS MYCOBACTERIAL DISEASE

C. Piersimoni
Regional Reference Mycobacteriology Laboratory, United Hospitals, Ancona, Italy
E-mail: piersim@tin.it

Nontuberculous mycobacteria (NTM) is the term indicating those *Mycobacterium* species that are different from *Mycobacterium tuberculosis* complex (MTC) and *Mycobacterium leprae* whose detection in clinical samples is almost invariably associated with disease. The most important features distinguishing NTM from MTC include a lower pathogenicity and the lack of human-to-human transmission. In addition, *in vitro* resistance to first-line antituberculous drugs is another important distinctive issue. The majority of the >120 NTM species recognised currently has been associated with disease in man or animals.

Epidemiology and pathogenesis

NTM are widely distributed in both natural and man-made environments; organisms can be found in soil and water with high isolation rates. Human disease is suspected to be acquired from environmental exposure and pulmonary infection is likely to depend on the aerosol route. Although much remains to be understood about the pathogenesis of NTM infections, the following is now well established:

- In HIV-infected patients, disseminated NTM infections occur only after the CD4+ T-lymphocyte count has dropped below $50 \cdot \mu L^{-1}$.
- In HIV-uninfected patients, NTM infections may be associated with specific mutations in interferon-γ and interleukin-12 synthesis and response pathways.

The most common clinical manifestation of NTM infection is pulmonary disease, but lymphatic, skin/soft tissue, osteoarticular and disseminated disease are also important.

Pulmonary disease

In immunocompetent subjects, NTM lung disease presents as one of the following clinical forms:

Cavitary lung disease This pattern, which closely resembles pulmonary TB, involves the upper lobes of older males usually affected by a pre-existing destructive or obstructive lung condition such as pneumoconiosis, chronic bronchitis with emphysema (frequently associated with long-lasting, heavy smoking) and bronchiectasis. Thin-walled cavities with scarce parenchymal infiltrate and a marked pleural thickening are characteristic. Signs

---

Key points

- Important features distinguishing NTM from *M. tuberculosis* complex include lower pathogenicity and lack of human-to-human transmission.
- Diagnosis of NTM disease requires both clinical and microbiological criteria to be met.
- Treatment is disappointing and is characterised by long duration and side-effects, leading to poor compliance.

and symptoms include chronic cough with sputum production and weakness. With advanced disease, dyspnoea, fever, weight loss and haemoptysis can also occur.

Nodular bronchiectasis This pattern (also known as *Lady Windermere's syndrome*) has been described in slender elderly females with structural chest abnormalities (pectus excavatum, scoliosis and mitral valve prolapse), but no evidence of pre-existing lung disease. Indolent productive cough and purulent sputum are the most common presenting symptoms, while constitutional symptoms and haemoptysis are not common unless extensive disease is present. The radiographic findings include small nodular infiltrates and cylindrical bronchiectasis, predominately located within the middle lobe and lingula.

Hypersensivity pneumonitis (HP) A syndrome indistinguishable from HP has been reported in subjects exposed to household water laden with *Mycobacterium avium* complex (MAC) organisms (hot tubs and medicinal baths). Full recovery usually occurs without any specific therapy (simply by avoiding further contact with contaminated solutions), but sometimes a combination therapy of steroids and antibiotics may be required.

In addition, NTM lung disease may be associated with the following conditions:

- HIV infection. Although NTM are frequently recovered from respiratory specimens of HIV-infected subjects, extrapulmonary or disseminated disease are more likely to occur. The most relevant exception to this generalisation is given by *Mycobacterium kansasii*.
- Immune reconstitution inflammatory syndrome.
- Transplantation including both solid-organ and haematopoietic stem cell transplants.
- Treatment with tumour necrosis factor-α antagonists.
- Cystic fibrosis.

Laboratory diagnosis

Mycobacterial culture remains the cornerstone with which to make a definitive diagnosis. Therefore, appropriate, high-quality specimens properly collected from all patients with suspected NTM disease have to be sent to a certified laboratory. Due to the ubiquitous occurrence of NTM in the environment, the recognition of disease as opposed to contamination of specimens or transient colonisation may be difficult. While smear-positive samples strongly suggest an active disease, a single positive culture (especially with small numbers of organisms) does not suffice to set such a diagnosis. In this context, the American Thoracic Society has recently updated the criteria for the diagnosis of pulmonary disease caused by NTM (table 1).

It is necessary to fulfil all the above elements to establish a correct diagnosis. Although these criteria are derived from experience with MAC, it is reasonable to believe they would work with other species provided that contamination of clinical specimens and medical devices with environmental NTM (pseudoinfection) has been excluded. Today, the combined use of automated liquid culture for detection and drug susceptibility testing (DST) plus the use of genetic probe technology for identification of mycobacteria

Table 1. American Thoracic Society criteria for diagnosis of pulmonary disease caused by NTM

Clinical criteria (both required):
Pulmonary symptoms, cavitary or noncavitary lung disease
Appropriate exclusion of other causes for the disease

Microbiological criteria (only one required):
Positive culture results from at least two separate expectorated sputum samples
Positive culture results from at least one bronchial wash or lavage
A transbronchial or lung biopsy showing granulomata and/or acid-fast bacilli (AFB) and positive culture for NTM
Biopsy showing granulomata and/or AFB and one or more sputa or bronchial washings that are culture-positive for NTM

Table 2. Clinical and radiographic features of pulmonary infections caused by the most frequently encountered NTM

Species	Pathogenicity; outcome	Radiographic findings	Treatment (time in months)
Mycobacterium avium complex	++; poor/fair	Upper lobe cavitations	Clarithromycin, ethambutol, rifampin (18)
		Middle lobe bronchiectasis	Clarithromycin, ethambutol, rifampin (18)
Mycobacterium kansasii	+++; good	Upper lobe cavitations	Rifampin, isoniazid, ethambutol (18)
Mycobacterium malmoense	+++; fair	Upper lobe infiltrates	Rifampin, ethambutol (24)
Mycobacterium xenopi	+; poor	Upper lobe cavitations and nodules	Clarithromycin, rifampin, ethambutol, moxifloxacin (18)
Mycobacterium szulgai	+++; good	Upper lobe cavitations	Rifampin, isoniazid, ethambutol, pyrazinamide (18)
Mycobacterium simiae	+; poor	Upper lobe cavitations and nodules	Clarithromycin, moxifloxacin cotrimoxazole (18)
Mycobacterium abscessus	++; poor	Multilobar interstitial and nodular lesions	Clarithromycin, amikacin, cefoxitin (1); surgical resection

+: number of + indicates degree of pathogenicity. Reproduced from PIERSIMONI and SCARPARO (2008), with permission from the publisher.

is mandatory in all laboratories wishing to perform mycobacteriology.

Treatment

Treatment regimens for NTM disease are still largely undefined and outcome remains disappointing despite considerable upgrading in mycobacteriology and the availability of some new antimicrobials. Treatment success is impaired by the long duration of regimens, their side-effects and drug interactions, which prevent patients from full compliance (table 2). In addition, although many NTM species may be susceptible *in vitro* to one or more antituberculous drugs, correlation between DST results and clinical outcome is poor.

References

- Clinical and Laboratory Standard Institute. Laboratory Detection and Identification of Mycobacteria. M48-A. Forbes, BA, CLSI, 2008.
- Field SK, Cowie RL. Lung disease due to the more common nontuberculous mycobacteria. *Chest* 2006; 129: 1653-1672.
- Fujita G, et al. Radiological findings of mycobacterial diseases. *J Infect Chemother* 2007; 13: 8-17.
- Glassroth J. Pulmonary disease due to nontuberculous mycobacteria. *Chest* 2008; 133: 243-251.
- Griffith DE, et al. An official ATS/IDSA statement: diagnosis, treatment, and prevention of nontuberculous mycobacterial diseases. *Am J Respir Crit Care Med* 2007; 175: 367-416.
- Mangione E, et al. Nontuberculous mycobacterial disease following hot tub exposure. *Emerg Infect Dis* 2001; 7: 1039-1042.
- National Committee for Clinical Laboratory Standards. Susceptibility Testing of Mycobacteria, Nocardiae, and Other Aerobic Actinomycetes. M24-A. Wayne, PA, NCCLS, 2003.
- Piersimoni C, Scarparo C. Pulmonary infections associated with non-tuberculous mycobacteria in immunocompetent patients. *Lancet Inf Dis* 2008; 8: 323-334.
- Prince DS, et al. Infection with *Mycobacterium avium* complex in patients without predisposing conditions. *N Engl J Med* 1989; 321: 863-868.
- Tortoli E. Impact of genotypic studies on mycobacterial taxonomy: the new mycobacteria of the 1990s. *Clin Microbiol Rev* 2003; 16: 319-354.

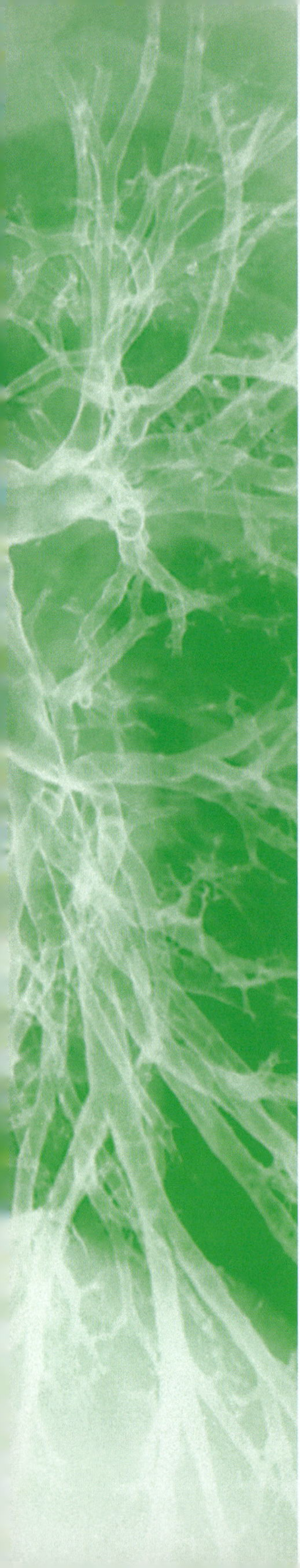

CHAPTER 9:

AIRWAY DISEASES

CHRONIC RHINITIS A. Bourdain and P. Chanez	**224**
ASTHMA B. Beghé and L.M. Fabbri	**227**
VOCAL CORD DYSFUNCTION A.H. Mansur	**236**
BRONCHITIS G. Rohde	**240**
GASTRO-OESOPHAGEAL REFLUX L. Dupont	**242**
COPD AND EMPHYSEMA E.G. Tzortzaki, K.D. Samara and N.M. Siafakas	**246**
BRONCHIECTASIS N. Ten Hacken	**252**
CYSTIC FIBROSIS A. Bush and J. Davies	**256**

CHRONIC RHINITIS

A. Bourdin[1] and P. Chanez[2]
[1] Department of Respiratory Disease, CHU Arnaud de Villeneuve, Montpellier, and [2] Service de Pneumo-Allergologie et Laboratoire d'Immunologie INSERM U600, Université de la Méditerranée, AP-HM Marseille, France
E-mail: pascal.chanez@univmed.fr

Rhinitis is one of the commonest human diseases. Its most important features are inflammation and structural changes of the nasal mucosa. The causes are heterogeneous and, if allergy and infections are dominant, it is often difficult to find a single common aetiology in chronic rhinitis. It is important to consider that rhinitis is often associated with sinusitis and lower airway diseases such as asthma. Rhinitis is a mild disease, but it interferes with sleep quality and daily life.

Epidemiology

Rhinitis is still increasing in prevalence in most countries. In some studies, 25–30% of the population is suffering from rhinitis, often linked to immunooglobulin (Ig)E sensitisation. It may increase with age, as demonstrated in both children and adults, and there is growing evidence that emerging countries are affected by an increase in prevalence. Thus, rhinitis is an important health problem worldwide. It affects health-related quality of life in both adults and children. It is usually a mild disease, but its direct and indirect costs are substantial. Absenteeism at school or at work is often reported by subjects suffering from rhinitis. Rhinitis is often associated with other IgE-related disease and the continuum linking upper and lower airways is well represented by the association of rhinitis and asthma, which frequently coexist: asthma is present in 20–50% of patients with allergic rhinitis. Rhinitis is present in up to 80% of asthma patients. Whether allergic rhinitis precedes, triggers or precipitates asthma is something that requires supportive data. Atopic status plays a potentially prominent role in this relationship, although it is not a prerequisite. The risk factors for rhinitis need to be better known and understood in order for preventive measures to be implemented.

Definition and clinical aspects of rhinitis

Allergic rhinitis is defined as inflammation of the nasal mucosa characterised clinically by nasal discharge, blockage, sneezing and itch, with two or more symptoms occurring for >1 h on most days. It can be further classified as intermittent (symptoms occurring on <4 days out of 7 or for <4 weeks per year) or persistent (symptoms occurring on ⩾4 days out of 7 or for ⩾4 weeks per year). The impact of chronic rhinitis on sleep, daily activities, work or school is a major determinant of quality-of-life impairment in patients. The perception of nasal symptoms is highly variable, a fact illustrated in patients suffering from chronic obstructive pulmonary

> **Key points**
>
> - The prevalence of rhinitis is increasing in most countries.
> - Asthma is present in 20–50% of allergic rhinitis patients, while up to 80% of asthma patients have rhinitis.
> - Treatment is anti-inflammatory and directed according to whether rhinitis is allergic or nonallergic.

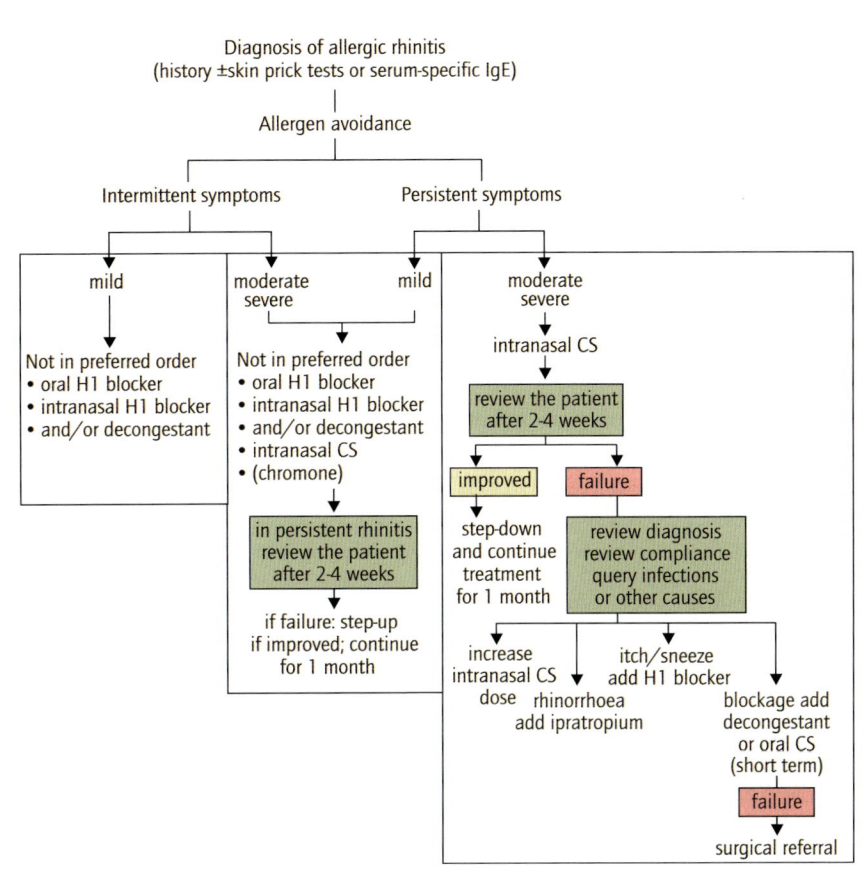

Figure 1. Treatment algorithm for allergic rhinitis. Ig: immunoglobulin; CS: corticosteroids. Reproduced from the ARIA guidelines, with permission from the publisher.

disease, where a discrepancy between nasal inflammation and symptoms has been demonstrated. From a clinical point of view, it is thus difficult to rely on patients' reports of symptoms as the only way to assess rhinitis.

Nonallergic rhinitis is difficult to differentiate clinically from allergic rhinitis. Exacerbations are usually associated with infections but several other triggers, including drugs, may cause recurrent symptoms.

Pathological and mechanistic aspects

Pseudostratified epithelium and a large highly developed vasculature cover the nasal wall. Tight junctions, peptidases and a large antioxidant apparatus are key features of the anatomical barrier of the nasal epithelium. The mucosal-associated lymphoid tissue is developed in the nose. Structural abnormalities including changes of the basement membrane have been reported in rhinitis. Inflammatory cells such as eosinophils, mast cells, T-cells and macrophages infiltrate the epithelium and submucosa. Mast cell-derived inflammatory mediators are overexpressed, such as histamine, chemokines and cytokines including interleukin (IL)-5, RANTES, IL-4, IL-13, granulocyte macrophage colony-stimulating factor. Most of these molecules trigger a local eosinophilic inflammatory process. Allergens, microorganisms and pollutants are potential triggers that can generate acute and chronic inflammatory reactions through the epithelium. The release of various mediators is responsible for most of the clinical symptoms reported by patients. Nasal hypersecretion, sneezing and itching are related to the release of vasoactive and proinflammatory mediators such as histamine and sulphido-leukotrienes. Persistent nasal obstruction is linked to the perpetuation of inflammatory reactions mostly related, in allergic rhinitis, to eosinophilic infiltration.

Effects of anti-inflammatory treatment

Intranasal corticosteroids and intranasal or oral antihistamines, have been shown to have effects on different aspects of inflammation in allergic rhinitis. Additionally, intranasal anticholinergic therapy provides relief for excessive rhinorrhoea, while leukotriene antagonists block the cysteinyl leukotriene receptor. Nasal obstruction improves significantly more with intranasal corticosteroids compared with most of the other pharmacological strategies. Specific immunotherapy using sublingual, oral or subcutaneous routes has been proven effective and safe in intermittent and persistent allergic rhinitis. Allergen avoidance is not effective in persistent allergic rhinitis. Several studies have demonstrated that the effective treatment of rhinitis decreases the burden of asthma as assessed by unscheduled visits to physicians and emergency rooms due to acute exacerbations.

Treatment should be directed according to the cause: nonallergic rhinitis should be treated by nasal decongestant and anticholinergic therapy. Allergic rhinitis should be treated according to the ARIA guidelines (fig. 1).

The term rhinitis covers a heterogeneous group of diseases. Allergic rhinitis and its associated diseases have been well defined and treatment is codified. Mucosal inflammation is the hallmark of rhinitis. Its natural history and its relationship with sinusitis and lower airways diseases need to be clarified. New treatments and management strategies are required, especially in the most chronic severe forms.

References

- Bousquet PJ, *et al.* ARIA (Allergic Rhinitis and its Impact on Asthma) classification of allergic rhinitis severity in clinical practice in France. *Int Arch Allergy Immunol* 2007; 143: 163–169.
- Carr WW, *et al.* Managing rhinitis: Strategies for improved patient outcomes. *Allergy Asthma Proc* 2008; 29: 349–357.
- Chanez P, *et al.* Comparison between nasal and bronchial inflammation in asthmatic and control subjects. *Am J Respir Crit Care Med* 1999; 159: 588–595.
- Lipworth BJ, White PS. Allergic inflammation in the unified airway: start with the nose. *Thorax* 2000; 55: 878–881.
- Raherison C, *et al.* How should nasal symptoms be investigated in asthma? A comparison of radiologic and endoscopic findings. *Allergy* 2004; 59: 821–826.
- Togias A. Rhinitis and asthma: evidence for respiratory system integration. *J Allergy Clin Immunol* 2003; 111: 1171–1183.

Weblink

- Allergic Rhinitis and its Impact on Asthma. www.whiar.org.

ASTHMA

B. Beghé and L.M. Fabbri
Dept of Oncology Haematology and Respiratory Diseases, Policlinico di Modena, University of Modena and Reggio Emilia, Italy
E-mail: leonardo.fabbri@unimore.it

Asthma is a chronic inflammatory disease of the airways, characterised clinically by recurrent respiratory symptoms: dyspnoea, wheezing, chest tightness and/or cough, almost always associated with reversible airflow limitation. Other characteristics of asthma are an exaggerated responsiveness of the airways to various stimuli, and in most cases a rather specific chronic inflammation of the airways characterised by an increased number of $CD4^+$ Th2 lymphocytes, eosinophils and methacromatic cells in the airway mucosa, and increased thickness of the reticular layer of the epithelial basement membrane.

Familial predisposition, atopy, and exposure to allergens and sensitising agents are important risk factors for asthma, even though the causes of asthma – the factors responsible for the development of asthma rather than its exacerbations – remain largely undetermined.

Asthma is a heterogeneous syndrome that, over the years, has been divided into many clinical subtypes, *e.g.* allergic asthma, adult-onset asthma that is usually nonallergic, occupational asthma, asthma in smokers and asthma in the obese.

Minimum requirements for the diagnosis of asthma

The diagnosis of asthma is based on clinical history and lung function tests, particularly peak expiratory flow (PEF) and spirometry, with assessment of variable and/or reversible airflow limitation. Allergy tests are also usually performed during the first assessment of a patient with suspected asthma to identify possible triggers of asthma and to guide their avoidance.

Asthma clusters in families, and its genetic determinants appear to be linked to those of other allergic immunoglobulin (Ig) E-mediated diseases. Thus, a personal or family history of asthma and/or allergic rhinitis, atopic dermatitis or eczema increases the likelihood of a diagnosis of asthma.

Symptoms and medical history

Most patients with asthma seek medical attention because of respiratory symptoms. A typical feature of asthma symptoms is their variability. One or more of the following symptoms: wheezing, chest tightness, and/or episodic shortness of breath are reported by >90% of patients with asthma. However, the presence of these symptoms is not diagnostic, because identical symptoms may be triggered

---

Key points

- Asthma is diagnosed based on clinical history and lung function testing. Allergy testing may also have a role.

- The differential diagnosis is extensive. In particular, COPD may be difficult to distinguish from asthma.

- The goal of pharmacological asthma treatment is to achieve and maintain control of symptoms and prevention of exacerbations.

- Asthma is a chronic, lifelong disease and must therefore be managed in partnership with the patient.

by different stimuli in nonasthmatics, *e.g.* by acute viral infections. In some asthmatics, wheezing and chest tightness are absent, and the only symptom the patient complains of is chronic cough ("cough-variant asthma").

Symptoms of asthma may be triggered or worsened by several factors, such as exercise, exposure to allergens, viral infections and emotions. Recurrent exacerbations of respiratory symptoms, worsening of lung function requiring change of treatment, unscheduled requests for medical assistance and sometimes hospitalisation are also among the characteristic clinical features of asthma.

Physical activity is an important trigger of symptoms (wheezing and/or cough) for most asthma patients, particularly children. For some, it is the only cause. Exercise-induced asthma usually develops not during exercise but 5–10 min afterwards, and it resolves spontaneously within 30–45 min. Prompt relief of symptoms after the use of inhaled β_2-agonist, or prevention by pre-treatment with an inhaled β_2-agonist before exercise, supports a diagnosis of asthma. Important aspects of personal history are exposure to agents known to worsen asthma in the home (some types of heating or cooking system, house dust mites), workplace conditions, air-conditioning, pets, cockroaches, environmental tobacco smoke or even the general environment, *e.g.* diesel fumes in traffic.

Since the respiratory symptoms of asthma are nonspecific, the differential diagnosis is quite extensive. The main goal for the physician is to consider and exclude other possible diagnoses (table 1). This is even more important if the response to a trial of therapy (bronchodilators) has been negative.

While respiratory symptoms suggest asthma, the *sine qua non* for the objective diagnosis of asthma is the presence of reversible airflow limitation in subjects with persistent airway obstruction, and/or airway hyperresponsiveness or increased PEF variability in subjects without airway obstruction.

Physical examination

In mild asthma, physical examination is usually normal under stable conditions but becomes characteristically abnormal during asthma attacks and when asthma is more severe or uncontrolled. Typical physical signs of asthma attacks are wheezing on auscultation, cough, expiratory rhonchi throughout the chest and signs of acute hyperinflation (*e.g.* poor diaphragmatic excursion at percussion, use of accessory muscles of respiration). Some patients, particularly children, may present with a predominant nonproductive cough (cough-variant asthma). In some asthmatics, wheezing – which usually reflects airflow limitation – may be absent or detectable only on forced expiration, even in the presence of significant airflow limitation; this may be due to hyperinflation or to very marked airflow limitation. In these patients, however, the severity of asthma is mostly indicated by other signs, such as cyanosis, drowsiness, difficulty in speaking, tachycardia, hyperinflated chest, use of accessory muscles and intercostal recession.

Lung function tests

Spirometry Lung function tests play a crucial role in the diagnosis and follow-up of asthma. Spirometric measurements – FEV_1 and slow vital capacity (VC) or forced vital capacity (FVC) – are the standard means for assessing airflow limitation. Spirometry is recommended at the time of diagnosis and for the assessment of the severity of both asthma and chronic obstructive pulmonary disease (COPD). It should be repeated to monitor the disease and when there is a need for reassessment, such as during exacerbations.

Measurements of residual volume and total lung capacity may also be useful in determining the degree of hyperinflation and/or enlargement of airspaces. Lung volumes may help in the differential diagnosis with COPD, but are not necessary for the diagnosis nor for the assessment of severity of asthma. In asthma, airflow limitation is usually reversible, either spontaneously or after

Table 1. Differential diagnosis of asthma

Localised pathology
 Inhaled foreign body
 Endobronchial tumour
 Vocal cord dysfunction

Diffuse airway pathology
 Chronic obstructive pulmonary disease
 Eosinophilic bronchitis
 Post-infectious airway hyperresponsiveness
 Cystic fibrosis
 Bronchiectasis
 Left ventricular failure

Other pathologies
 Gastro-oesophageal reflux
 Pulmonary embolism
 Pulmonary eosinophilia syndromes
 Drug-induced airway hyperresponsiveness

treatment, except for moderate/severe asthma with fixed airway obstruction (see below).

An important tool for the diagnosis and subsequent monitoring of asthma treatment is the PEF meter. If spirometry does not reveal airflow limitation, the home monitoring of PEF for 2-4 weeks may help to detect an increased variability of airway calibre, and thus to diagnose. Daily monitoring of PEF (at least in the morning at awakening and in the evening hours, preferably after bronchodilator inhalation) is also useful to assess the severity of asthma and its response to treatment, and it can help patients to detect early signs of asthma deterioration. Diurnal variability is calculated as follows:

(PEFmax − PEFmin) / [(PEFmax + PEFmin) / 2] × 100

A diurnal PEF variability of >20% is diagnostic of asthma, and the magnitude of the variability is broadly proportional to disease severity. PEF monitoring may be of use not only in establishing a diagnosis of asthma and assessing its severity but also in uncovering an occupational cause for asthma. When used in this way, PEF should be measured more frequently than twice daily, and special attention should be paid to changes occurring in and out of the workplace.

Reversibility to bronchodilators

Reversibility to bronchodilators (*i.e.* a >12% reversibility response and >200 mL in FEV_1 after bronchodilator) confirms the diagnosis of asthma. Poorly reversible airflow limitation is usually defined by the absolute reduction of post-bronchodilator FEV_1/FVC ratios to <0.7. However, because this parameter decreases with ageing, it should be confirmed with postbronchodilator FEV_1/VC values below the lower limit of normal. Reversibility is often not present at the time of examination,

Table 2. History, symptoms and results of pulmonary function tests in the differential diagnosis between asthma and COPD

	Asthma	**COPD**
Onset	Mainly in childhood	In mid to late adult life
Smoking	Usually nonsmokers	Almost invariably smokers
Chronic cough and sputum	Absent	Frequent (chronic bronchitis)
Dyspnoea on effort	Variable and reversible to treatment	Constant, poorly reversible and progressive
Nocturnal symptoms	Relatively common	Relatively uncommon
Airflow limitation	Increased diurnal variability	Normal diurnal variability
Response to bronchodilator	Good	Poor
Airway hyperresponsiveness	In most patients, with or without airflow limitation	In most patients with airflow limitation

Table 3. Ancillary tests in the differential diagnosis between stable asthma and COPD

Ancillary test	Asthma	COPD
Reversibility to bronchodilator and/or glucocorticosteroids	Usually present	Usually absent
Lung volumes Residual volume, total lung capacity Diffusing capacity	Usually normal or, if increased, reversible Normal	Usually irreversibly increased Decreased
Airway hyperresponsiveness	Increased	Might be increased but usually not measurable due to airflow limitation
Allergy tests	Often positive	Often negative
Imaging of the chest	Usually normal	Usually abnormal in advanced stages
Sputum	Eosinophilia	Neutrophilia
Exhaled nitric oxide	Increased	Usually normal

particularly in patients on treatment, and thus the absence of reversibility does not exclude the diagnosis. However, repeated testing of reversibility of both clinical features and functional abnormalities may be useful in obtaining the best level of asthma control achievable and/or the best lung function for individual patients. Achieving and maintaining lung function at the best possible level is one of the objectives of asthma management.

Airway hyperresponsiveness In patients who have symptoms consistent with asthma but who have normal lung function, bronchial provocation tests with methacholine, histamine or exercise are helpful in measuring airway hyperresponsiveness and thereby confirming or excluding the diagnosis of active asthma. These measurements are very sensitive, but poorly specific for a diagnosis of asthma. This means that while a negative test can be used to exclude a diagnosis of active asthma, a positive test does not always mean that a patient has asthma. While the measurement of airway hyperresponsiveness may be useful to confirm asthma in subjects with normal baseline lung function, it is not useful in presence of nonreversible airflow limitation, and thus in the differential diagnosis between asthma and COPD.

Arterial blood gases

In severe asthma and, more importantly, during acute exacerbations of asthma, the measurement of arterial blood gases while the patient is breathing air and/or after oxygen administration is essential for the diagnosis of chronic and/or acute respiratory failure. This test should be performed in all patients with clinical signs of acute or chronic respiratory and/or heart failure, and anyway in patients with a PEF <50%, those who do not respond to treatment and those with an arterial oxygen saturation ⩽92%.

Allergy tests

The presence of allergic disorders in a patient's family history should be investigated in all patients with symptoms of asthma. A history provides important information about the patient's lifestyle and occupation, both of which influence exposure to allergens and the time and factors possibly involved in onset and in exacerbations of asthma. Skin tests with all relevant allergens present in the geographic area in which the patient lives are the primary diagnostic tool in determining allergic status. Measurement of specific IgE is not usually more informative than a skin test, and is more expensive. Measurement of total IgE in serum has no value as a diagnostic test

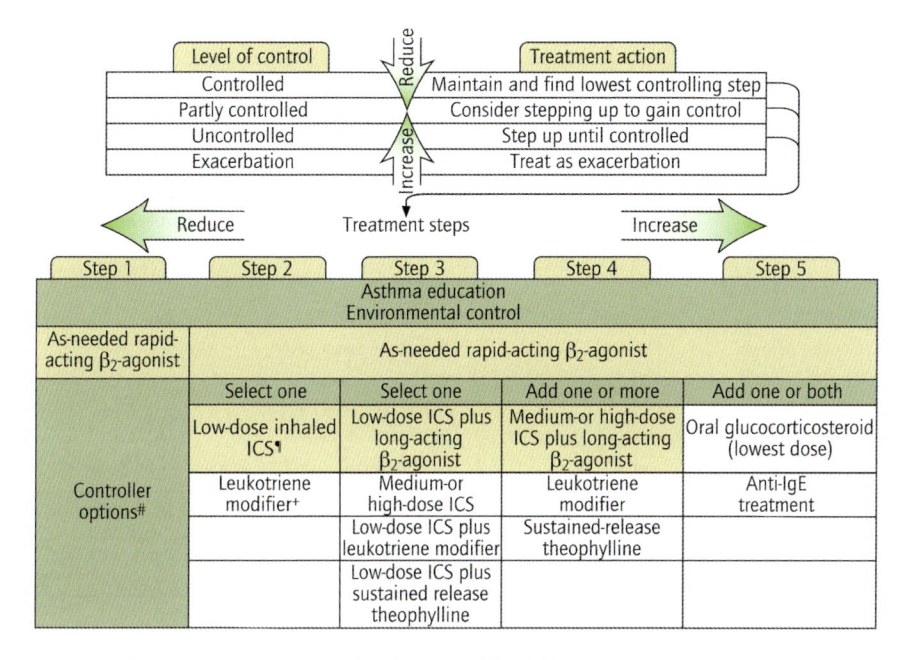

Level of control	Treatment action
Controlled	Maintain and find lowest controlling step
Partly controlled	Consider stepping up to gain control
Uncontrolled	Step up until controlled
Exacerbation	Treat as exacerbation

← Reduce — Treatment steps — Increase →

	Step 1	Step 2	Step 3	Step 4	Step 5
		Asthma education Environmental control			
	As-needed rapid-acting β_2-agonist	As-needed rapid-acting β_2-agonist			
		Select one	Select one	Add one or more	Add one or both
Controller options#		Low-dose inhaled ICS¶	Low-dose ICS plus long-acting β_2-agonist	Medium- or high-dose ICS plus long-acting β_2-agonist	Oral glucocorticosteroid (lowest dose)
		Leukotriene modifier+	Medium- or high-dose ICS	Leukotriene modifier	Anti-IgE treatment
			Low-dose ICS plus leukotriene modifier	Sustained-release theophylline	
			Low-dose ICS plus sustained release theophylline		

Figure 1. Asthma management approach based on control for children aged >5 yrs, adolescents and adults. Alternative reliever treatments include inhaled anticholinergics, short-acting oral β_2-agonists, some long-acting β_2-agonists, and short-acting theophylline. Regular dosing with short and long-acting β_2-agonist is not advised unless accompanied by regular use of an inhaled glucocorticosteriod. ICS: inhaled corticosteroids; IgE: immunoglobulin E. #: Preferred controller options are shown in shaded boxes; ¶: inhaled glucorticosteroids; +: Receptor antagonist or symthesis inhibitors. Reproduced from the Global Strategy for Asthma Management and Prevention, with permission.

for atopy. The main limitation of methods to assess allergic status is that a positive test does not necessarily mean that the disease is allergic in nature or that it is causing asthma, as some individuals have specific IgE antibodies without any symptoms and it may not be causally involved. The relevant exposure and its relation to symptoms must be confirmed by patient history.

Additional tests

While the diagnosis and assessment of severity of asthma and COPD can be fully established on the basis of clinical history and lung function tests (including arterial blood gases – see below), additional tests might be helpful to better characterise individual patients.

Imaging While chest radiography may be useful to exclude diseases that may mimic asthma, it is not required in the confirmation of the diagnosis and management of asthma. The utility of chest radiography is to exclude other conditions that may imitate or complicate asthma, particularly acute asthma. Examples include pneumonia, cardiogenic pulmonary oedema, pulmonary thromboembolism, tumours (especially those that result in airway obstruction with resulting peripheral atelectasis) and pneumothorax.

Assessment of airway inflammation

While airway biopsies and bronchoalveolar lavage may provide useful information in research protocols, they are considered too invasive for the diagnosis or staging of asthma. By contrast, noninvasive markers of airway inflammation have been increasingly used in research protocols, particularly to

Table 4. Levels of asthma control

Characteristic	Controlled (all of the following)	Partly controlled (any measure present in any week)	Uncontrolled
Daytime symptoms	None (twice or less per week)	More than twice per week	Three or more features of partly controlled asthma present in any week
Limitations of activities	None	Any	
Nocturnal symptoms/ awakening	None	Any	
Need for reliever/ rescue treatment	None (twice or less per week)	More than twice per week	
Lung function (PEF or FEV1)[#]	Normal	<80% predicted or personal best (if known)	
Exacerbations	None	≥1 per year[¶]	One in any week[+]

PEF: peak expiratory flow; FEV1: forced expiratory volume in 1 s. [#]: Lung function is not a reliable test for children aged ≤5 yrs; [¶]: any exacerbation should prompt a review of maintenance treatment to ensure it is adequate; [+]: by definition, an exacerbation in any week makes that an uncontrolled asthma week. Reproduced from the Global Strategy for Asthma Management and Prevention, with permission.

differentiate asthma from COPD and measure response to treatment.

Exhaled nitric oxide Exhaled nitric oxide (NO) is increased in atopic asthma, but less so in nonatopic asthma. It is reduced by glucocorticosteroids, but not by bronchodilators. Measurement of airway inflammation is not required for the diagnosis, assessment of severity and/or treatment of asthma in clinical practice.

Differential diagnosis between asthma and COPD

In most patients, the clinical presentation and particularly the history provide the strongest diagnostic criteria to distinguish asthma from COPD (table 2). Pulmonary function tests, particularly spirometry, that show a nearly complete reversibility of airflow limitation may help to confirm a diagnosis of asthma, and those that show poorly reversible airflow limitation may help to confirm the diagnosis of COPD (table 2). Differential diagnosis between asthma and COPD becomes more difficult in elderly patients, in whom some features may overlap, such as smoking and atopy and, more importantly, when the patient develops poorly reversible airflow limitation that responds only partially to treatment. In these cases, symptoms, lung function, airway responsiveness, imaging and even pathological findings may overlap and thus may not provide solid information for the differential diagnosis. Because the differential diagnosis mainly aims to provide better treatment, it is important in these cases to undertake an individual approach and to perform additional tests. Reversibility to corticosteroids alone or in combination with long-acting bronchodilators, measurements of lung volumes and diffusing capacity, analysis of sputum and exhaled NO, and imaging of the chest may demonstrate whether asthma or COPD is the predominant cause of airflow limitation (table 3). In contrast, reversibility to bronchodilator and assessment of airway hyperresponsiveness or skin testing may not be useful in these patients.

Comorbidities of asthma

The coexistence of chronic rhinitis, nasal polyposis and sinusitis may contribute to the severity of asthma. There is broad evidence to show that adequate treatment of these upper airway diseases is beneficial to asthma by

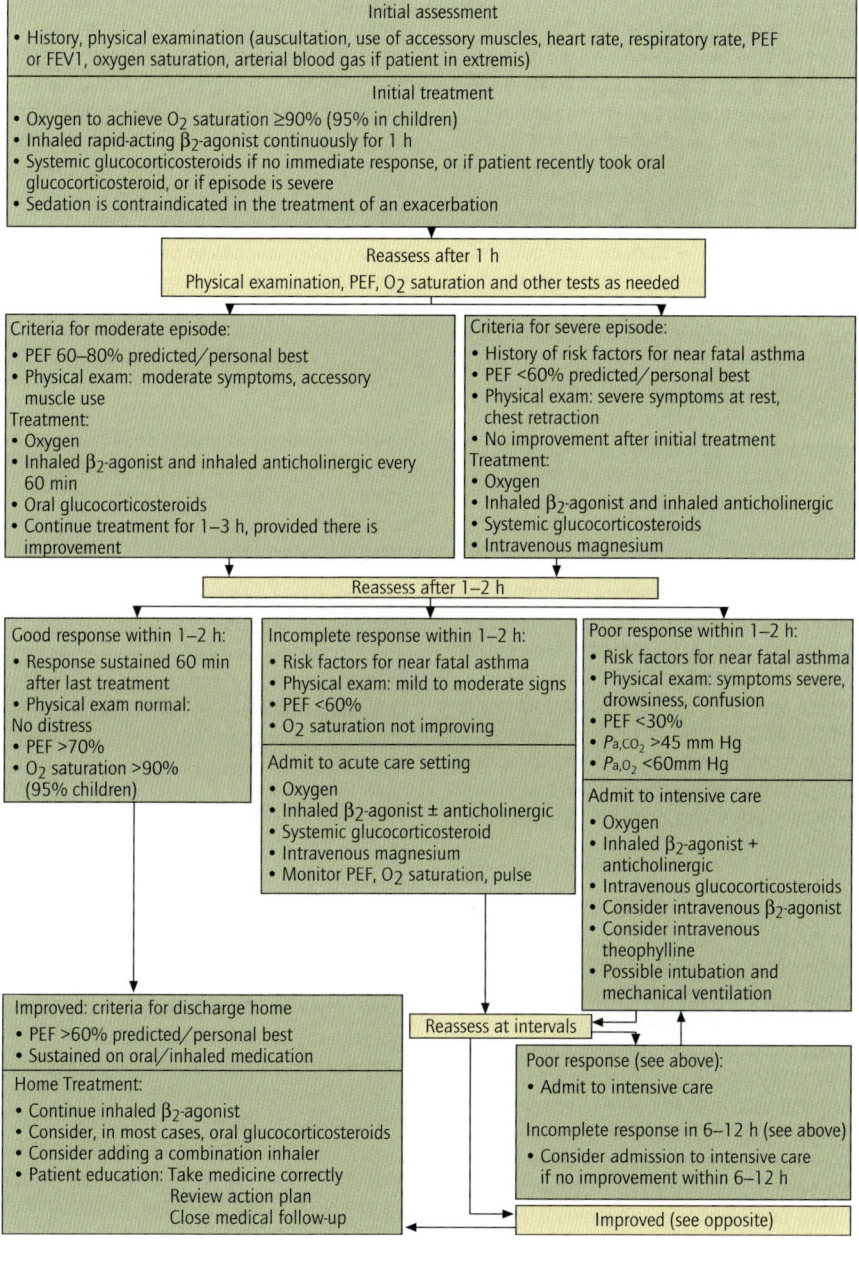

Initial assessment
- History, physical examination (auscultation, use of accessory muscles, heart rate, respiratory rate, PEF or FEV1, oxygen saturation, arterial blood gas if patient in extremis)

Initial treatment
- Oxygen to achieve O_2 saturation ≥90% (95% in children)
- Inhaled rapid-acting β_2-agonist continuously for 1 h
- Systemic glucocorticosteroids if no immediate response, or if patient recently took oral glucocorticosteroid, or if episode is severe
- Sedation is contraindicated in the treatment of an exacerbation

Reassess after 1 h
Physical examination, PEF, O_2 saturation and other tests as needed

Criteria for moderate episode:
- PEF 60–80% predicted/personal best
- Physical exam: moderate symptoms, accessory muscle use

Treatment:
- Oxygen
- Inhaled β_2-agonist and inhaled anticholinergic every 60 min
- Oral glucocorticosteroids
- Continue treatment for 1–3 h, provided there is improvement

Criteria for severe episode:
- History of risk factors for near fatal asthma
- PEF <60% predicted/personal best
- Physical exam: severe symptoms at rest, chest retraction
- No improvement after initial treatment

Treatment:
- Oxygen
- Inhaled β_2-agonist and inhaled anticholinergic
- Systemic glucocorticosteroids
- Intravenous magnesium

Reassess after 1–2 h

Good response within 1–2 h:
- Response sustained 60 min after last treatment
- Physical exam normal: No distress
- PEF >70%
- O_2 saturation >90% (95% children)

Incomplete response within 1–2 h:
- Risk factors for near fatal asthma
- Physical exam: mild to moderate signs
- PEF <60%
- O_2 saturation not improving

Admit to acute care setting
- Oxygen
- Inhaled β_2-agonist ± anticholinergic
- Systemic glucocorticosteroid
- Intravenous magnesium
- Monitor PEF, O_2 saturation, pulse

Poor response within 1–2 h:
- Risk factors for near fatal asthma
- Physical exam: symptoms severe, drowsiness, confusion
- PEF <30%
- P_{a,CO_2} >45 mm Hg
- P_{a,O_2} <60 mm Hg

Admit to intensive care
- Oxygen
- Inhaled β_2-agonist + anticholinergic
- Intravenous glucocorticosteroids
- Consider intravenous β_2-agonist
- Consider intravenous theophylline
- Possible intubation and mechanical ventilation

Improved: criteria for discharge home
- PEF >60% predicted/personal best
- Sustained on oral/inhaled medication

Home Treatment:
- Continue inhaled β_2-agonist
- Consider, in most cases, oral glucocorticosteroids
- Consider adding a combination inhaler
- Patient education: Take medicine correctly
  Review action plan
  Close medical follow-up

Reassess at intervals

Poor response (see above):
- Admit to intensive care

Incomplete response in 6–12 h (see above)
- Consider admission to intensive care if no improvement within 6–12 h

Improved (see opposite)

Figure 2. Management of asthma exacerbations in the acute care setting. PEF: peak expiratory flow; FEV1: forced expiratory volume in 1 s; P_{a,CO_2}: arterial carbon dioxide tension; P_{a,O_2}: arterial oxygen tension. Reproduced from the Global Strategy for Asthma Management and Prevention, with permission.

mechanisms not clearly understood. The "one airway" concept developed by the World Health Organization ARIA Group has drawn attention to the importance of treating the whole respiratory tract when managing asthma. Gastro-oesophageal reflux is also occasionally associated with asthma, both in adults and in children, but treatment of reflux usually has little overall effect on mild-to-moderate asthma. A frequent and quite important comorbidity of asthma in adults is COPD, most probably due to smoking, which is quite common in asthmatics. Smoking modifies the airway pathology of asthmatics to a COPD-like pattern and reduces the response to treatment. Comorbidities may become important in severe asthma, whereas they play a much less important role overall in the clinical manifestations of mild-to-moderate asthma.

Management

Considering its chronic nature and lifelong duration, asthma can be effectively managed only by developing a partnership between the patient and his or her doctor or health professional, that may provide the tools for a guided self-management (possibly written) plan including self-monitoring, and periodic review of treatment and level of asthma control. Education plays a major role in this partnership.

Long-term pharmacological treatment

The main goal of pharmacological asthma treatment is to achieve and maintain control of symptoms and prevention of exacerbations (table 4) using the safest treatment algorithm. While the initial treatment should be started according to the level of severity at the first visit, subsequently treatment should be adjusted according to the level of control achieved (fig. 1). Usually regular treatment is lowered only after a significant period of acceptable control, e.g. not <3 months. This means that monitoring of asthma is essential to maintain control and to establish the lowest step and dose of treatment. Step-up and step-down of treatment is not standardised, and thus should be tailored to the individual patient to achieve and maintain control with the minimum amount of medication.

Medications to treat asthma can be classified as controllers or relievers. Medications are preferably administered by inhalation, as it is more efficacious and has fewer side-effects. Controllers (inhaled glucocorticosteroids alone or in combination with long-acting β_2-agonists) are medications to be taken daily, over the long term, to keep asthma under clinical control. In asthma, long-acting β_2-agonists should be used only in combination with inhaled corticosteroids when the latter are insufficient to achieve control, and should be discontinued only when control is maintained for a sufficiently long time (e.g. $\geqslant$ 3 months).

Only in patients not controlled by full doses of inhaled glucocorticosteroids combined with long acting β_2-agonists may other secondary agents be considered (anti-leukotrienes, theophylline, systemic steroids, monoclonal anti-IgE antibodies in very specific cases).

Relievers (rapid-acting β_2-agonists alone or in combination in combination with inhaled steroids) are medications used on an as-needed basis that act quickly to reverse bronchoconstriction and relieve its symptoms. Ideally, if patients are adequately controlled, they should not need rescue medications.

Allergen immunotherapy may be considered in patients with asthma caused by specific allergens for which there are standardised extracts. Only patients with single or two similar allergen sensitivities whose role is confirmed by the history and who have preserved lung function are candidates for this treatment (which, however, has limited efficacy and is long and relatively expensive). Specific immunotherapy should be considered only after strict environmental avoidance and pharmacological interventions, including inhaled glucocorticosteroids, have failed to control the disease. Smoking asthmatics are resistant to anti-asthma medications and should be primarily treated for smoking addiction. Smokers with asthma may develop features of COPD.

Treatment of exacerbations

Shortness of breath, cough, wheezing, and/or chest tightness may develop or worsen recurrently in subjects with asthma even when they are under regular treatment. Milder exacerbations are usually managed by the patient with an increased as-needed use of rapid acting β_2-agonists alone or in combination with inhaled steroids. More severe exacerbations or exacerbations that do not respond to the increased use of rescue medications require repetitive administration of rescue medication and systemic, preferably oral, glucocorticosteroids, associated in the very severe cases with oxygen supplementation (fig. 2). Severe exacerbations require medical attention or even hospital admission.

Special considerations

Special considerations are required for patients with specific conditions and/or comorbidities, *e.g.* rhino/sinusitis and/or nasal polyps, aspirin-induced asthma particularly if associated with episodes of anaphylaxis, occupational asthma or obesity.

Additionally, patients with asthma should be informed that they may require specific medical attention in case of smoking addiction, pregnancy, surgery or infections (*e.g.* influenza epidemics).

References

- Boulet LP. Influence of comorbid conditions on asthma. *Eur Respir J* 2009; 33: 897–906.
- Bousquet J, *et al.* Allergic Rhinitis and its Impact on Asthma (ARIA) 2008 update (in collaboration with the World Health Organization, GA(2)LEN and AllerGen). *Allergy* 2008; 63: Suppl. 86, 8-160.
- Camargo CA, Jr., *et al.*:Managing asthma exacerbations in the emergency department: summary of the National Asthma Education and Prevention Program Expert Panel Report 3 guidelines for the management of asthma exacerbations. *J Allergy Clin Immunol* 2009; 124; Suppl., S5-S14.
- Global Strategy for Asthma Management and Prevention, Global Initiative for Asthma (GINA). Available from: http://www.ginasthma.org 2009.
- Global Strategy for Diagnosis, Management, and Prevention of COPD. Available from: http://www.goldcopd.org 2009.
- Maestrelli P, *et al.* Mechanisms of occupational asthma. J Allergy Clin Immunol 2009; 123: 531-542.
- Reddel HK, *et al.* An official American Thoracic Society/European Respiratory Society statement: asthma control and exacerbations: standardizing endpoints for clinical asthma trials and clinical practice. *Am J Respir Crit Care Med* 2009; 180: 59-99.
- Schatz M, Dombrowski MP. Clinical practice. Asthma in pregnancy. *N Engl J Med* 2009; 360: 1862-1869.
- Sin DD, Sutherland ER. Obesity and the lung: 4. Obesity and asthma. *Thorax* 2008; 63: 1018-1023.
- Thomson NC. Smokers with asthma: what are the management options? *Am J Respir Crit Care Med* 2007; 175: 749-750.

VOCAL CORD DYSFUNCTION

A.H. Mansur
Birmingham Heartlands Hospital, Birmingham, UK
E-mail: adel.mansur@heartofengland.nhs.uk

Vocal cord dysfunction (VCD) is characterised by paradoxical vocal cord adduction during inspiration and/or expiration, leading to symptoms of breathlessness and wheeze. It is a poorly understood condition that often co-exists with asthma and chronic cough and shares common triggers such as psychological factors, gastro-oesophageal reflux and rhinosinus disease. The management of VCD focuses on establishing the correct diagnosis, identification and treatment of underlying triggers, and speech therapy. Further research is required to define VCD, establish its natural history and develop evidence-based therapies.

Terminology

Numerous terms have been used to describe VCD. These include hysteric croup, Munchausen's stridor, pseudo-asthma, factitious asthma, upper airway dysfunction, functional upper airway obstruction, irritable larynx syndrome, emotional laryngeal wheeze, laryngeal hyper-responsiveness, and paradoxical vocal cord movement. Indeed, there is disagreement of what constitutes VCD, with some limiting it to an early description by CHRISTOPHER *et al.* (1983) of a conversion disorder meeting a strict definition of inspiratory adduction and posterior chinking of vocal cords, to those who use all encompassing VCD definition of all cases demonstrating paradoxical vocal cord movement (PVCM).

Epidemiology

While the true prevalence of VCD in the general population is unknown, it is more common in females, athletes, army recruits, and patients with asthma or chronic cough (table 1).

Pathogenesis

VCD was seen largely as a conversion disorder of psychogenic origin. The larynx is innervated by a complex neurological network, and the association between stress and comorbid psychology and VCD attacks strengthened this view. More recently it became apparent that PVCM "VCD" exists outside the conversion disorder prototype. Laryngeal closure is a normal physiological reaction to exposure to irritants (*e.g.* aspiration), but this reaction normally only lasts for few seconds. Acute (*e.g.* toxic fume inhalation) or recurrent irritation (*e.g.* repeated extreme cold air exposure) may lead to laryngeal hypersensitivity manifesting as vocal cord adduction and airflow limitation. Laryngeal hypersensitivity may form part of unified allergic airway syndrome with asthma and rhinitis. The association of laryngeal hypersensitivity with altered autonomic balance status maintained by central brain activity has been postulated to underlie development of VCD.

Clinical presentation

VCD presentation varies from cases with predominant throat symptoms, usually

Key points

- VCD is not well understood, and there is as yet no consensus definition.
- Classically, symptoms appear abruptly, resolve quickly and do not respond well to asthma medication.
- Long-term treatment is based around speech therapy and psychotherapy.

Table 1. Vocal cord dysfunction (VCD) prevalence in different patient groups.

Patient group	Prevalence %
Refractory asthma	5–10
Dyspnoea	2.8
Army recruits with stress-induced asthma	15
Olympic athletes	5
Childhood acute asthma[#]	14

[#]: presenting to emergency department. The reported mean age at VCD diagnosis is 14.5 yrs in children and 33 yrs in adults.

referred to ear, nose and throat (ENT) specialists, to asthma presenting to respiratory clinic, or angio-oedema presenting in an immunology clinic. Often the diagnosis of VCD is made after treatment for asthma has not been successful.

Patients may report rapid onset attacks of dyspnoea which may be preceded by intense coughing, sensation of strangulation or breathing through a straw, throat or upper chest tightness, dysphonia, or stridor. Classical VCD symptoms are of abrupt onset, resolve quickly and respond poorly to asthma medication.

Elucidation of triggers of VCD attacks is important for diagnostic and therapeutic purposes. Commonly associated triggers include exposure to cold air, exercise, inhalation of strong smells such as perfumes or chemical cleaning agents, smoke, cough, reflux, viral infections, allergens and emotional stress. Psychological morbidity and sexual abuse are experienced in some VCD sufferers. The physical examination of patients with VCD is usually unremarkable outside symptomatic attacks. During symptoms, examination may reveal stridor or wheeze originating at laryngeal level with clear chest auscultation. The severity of respiratory distress varies from mild to severe with tachypnoea, but oxygen saturation level is often normal. Extreme forms of VCD can lead to collapse and loss of consciousness usually leading to resolution of the attack or intubation. If intubated, the airway inflation pressure is characteristically normal.

Diagnosis

Flow–volume loops may show inspiratory loop truncation representing extra-thoracic airflow obstruction. The maximal inspiratory flow at 50% of the forced vital capacity (FVC)/maximal expiratory flow at 50% of the FVC ratio can be reduced due to predominant inspiratory flow limitation. An abnormally high forced inspiratory flow at 25% of the FVC/forced inspiratory flow at 75% of the FVC ratio would indicate an initially normal flow followed by rapid flow decline reflecting paradoxical vocal cord movement during inspiration. However, various studies reported the insensitivity of spirometry to diagnose VCD. Sensitivity of spirometry may be enhanced by histamine or other forms of airway challenge.

Impulse oscillometry can discriminate between central *versus* peripheral airway obstruction, and may be more sensitive than spirometry. Airway fluoroscopy and colour Doppler ultrasound imaging of vocal cords movement are other noninvasive tools that have not been standardised against laryngoscopy.

Laryngoscopy

VCD diagnosis is established by laryngoscopical demonstration of paradoxical vocal cord movement whilst the patient experiences spontaneous or induced symptoms. Agreed laryngoscopy standards have not been developed, with some advocating pre-procedure sedation and analgesia, whilst others recommend avoiding these measures. Following short periods of quiet breathing, specific manoeuvres such as repeating low and high pitched sounds, and forceful inspiration and expiration are conducted to induce an attack. Vocal cord movements are timed against respiratory cycle phases by putting a hand on the patient's chest. In VCD, the vocal cords adduct anteriorly leaving an open posterior glottic chink (fig. 1). The adduction occurs during inspiration or throughout the respiratory cycle. False-negative PVCM can be secondary to gag reflex or coughing. The larynx should also be inspected for signs of laryngo-pharyngeal reflux. VCD should be distinguished from vocal cord immobility due to paralysis, amyotrophic lateral sclerosis, cricoarytenoid joint dysfunction and Reinke's oedema. Laryngeal electromyography may help in differentiation. Normal laryngoscopy in the absence of symptoms does not exclude VCD. The presence of atypical features of asthma and/or VCD should prompt further investigations, such as CT of head–neck–thorax and bronchoscopy.

Investigations of causes of VCD

A careful history is essential to guide investigations. The presence of concomitant rhinitis/asthma or allergic airway disease needs to be assessed by lung function, skin allergy testing, blood/sputum eosinophils and exhaled nitric oxide. Gastro-oesophageal reflux disease symptoms or laryngeal refluxive changes on laryngoscopy should prompt further testing (*e.g.* oesophageal manometry and pH studies). Underlying psychological issues should be assessed.

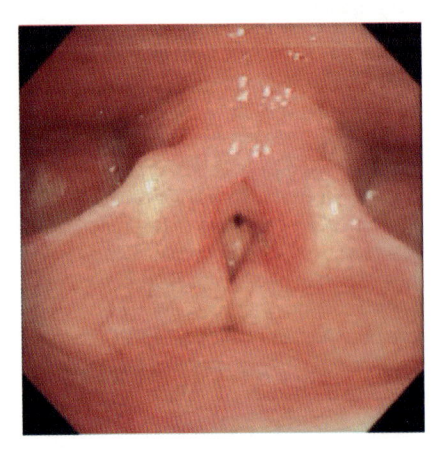

Figure 1. Laryngoscopy demonstrating inspiratory vocal cord adduction and posterior glottic chink.

Differential diagnosis

- Laryngeal oedema (angio-oedema).
- Allergic laryngitis.
- Subglottic stenosis.
- Laryngomalacia, tracheomalacia.
- Vocal cord paralysis.
- Systemic disease affecting larynx/upper airways (*e.g.* relapsing chondritis, Wegener's granulomatosis).

Treatment

The diagnosis and treatment is best conducted in a multidisciplinary team setting comprised of respiratory physician, speech therapist, ENT specialist and psychologist. The diagnosis is explained to the patient, preferably with support of imaging or illustration. The patient's good understanding of VCD is prerequisite to effective treatment. A management plan should be formulated that bear in mind co-existing asthma. Due to VCD under-recognition, patients should carry an alert card listing medication and treatment strategy.

Treatment of acute attacks

The treating physician should adopt a calm reassuring manner and ask patient to focus on expiration with an "S" sound that helps in diverting attention. A panting manoeuvre can abort acute attacks by inducing vocal cord abduction. Where hypoxaemia and hypercapnia has been excluded, sedation with benzodiazepines may help patient relaxation. Heliox gas mixture (*e.g.* 72% helium and 28% oxygen) can alleviate symptoms by enhancing upper airway laminar air flow. Intubation or tracheostomy should be avoided. In extreme cases presenting with an apparent life-threatening attack, the clinical decision will remain with the treating physician. If intubation is contemplated, prior inspection and documentation of the status of vocal cords is recommended.

Long-term treatment

Speech therapy forms the mainstay of VCD treatment with the primary aim of teaching patients to relax upper airways and control laryngeal area. It is conducted in four to six successive sessions to enable the patient to practice breathing techniques to abort or treat acute attacks. Patients are taught to exhale gently and avoid forceful inspiration in a rhythmic manner, followed by introduction of expiratory resistance by asking patient to produce sounds such as "S". The role of speech therapist extends to making diagnosis, identification and treatment of triggers and relaxation therapy.

Psychotherapy should form an integral part of VCD management, given the VCD link to adverse psychology. Psychotherapy can include relaxation therapy, management of stress and anxiety, and the development of coping strategies.

Other unproven therapies for VCD include inhaled anticholinergic drugs to abort exercise-induced VCD attacks, enhancing inspiratory resistance by a face mask device, continuous positive airway pressure, and injection of vocal cords by botulinum toxin A (botox). Tracheostomy has been used as a last resort in intractable cases.

Prognosis

The long-term outcome of VCD is unknown. VCD prognosis will probably depend on initial disease severity and associated morbidities. One study reported complete resolution of VCD within a 5-yr time frame, with symptoms disappearing within 6 months in many who had good response to speech therapy. However, intractable forms of the disease did not seem to improve over a 10-yr observation period.

Conclusion

VCD is a relatively uncommon condition that mimics and co-exists with asthma, and presents episodically thus making its diagnosis challenging and often delayed. Patients can become frequent healthcare users with substantial morbidity as result of erroneous diagnosis and toxic medication use. Establishing proper diagnosis and treatment can be effective and rewarding to both the patient and healthcare professionals.

References

- Ayres JG, Gabott PLA. Vocal cord dysfunction and laryngeal hyperresponsiveness: a function of altered autonomic balance? *Thorax* 2002; 57: 284–285.
- Belafsky PC, *et al*. Validity and reliability of the reflux symptom index (RSI). *J Voice* 2002; 16: 274–277.
- Christopher KL, *et al*. Vocal-cord dysfunction presenting as asthma. *New Engl J Med* 1983; 308: 1566–1570.
- Cukier-Blaj S, *et al*. Paradoxical vocal fold motion: a sensory-motor laryngeal disorder. *Laryngoscope* 2008; 118: 367–370.
- Doshi DR, Weinberger MM. Long-term outcome of vocal cord dysfunction. *Ann Allergy Asthma Immunol* 2006; 96: 794–799.
- Newman KB, *et al*. Clinical features of vocal cord dysfunction. *Am J Respir Crit Care Med* 1995; 152: 1382–1386.
- O'Connell M. Vocal cord dysfunction: ready for prime-time? *Ann Allergy Asthma Immunol* 2006; 96: 762–763.
- Ruppel GL. The inspiratory flow–volume curve: the neglected child of pulmonary diagnostics. *Respir Care* 2009; 54: 448–449.
- Sullivan MD, *et al*. A treatment for vocal cord dysfunction in female athletes: an outcome study. *Laryngoscope* 2001; 111: 1751–1755.
- Wood RP, Milgrom H. Vocal cord dysfunction. *J Allergy Clin Immunol* 1996; 98: 481–485.

BRONCHITIS

G. Rohde
Dept of Respiratory Medicine, Maastricht University Medical Centre, Maastricht, The Netherlands
E-mail: gernot.rohde@mumc.nl

Definition

Transient airway inflammation localised to the respiratory mucosa of the central airways and clinically characterised by cough and sputum production. Fever and dyspnoea can occur.

Symptoms

Cough is the cardinal symptom and is observed in 100% of cases. It usually persists for up to 2 weeks but in 26% it can stay for up to 8 weeks. Other symptoms include sputum production (90%), dyspnoea, wheezing (62%), rhonchi, chest pain, fever, hoarseness and malaise.

Epidemiology

Acute bronchitis is one of the most frequent human diseases worldwide, with children being most often affected. On average children contract bronchitis 2–6 times per year, and adults 2–3 times per year. The prevalence in UK is 44 cases per 1,000 adults per year. 82% of episodes occur during the cold months.

Aetiology/risk factors

Respiratory infections are the main trigger of acute bronchitis. However, in only 55% of cases can pathogens be detected. Respiratory viruses are the most frequent pathogens. Rhino-, adeno-, echo-, influenza-, parainfluenza-, entero- and coronaviruses, Coxsackie virus and respiratory syncytial viruses (RSV) represent the usual spectrum. Parainfluenza, entero- and rhinoviruses infect mainly in the autumn, while influenza, RSV and coronaviruses infect mainly in winter and early spring. Typical bacteria are *Streptococcus pneumoniae*, *Haemophilus influenzae* and *Moraxella catarrhalis*. Atypical bacteria (e.g. *Mycoplasma pneumoniae*, *Chlamydia pneumoniae*) and *Bordetella pertussis* also play a role.

Specific risk factors are not identified and it is currently not clear whether cigarette smoking increases the risk of acute bronchitis. There are epidemiological data showing that the frequency of bronchitis is increased after school holidays, which indicates that crowding facilitates dissemination of respiratory infections.

Prognosis

Acute bronchitis is usually a self-limiting disease. However there are only sparse data on prognosis and rate of complications. In a study investigating 653 previously healthy adulty with lower respiratory tract symptoms, 20% of patients had persistent sysmptoms. In 40% of these patients, there was reversible airway obstruction. In another study, a third of

> **Key points**
>
> - Respiratory viral infection is the most common cause of acute bronchitis.
> - Acute bronchitis is usually a self-limiting disease.
> - The diagnosis of acute bronchitis is purely clinical and in most cases symptomatic treatment is sufficient.
> - Chronic bronchitis is defined clinically as productive cough for 3 months in each of 2 successive years.

patients developed asthma or chronic bronchitis symptoms.

Diagnosis

Diagosis is purely clinical. Cough, sputum production optionally accompanied by dyspnoea and/or wheezing are suggestive. Tachycardia and tachypnoea are usually absent, and vital signs are normal. Complicated cases show fever; however, in these cases differential diagnosis like pneumonia or systemic influenza should be considered. Clinical signs of pneumonia (rales, egophony, dullness on percussion) should be absent. Acute bronchitis should be differentiated from asthma, which typically presents as progressive cough accompanied by wheezing, tachypnoea, respiratory distress and hypoxaemia. It should also be distinguished from bronchiectasis, a distinct phenomenon associated with permanent dilatation of bronchi and chronic cough. Laboratory investigations are not necessary. In more severe cases, sputum culture can be considered to guide antibiotic therapy.

Therapy

Therapeutic goals are reduction of symptoms and prevention of complications with as few side-effects as possible. Antibiotic therapy cannot be recommended generally, but in patients with fever and/or comorbidities, aminopenicillins or cephalosporins (second generation) can be administered. Dextromethorpham has been shown to reduce cough efficiently. In patients with dyspnoea and/or wheezing, short-acting bronchodilators can be beneficial.

Chronic bronchitis

Chronic bronchitis is defined clinically as chronic productive cough for 3 months in each of two successive years in a patient in whom other causes of productive chronic cough have been excluded. Cigarette smoking is by far the most important and preventable risk factor. Chronic bronchitis is a major component of chronic obstructive pulmonary disease.

References

- American Thoracic Society, Chronic bronchitis, asthma, pulmonary emphysema. A statement by the committee on diagnostic standards for non-tuberculous disease. *Am Rev Respir Dis* 1962; 85: 762-768.
- Anto JM, *et al.* Epidemiology of chronic obstructive pulmonary disease. *Eur Respir J* 2001; 17: 982-994.
- Boldy DA, *et al.* Acute bronchitis in the community: clinical features, infective factors, changes in pulmonary function and bronchial reactivity to histamine. *Respir Med* 1990; 84: 377-385.
- Chesnutt MS, Prendergast TJ. Lung. In: Tierney LM, ed. Current medical diagnosis and treatment, 41st Edn. New York, McGraw-Hill, 2002; pp. 269-362.
- Jonsson JS, *et al.* Acute bronchitis and clinical outcome three years later: prospective cohort study. *BMJ* 1998; 317: 1433-1440.
- Macfarlane JW, *et al.*, *Prospective study of the incidence, aetiology and outcome of adult lower respiratory tract illness in the community. Thorax* 2001; 56: 109-114.
- Wenzel RP, Fowler, III AA, Clinical practice. Acute bronchitis. *N Engl J Med* 2006; 355: 2125-2130.
- Williamson Jr HA. Pulmonary function tests in acute bronchitis: evidence for reversible airway obstruction. *J Fam Pract* 1987; 25: 251-256.

GASTRO-OESOPHAGEAL REFLUX

L. Dupont
Dept of Respiratory Medicine, University Hospital Gasthuisberg, KU Leuven, Belgium
E-mail: lieven.dupont@uz.kuleuven.ac.be

Gastro-oesophageal reflux disease (GORD) is an increasingly prevalent condition that affects up to 20% of the Western population. Transient lower oesophageal sphincter relaxations (TLOSRs) are now recognised as a major factor in the pathophysiology of GORD. Although GORD often causes typical symptoms such as heartburn or regurgitation, it may also present with atypical or extra-oesophageal symptoms, including respiratory and ear, nose and throat symptoms and disorders. Respiratory manifestations of GORD represent one of the most prevalent and challenging of these extra-oesophageal syndromes. The relationship between reflux and respiratory symptoms is frequently difficult to establish with a high degree of certainty and diagnostic, as well as therapeutic, management remains largely empirical. In contrast to oesophageal GORD manifestations, efficacy of acid-suppressive therapy in extra-oesophageal GORD symptoms has not been well established.

Key points

- GORD is a common disorder caused by the reflux of gastric contents into the oesophagus because of impaired function of the lower oesophageal sphincter and may result in oesophageal and extra-oesophageal symptoms.
- The relationship between reflux and respiratory symptoms or disorders is frequently difficult to establish with a high degree of certainty.
- Diagnostic, as well as therapeutic, management remains largely empirical.
- Treatment with PPI has been shown to improve cough in patients with acid GOR-induced cough but the effect of PPI remains disappointing when treating GOR in other respiratory diseases.
- Antireflux surgery was associated with improved allograft function after lung transplantation.

Pathophysiology

There are a number of potential mechanisms whereby GORD may aggravate or trigger respiratory disease. Direct aspiration of gastric refluxate into the airway occurs as a consequence of failure of the normal protective mechanisms to foreign material, i.e. reflex contraction of the upper oesophageal sphincter and closure of glottis and vocal cords is likely to be relevant in cystic fibrosis (CF) and rejection after lung transplantation. A vagally mediated oesophageal tracheobronchial reflex has been postulated to account for the association between acid reflux and cough or asthma. Oesophageal sensory stimulation can release tachykinins into the airways and may increase the bronchomotor responsiveness to airway stimuli bronchospasms. It has also been postulated that chronic exposure of the oesophageal mucosa to gastric juices can produce long-lasting hypersensitivity to a variety of stimuli that can cause the symptom even in the absence of increased oesophageal acid exposure or oesophagitis.

GOR in asthma and COPD

GORD is a common condition among patients with obstructive pulmonary diseases. Probably one-third of asthmatics present with GORD (prevalence range 10–84%) and some 50–60% of chronic obstructive pulmonary disease (COPD) patients have abnormally high oesophageal acid exposure times, which is more than the general population. There is no clear understanding of why this is true but it may be due to the fact that airway obstruction, diaphragmatic flattening, β_2-agonists and theophylline are able to promote oesophageal reflux. Often COPD or asthmatic patients with GORD do not have classic symptoms of GORD.

Recent randomised controlled data suggest that it is not a useful practice for mild-to-moderate asthmatic patients to treat asymptomatic GORD with proton pump inhibitors (PPIs) as it will not improve asthma control. Asthma outcome may only improve to some extent with PPI management among patients who present with severe difficult-to-control asthma and symptomatic GORD.

Reflux symptoms in COPD patients were associated with an increased number of COPD exacerbations and oxygen desaturation coincided with episodes of increased oesophageal acidity in 40% of patients with severe COPD and GORD. Uncontrolled data suggest that PPI treatment may decrease the number of COPD exacerbations.

GOR-induced cough

Studies have determined GOR to be a cause for chronic cough in up to 43% of patients referred for specialist evaluation. According to published guidelines GORD investigations are indicated in patients with chronic cough. Only a minority of patients with chronic cough and GORD have typical digestive symptoms and/or clear evidence of oesophagitis. The treatment of cough-associated reflux has been evaluated in many uncontrolled and a few controlled trials of drug therapy and antireflux surgery. A recent Cochrane systematic review retrieved 13 randomised, controlled trials of GORD treatment for cough in children and adults. Meta-analysis of the studies comparing PPI treatment (2 or 3 months) with placebo showed no difference between placebo and PPI (odds ratio 0.46, 95% CI 0.19–1.15) in the resolution of cough, although sensitivity analyses showed significant changes in cough scores in those receiving PPI in cross-over trials. Further randomised, parallel-design, placebo-controlled, double-blind trials are needed.

Based on these data two different management strategies of patients with suspected reflux-related cough can be proposed. The empirical strategy with PPI (usually double dose) given for at least 3 months is probably the most popular one but it should be underlined that this strategy is not supported by strong evidence. Appropriate initial selection of potential responders to GORD treatment could be done on the basis of the presence of typical reflux symptoms.

The second strategy consists of investigations, which should ideally detect both acidic and nonacidic reflux. Patients who failed to respond to empirical therapy should be investigated. In well-selected patients, antireflux surgery may be indicated for long-term control. This may also be the case for patients with refractory acidic or nonacidic reflux and a well-documented correlation between reflux episodes and cough.

GOR in advanced lung disease

The prevalence of increased GOR in CF is estimated to be between 35% and 81%. Acid GOR is most common, but weakly acidic GOR may also occur. Patients with CF have a high risk for gastric aspiration, as demonstrated by increased bile acids in saliva, sputum or in bronchoalveolar lavage fluid. Half of the CF patients with increased GOR or gastric aspiration do not present oesophageal symptoms like heartburn or regurgitation. The characteristics of GOR and material aspirated depend on the genotype with bile acids aspiration being more important in DF508 homozygotes. The causal relationship between GOR, aspiration and respiratory symptoms is not completely elucidated. Recent results suggest that patients with increased oesophageal acid exposure have more cough and a positive association between GOR and cough is associated with poorer lung function. Bile acid levels in sputum is correlated with elastase levels in sputum and forced expiratory volume in 1 s.

GOR may play a role in the pathogenesis and/or progression of idiopathic pulmonary fibrosis (specifically in acute exacerbation) as a recurrent inflammatory stimulus. Studies have found a high prevalence of reflux (36–87%) among patients with idiopathic pulmonary fibrosis. Pre-transplant patients with idiopathic pulmonary fibrosis undergoing antireflux surgery had reduced supplementary oxygen dependence compared with other pre-transplant patients with idiopathic pulmonary fibrosis. In addition, there are anecdotal cases of idiopathic pulmonary fibrosis disease stability following treatment for reflux. While it cannot be proven that disease stability was caused by control of reflux, they suggest that a subset of patients with idiopathic pulmonary fibrosis may benefit from antireflux therapy.

GOR and gastric aspiration have also been implicated as a potential nonalloimmune cause of lung allograft rejection (bronchiolitis obliterans syndrome (BOS)) after lung transplantation. Standard oesophageal pH recordings indicated an increased oesophageal acid exposure in >70% of lung transplant patients. Luminal gastric components such as pepsin and bile acids have been demonstrated in bronchial material of lung transplant recipients and were more prevalent in the lungs of patients with BOS. Aspiration of bile acids was related to weakly acidic reflux events and especially those occurring during the night were also associated with reduced concentration of pulmonary surfactant collectin proteins and reduced freedom from BOS. Aspiration even in the absence of an increased number of GOR events might therefore feature as a potential risk factor for the development of BOS after lung transplantation. Antireflux surgery was associated with improved allograft function.

Management of GORD

In general practice, most cases of GORD are diagnosed on the basis of typical symptoms and the response to inhibition of gastric acid secretion. Endoscopy, oesophageal manometry or acid instillation in the oesophagus (Bernstein test) have limited sensitivity and specificity for the diagnosis of GORD. 24-h oesophageal pH monitoring can provide useful information, in particular through assessment of the temporal association between symptoms and reflux events. The addition of impedance monitoring to pH monitoring further improves GOR diagnosis as it also detects nonacid (weakly acidic) reflux events and allows testing whilst the patient is on a PPI. Investigations of the routine diagnostic value of the measurement of pepsin and bile acid concentrations in saliva, sputum or BALF are in progress.

Medications interfering with acid production, especially the PPIs, are the cornerstone of GORD treatment. Acid-suppressive therapy is highly effective in the healing and maintenance of oesophagitis, but seems to be poorly effective when GORD is presumed to underlie extra-oesophageal symptoms. Symptoms that persist during standard acid suppressive therapy regimens have also been related to nonacid or weakly acidic reflux. There is little evidence that further intensification of acid suppression beyond high-dose PPI twice daily is of any benefit for these patients. Several attempts to improve symptoms in these patients through the addition of gastroprokinetic drugs have thus far not been successful. At present, the only alternative for these patients is a surgical fundoplication, but not all patients are eligible for surgery, the intervention is not without complications, and poor responders to PPI therapy are also less certain to experience symptom relief from surgery. Two classes of drugs, the γ-aminobutyric acid (GABA)-B agonists and the metabotropic glutamate receptor-5 antagonists are currently under evaluation for their ability to reduce TLOSRs and improve (weakly acidic) reflux and symptoms that are refractory to PPI therapy. Other pathways that are under investigation include mucosal protective agents, inhibitors of acid-sensitive ion channels, and endoscopic antireflux procedures.

References

- Asano K, Suzuki H. Silent acid reflux and asthma control. *N Engl J Med* 2009; 360: 1551-1553.
- Blondeau K, *et al.* Gastro-oesophageal reflux and aspiration of gastric contents in adult patients with cystic fibrosis. *Gut* 2008; 57: 1049-1055.
- Chang AB, *et al.* Systematic review and meta-analysis of randomised controlled trials of gastro-oesophageal reflux interventions for chronic cough associated with gastro-oesophageal reflux. *BMJ* 2006; 332: 11-17.
- Dupont LJ, D'Ovidio F. Emerging risk factors for bronchiolitis obliterans syndrome: gastro-oesophageal reflux and infections. *Eur Respir Mon* 2009; 45: 212-225.
- Galmiche JP, *et al.* Review article: respiratory manifestations of gastro-oesophageal reflux disease. *Aliment Pharmacol Ther* 2008; 27: 449-464.
- Pashinsky YY, *et al.* Gastroesophageal reflux disease and idiopathic pulmonary fibrosis. *Mt Sinai J Med* 2009; 76: 24-29.
- Rascon-Aguilar IE, *et al.* Role of gastroesophageal reflux symptoms in exacerbations of COPD. *Chest* 2006; 130: 1096-1101.
- Sweet MP, *et al.* Gastro-oesophageal reflux and aspiration in patients with advanced lung disease. *Thorax* 2009; 64: 167-173.

COPD AND EMPHYSEMA

E.G. Tzortzaki, K.D. Samara and N.M. Siafakas
Department of Thoracic Medicine, Medical School, University of Crete, Greece
E-mail: tzortzaki@med.uoc.gr

Chronic obstructive pulmonary disease (COPD) is a preventable and treatable disease with some significant extrapulmonary effects that may contribute to its severity in individual patients. Its pulmonary component is characterised by airflow limitation that is not fully reversible. The airflow limitation is usually progressive and associated with an abnormal inflammatory response of the lungs to noxious particles or gases. Cigarette smoking is by far the most common risk factor for the disease. COPD is a major cause of morbidity and mortality worldwide. It affects ~10% of the general population but its prevalence among smokers may reach 50%. According to an American Thoracic Society/European Respiratory Society Task Force, COPD is a preventable and treatable disease characterised by airflow limitation that is not fully reversible. The airflow limitation is usually progressive and is associated with an abnormal inflammatory response of the lungs to noxious particles or gases, primarily caused by cigarette smoking. Although COPD affects the lungs, it also produces significant systemic consequences. The cardinal symptoms of COPD - dyspnoea, cough and sputum production - are chronic and progressive.

COPD comprises pathological changes in four different compartments of the lungs (central airways, peripheral airways, lung parenchyma and pulmonary vasculature), which are variably present in people with the disease. Airflow limitation in COPD is caused by the presence of an abnormal inflammatory cellular infiltrate in the small airways, remodelling and thickening of the airway wall. The destruction of alveoli and enlargement of airspaces, which are anatomical hallmarks of emphysema, contribute to the loss of elastic recoil and the loss of outward traction on the small airways, leading to their collapse on expiration. This results in airflow obstruction, air trapping and hyperinflation. In general, the inflammatory and structural changes in the airways increase with disease severity and persist even after smoking cessation.

Chronic obstructive bronchitis and/or emphysema

COPD is a heterogeneous disease. Two main phenotypes are recognised: chronic bronchitis and emphysema.

Chronic bronchitis is characterised by cough and sputum production for at least 3 months in each of two consecutive years. The symptoms may precede the development of

---

Key points

- COPD is a heterogeneous disease, with two main phenotypes: chronic bronchitis and emphysema.
- A strong genetic component, in conjunction with environmental insult, probably accounts for the development of COPD.
- Smoking cessation is the single most effective intervention in COPD prevention and treatment.
- Bronchodilators are central to symptomatic treatment, backed up if necessary by other interventions.

Table 1. Spirometric classification of COPD severity based on post-bronchodilator forced expiratory volume in 1 s (FEV1)

At risk	FEV1/FVC >0.70
	FEV1 ⩾80% pred
Stage I: mild	FEV1/FVC <0.70
	FEV1 ⩾80% pred
Stage II: moderate	FEV1/FVC <0.70
	50% ⩽FEV1 <80% pred
Stage III: severe	FEV1/FVC <0.70
	30% ⩽FEV1 <50% pred
Stage IV: very severe	FEV1/FVC <0.70
	FEV1 <30% pred or FEV1 <50% pred plus chronic respiratory failure[#]

FVC: forced vital capacity; % pred: % predicted. [#]: respiratory failure is defined as an arterial partial pressure of oxygen <60 mmHg with or without arterial partial pressure of CO_2 >50 mmHg while breathing air at sea level. Respiratory failure may also lead to effects on the heart such as cor pulmonale (right heart failure). Clinical signs of cor pulmonale include elevation of the jugular venous pressure and pitting ankle oedema. Patients may have stage IV chronic obstructive pulmonary disease even if their FEV1 is >30% pred whenever these complications are present. At this stage, quality of life is significantly impaired and exacerbations may be life threatening. Reproduced from the Global strategy for the diagnosis, management, and prevention of chronic obstructive pulmonary disease, with permission.

airflow limitation by many years. Inflammation and secretions provide the obstructive component of the disease. In contrast to emphysema, chronic bronchitis is associated with a relatively undamaged pulmonary capillary bed. Emphysema is present to a variable degree but is usually centrilobular rather than panlobular. The body responds by decreasing ventilation and increasing cardiac output (ventilation/perfusion (V'/Q') mismatch) leading to hypoxaemia, polycythaemia and increased CO_2 retention, and eventually these patients develop signs of right heart failure.

The second major COPD phenotype is the emphysematous patient. Emphysema is defined by destruction of airways distal to the terminal bronchiole, gradual destruction of alveolar septae and of the pulmonary capillary bed, leading to decreased ability to oxygenate blood. The body compensates with lowered cardiac output and hyperventilation. This V'/Q' mismatch results in relatively limited blood flow through a quite well-oxygenated lung with normal blood gases and pressures. Eventually, due to low cardiac output, the rest of the body suffers from tissue hypoxia, pulmonary cachexia, muscle wasting and weight loss.

Stages of severity

Airflow limitation in COPD is best measured by spirometry, the most widely available and reproducible lung function test. A simple spirometric classification of disease severity into five stages has been established by the Global Initiative for Obstructive Lung Disease (GOLD) and the criterion for airflow obstruction is a forced expiratory volume in 1 s (FEV1)/forced vital capacity (FVC) ratio <0.7, regardless of age (table 1). The FEV1/FVC ratio in normal subjects declines with age, thus an alternative cut-off for diagnosing obstruction without over-diagnosing in younger subjects, is using values outside the 95% confidence intervals for predicted FEV1/FVC ratios ("below the lower limit of normal"). Newer publications on reference equations give explicit upper and lower limits of the normal range, or provide a method for its calculation. Normal values are most difficult to predict in older, shorter people, who may not be well represented in the reference population from which the prediction equation was derived.

Risk factors

Although smoking is the best-studied COPD risk factor, it is not the only one and there is consistent evidence from epidemiological studies that nonsmokers may develop chronic airflow obstruction (table 2). Other factors, such as indoor air pollution from burning biomass fuels for cooking and heating, are important causes of COPD in many developing countries, especially among women. Nevertheless, not all subjects exposed to a noxious agent develop COPD. Thus, a strong genetic component in relation with an environmental insult (gene–environment interaction) accounts, most probably, for the development of the disease (table 2). Familial clustering of COPD has been observed and twin studies have supported the concept of a genetic predisposition to COPD. Different strategies have been used to identify genes containing mutations or polymorphisms that contribute to the development of COPD due to smoking. Linkage analysis has revealed regions suggestive for COPD on chromosomes 1, 2 and 12. In addition, linkage of FEV1 and/or FEV1/FVC ratio with various loci in the genome has been reported (*i.e.* chromosomes 1, 2q, 4, 6, 8, 12p, 17, 18, 19 and 21). Among the candidate genes that have been studied in COPD are genes that regulate the production of proteases and antiproteases, genes that modulate the metabolism of toxic substances in cigarette smoke, genes involved with mucociliary clearance and genes that influence inflammatory mediators.

However, the genetic risk factor that is best documented is the hereditary deficiency of α_1-antitrypsin (α_1-AT), a serum protein made in the liver that is capable of inhibiting the activity of specific proteolytic enzymes, the serine proteases. The α_1-AT gene is located within the serpin cluster, on the chromosome 14q23.1-3. Neutrophil elastase is the main target of α_1-AT; if not inactivated by α_1-AT, neutrophil elastase destroys lung connective tissue, particularly elastin, and this leads to the development of emphysema. >90 phenotypes of α_1-AT have been described. The common gene variants are M, S and Z. M1, M2, M3, M4 are wild types found in 90% of the population. Different genotypes, ZZ, SZ, MZ, SS and MS, cause average serum α_1-AT concentration reduced to 16, 51, 83, 93 and 97%, respectively, of the wild-type MM genotype. ZZ homozygous have the most severe α_1-AT deficiency. Emphysema associated with α_1-AT deficiency is typically panlobular, characterised by uniform destruction of the pulmonary lobule. Cigarette smoking is the biggest risk factor for the development of emphysema and airflow obstruction in α_1-AT deficiency, and current smokers have an accelerated decline in FEV1, compared with ex-smokers and never-smokers and α_1-AT deficiency. Homozygous Z patients have a very low α_1-AT and generally show rapid decline in FEV1 even without smoking. In homozygous Z smokers, COPD is developed at a younger age. However, this homozygous state is rare in the general population (one in 5,000 live births) and thus as genetic risk factor can explain <1% of COPD.

Recently, epigenetic mechanisms, such as acquired somatic mutations, have been explored in COPD. Somatic mutations are not heritable, although the susceptibility to acquiring such mutations might be controlled by inherited genes. In normal conditions, cells are equipped with a number of repair pathways that remove the damage and restore DNA. However, increased and persistent oxidative stress (*e.g.* due to cigarette smoking) may inactivate the human DNA mismatch repair system leading to acquired mutations. Smoking-induced acquired somatic alterations have been detected in COPD patients.

Management

The overall approach to managing stable COPD is based on an individualised assessment of disease severity and response to various therapies. The patient who still smokes should be encouraged to quit. Smoking cessation is the single most effective intervention to reduce the risk of developing COPD and stop its progression, and can have a substantial effect on subsequent mortality.

The goals of therapy are to prevent and control symptoms, reduce the frequency and severity of exacerbations and improve exercise

Table 2. Risk factors for chronic obstructive pulmonary disease

Genes
Exposure to particles
Tobacco smoke
Occupational dusts, organic and inorganic
Indoor air pollution (heating and cooking with biomass fuel)
Outdoor air pollution
Lung growth
Oxidative stress
Sex
Age
Respiratory infections
Socioeconomic status
Nutrition
Reproduced from the Global strategy for the diagnosis, management, and prevention of chronic obstructive pulmonary disease, with permission.

tolerance, thus improving overall the quality of life (fig. 1). Bronchodilator medications are central to the symptomatic management of COPD. These drugs improve emptying of the lungs, tend to reduce dynamic hyperinflation and improve exercise performance. There is choice of β_2-agonists, anticholinergics and methylxanthines used either singly or in combination. Inhaled therapy is preferred and bronchodilators are prescribed on either an as-needed or a regular basis, although it is evident that regular treatment with long-acting bronchodilators is more effective and convenient than treatment with short-acting ones. Treatment with a long-acting inhaled anticholinergic drug reduces the rate of COPD exacerbations and improves the effectiveness of pulmonary rehabilitation. A combination of a short-acting β_2-agonist and an anticholinergic produces better and more sustained improvements in FEV1 than either drug alone. The addition of inhaled glucocorticosteroids is appropriate for symptomatic patients with COPD stage III and IV and repeated exacerbations according to the guidelines (fig. 1). This treatment does not modify the long-term decline of FEV1, but it has been shown to reduce the frequency of exacerbations and improve the health status of COPD patients. Recent data, however, based on a single large study of patients with FEV1 <60% pred, indicate that regular treatment with inhaled glucocorticosteroids can decrease the rate of decline of lung function. Long-term treatment with oral glucocorticosteroids should be avoided in COPD because side-effects such as steroid myopathy may contribute to muscle weakness, decreased functionality and respiratory failure in patients with advanced COPD. The regular use of mucolytic and antioxidant agents has been evaluated in COPD patients without significant overall benefit, although there has been a study reporting reduced frequency of exacerbations. The regular use of antibiotics, other than for treating infectious exacerbations of COPD is not recommended. The regular use of antitussive medications is also not recommended since cough, although a troublesome symptom, has a significant protective role. There has been some recent evidence regarding the use of statins and long-term macrolide treatment in decreasing COPD exacerbations, but these are not standard recommendations.

Influenza vaccination is strongly recommended for all COPD patients; it can reduce serious illness and death by ~50% and should be given once a year. Pneumococcal polysaccharide vaccine is recommended for COPD patients who are aged ⩾65 yrs.

Pulmonary rehabilitation aims at improving exercise capacity, reducing symptoms and overall improving quality of life. It is a multidisciplinary programme ideally involving several types of health professionals. COPD patients at all stages of disease appear to benefit from exercise training programmes, although benefit decreases after a rehabilitation programme ends. Pulmonary rehabilitation improves dyspnoea, improves quality-of-life scores, reduces the number of hospitalisations and days in hospital, reduces anxiety and depression related with COPD and improves survival. A comprehensive rehabilitation programme includes exercise training, education and nutrition counselling.

I: Mild	II: Moderate	III: Severe	IV: Very Severe
• FEV$_1$/FVC <0.70 • FEV$_1$ ≥80% pred	• FEV$_1$/FVC <0.70 • 50% ≤ FEV$_1$ <80% pred	• FEV$_1$/FVC <0.70 • 30% ≤ FEV$_1$ <50% pred	• FEV$_1$/FVC <0.70 • FEV$_1$ <30% pred or FEV$_1$ <50% pred plus chronic respiratory failure

Active reduction of risk factor(s); influenza vaccination →
Add short-acting bronchodilator (when needed) →

Add regular treatment with one or more long-acting bronchodilators (when needed); add rehabilitation

Add inhaled glucocorticosteroids if repeated exacerbations

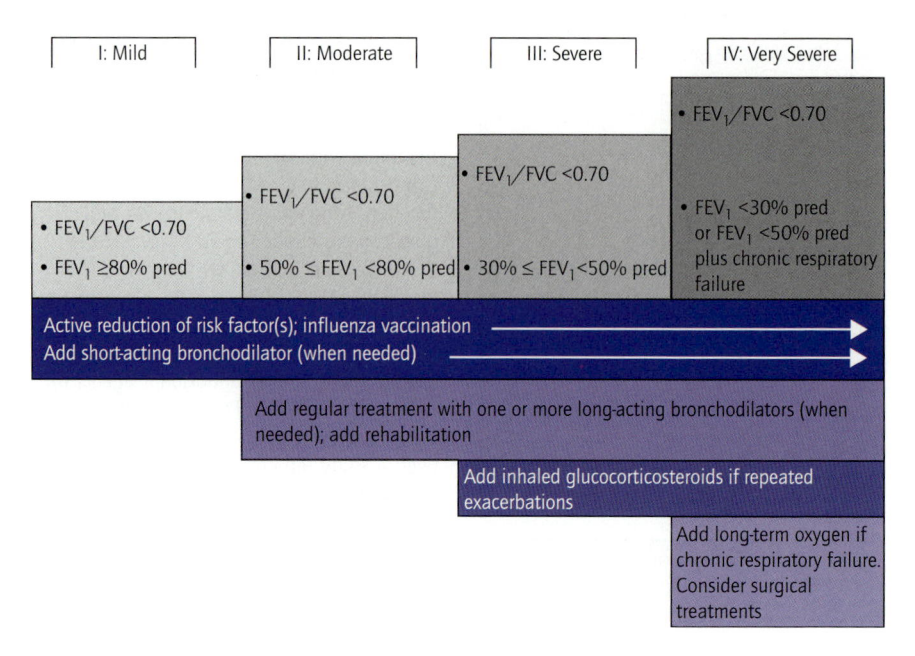

Add long-term oxygen if chronic respiratory failure. Consider surgical treatments

Figure 1. Chronic obstructive pulmonary disease (COPD) treatment by severity. FEV1: forced expiratory volume in 1 s; FVC: forced vital capacity; % pred: % predicted. Reproduced from the Global strategy for the diagnosis, management, and prevention of chronic obstructive pulmonary disease, with permission.

Nutritional status is an important factor in determining symptoms, respiratory function and prognosis in COPD. Both extremes (overweight and underweight) are detrimental. A reduction in body mass index, seen in ~25% of stage III and IV COPD patients, is an independent risk factor for mortality. Present evidence suggests a combination of nutritional support and exercise regimes, to induce anabolic action.

References

- Barnes PJ. Molecular genetics of chronic obstructive pulmonary disease. *Thorax* 1999; 54: 245-252.
- Blamoun AI, et al. Statins may reduce episodes of exacerbations and the requirement for intubation in patients with COPD: evidence from a retrospective cohort study. *Int J Clin Pract* 2008; 62: 1373-1378.
- Celli BR, et al. Airway obstruction in never smokers: results from the Third National Health and Nutrition Examination Survey. *Am J Med* 2005; 118: 1364-1372.
- Celli B, et al. Effect of pharmacotherapy on rate of decline of lung function in chronic obstructive pulmonary disease: results from the TORCH study. *Am J Respir Crit Care Med* 2008; 178: 332-338.
- Celli BR, et al. Standards for the diagnosis and treatment of patients with COPD: a summary of the ATS/ERS position paper. *Eur Respir J* 2004; 23: 932-946.
- Coventry PA. Does pulmonary rehabilitation reduce anxiety and depression in chronic obstructive pulmonary disease? *Curr Opin Pulm Med* 2009; 15: 143-149.
- DeMeo DL, Silverman EK. α1-Antitrypsin deficiency? 2: Genetic aspects of α1-antitrypsin deficiency: phenotypes and genetic modifiers of emphysema risk. *Thorax* 2004; 59: 259-264.
- Global Initiative for Chronic Obstructive Lung Disease. Global strategy for the diagnosis, management, and prevention of chronic obstructive pulmonary disease (2006). www.goldcopd.org. Updated: 2009. Date last accessed: April 14, 2010.
- Hersh CP, et al. Attempted replication of reported chronic obstructive pulmonary disease candidate gene associations. *Am J Respir Cell Mol Biol* 2005; 33: 71-78.

- Hogg JC. Pathophysiology of airflow limitation in chronic obstructive pulmonary disease. *Lancet* 2004; 364: 709-721.
- Molfino NA. Genetics of COPD. *Chest* 2004; 125: 1929-1940.
- Nici L, et al. Pulmonary rehabilitation: what we know and what we need to know. *J Cardiopulm Rehabil Prev* 2009; 29: 141-151.
- Samara KD, et al. Somatic DNA alterations in lung epithelial barrier cells in COPD patients: a case control study. *Pulm Pharmacol Ther* 2010; 23: 208-214.
- Seemungal TAR, et al. Long term erythromycin therapy is associated with decreased COPD exacerbations. *Am J Respir Crit Care Med* 2008; 178: 1139-1147.
- Silverman EK, Speizer FE. Risk factors for the development of chronic obstructive pulmonary disease. *Med Clin North Am* 1996; 80: 501-522.
- Stoller JK, Aboussouan LS. Alpha1-antitrypsin deficiency. *Lancet* 2005; 365: 2225-2236.
- Tager IB, et al. Household aggregation of pulmonary function and chronic bronchitis. *Am Rev Respir Dis* 1976; 114: 485-492.
- Tzortzaki EG, Siafakas NM. A hypothesis for the initiation of COPD. *Eur Respir J* 2009; 34: 310-315.
- Zheng JP, et al. Effect of carbocisteine on acute exacerbation of chronic obstructive pulmonary disease (PEACE study): a randomized placebo-controlled study. *Lancet* 2008; 371: 2013-2018.

BRONCHIECTASIS

N. ten Hacken
University Medical Center Groningen, Groningen, The Netherlands
E-mail: n.h.t.ten.hacken@long.umcg.nl

Bronchiectasis is a disorder characterised by abnormal bronchial wall thickening and luminal dilatation of the central and medium-sized bronchi due to a vicious circle of transmural infection and inflammation with mediator release. The prevalence varies between countries but seems to increase with age and is more common in females. Frequent symptoms are chronic cough and production of mucopurulent sputum. Less frequent are haemoptysis, pleuritic pain, recurrent fever, wheeze and dyspnoea. Exacerbations of bronchiectasis are characterised by increase in symptoms, i.e. increase in cough and change in purulence and volume of sputum associated with increase in malaise. These exacerbations are almost always associated with infections of bronchiectasis (table 1).

Underlying causes of bronchiectasis may be acquired or inherited, and include post-infective, mechanical obstruction, excessive immune response, deficient immune response, inflammatory pneumonitis, abnormal mucus clearance and fibrosis. Conditions associated with bronchiectasis include infertility, inflammatory bowel disease, connective tissue disorders, malignancy, diffuse panbronchiolitis, α_1-antitrypsin deficiency and mercury poisoning. In adults the aetiology is idiopathic in ~50%, and in children 25%; however, these figures may differ in time and between countries due to the availability of diagnostics and antibiotics (including vaccinations).

Work-up

The work-up of bronchiectasis comprises:

- blood tests: C-reactive protein, white blood count;
- differentiation, immunoglobulin (Ig)G, IgM, IgA, total IgE, IgG, aspergillus serology, α_1-antitrypsin;

Key points

- Diagnosis of bronchiectasis is based on the presence of daily production of mucopurulent phlegm and chest imaging that demonstrates dilated and thickened airways. HRCT scan is today the gold standard.

- The diagnosis of bronchiectasis should lead to the investigation and treatment of possible causes and associated conditions.

- Antibiotics form the mainstay of treatment of bronchiectasis. Acute exacerbations should be treated promptly with short courses of antibiotics.

- The continuous administration of antibiotics, mucolytics, anti-inflammatory agents and bronchodilators is not clear, but may be considered on an individual basis.

- Bronchopulmonary hygiene physical therapy techniques are widely used, yet there is not enough evidence to support or refute them.

- Surgery may be considered if the area of the bronchiectatic lung is localised and if the patient's symptoms are debilitating or life threatening (like massive haemoptysis).

Table 1. Microbiology of bronchiectasis

Bacterial
Haemophilus influenza
Pseudomonas aeruginosa
Moraxella catarrhalis
Streptococcus pneumoniae
Staphylococcus aureus

Mycobacterial
Avium-intracellulare complex
Kansasii
Fortuitum

Fungal
Aspergillus fumigatus

The pattern of microbiology is quite stable; however, resistance against antibiotics may increase in time. *Pseudomonas* is associated with more severe disease. Nontuberculous mycobacteria associates frequently with *Aspergillus*. Taken from ILOWITE *et al.* (2009).

- specific tests to identify underlying causes or contributing conditions dependent of the clinical setting;
- spirometry;
- sputum smear and cultures for bacteria, mycobacteria and fungi; and
- radiography of chest and sinus, if necessary a high-resolution computed tomography (HRCT) scan of the lung.

The chest radiograph is abnormal in most patients; however, a normal chest radiograph does not exclude bronchiectasis. HRCT is nowadays the "gold standard" for bronchiectasis. Characteristic findings include internal bronchial diameters 1.5 times greater than that of the adjacent pulmonary artery (signet ring sign, fig. 1), lack of bronchial tapering, visualisation of bronchi within 1 cm of the costal pleura, visualisation of the bronchi abutting the mediastinal pleura, and bronchial wall thickening. The distribution of bronchiectasis on HRCT scan may give diagnostic clues for allergic bronchopulmonary aspergillosis, cystic fibrosis (CF), primary ciliary dyskinesia, and idiopathic bronchiectasis. Severity of bronchiectasis on HRCT scan is poorly correlated with clinical indices.

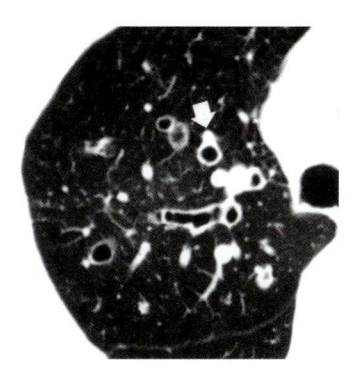

Figure 1. Signet ring sign. Cross-sectional computed tomography scan of the right lung in a patient with bronchiectasis. White arrow indicates a signet ring sign. Taken from OUELLETTE (1999).

Management

Management of bronchiectasis should aim at fast resolution and prevention of infective exacerbations, no sputum infections, optimal bronchial clearance, minimal respiratory symptoms, normal lung function, high quality of life and no treatment-related adverse effects. Obviously, the prompt recognition and treatment of the underlying cause(s) and/or condition(s) is important for both short- and long-term outcomes. For the specific treatment of CF-related bronchiectasis see next chapter on Cystic fibrosis. Unfortunately, there are only limited high-quality studies on the management of non-CF bronchiectasis. Several reviews list a large number of treatment options; however, due to small study samples, different study populations and outcome variables, and other methodological issues, it is difficult to draw definitive conclusions.

Acute exacerbations Antibiotic treatment is the mainstay of acute exacerbations and is targeted at likely organisms (table 1) or the results of sputum culture(s). A fluoroquinolone is recommended over 7–10 days in outpatients without history of recurrent exacerbations or sputum cultures (Barker, UpToDate; see Weblinks). Hospitalised patients may be treated with two *i.v.* antibiotics with efficacy for *Pseudomonas* (Barker, UpToDate; see Weblinks). Supportive management may consist of inhaled bronchodilators, systemic corticosteroids, and measures to improve bronchial clearance (physical therapy, hydration, mucolytic agents).

Prevention of exacerbations Prolonged use of antibiotics (>4 weeks) may be considered in patients who quickly relapse (>4-6 times per year) or demonstrate progressive lung function decline. Several treatment strategies are described:

- oral antibiotic 2-3 times daily,
- oral macrolide three times weekly,
- aerosolised tobramycin, gentamycin, colistin, ceftazidime, or aztreonam twice daily (aerosoled antibiotics in non-CF bronchiectasis are frequently not licensed or stopped because of side-effects),
- intravenous antibiotics, 2-3-week courses with 1-2-month intervals (Barker, UpTodate; see Weblinks).

A Cochrane review concluded that there is a small benefit on overall clinical response scores, but not on exacerbation rates. Clearly the indication for prolonged use of antibiotics should be based on a benefit–risk evaluation, also taking possible adverse effects into account.

Sputum and bronchial clearance Inhaled rhDNAse administered to stable non-CF bronchiectasis patients has been associated with increased exacerbation frequency and greater forced expiratory volume in 1 s decline and therefore should not be given. Oral bromhexine improved expectoration, quantity and quality of sputum, and auscultatory findings during acute infective exacerbations. Macrolides improved sputum production and sputum inflammatory markers. 12-day inhalation of mannitol improved the tenacity and hydration of sputum. Inhaled fluticasone improved sputum production and sputum inflammation, but not its microbiological profile. Nebulised 0.9 and 7% saline as an adjunct to physiotherapy improved sputum production, sputum viscosity and ease of sputum expectoration; however, 7% saline was superior to 0.9%. Two systematic reviews found insufficient evidence to either support or refute bronchial hygiene physical therapy.

Symptoms and quality of life
Haemoptysis is treated with bronchial embolisation; however, surgical resection is sometimes inevitable. Surgical resection may also be considered if the area of the bronchiectatic lung is localised and if the patient's symptoms are debilitating or life threatening. In this case, surgery can even be curative if there is absence of an ongoing underlying cause. Although surgery is widely used, there are no randomised controlled trials (RCTs). Inhaled fluticasone improved dyspnoea, sputum production, days without cough, β_2-agonist use and health-related quality of life.

Lung function RCTs on short-acting β_2-agonists, long-acting β_2-agonists, anticholinergic therapy, oral methyl-xanthines, leukotriene antagonists and oral corticosteroids were not selected in Cochrane reviews. Nevertheless, bronchodilator therapy may be considered if a patient has proven airway obstruction. Macrolides may improve methacholine reactivity, airway obstruction and carbon monoxide diffusion. However, if macrolides are considered, the presence of nontuberculous mycobacteria must be excluded first, and patients must be warned about ototoxicity.

Exercise tolerance Pulmonary rehabilitation is effective in improving exercise capacity and endurance, whereas simultaneous inspiratory muscle training may be important in the longevity of these training effects.

References

- Ilowite J, et al. Pharmacological treatment options for bronchiectasis: focus on antimicrobial and anti-inflammatory agents. Drugs 2009; 69: 407–419.

- Lynch DA, et al. Correlation of CT findings with clinical evaluations in 261 patients with symptomatic bronchiectasis. *AJR Am J Roentgenol* 1999; 173: 53-58.
- Nicotra MB, et al. Clinical, pathophysiologic, and microbiologic characterization of bronchiectasis in an aging cohort. *Chest* 1995; 108: 955-961.
- Ouellette H. The signet ring sign. *Radiology* 1999; 212: 67-68.
- Pasteur MC, et al. An investigation into causative factors in patients with bronchiectasis. *Am J Respir Crit Care Med* 2000; 162: 1277-1284.
- Rosen MJ. Chronic cough due to bronchiectasis: ACCP evidence-based clinical practice guidelines. *Chest* 2006; 129: Suppl. 1, 122S-131S.
- ten Hacken NH, et al. Bronchiectasis: Clinical Evidence Handbook (online), 2008. http://clinicalevidence.bmj.com/ceweb/conditions/rdc/1507/1507.jsp.
- ten Hacken NH, et al. Treatment of bronchiectasis in adults. *BMJ* 2007; 335: 1089-1093.

Weblinks

- Cochrane Library. Meta-analyses on bronchiectasis: anticholinergic therapy, oral methyl-xanthines, leukotriene receptor antagonists, short-acting beta-2-agonists, long-acting beta-2-agonists, oral steroids, inhaled steroids, mucolytics, inhaled hyperosmolar agents, prolonged antibiotics, surgery versus non-surgical treatment, bronchopulmonary hygiene physical therapy, nurse specialist care, and physical training. http://www3.interscience.wiley.com/cgi-bin/mrwhome/106568753/HOME.
- UpToDate. Clinical manifestations and diagnosis of bronchiectasis. Treatment of bronchiectasis. Author: AF Barker. http://www.utdol.com/home/index.html.

CYSTIC FIBROSIS

A. Bush and J. Davies
Imperial College and Royal Brompton Hospital, London, UK
E-mail: a.bush@rbht.nhs.uk

Key points

- Adult pulmonologists need to know about cystic fibrosis; it is common across Europe, patients are surviving into middle age and beyond, and new diagnoses are being made even in old age.

- Cystic fibrosis is now a true multisystem disease; to the well-known complications of chronic respiratory infection and malabsorbtion has been added conditions such as cirrhosis, insulin deficiency and diabetes, osteopenia, stress incontinence and infertility.

- Furthermore, with longevity is coming new complications, including the selection of resistant microorganisms and antibiotic allergy. Other organ systems will likely be affected in the aging cystic fibrosis population.

- Treatment of cystic fibrosis thus requires a dedicated multidisciplinary team, comprising physicians, specialist nurses, physiotherapists, dieticians, clinical psychologists and pharmacists.

- The increasing knowledge of the molecular pathophysiology of cystic fibrosis is leading the way in the development of genotype specific therapies, which will be a paradigm for other diseases.

The autosomal recessive condition cystic fibrosis (CF) is the most common inherited disease of white races; the prevalence varies across Europe. Although commonest in white people, it has been found in virtually every ethnic group. The gene, on the long arm of chromosome 7, encodes a multifunctional protein, cystic fibrosis transmembrane regulator (CFTR), which is active at the apical membrane of epithelial cells. Different classes of mutation have been described (fig. 1); severe mutations (classes I–III) are usually associated with pancreatic insufficient CF and a worse prognosis, whereas those with milder mutations (IV–VI) are more usually pancreatic sufficient. The combination of a mild and severe gene usually leads to a mild pancreatic phenotype; however, there is only a poor correlation between genotype and pulmonary phenotype. In many parts of Europe, the most common mutation is DF_{508}, but there are marked ethnic differences.

CFTR functions as a chloride channel and regulates other ion channels, such as the epithelial sodium channel (ENaC). Most of the morbidity and mortality of CF is due to chronic bronchial infection, but as adults survive longer, multisystem complications are becoming more important. The airways of the newborn with CF are effectively normal at birth, but from an early age, cycles of infection and inflammation supervene, leading ultimately to severe bronchiectasis and respiratory failure. The most popular hypothesis for the pathophysiology of CF lung disease is airway surface liquid dehydration due to uncontrolled activity of ENaC, possibly triggered by viral infection. Median survival is predicted to be ~50 yrs, longer for males. In parts of Europe there are now more adult than paediatric CF patients.

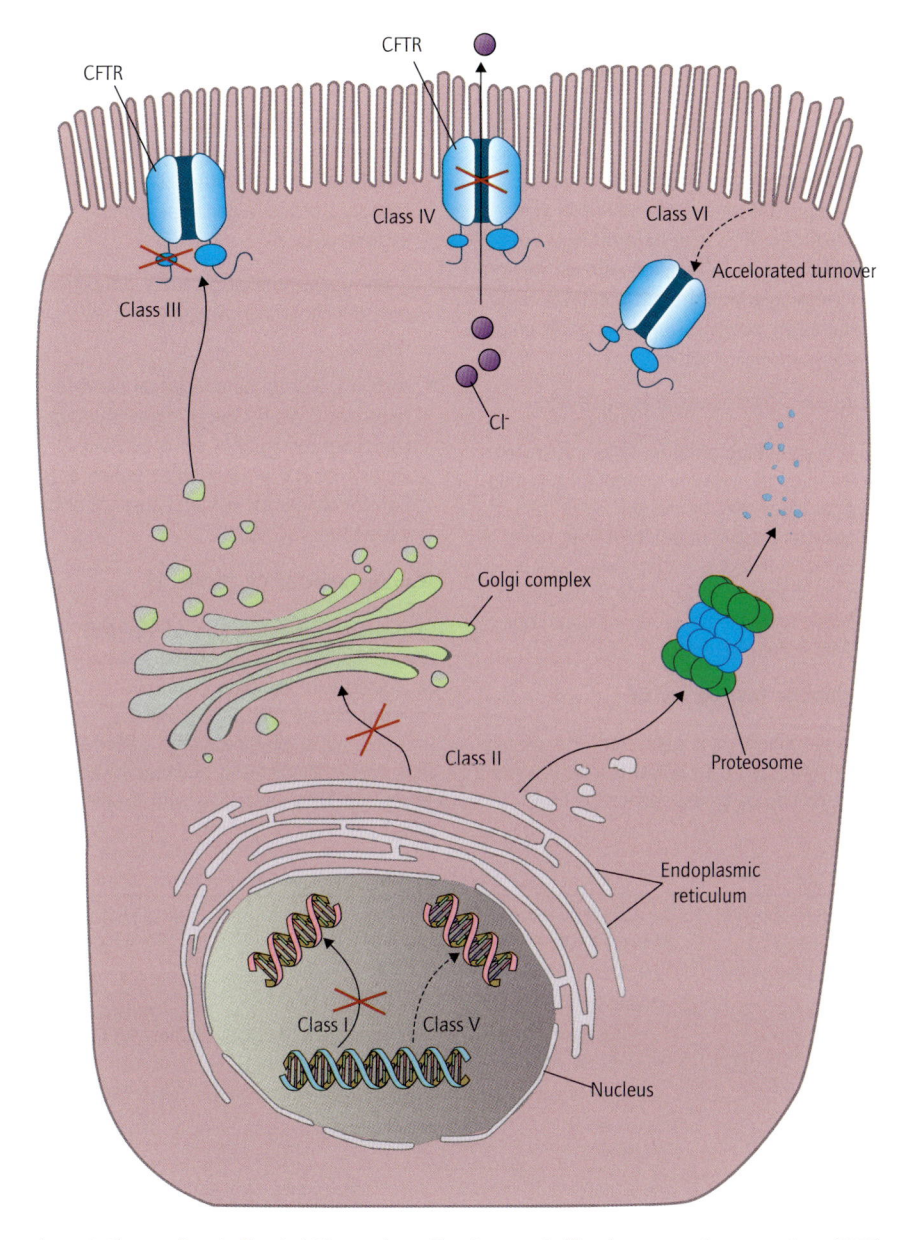

Figure 1. Classes of cystic fibrosis (CF) mutations. Class I: no cystic fibrosis transmembrane regulator (CFTR) synthesis (mutation, premature stop codon)(G542X); class II: CFTR processed incorrectly and does not reach apical cell membrane (DF$_{508}$); class III: CFTR reaches apical membrane, but channel regulation is abnormal (G551D); class IV: CFTR reaches apical membrane, but channel open time is reduced (R334W); class V: reduced CFTR synthesis (R117H); class VI: CFTR reaches apical cell membrane, but has a shortened half-life due to more rapid turnover (1811+1.6 kb A>G).

Adult physicians will encounter CF patients by two routes:

- referral from a paediatric clinic of an already diagnosed patient. Transition to a new and strange adult clinic from the familiar staff and surroundings of the paediatric clinic may be a difficult time, and needs to be handled with sensitivity. Increasingly, young adult handover clinics, staffed by paediatricians and adult physicians, are being set up.
- a new diagnosis made in adult life.

CF is usually diagnosed in early childhood, increasingly by newborn screening, but mild atypical cases may be missed. ~10–15% of CF patients present in adult life (see table 1). Conversely, always consider the possibility that the diagnosis of CF made in childhood is incorrect, and whether a repeat diagnostic work-up should be done.

Diagnostic testing for CF

Once the diagnosis is suspected, it is usually easily confirmed by a sweat test, which must be performed in an experienced centre.

Other diagnostic modalities that are employed include:

- Genetic testing: more than 1,300 variants are described, and rare ones are usually undetected in the routine clinical laboratory, so a negative genotype cannot exclude disease.
- Nasal transepithelial potential difference measurement: only available in a few centres.
- Ancillary testing: human faecal elastase (pancreatic insufficiency), high-resolution computed tomography for occult bronchiectasis, scrotal ultrasound or semen analysis for congenital bilateral absence of the vas deferens (CABVD).

Management of CF (table 2)

CF has now become a true multisystem disease. Treatment can only be optimally conducted with the help of a full multidisciplinary team (CF physician, specialist nurse, physiotherapist, dietician, clinical psychologist and pharmacist) and the help of ancillary specialists with expert

Table 1. Late presentation of cystic fibrosis (CF; such patients are usually but not invariably pancreatic sufficient)

Recurrent respiratory infections	Consider especially with 'suggestive' microorganisms such as *Staphylococcus aureus, Pseudomonas aeruginosa, Burkholderia cepacia*
Atypical 'asthma'	Especially if chronic productive cough, and a poor response to standard asthma therapy
Bronchiectasis	Especially if any extrapulmonary features, a positive family history, or infection with atypical microorganisms
Male infertility	Azoospermia due to congenital bilateral absence of the vas deferens (CABVD)
Electrolyte disturbance	Classically as acute heat exhaustion leading to sodium, chloride and potassium depletion
Atypical mycobacterial infection	Always consider the possibility of CF if these organisms are isolated from sputum
Acute pancreatitis	Typically seen in pancreatic sufficient CF
CF liver disease	Portal hypertension and variceal haemorrhage; liver cell failure is a late manifestation
Cascade screening	Diagnosis made in a relative leading to extended family screening

New diagnoses of CF have been made even in old age; CF diagnosis should always be considered.

Table 2. Management of cystic fibrosis (CF) lung disease

Disease stage	Pulmonary status	Aim	Management
Early (unusual but seen in adults with CF)	Pre-infection	Mucus clearance	Airway clearance techniques (physiotherapy and adjuncts; these include exercise and mucolytics, e.g. rhDNase, hypertonic saline)
	Intermittent isolation of *Pseudomonas aeruginosa*	Prevent infection	Segregation and cohorting to prevent cross-infection. Prophylactic antibiotics controversial; used against *Staphylococcus aureus* in the UK; avoid cephalosporins Influenza vaccination
		Eradication of infection. Energetic treatment is essential	High doses of appropriate antibiotics. *P. aeruginosa* eradication protocols include both topical (nebulised) and systemic (usually oral ciprofloxacin). Eradication achieved in 80–90%
Intermediate	Chronic infection with usual organisms (*P. aeruginosa*: eventually present in 80% of patients; *S. aureus* (methicillin resistant and sensitive), less usually *Haemophilus influenzae*)	Suppression of bacterial load and thus limitation of inflammatory response	Depends on organism: *P. aeruginosa*: nebulised high-dose tobramycin (300 mg *b.i.d.*) or colomycin Use the new, faster nebuliser devices, for example, e-Flow (PARI) and iNeb (Profile Pharma)
		Treat infective exacerbations	Oral or IV antibiotics (some centres use regular elective courses, but no evidence to prefer this over symptomatic use) Culture results usually guide choice, but no evidence that this improves outcome

Table 2. Continued

	Infection with less common organisms (*Burkholderia cepacia* complex, *Stenotrophomonas maltophilia*, *Achromobacter xylosoxidans*)	Eradication if early; suppression of bacterial load most commonly	No evidence for a role for corticosteroids except in treating ABPA, because of efficacy but adverse side-effect profile (oral) or lack of benefit (inhaled) Ibuprofen not much used in most of Europe; beware synergistic nephrotoxicity with intravenous aminoglycosides Azithromycin is useful, but mode of action unknown Confirm diagnosis in a reference laboratory; treat on an individual basis with specialist microbiological advice
	ABPA	Reduce allergic response Prevent bronchiectasis	Oral corticosteroids (long course often required), consider pulsed methyl prednisolone Addition of an antifungal agent common but evidence limited
	Nontuberculous *Mycobacterial* infection	Eradication or suppression (*Mycobacterium abscessus* may be very difficult to eradicate)	Diagnosis and management difficult; seek specialist advice, especially for *M. abscessus* infection Prolonged courses of multiple chemotherapies will be needed: ethambutol, rifampicin, azithromycin, amikacin, ciprofloxacin, moxifloxacin are among the agents used
	Lobar or segmental atelectasis (may be seen at any stage of CF)	Re-inflation of the lung	Intensive physiotherapy, with rhDNase and hypertonic saline as appropriate Intravenous antibiotics Fibreoptic bronchoscopy, consider endobronchial instillation of rhDNase if conventional management fails
Late	Major haemoptysis (may be seen also in those with well preserved lung function)	Prevent or halt acute bleeding	Admit for intravenous antibiotics and clotting studies; bronchoscopy not useful. Bronchial artery embolisation for ongoing bleeding; can consider the use of tranexamic acid. Lobectomy is a last resort
	Pneumothorax (carries a very bad prognosis)	Control air leak, prevent recurrence	Conservative management for trivial pneumothoraces, otherwise tube drainage. Early surgery and pleurodesis if does not respond rapidly
	End-stage respiratory failure	Optimise conventional treatment Refer for lung transplant	Oxygen therapy (no survival benefit demonstrated, unlike for COPD) Consider nasal ventilation as a bridge to transplantation

ABPA: allergic bronchopulmonary aspergillosis; COPD: chronic obstructive pulmonary disease.

Table 3. Management of gastrointestinal manifestations of cystic fibrosis (CF) in the adult

Organ	Manifestation	Management
Pancreas	Exocrine insufficiency: malabsorption, steatorrhoea	High-fat diet Supplementation with enteric-coated microsphere pancreatic enzymes and fat-soluble vitamins Fat absorption may be aided by alkaline environment (H_2-blockers or proton pump inhibitors) Gastrostomy feeds if in nutritional failure (parenteral nutrition only rarely required)
	Acute pancreatitis (pancreatic sufficient patients)	As for other causes; oral pancreatin powder (anecdotal evidence only)
Oesophagus	Gastro-oesophageal reflux (especially common post-lung transplant)	Proton pump inhibitors, prokinetic agents Surgery if refractory symptoms
Small bowel	Distal intestinal obstruction syndrome	Oral gastrografin (Schering) or klean prep (Norgine) Review dose of, and adherence to, pancreatic enzyme replacement therapy, perform 3-day faecal fat collection Consider pro-kinetic agents Severe acute cases, relieve with colonoscopy; laparotomy a last resort
	Coeliac disease (increased incidence in CF)	Gluten-free diet, as for isolated coeliac disease
	Crohn's disease (any part of the bowel)	Management as for isolated Crohn's disease, seek specialist gastroenterology advice
Colon	Constipation	Laxatives, high-fibre diet; must not be confused with distal intestinal obstruction syndrome
Rectum	Rectal prolapse	Rare in adults, usually related to uncontrolled fat malabsorption
Liver	Fatty liver (usually asymptomatic)	Liver ultrasound at least every 2 yrs
	Macronodular cirrhosis (variceal bleeding, splenomegaly, hypersplenism)	Ursodeoxycholic acid, taurine (seek specialist advice)
	Hepatocellular failure a late manifestation	Severe cases may need transplantation

DIOS: distal intestinal obstruction syndrome.

knowledge of CF (ear, nose and throat surgeon, obstetrician and endocrinologist). CF patients should be seen at least every 3 months by the core CF team. A large number of treatment guidelines have been published.

Respiratory tract disease The main issues are the prevention of infection where possible by cohort segregation of patients with particular infections, and the aggressive use of antibiotics; although conventional teaching is that airway infection occurs with a relatively

Table 4. Treatment of other manifestations of cystic fibrosis (CF) in the adult

Organ	Manifestation	Management
Upper airway	Nasal polyps (can cause obstructive sleep apnoea)	Topical steroids. Long courses of antibiotics Surgery if medical management fails, re-operation often needed
	Sinusitis	Most patients have asymptomatic changes on radiography or computed tomography scan, and require no treatment Topical steroids. Antibiotics Surgery if medical management fails, but results often disappointing. Some use sinus drainage tubes and repeatedly instil antibiotics into the sinuses
Endocrine pancreas	Insulin deficiency, which causes reduced lung function and nutrition before overt hyperglycaemia	Screen regularly with annual glucose tolerance test, or continuous glucose monitoring
	Frank diabetes; although there may be an element of peripheral insulin resistance, the main root cause is diminished insulin secretion	Have a low threshold for starting insulin Continue high-fat diet, adjust insulin doses accordingly Diabetic ketoacidosis is very rare Oral hypoglycaemic agents not to be used outside a randomised controlled trial
Sweat gland	Electrolyte depletion, often leading to acute collapse	Sodium and potassium chloride supplementation
Bones and joints	Osteopenia (cystic fibrosis transmembrane regulator is expressed in bones) Pathological fracture	Measure bone mineral density at least every 2 yrs Prevention: weight bearing exercise, high dairy intake, vitamin D and K therapy Treat with bisphosphonates if severe
	CF arthropathy (large or small joint)	Nonsteroidal anti-inflammatory agents, prednisolone; seek specialist rheumatological advice if more than mild
Male reproductive tract	Bilateral absence of vas deferens leading to male infertility	Sperm aspiration and *in vitro* fertilisation; genetic counselling prior to procedure
Female reproductive tract	Vaginal candidiasis	Topical anti-fungal agents
	Stress incontinence	Seek gynaecological advice
	Pregnancy (not an illness, but may be a major therapeutic challenge); women with severe CF may be subfertile, but normal conception is usual	Pre-pregnancy genetic counselling advisable Continue standard CF medications; close collaboration with obstetric unit; may need regular admissions to hospital for intravenous antibiotics Especially beware if low lung function prior to pregnancy, and CF related diabetes on insulin

Table 4. Continued

Late iatrogenic	Antibiotic allergy	Consider desensitisation in hospital
	Chronic renal failure	Related to multiple courses of intravenous aminoglycosides; use these agents appropriately sparingly
Miscellaneous	Vasculitis	Rare, usually responds to steroids, but seek specialist rheumatological advice
	Epithelial cancer	Small but definite increase in risk; careful clinical surveillance mandatory

narrow spectrum of microorganisms, recent work, including the use of molecular techniques, suggests that anaerobes in particular may be more important than previously thought. Sputum clearance using a choice of many chest physiotherapy techniques and the identification and aggressive management of late complications are also important. If the patient has poor lung function, early discussion with the local transplant centre is advisable. Routine respiratory care at every clinic visit should include spirometry and pulse oximetry, and sputum or cough swab culture.

Gastrointestinal disease (table 3) The main issues are to ensure optimal nutrition, and be alert to gastrointestinal causes of weight loss that are unrelated to pancreatic insufficiency. Bad nutrition is a very poor prognostic feature. CF patients have higher than normal energy requirements because of subclinical malabsorption and a higher energy consumption secondary to infection. Increased metabolic rate is thought by some to be part of the underlying defect. Weight should be measured, and body mass index calculated, 3-monthly.

Other organ system disease (table 4) It is important to be aware that new complications are being described as CF patients survive longer. A full systems review is essential at each clinic visit. Finally, the psychological aspects of CF and the effects of chronic illness and the burden of disease and its treatment should not be underestimated; see the poignant stories and poetry on the Breathing Room website.

Future developments

A large number of novel therapies are currently being trialled in CF. Gene therapy, using as vectors either liposomes, viruses or nanoparticles, has been the subject of proof of concept trials, and a large therapeutic trial is about to start. The age of genotype specific therapy dawned with the use of agents such as topical aminoglycosides or oral PTC_{124} to over-ride premature stop codons (class I mutations). Other approaches include the use of molecular chaperones ("correctors") to transport abnormal (class II mutations) CFTR to the apical cell membrane, and potentiators to improve activity when they reach this site. There is ongoing mutation-specific work to increase chloride channel activity of class III and IV mutations, as well as the use of compounds that activate alternative epithelial chloride channels. There is no doubt that we are on the verge of a CF treatment revolution. Most important, however, is to ensure that the basic therapy, which has so greatly improved prognosis, is not neglected here and now.

References

- Brenckmann C, Papaioannou A. Bisphosphonates for osteoporosis in people with cystic fibrosis. *Cochrane Database Syst Rev* 2001; 4: CD002010.
- Bush A. *In:* European Lung White Book. Sheffield, European Respiratory Society, 2003; pp. 89–95.
- Colombo C, *et al.* Liver disease in cystic fibrosis. *J Pediatr Gastroenterol Nutr* 2006; 43: Suppl. 1, S49–S55.
- Dodge JA, *et al.* Cystic fibrosis mortality and survival in the UK: 1947–2003. *Eur Respir J* 2007; 29: 522–526.

- Farrell PM, *et al*. Guidelines for diagnosis of cystic fibrosis in newborns through older adults: Cystic Fibrosis Foundation consensus report. *J Pediatr* 2008; 153: S4–S14.
- Festini F, *et al*. Isolation measures for prevention of infection with respiratory pathogens in cystic fibrosis: a systematic review. *J Hosp Infect* 2006; 64: 1–6.
- Flume PA, *et al*. Cystic fibrosis pulmonary guidelines: chronic medications for maintenance of lung health. *Am J Respir Crit Care Med* 2007; 176: 957–969.
- Flume PA, *et al*. Massive hemoptysis in cystic fibrosis. *Chest* 2005; 128: 729–738.
- Flume PA, *et al*. Pneumothorax in cystic fibrosis. *Chest* 2005; 128: 720–728.
- Kim RD, *et al*. Pulmonary nontuberculous mycobacterial disease: prospective study of a distinct preexisting syndrome. *Am J Respir Crit Care Med* 2008; 178: 1066–1074.
- Ledson MJ, *et al*. Prevalence and mechanisms of gastro-oesophageal reflux in adult cystic fibrosis patients. *J R Soc Med* 1998; 91: 7–9.
- Leus J, *et al*. Detection and follow up of exocrine pancreatic insufficiency in cystic fibrosis: a review. *Eur J Pediatr* 2000; 159: 563–568.
- MacDonald KD, *et al*. Cystic fibrosis transmembrane regulator protein mutations: 'class' opportunity for novel drug innovation. *Paediatr Drugs* 2007; 9: 1–10.
- McKone EF, *et al*. Effect of genotype on phenotype and mortality in cystic fibrosis: a retrospective cohort study. *Lancet* 2003; 361: 1671–1676.
- Nick JA, Rodman DM. Manifestations of cystic fibrosis diagnosed in adulthood. *Curr Opin Pulm Med* 2005; 11: 513–518.
- Onady GM, Stolfi A. Insulin and oral agents for managing cystic fibrosis-related diabetes. *Cochrane Database Syst Rev* 2005; 3: CD004730.
- Southern KW, *et al*. Macrolide antibiotics for cystic fibrosis. *Cochrane Database Syst Rev* 2004; 2: CD002203.
- Tarran R, *et al*. Normal and cystic fibrosis airway surface liquid homeostasis. The effects of phasic shear stress and viral infections. *J Biol Chem* 2005; 280: 35751–35759.
- Wood DM, Smyth AR. Antibiotic strategies for eradicating *Pseudomonas aeruginosa* in people with cystic fibrosis. *Cochrane Database Syst Rev* 2006; 1: CD004197.
- Yung MW, *et al*. Nasal polyposis in children with cystic fibrosis: a long-term follow-up study. *Ann Otol Rhinol Laryngol* 2002; 111: 1081–1086.

Weblinks

- www.ukneqas.org.uk/.
- www.genet.sickkids.on.ca/cftr/.
- www.thebreathingroom.org/cg.
- www.cfgenetherapy.org.uk.

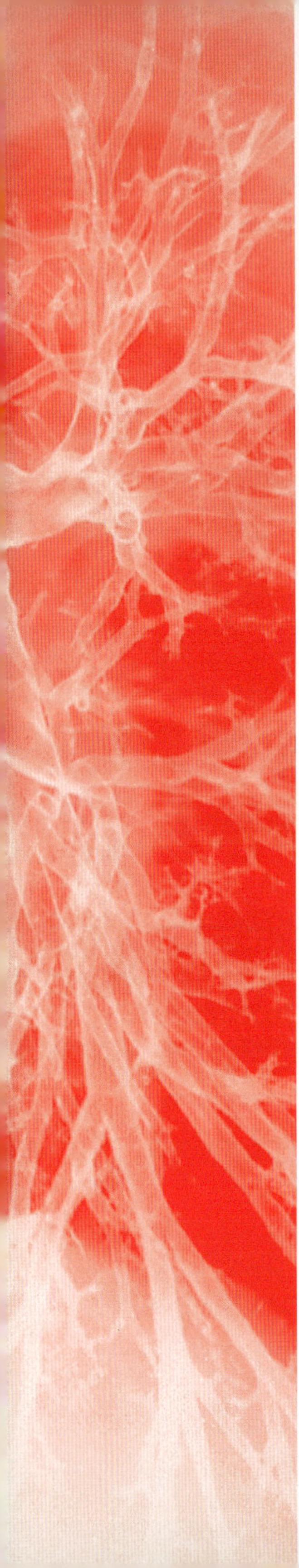

CHAPTER 10:

OCCUPATIONAL AND ENVIRONMENTAL LUNG DISEASES

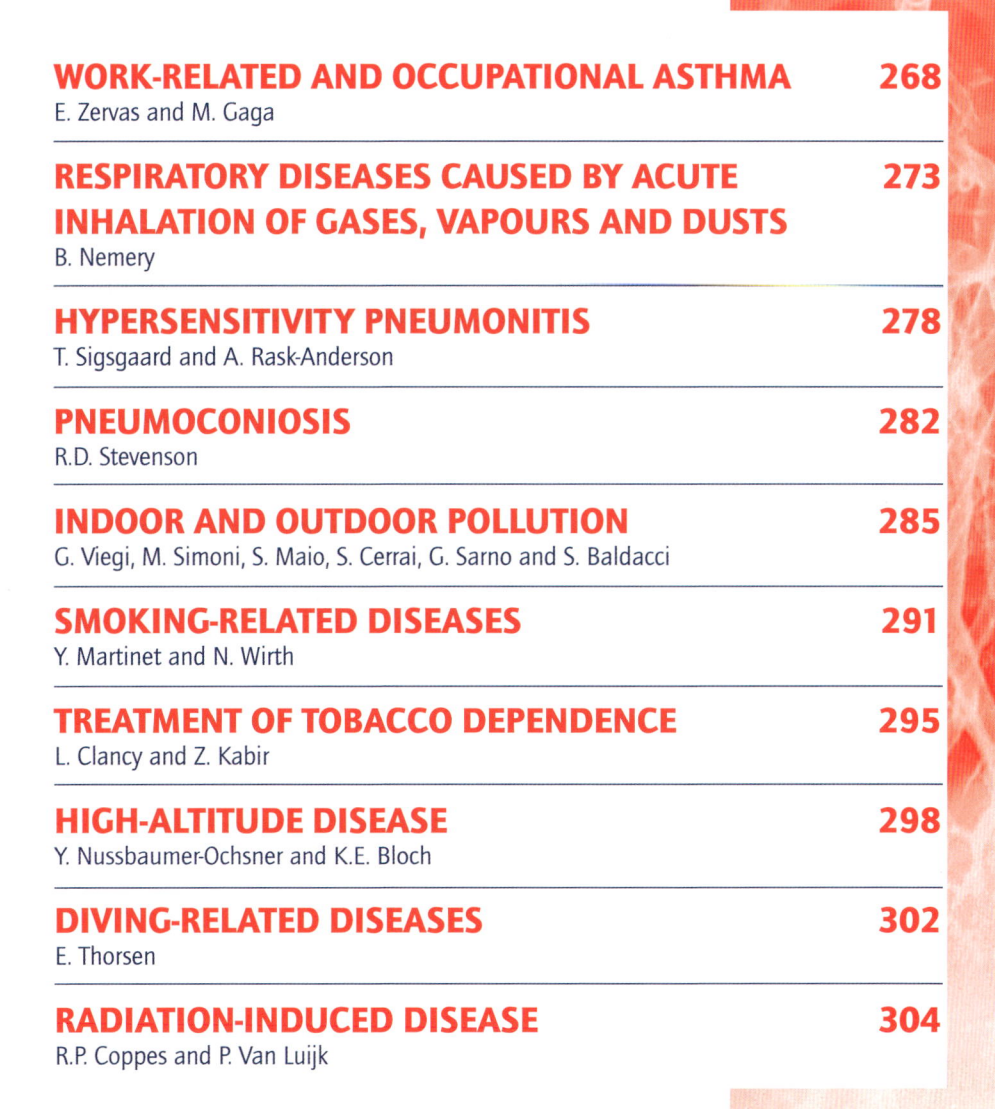

WORK-RELATED AND OCCUPATIONAL ASTHMA E. Zervas and M. Gaga	**268**
RESPIRATORY DISEASES CAUSED BY ACUTE INHALATION OF GASES, VAPOURS AND DUSTS B. Nemery	**273**
HYPERSENSITIVITY PNEUMONITIS T. Sigsgaard and A. Rask-Anderson	**278**
PNEUMOCONIOSIS R.D. Stevenson	**282**
INDOOR AND OUTDOOR POLLUTION G. Viegi, M. Simoni, S. Maio, S. Cerrai, G. Sarno and S. Baldacci	**285**
SMOKING-RELATED DISEASES Y. Martinet and N. Wirth	**291**
TREATMENT OF TOBACCO DEPENDENCE L. Clancy and Z. Kabir	**295**
HIGH-ALTITUDE DISEASE Y. Nussbaumer-Ochsner and K.E. Bloch	**298**
DIVING-RELATED DISEASES E. Thorsen	**302**
RADIATION-INDUCED DISEASE R.P. Coppes and P. Van Luijk	**304**

WORK-RELATED AND OCCUPATIONAL ASTHMA

E. Zervas and M. Gaga
Athens Chest Hospital, Asthma Centre and 7th Respiratory Medicine Dept, Sotiria Hospital, Athens, Greece
E-mail: minagaga@yahoo.com

Definition

Work-related asthma (WRA) is the most common form of occupational lung disease, causing significant morbidity and disability.

Key points

- The burden of work-related asthma (WRA) is still very high, accounting for one in ten cases of adult asthma, and causing morbidity, disability and high costs.

- Prevention is very important. Health officials, work managers and doctors must be aware of the problem, strict measures for exposures to known sensitisers should always be followed, conditions at work examined and, when necessary, amended.

- Better education of workers and managerial staff as well as medical professionals is key to the prevention and prompt diagnosis and management of WRA and occupational asthma (OA). When WRA is diagnosed, prompt management is required and consists of removing or reducing exposure through elimination or substitution of causative agents and, where this is not possible, by effective control of exposure.

- Pharmaceutical treatment of OA follows the general asthma guidelines.

WRA accounts for 9–15% of cases of asthma in adults of working age.

WRA may be categorised into: occupational asthma (OA), which refers to asthma caused specifically by exposure to an agent present at the workplace; and work-aggravated or work-exacerbated asthma (WEA), in which pre-existing asthma is exacerbated by conditions in the work environment. The American College of Chest Physicians consensus document and British Occupational Health Research Foundation guidelines therefore define WRA to include OA (i.e. asthma induced by sensitiser or irritant work exposures) and WEA (i.e. pre-existing or concurrent asthma worsened by work factors).

OA can occur in workers with or without prior asthma and can be subdivided into: 1) sensitiser-induced OA, characterised by a latency period between first exposure to a respiratory sensitiser at work and the development of symptoms; and 2) irritant-induced OA that occurs typically within a few hours of a high-concentration exposure to an irritant gas, fume or vapour at work. When the causal exposure consists of a single inhalation incident, the condition is commonly called reactive airways dysfunction syndrome.

In clinical practice, it is often difficult to differentiate between "true" OA and aggravation of pre-existing asthma. Conversely, aggravation of symptoms related to work exposure, even in the absence of new sensitisation, requires individual and collective measures at the workplace, similar to OA. A recent consensus definition therefore is that

"OA is defined as asthma induced by exposure in the working environment to airborne dusts, vapours or fumes, with or without pre-existing asthma" (FRANCIS (2007)). Physicians involved in adult asthma care need to be aware of the high prevalence of WRA and the importance of inducing or exacerbating factors at work.

Sensitising and triggering agents

More than 250 agents causing OA have been described and are categorised into high molecular weight (HMW) and low molecular weight (LMW) agents, according to whether their molecular weight is above or below 1 kD. HMW agents are usually proteins of animal and vegetal origin such as flour, laboratory animal proteins and enzymes. LMW agents include a wide variety of chemicals, such as acid anhydrides, platinum salts and reactive dyes. Sensitisation to most HMW and some LMW factors is through an immunoglobulin (Ig)E mechanism and can be tested by skin tests. An immunological mechanism is suspected for LMW agents but has not been demonstrated, and an antigen-specific immune response cannot easily be tested in most affected workers.

The most frequently reported agents of occupational asthma are:

- Isocyanates
- Flour and grain dust
- Colophony and fluxes
- Latex
- Animal and plant proteins
- Aldehydes
- Wood dust
- Metal salts

Epidemiological studies have demonstrated that the level of exposure is the most important determinant of OA. This implies that preventive measures should be aimed at reducing workplace exposure. Prevention through elimination/reduction of exposure is the most effective approach for reducing the burden of OA. However, the relationship between the levels of exposure and the induction of OA is not always clear and the methodology of exposure assessment requires standardisation. Atopy increases the risk of developing OA in workers exposed to various sensitisers including enzymes, bakery allergens, laboratory animals, crab, prawn and acid anhydrides. The latent interval between first exposure and the onset of symptoms varies depending on the agent, the level of exposure/management and biological variability of exposure. The latent interval can extend to many years; however, the risk of OA appears to be highest soon after first exposure to laboratory animal allergens, isocyanates, platinum salts and enzymes. See table 1 for a list of agents frequently identified by inhalational challenge.

Diagnosis

The clinical presentation and symptoms of OA are no different from non-OA. Patients experience attacks of breathlessness, wheezing, cough, chest tightness and limitations in their daily activities. In any working adult patient presenting with such symptoms, the diagnosis of WRA should be considered. In individuals with suspected WRA, the physician should obtain a history of job duties and possible exposures, the use of protective devices and the presence of respiratory disease in co-workers. Table 2 shows examples of occupations/industries with sentinel health events for sensitiser-induced OA.

Symptoms may get worse when the patient enters the work environment, but very often the patients experience delayed symptoms and therefore may get worse after leaving work. A clinically useful approach, therefore, is not asking whether the patients experience worsening of their symptoms when at work but rather whether they feel better after a weekend or a holiday away from work. However, this is difficult to describe, as most people feel rested and happier at the end of a holiday. The diagnosis requires first spirometry, with a positive bronchodilation test and/or histamine, methacholine or

Table 1. Low molecular weight (LMW) and high molecular weight (HMW) agents frequently identified by inhalational challenge

LMW agents
Isocyanates
HDI
MDI
TDI
Metals
Plicatic acid (white or red cedar)
Wood dust
Hairdresser products
Epoxy
Gums
Dyes and fabrics
Chemicals
Perfume
HMW agents
Flour
Plants and grain dust
Seafood/fish
Latex
Animal-derived allergens
Leather
Enzymes
Talc

HDI: hexamethylene diisocyanate; MDI: methylene diphenyl diisocyanate; TDI: toluene diisocyanate. Data derived from DUFOUR (2009).

exercise testing of airway hyperresponsiveness for the confirmation of asthma. Furthermore, the patient should be asked to record symptoms, use of medication and peak expiratory flow (PEF) measurements when working and off work. PEF should be measured at least four times a day for a period of a month while times on and off work should be noted (the recommendation is at least 2 weeks on and 2 weeks off work). The sequential self-measurements of PEF can be complemented by repeated measurements of provocative concentration of histamine or methacholine causing a 20% fall in forced expiratory volume in 1 s. Allergic sensitisation to some inducers such as animal proteins can be examined by skin prick testing or *in vitro* assays of specific IgE. When the diagnosis cannot be confirmed by serial PEF measurements and skin tests or IgE assays, the "gold standard" for diagnosing sensitiser-induced OA is a specific bronchial provocation test (specific inhalation challenge), which may demonstrate a direct relationship between exposure to a test agent and an asthmatic response. The response may be early or late and may carry a risk to the patient of a severe reaction. Therefore, these tests should be performed only when necessary and only in specialised centres under medical supervision.

Management

Ideally, causal agents should be eliminated from the workplace, an option that is not often available. The second-best option is to remove the workers from exposure; however, many patients cannot quit their job. In such cases, the early institution of preventive measures, including the replacement of specific reagents where possible, the strict monitoring of exposure levels, and the use of extractor fans and masks, is necessary. The EU has allocated a high priority to safeguarding the health and safety of workers. Existing EU health and safety legislation aims to minimise the health risks from dangerous substances in the workplace, placing the emphasis on their elimination and substitution in order to protect workers. There are four important directives in this field, containing the basic provisions for health and safety at work, and further defining the risks related to exposure to chemical agents, to biological agents and to carcinogens at work. Medical surveillance programmes are very important and may include symptom questionnaires, spirometry and skin prick testing at regular intervals (*e.g.* every 6 or 12 months), as well as monitoring of exposure levels.

Once OA has developed, recovery is directly dependent on the duration and level of exposure to the causative agent. Depending on the severity of the case, the condition of the patient can substantially improve during the first year after removal from exposure. Conversely, asthma may persist even after removal from exposure to the causative workplace agent. The likelihood of improvement or resolution of symptoms or

Table 2. Examples of occupations/industries with sentinel health events for sensitiser-induced occupational asthma

Industry, process or occupation	Selected agents
Jewellery, alloy and catalyst makers	Platinum
Polyurethane, foam coatings, adhesives production and end-use settings (e.g. spray painters, and foam and foundry workers)	Isocyanates
Alloy, catalyst, refinery workers	Chromium, cobalt
Solderers	Soldering flux (colophony)
Plastics industry, dye, insecticide makers, organic chemical manufacture	Phthalic anhydride, trimetallic anhydride (used in epoxy resins)
Foam workers, latex makers, biologists, and hospital and laboratory workers	Formaldehyde
Printing industry	Gum arabic, reactive dyes and acrylates
Metal plating	Nickel sulphate and chromium
Bakers	Flour, amylase and other enzymes
Woodworkers and furniture makers	Red cedar (plicatic acid) and other wood dusts
Laboratory workers and animal researchers	Animal proteins
Detergent formulators	Detergent enzymes such as protease, amylase, and lipase
Seafood (crab, snow crab and prawn) workers	Crab, prawn and other shellfish proteins
Healthcare workers and nurses	Psyllium, natural rubber latex, glutaraldehyde, methacrylates, antibiotics and detergent enzymes
Laxative manufacture and packing	Psyllium
Hairdressers and manicurists	Persulphates and acrylates (artificial nails)

Reproduced from TARLO (2008), with permission from the publisher.

preventing deterioration is greater in workers who have no further exposure to the causative agent, have relatively normal lung function at diagnosis, and those who have shorter duration of symptoms prior to diagnosis and prior to avoidance of exposure.

Trigger avoidance is pivotal in preventing asthma symptoms and progression of severity. Nevertheless, pharmacological treatment is also required to control symptomatic patients. Pharmacological treatment follows the general asthma treatment guidelines, and inhaled steroids and β-agonists are the cornerstone of management. Treatment follows a stepwise approach, based on asthma control and severity and the approach is identical to that of non-OA.

Socioeconomic impact of WRA

The economic impact of WRA is due not only to direct healthcare costs but also to indirect costs from impaired work productivity and compensation/rehabilitation costs, as well as to the intangible costs from impaired quality of life. Income loss is more likely when avoidance of exposure leads to a change of job and this income loss is not offset by compensation. In many European countries, compensation does not include rehabilitation or retraining, perhaps accounting for the relatively high proportion (30%) of workers who continue to be exposed to the causative agent.

Moreover, when considering the cost of OA and/or compensation, it is not only lung function impairment and optimal asthma treatment that need to be taken into account, but also psychogenic factors. These can play an important role in the quality of life of OA patients, and significant prevalence of anxiety and depression has been shown in that population.

References

- Ameille J, et al. Consequences of occupational asthma on employment and financial status: a follow-up study. *Eur Respir J* 1997; 10: 55–58.
- Dufour M-H, et al. Comparative airway response to high- versus low-molecular weight agents in occupational asthma. *Eur Respir J* 2009; 33: 734–739.
- Dykewicz MS. Occupational asthma: current concepts in pathogenesis, diagnosis, and management. *J Allergy Clin Immunol* 2009; 123: 519–528.
- Francis HC, et al. Defining and investigating occupational asthma: a consensus approach. *Occup Environ Med.* 2007; 64: 361–365.
- Larbanois A, et al. Socioeconomic outcome of subjects experiencing asthma symptoms at work. *Eur Respir J* 2002; 19: 1107–1113.
- Moscato G, et al. Diagnosing occupational asthma: how, how much, how far? *Eur Respir J* 2003; 21: 879–885.
- Mullan RJ, Murthy LI. Occupational sentinel health events: an up-dated list for physician recognition and public health surveillance. *Am J Ind Med* 1991; 19: 775–799.
- Nemery B. Occupational asthma for the clinician. *Breathe* 2004; 1: 25–32.
- Newman Taylor AJ, Nicholson PJ, eds, Guidelines for the prevention, identification and management of occupational asthma: evidence review and recommendations. London, British Occupational Health Research Foundation, 2004. Available from http://www.bohrf.org.uk/downloads/asthevre.pdf.
- Newman Taylor AJ. Occupational asthma. *Thorax* 1980; 35: 241–245.
- Tarlo SM, et al. An official ATS proceedings: asthma in the workplace: the Third Jack Pepys Workshop on Asthma in the Workplace: answered and unanswered questions. *Proc Am Thorac Soc* 2009; 6: 339–349.
- Tarlo SM, et al. Diagnosis and management of work-related asthma: American College of Chest Physicians Consensus Statement. *Chest* 2008; 134: Suppl. 3, 1S–41S.
- Vandenplas O, Malo JL. Definitions and types of work-related asthma: a nosological approach. *Eur Respir J* 2003; 21: 706–712.

RESPIRATORY DISEASES CAUSED BY ACUTE INHALATION OF GASES, VAPOURS AND DUSTS

B. Nemery
Research Unit of Lung Toxicology, Occupational, Environmental and Insurance Medicine, K.U. Leuven, Leuven, Belgium
E-mail: Ben.Nemery@med.kuleuven.be

Acute inhalation injury may occur in the workplace, but also at home or in the community, *e.g.* as a result of fires and explosions, volcanic eruptions, industrial disasters, and accidents involving trains or trucks transporting chemicals. Inhalation accidents may be of catastrophic proportions, as occurred with the release of methyl isocyanate in Bhopal, India, in 1984. Mass casualties with inhalation injuries may also result from chemical warfare, and from conventional warfare or terrorist actions involving explosions, fires and building destructions.

The clinical presentation and severity of inhalation injury range from self-limited inhalation fever to life-threatening chemical pneumonitis with lung oedema and evolution to acute respiratory distress syndrome (ARDS) and multiorgan failure. Following inhalation injury, the lesions may heal completely or there may be persisting structural or functional sequelae.

Inhalation fever

Inhalation fever is the name given to a group of nonallergic, noninfectious flu-like clinical syndromes caused by the acute inhalation of metal fumes, organic dusts or some plastic fumes.

Metal fume fever is caused by a single exposure to high amounts of some metallic fumes, most notably those emitted when heating zinc. Organic dust toxic syndrome (ODTS) is caused by the inhalation of large quantities of agricultural and other dusts of biologic origin (bio-aerosols), which are generally heavily contaminated with toxin-producing microorganisms. Polymer fume fever occurs after exposure to the fumes of heated fluorine-containing polymers.

Key points

- An influenza-like response ("inhalation fever") may follow the inhalation of high quantities of zinc fumes ("metal fume fever") or organic aerosols ("organic dust toxic syndrome").

- After inhalalation of poorly water-soluble agents, such as nitrogen dioxide, phosgene or cadmium fumes, pulmonary oedema becomes clinically manifest only 4–12 h after exposure.

- Acute inhalation injury may be followed by various structural lesions in the airways, but also by asthma. Such asthma induced by a single inhalation injury is called acute irritant-induced asthma, or RADS.

The clinical features of the inhalation fevers are those of a beginning influenza. The actual exposure may or may not have been experienced as irritant for the eyes and respiratory tract. 4–8 h after the exposure, the subject begins to feel unwell with fever (up to 40°C), chills, headaches, malaise, nausea and muscle aches. Respiratory symptoms are usually mild and consist mainly of cough and/ or sore throat, but occasionally subjects may have more severe responses with dyspnoea.

The diagnosis of inhalation fever rests essentially on the recent exposure history and the clinical condition, and when these clearly point to inhalation fever, no sophisticated investigations are required. In general, chest auscultation and chest radiograph are normal, but in more severe cases crackles may be heard and there may be transient infiltrates on chest radiograph. Pulmonary function is often within normal limits; in severe cases there may be a decrease in diffusing capacity and arterial hypoxaemia. Increased peripheral blood leukocytosis, with a rise in neutrophils, is a consistent finding until 24 h after the exposure; other blood tests should be normal, except for indices of an inflammatory response. Bronchoalveolar lavage studies have shown pronounced and dose-dependent increases in polymorphonuclear leukocytes on the day after exposure to zinc fumes or organic dust.

Inhalation fever must not be confused with other more serious conditions, including chemical pneumonitis, which in its early phases could be mistaken for inhalation fever. A differential diagnosis must also be made with various types of infectious pneumonias and with acute extrinsic allergic alveolitis.

Inhalation fever is a self-limited syndrome and recovery normally takes place after a night's rest. Tolerance exists against re-exposures occurring shortly after a bout of metal fume fever or ODTS.

Acute chemical pneumonitis

Major causes The response to acute chemical injury in the respiratory tract is rarely compound-specific (table 1). The main agents that may cause acute inhalation injury are as follows:

- Water-soluble irritants, such as ammonia (NH_3), sulphur dioxide (SO_2), hydrochloric acid (HCl), formaldehyde, acetic acid, have good warning properties and mainly affect the upper respiratory tract, unless massive quantities have been inhaled.

- Gases of intermediate water solubility, such as chlorine (Cl_2) and hydrogen sulphide (H_2S), penetrate deeper into the bronchial tree. Accidental release of gaseous chlorine is one of the most frequent causes of inhalation injury, not only in industry, but also in the community as a result of transportation accidents, the use of chlorine for disinfecting swimming pools, or the mixing of bleach (NaClO) with acids; mixing bleach with ammonia leads to the release of volatile and irritant chloramines (including trichloramine, NCl_3). Hydrogen sulphide (H_2S), which is formed by the putrefaction of organic material in sewage drains, manure pits or ship holds, and is also a frequent contaminant in the petrochemical industry, does not only cause mucosal irritation, but it also leads to chemical asphyxia by mechanisms that are somewhat similar to those of cyanide.

- Poorly water-soluble agents, such as nitrogen dioxide (NO_2), phosgene ($COCl_2$), ozone (O_3), mercury vapours (Hg), cadmium oxide (CdO) fumes, are particularly hazardous because they cause little sensory irritation and are, therefore, hardly noticed, and they reach the distal airways thus potentially causing noncardiogenic pulmonary oedema, which develops over the course of several hours.

- Exposure to organic solvents is rarely a cause of toxic pneumonitis. However, exposure to very high concentrations of solvent vapours in confined spaces (*e.g.* in chemical tanks) may cause chemical

Table 1. Possible causes of toxic tracheo-bronchitis or pneumonitis

Irritant gases
  High water-solubility: NH_3, SO_2, HCl, *etc.*
  Moderate water-solubility: Cl_2, H_2S, *etc.*
  Low water-solubility: O_3, NO_2, $COCl_2$, *etc.*

Organic chemicals
  Organic acids: acetic acid, *etc.*
  Aldehydes: formaldehyde, acrolein, *etc.*
  Isocyanates: methylisocyanate (MIC), toluene diisocyanate (TDI)
  Amines: hydrazine, chloramines, *etc.*
  Riot control agents (CS) and vesicants (mustard gas)
  Organic solvents
  Leather treatment sprays
  Some agrochemicals (paraquat, cholinesterase inhibitors)

Metallic compounds
  Mercury vapours
  Metallic oxides: CdO, V_2O_5, MnO, Os_3O_4, *etc.*
  Halides: $ZnCl_2$, $TiCl_4$, $SbCl_5$, UF_6, *etc.*
  $Ni(CO)_4$
  Hydrides: B_2H_5, LiH, AsH_3, SbH_3

Complex mixtures
  Fire smoke
  Pyrolysis products from plastics
  Solvent mixtures
  Spores and toxins from microorganisms

pneumonitis and pulmonary oedema, often in victims who have been unconscious. Pneumonia and respiratory distress syndrome caused by loss of alveolar surfactant may also result from the aspiration of solvents or fuels ingested unintentionally (*e.g.* from siphoning petrol) or intentionally (*e.g.* by "fire eaters"). Severe acute respiratory illness may also be caused by spraying solvent-propelled fluorocarbon-containing water-proofing agents and leather conditioners.

- Some agrochemicals (such as paraquat and organophosphate or carbamate insecticides) may cause toxic pneumonitis after ingestion or dermal exposure.
- The commonest cause of toxic pneumonitis is smoke inhalation caused by domestic, industrial or other fires. Respiratory morbidity is often the major complication in burn victims. It may be caused by direct thermal injury (particularly if hot vapours have been inhaled), but more generally the lesions are caused by chemical injury. The toxic components of smoke include gaseous asphyxiants (CO, HCN) and irritants, as well as particulates.

Clinical presentation Depending on the circumstances of the accident, there may be thermal or chemical facial burns. Signs of mucosal irritation include cough, hoarseness, stridor or wheezing, retrosternal pain, discharge of bronchial mucus, possibly with blood, mucosal tissue and soot. Auscultation of the chest may or may not be abnormal, with wheezing, rhonchi or crepitations. Mucosal oedema, haemorrhage and ulcerations may be visible in the air passages. Victims of inhalation accidents with poorly soluble agents may feel – and look – perfectly well initially, but then experience progressive dyspnoea, shallow breathing, cyanosis, frothy pink sputum and eventually ventilatory failure. A clinical picture of ARDS may thus develop gradually over 4–72 h, even after a period of clinical improvement.

Pulmonary function can be used to monitor ambulatory subjects who have been exposed. Arterial blood gases show varying degrees of hypoxaemia and respiratory acidosis, depending on the severity of the injury. The chest radiograph is usually normal if only the conducting airways are involved, but there may be signs of peribronchial cuffing. After exposure to deep lung irritants the chest radiograph is unremarkable in the first hours after presentation, but signs of interstitial and alveolar oedema may become visible and, with time, patchy infiltrates, areas of atelectasis and even "white lungs" may develop. These changes may be due to tissue damage and organisation or they may reflect superimposed infectious (broncho)pneumonia.

In some instances, particularly in the later stages of chemical pneumonitis, there may be pathological (and radiological) features of organising pneumonia with or without bronchiolitis obliterans. Following resolution of the acute pulmonary oedema, a relapse in the clinical condition may occur after 2-6 weeks with dyspnoea, cough, fine crackles, a radiographic picture of miliary nodular infiltrates, arterial hypoxaemia and a restrictive or mixed impairment, with low diffusing capacity. This relapse phase has been attributed to bronchiolar scarring with peribronchiolar and obliterating fibrosis of the bronchioli.

Management At the scene of the accident, appropriate medical intervention includes removal from exposure, resuscitation and supportive treatment. In some instances, emergency personnel must also be protected from chemicals that remain present on victims or their clothes and decontamination procedures must be available. For some types of exposures asymptomatic persons must remain under observation for 24 h; they should not exercise, nor should they be overfilled by intravenous fluids. Oxygen treatment should be given as required by the level of arterial oxygen saturation.

The further management of acute inhalation injury will be governed by the severity of the patient's condition and will involve intensive care treatment with intubation and artificial ventilation, as required. Antibiotics are only to be given if there are signs of infection. In victims of smoke injury, bronchoscopic removal of soot from the airways may be necessary. The administration of (systemic) corticosteroids is probably justified to prevent complications arising from (excessive) inflammation, such as bronchiolitis obliterans, although there are no controlled studies on this issue.

Physicians treating victims in the early days after the incident must document accurately the clinical condition and all relevant data in these patients. Documentation of the damage by bronchoscopy and high-resolution computed tomography may be justified. Repeated measurements of ventilatory function and arterial blood gases must be carried out, and victims of acute inhalation injury should never be discharged without a comprehensive assessment of their pulmonary function.

Subacute toxic pneumonitis

Although the concept of chemical-induced lung injury is used only for disorders resulting from a single, acute exposure to a toxic chemical, the term "subacute toxic pneumonitis" may be used to refer to lung injury caused by repeated peaks of toxic exposures or a more prolonged toxic exposure over weeks to months. This is the case with exogenous lipoid pneumonitis, which may be caused by inhalation of natural or synthetic mineral oils, and with pulmonary alveolar proteinosis, which may be caused by heavy exposure to silica ("acute silico-proteinosis") and possibly by other agents.

The "Ardystil syndrome" is an example of subacute toxic pneumonitis. This outbreak of severe organising pneumonia occurred in 1992 in Spain, and involved several workers from factories where textiles were air-sprayed with dyes.

Another recently described form of subacute toxic lung injury is "popcorn worker's lung". This severe lung disease, characterised as bronchiolitis obliterans, occurred in subjects occupationally exposed to vapours of butter flavouring (containing diacetyl) used for making microwave-popcorn and other food.

Possible sequelae of acute inhalation injury

Following acute inhalation injury, there is often complete recovery. However, this is not always the case. Various persistent anatomical lesions such as constrictive bronchiolitis, bronchiectases, bronchial strictures or polyps, may be identified by imaging studies or through bronchoscopy.

Moreover, even in the absence of such structural sequelae or in the absence of significant defects in basal spirometry, a state of permanent nonspecific bronchial hyperreactivity may be observed. This condition of adult-onset, nonallergic asthma known as "reactive airways dysfunction syndrome" (RADS) or "acute irritant-induced asthma" occurs in a proportion of survivors of inhalation injury. Observations in fire-fighters and other personnel involved in rescue operations during and following the collapse of the World Trade Center on September 11, 2001, suggest that RADS may occur even without the occurrence of clinically serious injury.

References

- Blanc P, Boushey HA. The lung in metal fume fever. *Semin Respir Med* 1993; 14. 212-225.
- Douglas WW, Colby TV. Fume-related bronchiolitis obliterans. *In*: Epler GR, ed. Diseases of the bronchioles. New York, Raven Press, 1994; pp. 187-213.
- Das R, Blanc PD. Chlorine gas exposure and the lung: a review. *Toxicol Indust Health* 1993; 9: 439-455.
- Kreiss K, *et al*. Clinical bronchiolitis obliterans in workers at a microwave-popcorn plant. *N Engl J Med* 2002; 347: 330-338.
- Moya C, *et al*. Collaborative Group for the Study of Toxicity in Textile Aerographic Factories. Outbreak of organising pneumonia in textile printing sprayers. *Lancet* 1994; 344: 498-502.
- Nemery B. Late consequences of accidental exposure to inhaled irritants : RADS and the Bhopal disaster. *Eur Respir J* 1996; 9: 1973-1976.
- Nemery B. Reactive fallout of World Trade Center dust. *Am J Respir Crit Care Med* 2003; 168: 2-3.
- Nemery B. Toxic Pneumonitis. *In:* Hendrick DJ, et al., eds. Occupational Disorders of the Lung. Recognition, Management, and Prevention. London, WB Saunders, Harcourt Publishers, 2002; pp. 201-219.
- Olson KR, Shusterman DJ. Mixing incompatibilities and toxic exposures. *Occup Med* 1993; 8: 549-560.
- Shusterman DJ. Polymer fume fever and other fluorocarbon pyrolysis-related syndromes. *Occup Med* 1993; 8: 519-531.

HYPERSENSITIVITY PNEUMONITIS

T. Sigsgaard[1] and A. Rask-Andersen[2]
[1] Aarhus University, Aarhus, Denmark
[2] Uppsala University, Uppsala, Sweden
E-mail: sigsgaard@dadlnet.dk

Hypersensitivity pneumonitis (HP), also known as allergic alveolitis, is an immunologically mediated inflammatory lung disease in the lung parenchyma induced by the inhalation of a variety of organic or inorganic antigens and characterised by hypersensitivity to the antigens. The disease is usually named colourfully after the environment in which it occurs (*e.g.* farmer's lung and bird fancier's lung) and has been reported from over 30 different occupations and environments.

Key points

- Hypersensitivity pneumonitis (HP) is an immunologically mediated inflammatory lung disease in the lung parenchyma induced by the inhalation of a variety of organic or inorganic antigens and characterised by hypersensitivity to the antigens,

- The disease is usually named after the environment in which it occurs.

- The main characteristic of HP is a massive lymphocytic inflammation with accumulation of activated T-lymphocytes in the lung interstitium.

- The only treatment for allergic diseases such as HP is to avoid exposure to the offending allergen and if the exposure ceases, the symptoms usually subside rapidly, but the lung function impairment may persist.

Regardless of the causative agents or environmental setting, the pathogenesis and clinical manifestations of the disease are similar. The hallmark of the disease is a massive lymphocytic inflammation with accumulation of activated T-lymphocytes in the lung interstitium.

Epidemiology

In a large, general-population-based cohort of HP patients from the UK, the overall incidence rate was approximately one per 100,000 population, and in Japan the summer-type HP occurs every year in approximately one per million population. Most other studies have focused on the risk of developing clinical disease among subsets of the population with high levels of exposure to particular antigens. For example, the incidence of farmer's lung in Sweden in the 1980s was ~20 per 100,000 person-yrs. However, there has been a decrease in the incidence of farmer's lung due to changes in farming practice (hay making replaced by silage bags). A recent study from North America showed that the most common cause was bird or hot-tub exposure.

Risk factors

The first reported HP was farmer's lung, caused by inhalation of microorganisms from infested crops. The disease was first described among farmers in the Nordic parts of the globe; however, it has since been described in a range of farming operations all over the world, making farming-like operations with decaying organic material one of the important exposures to look for when confronted with a case of HP. One of the most common appearances of HP is bird fancier's lung, caused by exposure to birds, *e.g.* pigeons or parakeets. Among pigeon breeder's HP, intestinal mucin, a high molecular weight glycoprotein, has been identified as a major antigen.

Host factors

Smoking seems to give protection towards HP, although the disease has been described in a few smokers. The reason behind this protection might be the downregulation of the immune system by tobacco smoke and nicotine.

Virus infection seems to increase the susceptibility of mice towards the antigens, and a higher number of virus antigens have been found in the bronchial lavage of HP patients.

Pathological mechanism

Although HP is a well known disease, the pathogenesis is still only partly understood. When PEPYS (1978) found precipitating antibodies to mould antigen in many cases, it was believed for many years that the immune complexes were the basis of the lung changes. It is now believed that the cellular immune response is driving the disease. Following inhalation of antigen, a complex formed by soluble antigens and immunoglobulin G antibodies triggers the complement cascade and alveolar macrophage activation is induced, resulting in an increase in macrophages. These cells secrete cytokines and chemokines that attract neutrophils in alveoli and small airways. The number of T-lymphocytes is also increased, with a predominance of the CD8+ T-lymphocytes subset, resulting in a decrease in the CD4+/CD8+ ratio (in contrast to what is seen in sarcoidosis). Different upregulatory mechanisms result in a stronger interaction between macrophages and T-cells and a more effective antigen-presenting capacity.

Symptoms and findings

The predominant symptoms in HP are tiredness, dyspnoea, fever, shivering, flu-like feeling, cough, muscle and joint aches and headache. Radiography of the thorax shows diffuse, fine, nodular shadows, either general or predominantly in the bases. In the early stages the changes can be difficult to detect, but widespread patchy opacities may also be seen. Lung function is decreased, with a typical restrictive pattern and a decreased diffusing capacity.

Environmental assessment

The origin of the disease is an adverse reaction towards an occupational or environmental factor, so it is imperative to search the patient's environment for this exposure, and to minimise further contact to the offending agent. Often it is obvious what the reason might be, *e.g.* a mouldy hay problem occurring after a wet harvest season. In some instances the causal agent might be difficult to find and techniques for the assessment of microorganisms should be employed in order to assess the exposure to which the patient is exposed.

Diagnosis

The diagnosis of HP relies on an array of nonspecific clinical symptoms and signs developed in an appropriate setting, with demonstration of bilateral patchy infiltrates on chest radiographs, and serum precipitating antibodies against offending antigens. Several different diagnostic criteria for HP have been proposed; all have significant problems that limit their utility. After studying a total of 661 HP patients with a stepwise logistic regression, a panel of clinical experts identified six significant predictors of HP.

Diagnostic criteria of extrinsic hypersensitivity pneumonitis:

- Exposure to a known offending antigen
- Symptoms occurring 4–8 h after exposure
- Positive precipitating antibodies to the offending antigen
- Inspiratory crackles on physical examination

Table 1. Types of hypersensitivity pneumonitis (HP) and typical causative exposures and antigens

HP type	Exposure	Antigen
Farmer's lung	Mouldy hay	Saccharopolyspora rectivirgula
Bagassosis	Mouldy bagasse	Thermoactinomyces sacchari
Mushroom worker's lung	Mushroom spores, mushroom compost	Thermophilic actinomycetes
Malt worker's lung	Mouldy barley	Aspergillus clavatus, Faenia rectivirgula
Humidifier/air-conditioner lung	Contaminated water reservoirs	Thermophilic actinomycetes
Grain handler's lung	Mouldy grain	Saccharopolyspora rectivirgula, Thermoactinomyces vulgaris
Cheese worker's lung	Cheese mould	Penicillium casei
Paprika splitter's lung	Paprika dust	Mucor stolonifer
Compost lung	Compost	Aspergillus spp.
Peat moss worker's lung	Peat moss	Monocillium spp., Penicillium citreonigrum
Suberosis	Mouldy cork dust	Penicillium frequentans
Maple bark stripper's lung	Mouldy wood bark	Cryptostroma corticale
Wood pulp worker's lung	Mouldy wood pulp	Alternaria spp.
Wood trimmer's disease	Mouldy wood trimmings	Rhizopus spp.
Japanese summer-type HP	Indoor air	Trichosporon cutaneum
Metal grinding	Metalworking fluids	Mycobacteria
Hot-tub lung	Mist from hot tubs	Mycobacteria
Bird breeder's lung	Pigeons, parakeets, fowl, rodents	Avian or animal proteins
Mollusc-shell hypersensitivity	Sea snail shells	Shell dust
Chemical worker's lung	Manufacture of plastics, polyurethane foam, rubber	Trimellitic anhydride, diisocyanate, methylene diisocyanate

- Recurrent episodes of symptoms
- Weight loss

However, diagnosing HP often poses challenges, even to expert clinicians. Additional investigations (including surgical biopsy) are indicated in patients with interstitial diseases in whom the diagnosis remains unclear after initial assessment.

Treatment

The only treatment for allergic diseases is to avoid the exposure to the offending allergen. This can be done in many circumstances, e.g. when the occurrence is sporadic and not part of the daily work of the patient. However, in some cases, e.g. farmers, it might be difficult to avoid the exposure totally for a range of different reasons. Under such circumstances respiratory protection can be used to minimise the exposure as much as possible.

It has been discussed whether medical treatment has an effect on the outcome of HP. Cortisone has been found to reduce interleukin-8 synthesis. Cortisone treatment seems to improve the radiological findings and should be given to severely ill patients to ameliorate symptoms, but no apparent benefit is derived from long-term treatment. The cortisone treatment should be given for about 2 months.

Prognosis

If the exposure ceases, the symptoms usually subside rapidly, but the lung function impairment may persist for a longer period and become permanent, with a restrictive pattern and decreased diffusing capacity. Repeated attacks increase the risk of sequelae. It is therefore important to treat the patient as soon as possible in order to avoid more damage to the lung parenchyma than is already the case at the time of diagnosis.

Differential diagnosis

Infectious lung diseases, both of virological and bacteriological origin, as well as other lung diseases such as sarcoidosis, have to be ruled out. Another differential diagnosis is the organic dust toxic syndrome (ODTS) also known as "inhalation fever" or "toxic pneumonitis": acute, febrile, noninfectious, flu-like, short-term reactions that can be produced by inhalation of bio-aerosols and organic dusts as well as plastic hardeners and metal (zinc) fumes. Symptoms are caused by the release of inflammatory cytokines from the lungs caused by an inhalatory overexposure to aerosols. ODTS is quite a common condition, but the prognosis is good and most people have recovered totally without any sequels after 24 h. No treatment is required if the exposure is terminated.

References

- Ando M, *et al*. Japanese summer-type hypersensitivity pneumonitis. Geographic distribution, home environment, and clinical characteristics of 621 cases. *Am Rev Respir Dis* 1991; 144: 765-769.
- Arya A, *et al*. Farmer's lung is now in decline. *Ir Med J* 2006; 99: 203-205.
- Bourke SJ, *et al*. Hypersensitivity pneumonitis: current concepts. *Eur Respir J* 2001; 18: Suppl. 32, 81s-92s.
- Hanak V, *et al*. Causes and presenting features in 85 consecutive patients with hypersensitivity pneumonitis. *Mayo Clin Proc* 2007; 82: 812-816.
- Lacasse Y, *et al*. Clinical diagnosis of hypersensitivity pneumonitis. *Am J Respir Crit Care Med* 2003; 168: 952-958.
- Malmberg P, *et al*. Incidence of organic dust toxic syndrome and allergic alveolitis in Swedish farmers. *Int Arch Allergy Appl Immunol* 1988; 87: 47-54.
- Pepys J. Antigens and hypersensitivity pneumonitis. *J Allergy Clin Immunol* 1978; 61: 201-203.
- Solaymani-Dodaran M, *et al*. Extrinsic allergic alveolitis: incidence and mortality in the general population. *QJM* 2007; 100: 233-237.

PNEUMOCONIOSIS

R.D. Stevenson
Glasgow Royal Infirmary and University of Glasgow, Glasgow, UK
E-mail: robstevenson@doctors.org.uk

Asbestos, coal and silica exposures are the main causes of pneumoconiosis relevant to current clinical and medico-legal practice. Although these exposures have greatly diminished in recent years, many patients still present to pneumologists with disease resulting from exposure that occurred in previous years. This article will consider the effects of dust inhalation both on lungs and pleura.

Asbestos

The mining and use of amphibole forms of asbestos, mainly crocidolite and amosite, has ceased worldwide, but chrysotile, the serpentine form, is still used in Africa, South America and Asia, both because of a lack of cheaper substitutes and because it is less harmful than the amphiboles. Some ceiling boards still contain chrysotile and people who live near chrysotile mines experience environmental exposure. There is a high incidence of mesothelioma in women who lived in the chrysotile mining region of Quebec, Canada, where contamination of chrysotile by the amphibole tremolite increases toxicity.

Pleural plaques Pleural plaques, which are discrete areas of thickening on the parietal pleura, are the commonest manifestation of asbestos exposure. They are usually discovered incidentally on plain chest radiographs or computed tomography scans. They do not become evident radiographically in <15 yrs from first exposure. Previously, plaques were thought to have no effect on lung function, but a recent statement from the American Thoracic Society claimed that studies of large cohorts showed a reduction in lung function attributable to pleural plaques.

Key points

- Pleural plaques are benign and do not predispose to malignancy.
- Asbestosis is a disappearing disease.
- Diffuse pleural thickening is the sequel to benign asbestos pleurisy and may cause restricted ventilation.
- New cases of coal workers' pneumoconiosis are still occurring.
- Silicosis increases the risk of both TB and lung cancer.

However in the majority of cases, any such effect is unlikely to be of clinical significance. Some studies have suggested that plaques predispose to the development of mesothelioma, but the consensus view is that they are not pre-malignant. Until recently in the UK, pleural plaques were accepted as justifying compensation. However, in 2007, the House of Lords ruled that plaques did not constitute an injury and that compensation would no longer be awarded to affected individuals.

Benign asbestos pleurisy and diffuse pleural thickening Asbestos pleurisy was first described in 1964. Many episodes are asymptomatic but some patients experience pain, fever and dyspnoea. Typically the pleurisy is associated with a blood-stained effusion but some cases are of "dry pleurisy". Spontaneous recovery is usual although recurrence on the other side is common. Asbestos pleurisy may occur after a latency of <10 yrs, but in another study the mean latency was 26 yrs.

Diffuse pleural thickening (DPT) involves the visceral pleura and may be unilateral or bilateral. It is now thought to follow earlier episodes of benign pleurisy. The fibrosis may be extensive and cause restricted ventilation. It may be difficult to distinguish from confluent pleural plaques but in DPT, obliteration of the costo-phrenic angle has usually occurred and this does not happen with plaques.

Asbestosis Asbestosis is diffuse interstitial pulmonary fibrosis secondary to severe asbestos exposure. In the USA, it is becoming a disappearing disease because of the great reduction in exposure. Disease progression was a feature of severe disease after heavy exposure, but after mild exposure, the disease tends to become quiescent. It is therefore very rare nowadays to see patients with severe asbestosis.

The relevance of asbestosis in current practice is almost entirely medico-legal. Patients with pulmonary fibrosis and a history of asbestos exposure seek compensation, but many of them had limited exposure and have coincidentally developed idiopathic pulmonary fibrosis of the usual interstitial pneumonia (UIP) sub-type. The two important distinguishing features are the more progressive nature of UIP in terms of radiographic changes and declining lung function and the presence of pleural plaques which occur in ~95% of patients with asbestosis.

An international meeting was held in Helsinki in 1997 and criteria for the diagnosis of asbestosis were developed, which in addition to radiological features, included data on analysis of lung tissue for asbestos bodies and fibres.

There is agreement that asbestosis increases the risk of lung cancer but there is still no consensus about whether asbestos exposure in the absence of asbestosis also increases the cancer risk.

Coal workers' pneumoconiosis

Populations at risk Over the past 30 yrs, the prevalence of coal workers' pneumoconiosis (CWP) has fallen consistently as the numbers of coal miners and the dust levels in mines have decreased. Nevertheless, mining is still a major industry in many parts of eastern Europe, India, China, South America and Africa. Increased mechanisation results in higher dust levels. New cases of CWP are still being diagnosed in miners who have worked exclusively under current exposure limits. The risk of CWP depends on the total dust burden and is also related to the coal rank, which is based on carbon content. Anthracite has a higher rank than bituminous. Therefore, this disease is not disappearing as definitely as asbestosis and continued vigilance is necessary in assessing respiratory symptoms in miners.

Clinical features Simple CWP is a radiological and pathological diagnosis. The characteristic lesion is the coal macule, which is a centrilobular accumulation of macrophages. This lesion causes no signs or symptoms and dyspnoea in a patient with simple CWP must prompt a search for another diagnosis. This may be associated emphysema due to coal dust or smoking, or the development of progressive massive fibrosis, but it may also be a treatable disease unrelated to CWP.

It is now accepted that CWP causes bronchitis due to coal dust resulting in cough and mucus production. In addition, CWP is recognised as being associated with airflow obstruction independent of smoking. *Post-mortem* examination suggests that coal mine dust causes centrilobular emphysema, especially when pneumoconiosis is present. In the UK, chronic bronchitis and emphysema are classified as an occupational disease for which industrial injuries benefit can be paid.

Silicosis

Prevalence Silicosis is a major worldwide disease even in developed countries. It affects miners and workers in the construction industry and foundries. There is some evidence that prevalence in South Africa is rising. A recent study claimed that exposure over a working lifetime to the commonly used standard of 0.1 mg·m^{-3} results in significant radiological silicosis with death both from silicosis and from lung cancer.

Clinical features Like CWP, uncomplicated silicosis is not associated with signs or symptoms. Dyspnoea usually indicates the development of progressive massive fibrosis or tuberculosis but may reflect associated airway disease or emphysema. Silicosis often continues to progress after exposure has ceased.

Lung cancer Traditionally lung cancer was not associated with silicosis, but recent authoritative reviews have concluded that the data are sufficient to support an association between silicosis and lung cancer. It remains unclear whether the increased risk derives from exposure to silica or requires the presence of silicosis.

Tuberculosis It is well known that silicosis predisposes to tuberculosis which may be two- to 30-fold more common than in controls without silicosis. HIV status adds a further complication. In black South African gold miners, HIV infection increased tuberculosis incidence by five times, whereas silicosis increased incidence by three times. When HIV and silicosis were both present, the tuberculosis incidence increased multiplicatively by 15 times. In addition to tuberculosis, patients with silicosis have an increased incidence of infection with environmental mycobacteria and also of extrapulmonary tuberculosis.

Chronic obstructive pulmonary disease Emphysema is a common feature of long-term silica exposure and along with bronchitis may develop with or without radiological signs of silicosis. Smoking may potentiate the effect of silica on airflow obstruction.

References

- al Jarad N, *et al.* Bronchoalveolar lavage and 99mTc-DTPA clearance as prognostic factors in asbestos workers with and without asbestosis. *Respir Med* 1993; 87: 365–374.
- American Thoracic Society Committee of the Scientific Assembly on Environmental and Occupational Health, Adverse effects of crystalline silica exposure. *Am J Respir Crit Care Med* 1997; 155: 761–768.
- Asbestos, asbestosis, and cancer: the Helsinki criteria for diagnosis and attribution.:: Scand J Work Environ Health 1997; 23: 311–316.
- Coggon D, Newman Taylor A. Coal mining and chronic obstructive pulmonary disease: a review of the evidence. *Thorax* 1998; 53: 398–407.
- Copley SJ, *et al.* Asbestosis and idiopathic pulmonary fibrosis: comparison of thin-section CT features. *Radiology* 2003; 229: 731–736.
- Corbett EL, *et al.* HIV infection and silicosis: the impact of two potent risk factors on the incidence of mycobacterial disease in South African miners. *AIDS* 2000; 14: 2759–2768.
- Martensson G, *et al.* Asbestos pleural effusion: a clinical entity. Thorax 1987; 42: 646–651.
- 't Mannetje A, *et al.* Exposure-response analysis and risk assessment for silica and silicosis mortality in a pooled analysis of six cohorts. *Occup Environ Med* 2002; 59: 723–728.

INDOOR AND OUTDOOR POLLUTION

G. Viegi[1,2], M. Simoni[1], S. Maio[1], S. Cerrai[1], G. Sarno[1] and S. Baldacci[1]
[1] Pulmonary Environmental Epidemiology Unit, Institute of Clinical Physiology, National Research Council, Pisa and
[2] Institute of Biomedicine and Molecular Immunology "A. Monroy", National Research Council, Palermo, Italy
E-mail: viegig@ifc.cnr.it

Air pollution is a well-established hazard to human health. Air quality is particularly important for subpopulations that are more susceptible (*i.e.* children, the elderly, subjects with cardiorespiratory diseases or those who are socioeconomically deprived) or at higher risk of specific exposures (workers exposed to inorganic dust, wood dust, fumes, gases and cleaning agents). Children are particularly vulnerable since they inhale a higher volume of air per body weight than adults, the lungs are growing, the immune system is incomplete, and defence mechanisms are still evolving. Air pollution can affect the cells in the lung by damaging those that are most susceptible, and if the damaged cells are important in the development of new functional parts of the lung, the lung may not achieve its full growth and function as a child matures to adulthood. This can lead to enhanced susceptibility during adulthood to the effects of ageing and infections as well as to pollutants. Air pollution is mostly produced by human activities. Other pollutants derive from natural sources, such as biological allergens (*e.g.* acarids, house dust mites, pets, moulds), and natural phenomena (*e.g.* volcanic activity, forest fires).

Key points

- Recent epidemiological studies have clearly shown that outdoor and indoor air pollution affects respiratory health worldwide, causing an increase in the prevalence of respiratory symptoms/diseases (*i.e.* COPD, asthma, hay fever, lung function reduction) and of mortality, both in children and in adults.

- Rapid industrialisation and urbanisation have increased air pollution and, consequently, the amount of exposed people.

- Conservative estimates show that between 1.5 and 2 million deaths per year could be attributed to indoor air pollution in developing countries.

- The abatement of the main risk factors for respiratory diseases and the support of health care providers and general community to public health policy for improving outdoor/indoor air quality can achieve huge health benefits.

Outdoor pollution

The most important outdoor pollutants derive from fossil fuel combustion. Primary pollutants directly emitted into the atmosphere are carbon monoxide (CO), sulphur dioxide (SO_2), nitrogen dioxide (NO_2) and particulates (PM). Ozone (O_3) is a secondary pollutant, mainly produced by chemical reaction of NO_2 and hydrocarbons in the presence of sunlight at warm temperature. Rapid industrialisation and urbanisation in many parts of the world have increased air pollution and, consequently, the number of people exposed to it. In China, for instance, rapid economic development has led to severe environmental degradation, particularly due to coal combustion (it provides 70–75% of energy) and vehicular traffic. Chinese mortality and morbidity associated to outdoor pollution are very high: more than 300,000 deaths and 20 million cases of respiratory illnesses annually. The main effects of the more common outdoor pollutants are summarised in table 1.

Exposure–response relationships for outdoor pollutants, especially PM, have been confirmed by epidemiological studies in recent decades. Short-term exposure, due to acute increase in air pollution, may cause premature mortality and increase hospital admissions for exacerbations of chronic obstructive pulmonary disease (COPD) or asthma. Long-term cumulative health effects of chronic exposure comprise an increase in morbidity and mortality for cardiovascular and respiratory diseases, including COPD and lung cancer, and impaired development of the lungs in children. In COPD patients, continued exposure to noxious agents promotes a more rapid decline in lung function and increases the risk of repeated exacerbations. Air pollution can harm the foetus if the mother is exposed to high levels during pregnancy (*i.e.* intra-uterine growth retardation), and it can increase respiratory neonatal mortality. PM, NO_2 and O_3 are the most important pollutants today. The health effects of PM are more serious for fine (aerodynamic diameter <2.5 μm, PM2.5) and ultrafine (aerodynamic diameter <0.1 μm, PM0.1) particles, as they penetrate deeper into the airways of the respiratory tract, reaching the alveoli. Vehicular exhausts are responsible for small-sized airborne PM air pollution in urban

Table 1. Major outdoor pollutants and related health effects

Pollutant	Major sources	Health effects
Particulate matter	Vehicular traffic Wood stoves Organic matter/fossil fuel combustion Power plants/industry Wind-blown dust from roads, agriculture and construction Bush fires/dust storms	Lung cancer Premature death Mortality from cardiorespiratory diseases Reduced lung function Lower airways inflammation Upper airways irritation
Nitrogen dioxide	Vehicular traffic Power plants/industry	Exacerbation of asthma Airway inflammation Bronchial hyperresponsiveness Increased susceptibility to respiratory infection
Ozone	Sunlight: chemical reaction between other pollutants Vehicular traffic Power plants/industry Consumer products	Lung tissue damage Reduced lung function Reduced exercise capacity Exacerbation of asthma Upper airway and eye irritation
Carbon monoxide	Organic matter/fossil fuel combustion Vehicular traffic Wood stoves	Death/coma at very high levels Headache, nausea, breathlessness Confusion/reduced mental alertness Bronchial hyperresponsiveness
Sulphur dioxide	Coal/oil burning power plants Industry/refineries Diesel engines Metal smelting	Exacerbation of respiratory diseases including asthma Respiratory tract irritation

areas. A recent Chinese study showed that long-term exposure to PM2.5 increases the risk of mortality from lung cancer by 15–21% per 10 $\mu g \cdot m^{-3}$ increase. O_3 significantly increases annual mortality rates from respiratory causes, as demonstrated by a very large cohort study performed in the USA (~450,000 subjects from 96 metropolitan areas). Even in Sweden, with overall low levels of traffic-related air pollution, adults living near a road with higher traffic show significantly higher risk for diagnosis of asthma (OR 1.40, 95% CI 1.04–1.89) and COPD (OR 1.64, 95% CI 1.11–2.40) and for related symptoms. In Italy, the current authors have recently reported that people living in an urban area show a higher risk of having increased bronchial responsiveness (OR 1.41, 95% CI 1.13–1.76) than people living in a rural area.

The role of air pollution in the epidemics of allergies is still debated, even if experimental studies have suggested that the effects of air pollutants on the development and worsening of allergies are biologically plausible. Asthma shows a strong familial association, but genetic factors alone are unlikely to account for the rapid rise in its prevalence seen in recent decades. The rapid increase in the burden of atopic diseases occurred along with rapid urbanisation/industrialisation. Thus, genetic and environmental factors may interact to cause asthma. A growing number of studies shows significant associations of traffic with new-onset asthma, or asthma symptoms/exacerbations, in children. A recent study on a very large sample of German children shows significantly higher risk for asthmatic bronchitis (OR 1.56, 95% CI 1.03–2.37), hayfever (OR 1.59, 95% CI 1.11–2.27) and allergic sensitisation to pollen (OR 1.40, 95% CI 1.20–1.64), in children living near busy streets. Another recent study on 70,000 children, in the USA, indicates that the risk for respiratory allergy/hayfever increases with increasing summer O_3 levels (OR 1.20, 95% CI 1.15–1.26 per 10 ppb increment) and increasing PM2.5 levels (OR 1.23, 95% CI 1.10–1.38 per 10 $\mu g \cdot m^{-3}$ increment). A study on asthmatic children in Mexico City suggests that recent exposure to NO_2 and O_3 may reduce the efficacy of short-acting β-agonists in producing bronchodilation.

Furthermore, European Community Respiratory Health Survey data suggest that NO_2 traffic-related pollution causes asthma symptoms and possibly asthma incidence in adults.

Indoor pollution

Indoor environments contribute significantly to human exposure to air pollutants. People spend most of their time indoors: up to 90% in industrialised countries. Further, levels of some pollutants are higher inside than outside buildings. Even at low concentrations, indoor pollutants may have an important biological impact because of long exposure periods (*e.g.* at home/school, in working places). Conservative estimates show that 1.5–2 million deaths per year could be attributed to indoor air pollution. There is consistent evidence that exposure to indoor pollutants increases the risk of several respiratory/allergic symptoms/diseases (table 2). Relevant indoor pollution sources are environmental tobacco smoke (ETS), a common source of indoor PM, biomass (wood/coal) fuel use and mould/damp.

ETS is associated with increased risk of acute respiratory or irritation symptoms, infectious diseases, chronic respiratory illnesses, lung function reduction and even lung cancer. It has been estimated to be a significant pooled risk for chronic cough in never-smokers heavily exposed to ETS, both in males (OR 1.60, 95% CI 1.22–2.10) and females (OR 1.68, 95% CI 1.17–2.34). In nonsmoking males, the mortality risk for respiratory diseases is about double for those living with smokers than for those who do not. A few studies performed worldwide suggest higher risk for ETS exposure in females than in males. In China, about 80% of the cardiorespiratory burden caused by ETS exposure concerns women, and the number of deaths from ETS due to cardiovascular diseases and lung cancer in women is about two-thirds of that from active smoking. The induction period of lung cancer being long, its risk is probably related to cumulative lifetime ETS exposure. Meta-analyses on spousal ETS exposure estimated a

287

Table 2. Major indoor pollutants and related health effects

Pollutant	Major sources	Health effects
Particulate matter	Wood stoves Organic matter/fossil fuel combustion for heating/cooking Environmental tobacco smoke	Lung cancer Premature death Mortality from cardiorespiratory diseases Reduced lung function Lower airways inflammation Upper airways irritation
Nitrogen dioxide	Unvented gas/kerosene appliances	Exacerbation of asthma Airway inflammation Bronchial hyperresponsiveness Increased susceptibility to respiratory infection
Carbon monoxide	Organic matter/fossil fuel combustion for heating/cooking Wood stoves Unvented gas/kerosene appliances Environmental tobacco smoke	Death/coma at very high levels Headache, nausea, breathlessness Confusion/reduced mental alertness Low birth weight (foetal exposure) Bronchial hyperresponsiveness
Volatile organic compounds	Building materials and products such as new furniture, solvents, paint, adhesives, insulation Cleaning activities and products Office materials	Lung cancer Asthma, dizziness, respiratory and lung diseases Chronic eye, lung or skin irritation Neurological and reproductive disorders

pooled risk for lung cancer of OR 1.23 (95% CI 1.13–1.34). ETS exposure is a risk factor for new-onset asthma among both nonsmoking adults and children; it exacerbates pre-existing asthma and increases symptom burden and morbidity. In children, ETS also increases the risk of sudden infant death syndrome, middle-ear disease, lower respiratory tract illnesses, wheeze and cough.

About half of the world's population burns biomass for cooking, heating and lighting, in open fires or with inefficient stoves, and in poorly ventilated rooms, especially in developing countries. There is very high production of PM and CO. Indoor air pollution from biomass fuels is strongly poverty-related and represents an important risk factor for acute respiratory illness morbidity and mortality, especially in children and women. The evidence that biomass use increases the risk of COPD in women is very strong (about threefold higher risk in those exposed than in those unexposed). Besides COPD, observed health effects include weakening of the immune system, impaired lung function and lung cancer.

Based on meta-analyses, building dampness and mould are associated with approximately 30–50% increases in respiratory and asthma-related health outcomes. In adults, a pooled risk for cough by indoor mould/dampness was estimated at OR 2.10, 95% CI 1.27–3.47. There is also evidence on the association of mould exposure with new-onset sthma, and worsening of pre-existing asthma (wheezing, cough, shortness of breath) in both children and adults. Allergic symptoms are commonly related to mould exposure (sneezing, nose/mouth/throat irritations, nasal stuffiness/ runny nose, red/itchy/watery eyes). In children, a population attributable risk for asthma of 6.7% has been estimated.

Finally, exposure to VOCs may result in a spectrum of illnesses ranging from mild (irritations) to very severe effects, including cancer. Many studies indicate that the effects are related to very low levels of exposure. VOC exposure also seems a significant risk factor for asthma (especially benzene, ethylbenzene and toluene).

Biological mechanisms

Many recent studies have shown that oxidative stress, induced by air pollutants, plays a central role in the impact of air pollution. The first contact of inhaled ambient pollutants is with the fluid layer that covers the respiratory epithelium, and the responses following the exposure are mediated through oxidation reactions occurring within this fluid air–lung interface. These reactions can result in oxidative stress and consequent increased production of inflammatory mediators from human airway epithelial cells. Oxidative stress is a situation in which the oxidant–antioxidant balance is disturbed. This imbalance can occur when the generation of oxidant molecules (free radicals) exceeds the available antioxidant defences.

The three pollutants of most concern that can cause oxidative stress include NO, which is a free radical, PM_{10}, and O_3. The majority of human genetic association studies of air pollutants have examined O_3 exposure. O_3 is a powerful oxidant and reacts with the bronchial epithelium lining fluid to generate free radicals. It depletes levels of protective antioxidants and increases the production of inflammatory mediators.

The size and the surface of PM determine the potential to elicit oxidative damage. In general, the smaller the size of PM the higher the toxicity through mechanisms of oxidative stress and inflammation. Nanoparticles (ultrafine particles with diameter <100 nm) are more toxic and inflammogenic than fine particles. They generate reactive oxygen species to a greater extent and exacerbate pre-existing respiratory and cardiovascular disease, also through a dose–response effect.

Pulmonary impairment related to pollutants exposure may be higher in individuals who are genetically at risk for greater susceptibility to oxidative stress. The formation of reactive oxygen species is an important aspect of the inflammatory process of asthma, and genetic aberrations associated with antioxidants might explain the reason why some people with asthma seem at higher risk of exacerbations due to air pollution exposure.

Conclusion

Outdoor and indoor pollution greatly affect respiratory health worldwide as shown by many recent epidemiological studies.

Patient education about the importance of good indoor air quality in the home and workplace is essential. The support of healthcare providers and the general community for public health policy aimed at improving outdoor air quality through programmes to abate/reduce polluting emissions is also important. Moreover, there is evidence that increased antioxidant intake may protect against the effects of air pollution.

Hopefully, these actions will reduce the negative effects of air pollution on the respiratory health status and quality of life of the general population, in particular of the more susceptible individuals.

References

- Effects of air pollution on children's health and development – a review of the evidence. Geneva, World Health Organization, 2005. Available at: http://www.euro.who.int/__data/assets/pdf_file/0010/74728/E86575.pdf.
- Groneberg-Kloft B, *et al*. Analysis and evaluation of environmental tobacco smoke exposure as a risk factor for chronic cough. *Cough* 2007; 3: 6.
- Hernández-Cadena L, *et al*. Increased levels of outdoor air pollutants are associated with reduced bronchodilation in children with asthma. *Chest* 2009; 136: 1529–1536.
- Maio S, *et al*. Urban residence is associated with bronchial hyper-responsiveness in Italian general population samples. *Chest* 2009; 135: 434–441.
- Parker JD, *et al*. Air pollution and childhood respiratory allergies in the United States. *Environ Health Perspect* 2009; 117: 140–147.
- Simoni M, *et al*. Mould/dampness exposure at home is associated with respiratory disorders in Italian children and adolescents: the SIDRIA-2 Study. *Occup Environ Med* 2005; 62: 616–622.
- Valavanidis A, *et al*. Airborne particulate matter and human health: toxicological assessment and importance of size and composition of particles for oxidative damage and carcinogenic

mechanisms. *J Environ Sci Health C Environ Carcinog Ecotoxicol Rev* 2008; 26: 339-62.
- Viegi G, *et al.* Definition, epidemiology and natural history of COPD. *Eur Respir J* 2007; 30: 993-1013.
- Viegi G, *et al.* Indoor air pollution and airway disease. *Int J Tuberc Lung Dis* 2004; 8: 1401-1415.
- Yang IA, *et al.* Genetic susceptibility to the respiratory effects of air pollution. *Thorax* 2008; 63: 555-563.

SMOKING-RELATED DISEASES

Y. Martinet and N. Wirth
University of Nancy, Henri Poincaré, Nancy, France
E-mail: y.martinet@chu-nancy.fr

Tobacco use is by far the single largest avoidable cause of chronic illness and premature death worldwide. Smokers die of cancer of the lung and of other organs as well as of respiratory and cardiovascular diseases. In the European Union (EU), tobacco use kills at least 650,000 people (more than one in seven of all deaths) each year. Nearly 50% of these deaths involve diseases of the respiratory system, mainly lung cancer and chronic obstructive pulmonary disease (COPD). Given the relatively long period between time of smoking initiation ("first puff") and time of onset of smoking-related lung disease ($\geqslant =10$ yrs), young people who start smoking often disregard future health risks of tobacco use. Unfortunately, while male smoking is declining in most European countries, female smoking rates are still on the rise in some parts of the EU, and in most other countries of the world, due to tobacco industry activism.

Key points

- Tobacco use is responsible for more than one in seven out of all deaths in the EU.
- About 50% of tobacco-related deaths are due to lung cancer and COPD.
- Female smoking is still on the rise in some parts of the EU.
- Preventing tobacco use and treating tobacco addicts should be given top priority.

Tobacco smoke

Almost all tobacco-associated lung cancer and respiratory diseases result from smoke inhalation. In this respect, studies have shown that people who only use oral tobacco (such as Swedish snus, for example) during their lifetime are at no greater risk of developing these diseases than nonsmokers; however, the use of oral tobacco is related to several health problems, such as gum and pancreatic cancer and, possibly, cardiovascular diseases. Given that cigarette smoking is by far the most common method of tobacco consumption, the following data mainly concern diseases related to active cigarette smoking.

Cigarette smoke is composed of >4,000 substances, including nicotine, chemical poisons, toxic gases, small particles and carcinogens. The nicotine present in tobacco leaves is highly addictive but has little toxicity on the respiratory tract. Thus, people smoke for the psychoactive effects of nicotine, but die from the high toxicity of the other components present in smoke. Even if tobacco smoke composition varies slightly (due to tobacco type, substances added during manufacturing, filter type) the health risks and effects of tobacco smoking are quite constant from one cigarette brand to another. Furthermore, previously labelled "low tar/low nicotine" cigarettes have been shown to be as hazardous as "regular" ones. Likewise, hand-rolled cigarette, bidi, and water-pipe smoking are at least as dangerous as cigarette smoking. Finally, while pipe and cigar smoke is more toxic than cigarette smoke, cigar and pipe smokers are seldom deep inhalers. This explains the lower incidence of respiratory disease in these "noninhaling" smokers. Nevertheless, this rate is still higher than in nonsmokers.

Cannabis smoke

In respect to effects on the respiratory tract, cannabis smoking is at least as dangerous as tobacco smoking. Moreover, since cannabis is usually smoked mixed with tobacco, young people often become addicted to tobacco for life, even occasional users merely seeking to experience the relaxing effects of tetrahydrocannabinol. This co-consumption of cannabis and tobacco complicates characterisation of the specific health effects of cannabis smoking. Nevertheless, it has been shown that cannabis smoking causes lung cancer and COPD.

Lung cancer

Lung cancer is the most frequent cause of death due to tobacco use: 85-90% of the 225,000 lung cancer deaths occurring each year in the EU are the consequence of tobacco smoking. Lung cancer is one of the deadliest cancers, with 5-yr survival rates ranging from 10-15%. Lung cancer incidence and mortality increase roughly in proportion to the first power of smoking intensity (number of cigarettes smoked per day) and, most importantly, to the second power of smoking duration (total number of years of smoking). Tobacco smoking results in all major histological types of lung cancer. Lung cancer risk is similar in males and females with comparable smoking histories. With such a highly specific cause and terrible prognosis, the best "treatment" of lung cancer is to avoid it through tobacco smoking prevention and treatment. Indeed, the relative risk of lung cancer steadily decreases when smokers give up smoking. For example, in the UK, for males who stopped smoking at ages 30, 40, 50 and 60, the risk of lung cancer by age 75 yrs was 2, 3, 6 and 10%, respectively; whereas for males who smoked up to 75 yrs of age this cumulative risk reached 16%. In the same way, an increase in overall tobacco consumption by a population is followed by an increase of lung cancer incidence, while a fall in consumption is followed by a drop in lung cancer incidence, as shown for males in France between 1950 and 2006 (fig. 1).

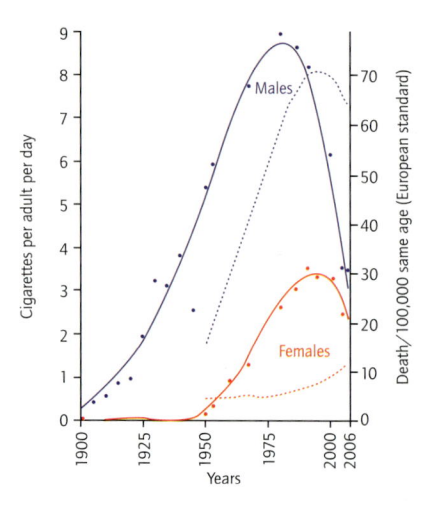

Figure 1. Trends in cigarette smoking (---) and death by lung cancer (······) by sex in France, 1950-2006. Modified from HILL *et al.* (2010).

COPD and asthma

In 2000, ~30% of the 371,000 deaths from nonmalignant respiratory diseases occurring in the EU were caused by cigarette smoking. Among these cases, COPD was the most frequent cause of death. Nearly two-thirds of these COPD deaths were caused by tobacco smoking. The COPD mortality rate is roughly 20 times higher among heavy smokers (male or female) than nonsmokers. According to international guidelines for COPD classification (American Thoracic Society,

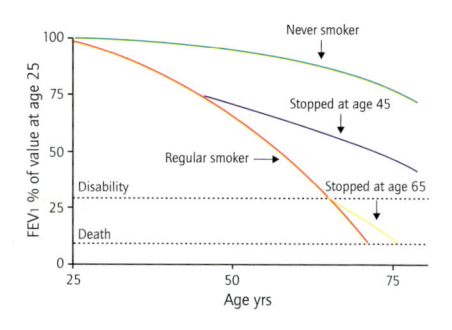

Figure 2. Loss of forced expiratory volume in 1 s (FEV_1) in never-smokers, regular smokers and smokers giving up at ages 45 and 65 yrs. Modified from FLETCHER and PETO (1977).

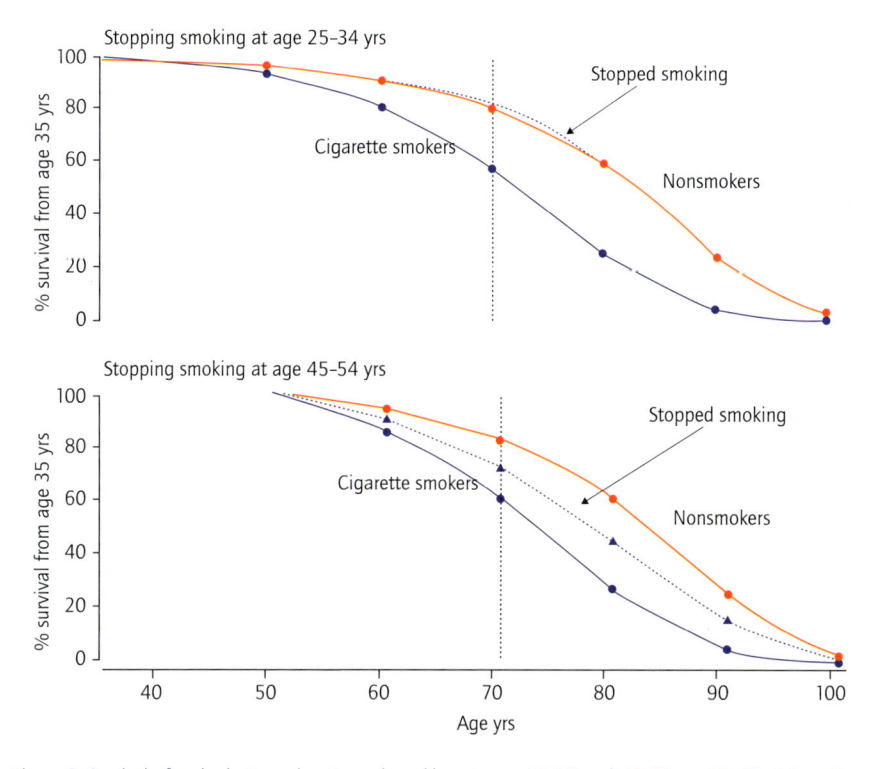

Figure 3. Survival of male doctors who stopped smoking at ages 25–34 and 45–54 yrs. Modified from Doll et al. (2004).

European Respiratory Society), up to 60% of current smokers aged >65 yrs suffer from COPD. Measurement of forced expiratory volume in 1 s (FEV_1) and of its decline is the best marker of airflow limitation in COPD, and FEV_1 value is directly related to COPD morbidity and mortality. Physiological decline of FEV_1 with age is accelerated by tobacco smoking, whereas, in contrast, smoking cessation slows lung function decline in smokers (fig. 2). Cessation also improves COPD patient quality of life, and is the only measure that definitively improves COPD patient survival. Asthmatic patients who smoke have a higher risk of hospitalisation for their disease and experience more severe symptoms with poor clinical control and poorer quality of life. Finally, active cigarette smoking is a direct cause of asthma onset, and causes more severe symptoms and lung function decline.

Respiratory infectious diseases

Bronchial and lung infectious diseases, including tuberculosis, acute bronchiolitis, pneumonia, the common cold, and influenza are more frequent and more severe in smokers.

Interstitial lung diseases

Several interstitial lung diseases, namely, respiratory bronchiolitis-associated interstitial lung disease, desquamative interstitial pneumonia, and pulmonary Langerhans' cell histiocytosis are strongly associated with cigarette smoking.

Passive smoking

In addition to its direct harmful effects on active smokers, exposure to tobacco combustion products from smoking is dangerous to nonsmokers, as environmental tobacco smoke is highly toxic. In the EU, in

2002, an estimated 79,449 deaths were attributable to passive smoking from various diseases caused by second-hand smoking, including lung cancer (13,241 deaths), chronic non-neoplastic respiratory disease (5,275 deaths), ischaemic heart disease (32,342 deaths), and stroke (28,591 deaths).

Furthermore, COPD, asthma, and several infectious diseases are more severe in nonsmokers exposed to passive smoking.

Conclusion

Since current treatments of lung cancer and COPD are poorly efficient, it is obvious that preventing tobacco use through tobacco control and treating tobacco addiction are by far the most efficient means to prevent and "cure" these respiratory diseases. This conclusion is also true for most other diseases related to cigarette smoking. Indeed, the overall impact of smoking cessation on survival is significant for all smokers at any age, as shown in fig. 3.

References

- Arcavi L, Benowitz NL. Cigarette smoking and infection. Arch Intern Med 2004; 164: 2206–2216.
- Doll R, et al. Mortality in relation to smoking: 50 years' observations on male British doctors. Br Med J 2004; 328: 1519–1528.
- Flanders WD, et al. Lung cancer mortality in relation to age, duration of smoking, and daily cigarette consumption: results from Cancer Prevention Study II. Cancer Res 2003; 63: 6556–6562.
- Fletcher C, Peto R. The natural history of chronic airflow obstruction. Br Med J 1977; 1: 1645–1648.
- Foulds J, Kozlowski L. Snus – what should the public-health response be? Lancet 2007; 369: 1976–1978.
- Hill C, et al. Assessment of the Lung Cancer Epidemic Due to Smoking. BEH 19–20. Saint Maurice (France), Institut de Veille Sanitaire, 2010.
- Lifting the smokescreen: 10 reasons for a smokefree Europe. Brussels, European Respiratory Society Journals Ltd, 2006.
- Mannino DM, et al. The natural history of chronic obstructive pulmonary disease. Eur Respir J 2006; 27: 627–643.
- Ryu JM, et al. Smoking-related interstitial lung diseases: a concise review. Eur Respir J 2001; 17: 122–132.
- Tobacco or health in the European Union. Past, present and future. Brussels, Commission of the European Communities, 2004.

TREATMENT OF TOBACCO DEPENDENCE

L. Clancy and Z. Kabir
Tobacco Free Research Institute, Dublin, Ireland
E-mail: lclancy@tri.ie

Tobacco dependence is a disease that would be of little consequence if it were not for adverse effects of smoking. Instead it causes 30–40% of all cancers and is the principal cause of lung cancer. It is the biggest cause of preventable respiratory disease, even if lung and other respiratory cancers are excluded: smoking is linked causally or as an important risk factor to chronic obstructive pulmonary disease (COPD), emphysema, asthma and respiratory infections including tuberculosis. Nevertheless, to speak of smoking as an occupational or environmental disease is perhaps not entirely accurate. Without doubt, however, smoking prevalence has a strong occupational bias. Exposure to second-hand smoke at work is also a significant occupational hazard. This situation has been greatly improved by the enactment of smoke-free laws in many countries, especially within the European Union. Second-hand smoke remains, however, the most significant indoor pollutant, especially in homes and motor cars.

Treating tobacco dependence is an important issue for respiratory physicians. An interest in the prevention of dependence through tobacco control mechanisms should also be a priority.

Prevention

As always, prevention is the primary intervention to be considered. The mechanisms for tobacco control are well established and incorporated in the Framework Convention for Tobacco Control (FCTC), which is the first medical treaty of the World Health Organization (WHO) and has been ratified by 168 countries. The WHO has also proposed a strategy, MPOWER, for these mechanisms' implementation and monitoring. It is clearly stated in the FCTC that price is the most effective tobacco control measure but that interventions such as workplace restrictions on smoking, protection from exposure and product regulation by various means are important. It is also agreed that proper information about the dangers of smoking needs to be made known. The value of health warnings, especially graphic image warnings is emphasised and there is a realisation that packaging and labelling are important methods of advertising for the tobacco industry. This is especially so in countries where direct advertising and

> **Key points**
>
> - Tobacco dependence is a disease and is an important issue for respiratory physicians.
> - The prevention of tobacco dependence through tobacco control mechanisms is a priority.
> - Effective and cost-effective treatments for tobacco dependence exist in the form of motivational support and pharmacotherapy.
> - The treatment of tobacco dependence benefits from knowledge, experience and training, which is not provided in medical schools at undergraduate level, and that should be a priority.

promotion and sponsorship are banned. However the role of treating smoking in the plan, although regarded as important, is left unclear. The reasons for this are many and include considerations of availability, cost, efficacy and efficiency. This is not surprising but is challenging. Even more challenging is the fact that the costs of other evidence-based interventions are usually much smaller than those of treatment. This may also be true of some other diseases, for which treatments are much better developed. The cost-effectiveness of treatment of tobacco dependence as a disease in patients without other diseases may not be obvious: the time lag between the treatment and the prevention of serious physical disease may obscure comparisons with the treatments of other diseases. However, effective treatments are available, are very cost-effective and compare very well with treatment of other diseases in this regard. Despite this, interest in supplying this service seems to be low among policymakers. Smoking was, and to some extent still is, not accepted as a disease by many people. This is in no small part due to the tobacco industry. For generations, it denied that smoking was harmful and addictive and emphasised the free choice argument and the apparent glamour of smoking. It is now becoming widely accepted that smoking is a disease and that it is based on addiction. It is very difficult to treat but the rewards for treating it successfully are enormous.

One-third of the population of the world smokes. If this disease is to be tackled by treating all smokers, the implications are daunting: treatment alone will probably never become the appropriate response to this epidemic, unless much better and cheaper treatments can be developed to make this possible in the future. At present treatment has a defined role. Its importance in tobacco control will vary from time to time and from country to country depending on the stage of implementation of tobacco control policies. Our first responsibility as doctors is probably to know what treatments exist, then to examine the evidence base for their

usefulness and consider how they could be made available to our patients.

Evidence-based treatments

Effective and cost-effective treatments for smoking exist. The two treatment modalities proven to be effective consist of motivational support, in the form of counselling, and pharmacotherapy. Present knowledge suggests that a combination of the two is more effective than either alone. The duration of counselling seems to be important. Within limits, longer seems better – for instance, brief intervention by a general practitioner of some 3 min increases success rates by ~2.5% when compared with those who did not receive such advice. Sessions lasting ~10 min and repeated three to four times at intervals according to present knowledge seem to be near optimal, but these considerations need further defining and application.

As regards pharmacological therapies, a number of preparations have been shown to have measurable success rates. These include nicotine replacement therapy (NRT), which approximately doubles success rate. Varenicline and buproprion also have established success rates. Varenicline seems to be more effective than NRT, while buproprion's success rate is similar to that of NRT. The use of these preparations and their safety profiles need to be studied carefully. They provide the clinician with pharmacotherapy which has proven efficacy and should be used knowledgably by physicians. TØNNESEN (2009) recently reviewed the evidence for smoking cessation, concluding that with the most optimal drugs and counselling a 1-yr abstinence rate of ~25% can be expected in smoking cessation. This compares very favourably with the treatment of any other chronic relapsing disease. CAPONNETTO and POLOSA (2008) recently outlined the predictors of success and failure in treatment. Factors which influence outcomes include degree of nicotine dependence, age at initiation, how many cigarettes are smoked per day, social support and family circumstances, such as a nonsmoking partner, sex and comorbidities such as alcoholism and depression. They also point out the complex relationship with previous attempts and of course the importance of motivation to quit.

In addition, evidence suggests that quit attempts are more frequent in subjects with high baseline body-mass index and low weight concerns. Innovative approaches, such as brief isometric exercise and the cognitive technique of body scanning, may be effective for reducing desire to smoke and withdrawal symptoms in temporarily abstaining smokers.

Conclusion

The treatment of tobacco dependence benefits from knowledge, experience and training. This is not provided in medical schools at undergraduate level. We expect that the structure of training for the management of this disease and particularly its treatment will improve and increase in the short term. Knowledge of general tobacco control principles will also need attention if we are to succeed in this important endeavour.

References

- Caponnetto P, Polosa R. Smoking cessation: tips for improving success rates. *Breathe* 2008; 5: 16-24.
- Cromwell J, et al. Cost-effectiveness of the clinical practice recommendations in the AHCPR guideline for smoking cessation. *JAMA* 1997; 278: 1759-1766.
- Fagerstrom KO, Jimenez-Ruiz CA. Pharmacological treatments for tobacco dependence. *Eur Respir Rev* 2008; 17: 192-198.
- Goodman P, et al. Effects of the Irish smoking ban on respiratory health of bar workers and air quality in Dublin pubs. *Am J Respir Crit Care Med* 2007; 175: 840-845.
- Raw M, et al. A survey of tobacco dependence treatment guidelines in 31 countries. *Addiction* 2009; 104: 1243-1250.
- Rigotti NA, et al. Smoking cessation interventions for hospitalized smokers: a systematic review. *Arch Intern Med* 2008; 168: 1950-1960.
- Tønnesen P, et al. Smoking cessation in patients with respiratory diseases: a high priority, integral component of therapy. *Eur Respir J* 2007; 29: 390-417.
- US Department of Health and Human Services. The health consequences of involuntary exposure to tobacco smoke: a report of the Surgeon General. Atlanta: Department of Health and Human Services, 2006.
- Ussher M, et al. Effect of isometric exercise and body scanning on cigarette cravings and withdrawal symptoms. *Addiction* 2009; 104: 1251-1257.

Weblink

- World Health Organization. WHO Report on the Global Tobacco Epidemic, 2009: Implementing smoke-free environments. www.who.int/tobacco/mpower/en/.

HIGH-ALTITUDE DISEASE

Y. Nussbaumer-Ochsner and K.E. Bloch
Pulmonary Division, University Hospital of Zurich, Switzerland
E-mail: konrad.bloch@usz.ch

Physiological response to altitude

The low barometric pressure at altitude results in a reduced inspiratory and arterial oxygen tension. The immediate physiological response comprises a rise in heart rate and pulmonary arterial pressure. Chemoreceptor-mediated hyperventilation tends to mitigate hypoxaemia but the associated hypocapnia with an arterial carbon dioxide tension close to the apnoeic threshold promotes ventilatory instability with periods of hyperpnoea alternating with central apnoea/hypopnoea. This pattern, termed high-altitude periodic breathing, is observed in healthy subjects at altitudes >2,000 m mostly during sleep. It may cause intermittent dyspnoea and sleep disturbances (figs 1 and 2).

Prolonged altitude exposure triggers various acclimatisation mechanisms including an increased chemoreceptor sensitivity to hypoxia and hypercapnia, enhanced erythropoesis and alterations in the endocrine system, metabolism and in fluid balance.

The reduced air density at altitude lowers airflow resistance. Vital capacity is slightly reduced due to respiratory muscle weakness and pulmonary congestion. Oxygen uptake through the lungs is affected by a reduced alveolar–capillary oxygen gradient and a reduced transit time of blood through pulmonary capillaries due to increased cardiac output. This causes diffusion limitation leading to hypoxaemia especially during exercise.

High-altitude-related disease

Acute mountain sickness (AMS) is the most common altitude-related illness. It affects 10–40% of lowlanders ascending to 3,000 m and 40–60% at 4,500 m. A lack of prior acclimatisation, rapid ascent, high sleeping altitude and individual susceptibility predispose to AMS. Symptoms start within 6–12 h after arrival at altitude and include headache, loss of appetite, nausea or vomiting, weakness, fatigue and insomnia. The diagnosis relies on the constellation of typical symptoms in the setting of altitude exposure. Different scores (*e.g.* the Lake Louise Score) help to establish the diagnosis and to grade AMS severity. If additional neurological signs such as ataxia, cognitive deficits and impaired vigilance develop, a

Key points

- A low barometric pressure at altitude results in reduced inspired and arterial oxygen partial pressures.
- Hypoxaemia triggers adaptive physiological repsonses termed acclimatisation.
- Respiratory acclimatissation includes hyperventilation and periodic breathing, which typically prevails ?during sleep.
- Acute mountain sickness, high-altitude cerebral oedema and high-altitude pulmonary oedema may affect travellers after rapid ascent to altitude. Chronic mountain sickness occurs in long-term residents of high mountain areas.
- Treatment of high-altitude related illness consists of descent, supplemental oxygen and drugs.

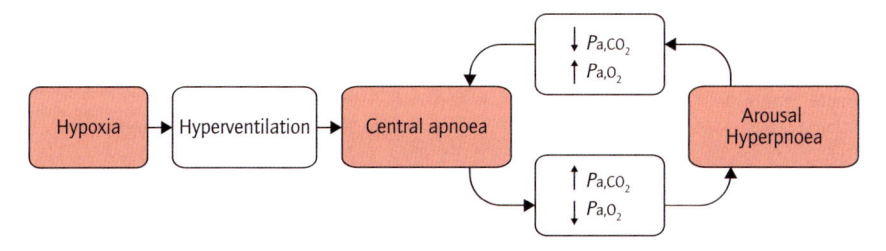

Figure 1. Mechanisms of high-altitude periodic breathing.

potentially life-threatening high-altitude cerebral oedema (HACE) must be considered. Treatments of AMS include descent to lower altitude, analgesics for headache and acetazolamide. More severe forms of AMS and HACE require dexamethasone and oxygen if available. Inflatable hyperbaric bags simulating descent to 1,500–2,500 m are also used.

High-altitude pulmonary oedema (HAPE) is a noncardiogenic and noninflammatory oedema resulting from excessive elevation of pulmonary capillary pressure, uneven distribution of blood flow and impaired alveolar fluid clearance. HAPE is rare below 3,500 m but occurs in 2–4% of mountaineers within hours to 4 days after arrival at 4,500 m. It is promoted by rapid ascent, physical exertion and individual susceptibility. Manifestations of HAPE include excessive dyspnoea, dry cough, tachycardia, cyanosis, pulmonary crackles and low-grade fever. Chest radiography shows interstitial or alveolar opacities but a normal-sized heart. Descent, supplemental oxygen or both are nearly always successful in HAPE. If oxygen is not available or descent not possible, pharmaceuticals become necessary (table 1). Pulmonary vasodilators such as nifedipine or phosphodiesterase inhibitors (sildenafil) lower pulmonary artery pressure. If descent is

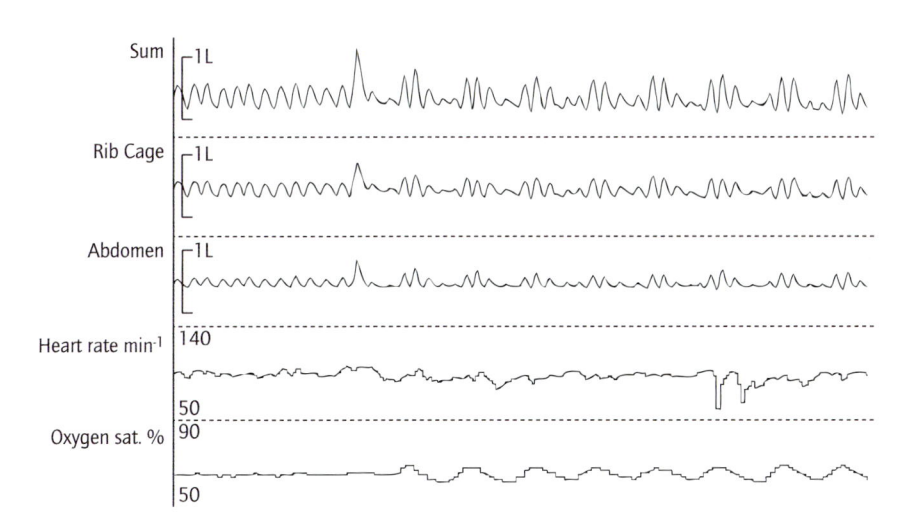

Figure 2. Periodic breathing associated with oscillations in oxygen saturation and heart rate recorded in a 28-yr-old women resting after a climb at 6,850 m. Modified from BLOCH *et al.* (2010), with permission from the publisher.

Table 1. Prevention and treatment of high-altitude disease

Disease	Prevention	Treatment
Acute mountain sickness (AMS)	Acclimatisation Slow ascent Acetazolamide $2 \times 125\text{-}250$ mg·day^{-1}, starting 24 h before ascent or dexamethasone 2×4 mg·day^{-1} 24 h before ascent	Analgesics, antiemetics Acetazolamide 2×250 mg·day^{-1} More severe forms: descent oxygen 2-6 L·min^{-1} Dexamethasone (initially mg $i.v.$, then 4×4 mg·day^{-1} $p.o.$) Acetazolamide (2×250 mg·day^{-1}), eventually in combination with dexamethasone Portable hyperbaric chamber
High-altitude cerebral oedema (HACE)	As for AMS	Immediate descent. If not possible: Oxygen (2-6 L·min^{-1}), Portable hyperbaric chamber Dexamethasone (initially 8 mg $i.v.$, then 4×4 mg·day^{-1} $p.o.$) Check for accompanying HAPE, acetazolamide if descent delayed
High-altitude pulmonary oedema (HAPE)	Acclimatisation Slow accent Avoid overexertion Nifedipine 30-60 mg·day^{-1} (extended-release formulation)	Immediate descent. If not possible: Oxygen 2-6 L·min^{-1} until oxygen saturation >90% or hyperbaric chamber Nifedipine 10-20 mg initially, switch to an extended-release formulation (nifedipine 30/60 mg) depending on blood pressure Treat accompanying AMS by dexamethasone

impossible and oxygen unavailable a hyperbaric bag may be life-saving.

Table 1 summarises prevention and treatment of altitude related diseases.

Chronic mountain sickness, a condition observed in long-term high altitude residents, is characterised by severe hypoxaemia, excessive erythrocytosis and pulmonary hypertension. Affected people suffer from fatigue, dizziness, headache and confusion. Descent to low altitude leads to prompt relief.

Patients with lung disease at altitude

Little is known about the risks of altitude exposure in patients with pre-existing lung disease. Recommendations are largely based on anecdotal evidence.

Chronic obstructive pulmonary disease
In patients with impaired gas exchange, arterial oxygen tension may drop to low levels at altitude so that the use of supplemental oxygen should be considered. It seems reasonable that patients with severe disease (forced expiratory volume in 1 s <50% predicted) with an arterial oxygen saturation <95% at low altitude should have an individual assessment before travelling to altitude. Acetazolamide should be used with caution in patients with severe airflow obstruction since carbon dioxide retention may lead to worsened dyspnoea or respiratory failure.

Asthma
A reduced allergen burden with increasing altitude can be expected at >1,500 m. Conversely, inhalation of cold air may worsen asthma, especially in combination with exercise or hypoxia-induced hyperventilation. Asthma patients with controlled disease are advised to take their usual medications when travelling to altitude, to avoid

strenuous exercise in a cold environment and to treat any exacerbation appropriately. Patients with uncontrolled, severe asthma should be cautioned against travelling to altitude.

Obstructive sleep apnoea syndrome Untreated patients residing at sea-level and travelling to moderate altitude (2,500 m) revealed an exacerbation of sleep apnoea with pronounced hypoxaemia and frequent central events. Sleep quality was worse at altitude and daytime testing revealed impaired vigilance and elevated blood pressure. Combined treatment with continuous positive airways pressure ventilation and acetazolamide seems advisable.

Pulmonary hypertension In general, patients with more than mild pre-existing pulmonary hypertension should be counselled against high-altitude travel because pre-existing pulmonary hypertension may predispose to HAPE. In patients not on medical therapy, prophylaxis with nifedipine and supplemental oxygen should be considered.

Conclusions

Physiological adaptation allows humans to tolerate exposure to even very high altitudes. Rapid ascent, inappropriate time for acclimatisation, strenuous physical exertion and individual susceptibility predispose to high-altitude-related illnesses, which may be prevented with appropriate precautions.

References

- Basnyat B, Murdoch DR. High-altitude illness. *Lancet* 2003; 361: 1967–1974.
- Bloch KE, *et al*. Nocturnal periodic breathing during acclimatization at very high altitude at Mt. Muztagh Ata (7546m). *Am J Respir Crit Care Med* 2010; Epub ahead of print. DOI: 10.1164/rccm.200911-16940.
- Imray C, *et al*. Acute mountain sickness: pathophysiology, prevention, and treatment. *Prog Cardiovasc Dis* 2010; 52: 467–484.
- Luks AM, Swenson ER. Travel to high altitude with pre-existing lung disease. *Eur Respir J* 2007; 29: 770–792.
- Maggiorini M. Prevention and treatment of high-altitude pulmonary edema. *Prog Cardiovasc Dis* 2010; 52: 500–506.
- Nussbaumer-Ochsner Y, *et al*. Exacerbation of sleep apnoea by frequent central events in patients with the obstructive sleep apnoea syndrome at altitude: a randomised trial. *Thorax* 2010; 65: 429–435.
- Nussbaumer-Ochsner Y, Bloch KE. Lessons from high-altitude physiology. *Breathe* 2007; 4: 123–132.

DIVING-RELATED DISEASES

E. Thorsen
University of Bergen, Bergen, Norway
E-mail: einar.thorsen@helse-bergen.no

Professional divers are engaged in underwater construction and inspection, and compressed air workers (Caisson workers) work at increased ambient pressure in a dry environment, mostly in tunnel construction. Military forces, police and fire brigades have teams of divers for specialised underwater operations. Recreational divers make up by far the largest group of divers. The physical environment in which these divers are operating is different, but common to all groups is exposure to increased ambient pressure and the exposure factors associated with pressure.

Pulmonary limitations at depth

Gas density increases proportionately with ambient pressure when air is used as the gas breathed. Airway resistance is proportional to gas density and maximal expiratory flow rates are inversely proportional to the square root of gas density. This means that at a depth of 30 m, when relative gas density is four times that of air at atmospheric pressure, maximal expiratory flow rates and maximal voluntary ventilation are reduced by 50%. Most experimental data are close to this theoretical relationship, as illustrated in fig. 1.

When diving to depths >50 m, the gas breathed is often a mixture of helium and oxygen to compensate for the mechanical limitations of ventilatory capacity due to gas density. The partial pressure of oxygen in these gas mixtures is usually 30–50 kPa, corresponding to a fraction of oxygen of 2–5% at depths of ⩾100 m.

Physical work under water is demanding. A normal ventilatory capacity and physical work capacity evaluated by exercise testing are required. External resistance and static load related to breathing apparatus and submersion adds to the increased load imposed by gas density. The gas breathed at depth has to be dry to prevent icing in the pressure regulators and evaporative heat loss is high. The gas breathed has the temperature of ambient water and, because of increased gas density, convective heat loss is increased. Subjects with bronchial hyperreactivity may be at increased risk of bronchoconstriction at depth. There are, however, no definite studies confirming this risk as subjects with asthma traditionally have been excluded from diving.

Pulmonary barotrauma

Intra-alveolar gas volume will expand during decompression. If there is any obstruction to the free flow of gas out of the alveoli or a decrease in lung compliance, there will be an increase in intra-alveolar pressure imposing a risk for lung rupture or pulmonary barotrauma. Any processes in the lung associated with airway obstruction or

---

Key points

- Normal lung function and physical work capacity are required for underwater work.
- Normal lung function is required to reduce the risk of pulmonary barotrauma.
- Cumulative diving exposure is associated with a long-term reduction in lung function of an obstructive pattern, which at some time in the career may preclude further diving.

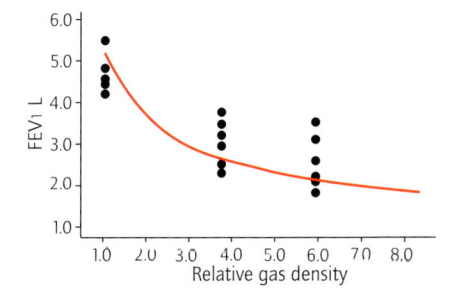

Figure 1. The theoretical relationship between gas density and forced expiratory volume in 1s (FEV1: red line), and some experimental data. The relative gas density of air at atmospheric pressure is 1.

decreased compliance locally or generally are considered to increase the risk. Lung rupture may cause pneumothorax, pneumopericardium, mediastinal emphysema and most seriously arterial gas embolism, which may be fatal. A pneumothorax or pneumopericardium encountered at depth may be fatal because of an increase in the transpulmonary pressure difference during decompression that obstructs venous return. The lowest pressure drop associated with diving causing pulmonary barotrauma described in the literature was <20 kPa (or 200 cmH$_2$O). The volume expansion for a given pressure reduction is larger close to the surface (Boyle-Mariotte's law).

Pulmonary effects of a single dive

A dive is associated with exposure to hyperoxia and a decompression stress, and both are related to ambient pressure and time. Hyperoxia at partial pressures of oxygen >40 kPa has well known toxic effects on the lung causing acute reductions in diffusion capacity, vital capacity and maximal expiratory flow rates. The decompression stress is related to the amount of inert gas dissolved in the tissues during the bottom phase of the dive and the rate of decompression. Supersaturation resulting in formation of venous gas bubbles has been demonstrated when the tension of inert gas in the tissues exceeds ambient pressure by ~30 kPa. Venous gas microemboli have been shown to be common with the decompression procedures routinely used in commercial and military diving operations.

The venous gas microemboli are filtered in the pulmonary circulation and are associated with inflammatory responses that add to toxic effects of hyperoxia. Venous gas microemboli may be shunted over to the systemic circulation through intrapulmonary and intracardiac shunts. A patent foramen ovale is present in 20–30% of the general population. Local circulatory disturbances due to gas bubbles that are either formed *in situ* or transported by the systemic circulation to other areas like joints, skin, brain and spinal cord may cause decompression sickness.

The combination of added static and dynamic respiratory load, immersion and exercise results in a large increase in pulmonary arterial pressure. Undue breathlessness after diving, or even swimming only, may be related to pulmonary oedema.

Long-term effects of diving

The exposure to hyperoxia and the accumulation of gas microemboli in the lung are associated with inflammatory responses. Several cross-sectional studies of divers' lung function indicate that residual effects of single dives accumulate to a long-term effect characterised by an obstructive spirometric pattern and a reduction in diffusion capacity. There are only a few longitudinal studies of divers' lung function, but these studies confirm the findings in the cross-sectional studies by demonstrating a negative relationship between cumulative diving exposure and maximal expiratory flow rates and forced expired volume in 1 s.

References

- Lundgren CEG, Miller JN, eds. The Lung at Depth. New York, Marcel Dekker Inc., 1999.
- Brubakk AO, Neumann TS, eds. Bennett and Elliott's Physiology and Medicine of Diving. Edinburgh, Saunders, Elsevier Science Ltd, 2003.
- Tetzlaff K, Thorsen E. Breathing at depth: physiologic and clinical aspects of diving while breathing compressed gas. *Clin Chest Med* 2005; 26: 355–380.

RADIATION-INDUCED DISEASE

R.P. Coppes and P. van Luijk
University Medical Center Groningen, University of Groningen, Groningen, the Netherlands
E-mail: r.p.coppes@med.umcg.nl

Radiotherapy plays an important role in the treatment of tumours located in the thoracic area. The cure rate for these tumours is, however, limited by the low radiation dose that can be tolerated by the lungs. The presently set dose already results in pulmonary complications in about one-fifth of patients.

Radiation-induced lung injury develops in an early inflammatory phase termed radiation pneumonitis (RP) followed by a late fibroproductive phase (fig. 1). These phases lead to compromised lung perfusion, increased vascular resistance, reduced gas-exchange interphase between air and blood, and suboptimal blood oxygenation. Symptoms range from dyspnoea on effort to respiratory failure, oxygen dependency, right heart failure and death.

Key points

- Radiotherapy for tumour treatment results in pulmonary complications in about 20% of patients.
- Radiation-induced lung injury develops from an early, inflammatory phase to a late fibrotic phase.

Several inflammatory responses contribute to RP. Acute alveolar and interstitial inflammation and loss of type I epithelial induces proliferation of type II epithelial cells. This leads to a cascade of induction of inflammatory cytokines (fig. 1), potentially aggravated by chemotherapeutic agents. Subsequently, an influx of inflammatory cells,

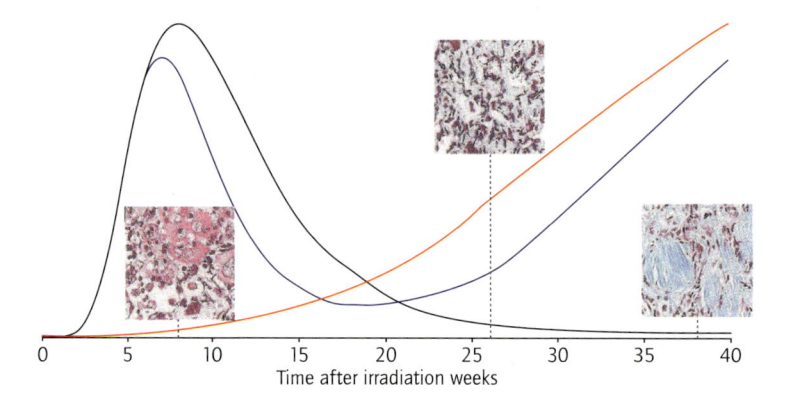

Figure 1. Radiation-induced lung injury develops in an early inflammatory and late fibrotic phase. Black line: pneumonitis; red line: fibrosis; blue line: cytokine response.

such as leukocytes, lymphocytes, neutrophils and macrophages, is induced. Though macrophages are a hallmark, T-lymphocytes and matured dendritic cells also play an important role in RP.

Radiation-induced lung disease is a consequence of:

- loss of type I epithelial and endothelial cells
- inflammatory responses
- malfunction of microvasculature
- lung fibrosis.

In addition, malfunction of the microvasculature due to endothelial injury and subsequent increased permeability with protein exudation contributes to the develoment of RP. Depending on the irradiated region and volume, the inflammatory response may affect only pulmonary blood vessels (low dose, large volumes) or vessels and parachyma (high dose, low volumes) to induce complications.

Following or even without prior symptomatic pneumonitis, chronic radiation-induced pulmonary fibrosis (RF) may develop depending on the irradiated lung volume.

RF is caused by accumulation of collagen and other extracellular matrix fibres in the interstitium under persistent cytokine stimuli in combination with arterio-capillary sclerosis.

References

- Johnston CJ, et al. Inflammatory cell recruitment following thoracic irradiation. *Exp Lung Res* 2004; 30: 369-382.
- Marks LB, et al. Radiation-induced lung injury. *Semin Radiat Oncol* 2003; 13: 333-345.
- McBride WH, et al. A sense of danger from radiation. *Radiat Res* 2004; 162: 1-19.
- Novakova-Jiresova A, et al. Changes in expression of injury after irradiation of increasing volumes in rat lung. *Int J Radiat Oncol Biol Phys* 2007; 67: 1510-1518.
- Novakova-Jiresova A, et al. Pulmonary radiation injury: identification of risk factors associated with regional hypersensitivity. *Cancer Res* 2005; 65: 3568-3576.
- Rodemann HP, Bamberg M. Cellular basis of radiation-induced fibrosis. *Radiother Oncol* 1995; 35: 83-90.
- Rübe CE, et al. Increased expression of pro-inflammatory cytokines as a cause of lung toxicity after combined treatment with gemcitabine and thoracic irradiation. *Radiother Oncol* 2004; 72: 231-241.

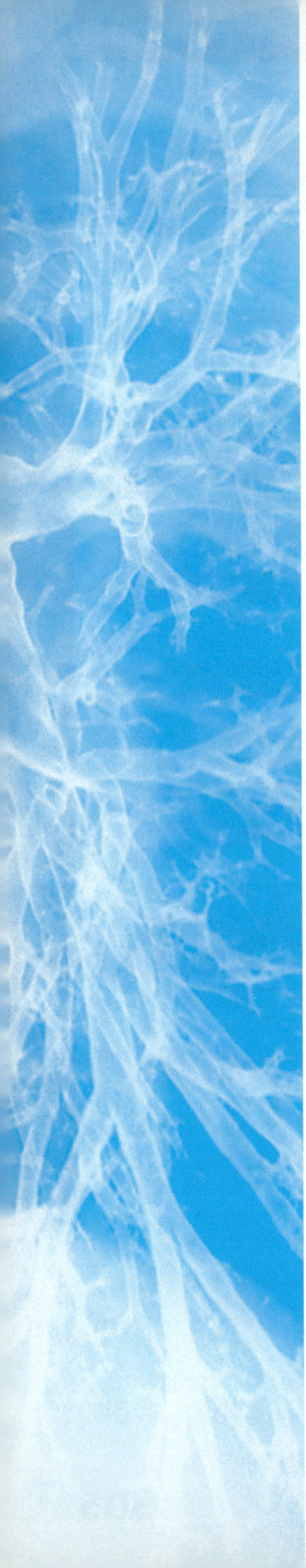

CHAPTER 11:

INTERSTITIAL LUNG DISEASE

SARCOIDOSIS — 308
U. Costabel

IDIOPATHIC INTERSTITIAL PNEUMONIAS — 311
D. Olivieri, S. Chiesa and P. Tzani

EOSINOPHILIC DISEASES — 319
A. Menzies-Gow

DRUG-INDUCED RESPIRATORY DISEASE — 322
Ph. Camus

SARCOIDOSIS

U. Costabel
Dept Pneumology/Allergy, Ruhrlandklinik, Essen, Germany
E-mail: ulrich.costabel@ruhrlandklinik.uk-essen.de

Sarcoidosis is a multisystem granulomatous disorder of unknown aetiology, which commonly affects young and middle-aged adults. The disease frequently presents with bilateral hilar lymphadenopathy, pulmonary infiltration, and ocular and skin lesions. Any organ of the body may be involved. The prevalence rates of Sarcoidosis vary widely, from <1 case to 40 cases per 100,000 population. Sarcoidosis is common in Scandinavia, Central Europe, the USA and Japan. It is less frequently seen in other Asian countries, Central and South America, and Africa. Sarcoidosis in Afro-Americans is more severe, while Caucasians are more likely to present with asymptomatic disease. Overall mortality is 1–5%.

The cause of sarcoidosis remains unknown. Available evidence strongly supports the hypothesis that the disease develops when a specific environmental exposure with antigenic properties occurs in a genetically susceptible individual. Potential aetiologic agents include mycobacteria and *Propionibacterium acnes*. Sarcoidosis susceptibility or chronicity has been associated with a number of human leukocyte antigen alleles. Some genetic associations have been found with specific disease subsets, most notably with Löfgren's syndrome. A polymorphism of the BTNL2 gene has been linked with sarcoidosis. The immunological abnormalities are characterised by the accumulation of activated T-cells of the T-helper cell type 1 and macrophages at sites of ongoing inflammation.

Clinical presentation

The clinical presentation of sarcoidosis varies widely. 30–50% of patients are asymptomatic at the time of diagnosis. Symptoms of sarcoidosis are largely nonspecific. Low-grade fever (sometimes up to 40°C), weight loss (usually limited to 2–6 kg during the 10–12 weeks before presentation), night sweats and arthralgias can be found in about 20–30% of patients. Sarcoidosis is an important and frequently overlooked cause of fever of unknown origin. Fatigue and skeletal muscle weakness are more common; present in ⩽70% of patients when carefully looked for. According to their initial presentation, sarcoidosis patients can be divided into two

---

Key points

- Sarcoidosis is a multisystem granulomatous disorder of unknown aetiology, which commonly affects young and middle-aged adults.

- Prevalence of sarcoidosis varies from <1 case to 40 cases per 100,000 population, and overall mortality is 1–5%.

- Clinical presentation varies widely, though fever, fatigue and skeletal muscle weakness are often noted.

- Decision to treat should be carefully assessed based on benefit to the patient and disease severity; treatment should mainly be considered if symptoms develop or lung function deteriorates.

- The clinical course of sarcoidosis can be unpredictable, so regular monitoring of signs of disease progression is advised.

distinct subgroups: acute and chronic. The acute form can present as classical Löfgrens syndrome, which is characterised by fever, bilateral hilar lymphadenopathy, ankle arthritis and erythema nodosum. The chronic form shows an insidious onset, and organ-related symptoms predominate, such as cough, dyspnoea, and chest pain.

Diagnostic approach

The criteria of the American Thoracic Society (ATS), European Respiratory Society (ERS), and the World Association of Sarcoidosis and Other Granulomatous Disorders (WASOG) for the diagnosis of sarcoidosis include:

- The presence of a consistent clinical and radiological picture
- Histological evidence of non-caseating granulomas
- Exclusion of other conditions capable of producing a similar histological or clinical picture

The initial diagnostic work-up for patients with suspected sarcoidosis involves careful baseline assessment of disease distribution and severity by organ, with emphasis on vital target organs (table 1). Specifically, the diagnostic assessment should attempt to accomplish four goals:

- Provide histological confirmation of the disease
- Assess the extent and severity of organ involvement
- Assess whether the disease is stable or is likely to process
- Determine whether therapy will benefit a patient

Granuloma alone are never diagnostic proof of sarcoidosis.

An important step is choice of site for a proper biopsy. Transbronchial lung biopsy is the recommended procedure in most cases, with the diagnostic yield reaching 80%. This can be combined with transbronchial needle aspiration, which has the highest yield when guided by endobronchial ultrasound, and with biopsy of the bronchial mucosa. Other easily accessible sites for biopsy are the skin, lip, or superficial lymph nodes. In patients without biopsy, clinical and/or radiological features alone may be diagnostic in stage I (reliability of 98%) or stage II (89%), but are less accurate in stage III (52%) or stage 0 (23%). The classical Löfgren's syndrome may not require biopsy proof. Bronchoalveolar lavage and studies of lymphocyte subpopulations showing an increase in the CD4/CD8 ratio may be helpful. Elevated serum angiotensin-converting enzyme and calcium levels may lend support to the diagnosis.

The chest radiogram is described in 4 stages (table 2). Computed tomography scanning describes much greater detail of mediastinal and parenchymal abnormalities, but is not an essential of baseline study. It is indicated when clinical presentation and/or chest radiographic findings are unclear or to detect complications of the lung disease.

Natural history and prognosis

The disease course is highly variable. Spontaneous remissions occur in nearly two thirds of patients. Serious extrapulmonary involvement (cardiac, central nervous system, hepatic) occurs in 4–7% of patients at time of presentation. Incidence becomes higher as the disease evolves. Adverse prognostic factors include lupus pernio, chronic uveitis, age at onset >40 yrs, chronic hypercalcaemia, nephrocalcinosis, African ethnic origin, progressive pulmonary sarcoidosis, nasal mucosal involvement, cystic bone lesions, neural sarcoidosis, cardiac sarcoidosis, and chronic respiratory insufficiency.

Treatment and follow-up

The indication to treat a patient depends on many factors, the most important being whether or not the patients is symptomatic. Except for life- and sight-threatening organ involvement, it should be carefully considered whether the patient might benefit from treatment. For asymptomatic pulmonary

Table 1. Initial evaluation for sarcoidosis

History (occupational and environmental exposure, symptoms)
Physical examination
Chest radiography
Pulmonary function tests: vital capacity, FEV1, carbon monoxide diffusion capacity
Peripheral blood counts
Serum chemistries: calcium, liver enzymes, creatinine, ACE
Urine analysis
Electrocardiography
Eye investigation
Tuberculin skin test
Selection of site for biopsy

FEV1: forced expiratory volume in 1 s; ACE: angiotensin-converting enzyme.

patients, a watch-and-wait approach is appropriate; treatment should mainly be considered if symptoms develop or lung function deteriorates. The goal of treatment is to make the patient asymptomatic and to restore or preserve organ function. Initial therapy is still based on corticosteroids. For pulmonary sarcoidosis, the initial prednisone dose is 20–40 mg; higher doses may be needed for cardiac or neural sarcoidosis. The dose is slowly tapered to 5–10 mg per day; treatment should be continued for a minimum of 12 months. Patients with Löfgren's syndrome do not require therapy with corticosteroids.

For patients with chronic disease requiring years of therapy, alternatives to corticosteroids include methotrexate, azathioprine and hydrocloroquine, all given usually in combination with low dose corticosteroids. For refractory sarcoidosis patients, new therapeutic approaches have begun to emerge through the use of immuno-modulatory agents. Based on current understanding of pathogenic mechanisms, these are tumour necrosis factor-α-blocking drugs, such as infliximab, thalidomide, and pentoxyfyllin.

Because the clinical course of sarcoidosis can be unpredictable, regular monitoring for signs of disease progression is necessary, using the least invasive and most sensitive tools. For pulmonary sarcoidosis, this is spirometry and diffusion capacity. For stable stage I disease, follow-up every 6–12 months is usually adequate; more frequent evaluations (every 3–6 months) are advised for stage II, III or IV sarcoidosis. All patients should be monitored for a minimum of 3 yrs after therapy is discontinued. Follow-up needs to be more vigilant after corticosteroid-induced remissions, due to the high rate of relapses in this context, ranging 15–70%.

References

- Drent M, Costabel U, eds. Sarcoidosis. *Eur Respir Mon* 2005; 32.
- Grutters JC, et al. Sarcoidosis. In: du Bois RM, Richeldi L, eds. Interstitial lung diseases. Eur Respir Mon 2009; 46: 126–154.
- Hunninghake GW, et al., ATS/ERS/WASOG statement on sarcoidosis. *Sarcoidosis Vasc Diffuse Lung Dis* 1999; 16: 149–173.

Table 2. Chest radiographic stages

Stage	Findings	Frequency
0	Normal	5–10%
I	BHL	50%
II	BHL and parenchymal infiltrates	25%
III	Parenchymal infiltrates without BHL	15%
IV	Sign of fibrosis	5–10%

BHL: bilateral hilar lymphadenopathy

IDIOPATHIC INTERSTITIAL PNEUMONIAS

D. Olivieri, S. Chiesa and P. Tzani
Cardiopulmonary Dept, Section of Respiratory Diseases, University Hospital, Parma, Italy
E-mail: dario.olivieri@unipr.it

Idiopathic interstitial pneumonias (IIPs) represent a heterogeneous group of disorders with different clinical and histological features and prognoses. They are considered as inflammatory disorders of the interstitium without extrapulmonary involvement.

The most recent American Thoracic Society (ATS) and European Respiratory Society (ERS) classifications of IIPs include seven different diseases identified by a typical histological pattern; each histological pattern meets precise clinical and radiological features and corresponds to a particular prognosis.

Epidemiology

The incidence of IIPs has been estimated at 7–11 cases per 100,000 persons while the prevalence ranges between 27–29 cases per 100,000 persons. The disease typically affects adults, peaking after the sixth decade of life, with a higher incidence in males and smokers. There is a familial variant of idiopathic pulmonary fibrosis (IPF), which accounts for 0.5–3% of cases of IIPs; this form is indistinguishable from the nonfamilial forms, except that patients tend to be younger in the former.

Clinical features and treatment

The IIPs include IPF, nonspecific interstitial pneumonia (NSIP), cryptogenic organising pneumonia/bronchiolitis obliterans organising pneumonia (COP/BOOP), acute interstitial pneumonia (AIP), respiratory bronchiolitis/interstitial lung disease (RB/ILD), desquamative interstitial pneumonia (DIP)/alveolar macrophage pneumonia (AMP) and lymphoid interstitial pneumonia (LIP) (table 1).

Some of these entities have been well identified clinically, as well as the appropriate corresponding treatments. In particular, when the inflammatory component dominates, such as in DIP/AMP, AIP and COP/BOOP, prompt corticosteroid therapy may lead to a significant improvement and sometimes to complete resolution of the disease.

LIP and AIP require prompt intervention by the haematology and intensive care units (ICU) respectively, because of their particular onset and the necessity of a specific therapeutical approach.

Nowadays the terms IPF and NSIP should be used only for chronic fibrosing interstitial

---

Key points

- IIPs represent a heterogeneous group of disorders with different clinical and histological features and prognoses.

- The most recent ATS and ERS classifications of IIPs include seven different diseases identified by a typical histological pattern: NSIP, COP/BOOP, AIP, RB/ILD, DIP/AMP and LIP.

- The terms IPF and NSIP should only be used for chronic fibrosing interstitial pneumonia of unknown cause limited to the lungs. The prognosis in IPF is worse with a histological pattern of UIP.

Table 1. Classification of idiopathic interstitial pneumonias

IPF/UIP	Idiopathic pulmonary fibrosis/usual interstitial pneumonia
DIP/AMP	Desquamative interstitial pneumonia/alveolar macrophage pneumonia
RB/ILD	Respiratory bronchiolitis/interstitial lung disease
AIP	Acute interstitial pneumonia
COP/BOOP	Cryptogenic organising pneumonia/bronchiolitis obliterans organising pneumonia
NSIP	Nonspecific interstitial pneumonia
LIP	Lymphoid interstitial pneumonia

pneumonia of unknown cause limited to the lungs. This distinction is particularly relevant because of the different clinical aspects and therapeutic approaches. Moreover, the prognosis is worse in these forms and particularly in IPF with a histological pattern of usual interstitial pneumonia (UIP).

Desquamative interstitial pneumonia/alveolar macrophage pneumonia

DIP is characterised by its insidious onset, with a worsening dry cough and progressive dyspnoea. There is a strong correlation between this disease and cigarette smoking. The term "desquamative" originated from the belief that the principal histological feature was desquamation of epithelial alveolar cells; in fact, intra-alveolar macrophage accumulation and the presence of hyperplastic epithelial cells seem to be the dominant aspects of the disease. Radiological features include ground-glass opacities with a lower zone predilection. The pathogenesis is unclear and the clinical course may vary: most patients improve with steroid treatment, but some may develop fibrosis.

Respiratory bronchiolitis/interstitial lung disease

This form affects primarily current or former smokers, especially males. Symptoms are mild and aspecific. The principal histological aspect is the presence of clusters of brown macrophages in the respiratory bronchioles, alveolar ducts and peribronchial alveolar space. Usually, smoking cessation leads to a complete resolution of the lesions. Steroid treatment may be necessary.

Acute interstitial pneumonia

AIP is a rare fulminating form of lung injury, with clinical and radiological findings similar to those seen in acute respiratory distress syndrome (ARDS). The disease evolves through three phases. First the exudative phase (from the onset to the 7th day) showing oedema, hyaline membranes and acute interstitial inflammation. The proliferative phase (30th day) is then characterised by hyperplasia of type 2 pneumocytes. Finally, the organising phase shows loose organising fibrosis mostly with type II alveolar septa. Hypoxaemia develops early and progresses rapidly to respiratory failure, which may be refractory to supplemental oxygen, whereby AIP requires prompt treatment in the ICU.

Cryptogenic organising pneumonia/bronchiolitis obliterans organising pneumonia

COP/BOOP is a rare form of IIP of unknown aetiology. Features of the organising pneumonia pattern are organisation within alveolar ducts and alveoli, with or without organisation in bronchioles. The clinical onset is aspecific and includes dyspnoea, dry cough, fever and inspiratory crackles. Radiological aspects are bilateral diffuse alveolar opacities with a lower zone predilection and peripheral predominance. The characteristic histopathological lesion includes an excessive proliferation of granulation tissue within small airways and alveolar ducts associated with chronic inflammation in the surrounding alveoli. Systemic steroid therapy is the gold standard treatment when other causes of bronchiolitis (*i.e.* infective bronchiolitis) are excluded.

Lymphoid interstitial pneumonia

LIP is more common in children than adults. The aetiology is unknown. Up to three quarters of patients present a monoclonal increase in gammaglobulin, whereas in childhood hypogammaglobulinemia may occur. LIP is associated with Sjögren's Syndrome in a quarter of cases. LIP is defined as an interstitial lymphoid infiltrate including lymphocytes, plasma cells and histiocytes, with associated type II cell hyperplasia and the presence of interstitial mononuclear cells and the formation of noncaseating granulomas. In LIP the infiltrate is characterised by the presence of polyclonal lymphocytes (T and B); by contrast, in the lymphomas the infiltrate is usually monoclonal. Radiological aspects are bilateral interstitial linear or nodular opacities; honeycombing may appear in the advanced phase of the disease. Spontaneous resolution is possible, but steroid and/or immunosuppressive therapy may be necessary.

Idiopathic pulmonary fibrosis/usual interstitial pneumonia and nonspecific interstitial pneumonia

Pathogenesis The pathogenetic mechanisms of IPF (pattern UIP) and NSIP are not completely clear. There are various hypotheses relative to the initial stimulus responsible for the pathogenetic process, such as exposure to toxic substances or viral infections. Regardless of the initial cause, the inflammatory–fibrotic process in UIP is characterised by injury to the alveolar epithelial cells, destruction of the subepithelial basement membrane, and the subsequent abnormal cicatrisation with increased fibroblastic response and excessive deposition of collagen and extracellular matrix.

The interplay between inflammatory and mesenchymal cells is regulated by a number of cytokines produced by fibroblasts and epithelial cells; the most important of these mediators are the transforming growth factor (TGF)-β, tumour necrosis factor (TNF)-α, platelet-derived growth factor, connective tissue growth factor, integrin-mediated intercellular adhesion molecules, proteases and oxygen radicals. Deficiency of interferon-γ may contribute to activating and perpetuating the fibroblastic process. As far as the histological aspect is concerned, the presence of fibroblastic foci is typical in UIP; the fibroblastic foci are formed by mesenchymal cells similar to myofibroblasts. Under the influence of TGF-β the cells increase the production of collagen, vimentin and actin, leading to an excessive deposition of extracellular matrix.

In the rare familial form, the transmission mode is unknown. It is likely to be autosomal dominant with variable penetration in two thirds of patients. Familial IPF has been associated with altered α_1-antitrypsin inhibitor alleles on chromosome 14. Genetic polymorphism for interleukin (IL)-1 receptor antagonists or TNF-α may be involved.

Physiology The physiological aberrations in IPF are typical of a restrictive pattern and include reduced lung volumes (vital capacity and total lung capacity), and normal or increased expiratory flow rates. Transfer factor of the lung for carbon dioxide ($T_{L,CO}$) is typically reduced, indicating damage to the interstitium causing impaired gas exchange. A further consequence of this alteration is hypoxaemia, which is exacerbated with exercise. Late in the course of the disease severe hypoxaemia may be observed also at rest; hypercapnia may be present as well.

Clinical features and diagnosis The initial insidious symptoms of IPF/UIP and NSIP are an insistent nonproductive cough and progressive dyspnoea. In most patients, physical examination reveals end-inspiratory crackles (velcro-type). The course of the disease may vary, in relation to the types of IIP. As far as UIP is concerned, prognosis is extremely severe; the course of the disease is rapid, even if some patients stabilise after an initial period of decline. Respiratory failure appears in 3–8 yrs and mean survival from the onset of the disease is approximately 3–5 yrs. During the late phases of the disease, patients often show cor pulmonale. Respiratory failure is the main cause of death, followed by pulmonary embolism and heart failure.

Diagnosis of IPF and NSIP is the result of an integrated and multidisciplinary process, requiring cooperation among clinicians, radiologists and pathologists. International guidelines state that histology is necessary for diagnosis. A surgical lung biopsy has a higher diagnostic value compared to a transbronchial biopsy or bronchoalveolar lavage. However, it is an invasive approach with potential risks, and sometimes patients may present clinical and physiological contraindications to surgery. In some cases, an acute exacerbation of the disease follows surgery, leading to a general decline.

The most recent ATS/ERS guidelines present new clinical diagnostic criteria, which increase the likelihood of a correct diagnosis of IPF in the immunocompetent adult, in the presence of all the major criteria as well as at least three minor criteria, even without histological data (table 2).

High resolution computed tomography (HRCT) has become a crucial tool for the diagnostic process and allows an accurate and objective follow-up of the disease. HRCT scans consistent with IIP represent one of the major ATS/ERS guidelines diagnostic criteria. In particular, the HRCT scans in the case of UIP show a heterogeneous distribution with predilection for the peripheral, especially subpleural and basilar regions of the lung. The main radiological feature in UIP is honeycombing, that is cystic radiolucencies as expression of severe and irreversible fibrotic conversion of the parenchyma. Secondary features include coarse reticular opacities, thickened bronchial walls, bronchiectasis and bronchioloectasis.

NSIP is characterised by the presence of ground-glass areas, signifying an active inflammatory process. The main aspects to be considered for differential diagnosis between UIP and NSIP are the geographic and temporal histological and radiological heterogeneity, the high concentration of fibroblastic foci and honeycombing in the UIP form.

Natural history and exacerbations The course of the disease is characterised by a progressive decline in pulmonary function, leading to a worsening general condition and ultimately death. A subset of patients, particularly in cases of UIP, develops an accelerated and usually fatal course, showing an extremely rapid decline; this condition is known as an acute exacerbation.

Table 2. American Thoracic Society/European Respiratory Society criteria for diagnosis of IPF

Major criteria
Exclusion of other known causes of IIP (environmental/professional exposures, drug toxicities, connective tissue diseases)
Abnormal lung function: restrictive pattern and impaired gas exchange
Bibasilar reticular abnormalities and ground glass opacities on HRCT scans
Transbronchial lung biopsy or BAL not consistent with other diseases
Minor criteria
Age >50 yrs
Duration of illness >3 months
Insidious onset of dyspnoea on exertion
Bibasilar inspiratory crackles ("velcro"-type)

The criteria for defining an exacerbation are:

- progressive dyspnoea during the last 30 days
- new pulmonary infiltrates in chest radiographs
- worsening of hypoxaemia with a reduction in oxygen partial pressure >10 mmHg
- absence of pulmonary infection supported by negative bronchoalveolar lavage (BAL)
- absence of any other cause, such as heart failure, pulmonary embolism or conditions which may cause acute lung damage.

Diagnosis of exacerbation may be controversial, despite the codification of the diagnostic criteria; ground-glass opacities are not specific for IPF and NSIP and may be present in cases of infection. Nonintubated patients in the acute phase of the disease often cannot undergo BAL because of their unstable conditions and they are treated with antibiotics for precautionary measure. Lung biopsy shows diffuse alveolar damage, however the invasiveness of the procedure is a limiting factor and only few well-selected patients undergo surgical lung biopsy. It is our duty to mention the correlation between surgical lung biopsy or lung resection and acute exacerbation, however unclear, as far as causality is concerned. Risk factors involved in this accelerated phase may be a high concentration of oxygen (100%), hyperexpansion of the lung parenchyma and the use of mechanical ventilation in the postoperative phase.

Generally, the factors responsible for the exacerbations are still unknown; clinical presentation in some patients (fever, influenza-like symptoms, neutrophilia in BAL) may be consistent with a viral infection, however the pathogen has not been identified.

Treatment Poor understanding of the pathogenetic mechanisms underlies the ineffectiveness of the current treatment options. Initially, a pathogenetic theory considered IPF and NSIP as inflammatory processes justifying the use of anti-inflammatory drugs, such as corticosteroids, which were considered first-line drugs. Later, cytotoxic and immunosuppressive agents were used, usually in combination with corticosteroids.

The most recent revelations from the pathogenetic field identify the initial phase of the disease as injury to the alveolar epithelial cells and destruction of the subepithelial basement membrane, leading to abnormal wound healing with a vigorous fibroblastic response and excessive deposition of collagen and extracellular matrix. This new pathogenetic theory suggests a primary role for fibroblast deregulation. Thus, the fibroproliferative process became the therapeutic target, and new drugs which arrest the proliferation of fibroblasts and the depostition of extracellular matrix are being testing.

Established treatment Corticosteroids have been considered the mainstay of IPF treatment for decades, although there are no randomised placebo-controlled trials using corticosteroids alone. The ATS/ERS international consensus statement concludes that existing therapies are of unproven benefit.

In the past, high doses of prednisone or prednisolone (1 mg$\cdot$kg$^{-1}\cdot$day^{-1}), considering ideal body weight) for 4–6 weeks, with a gradual taper, were used. Given the high risk of systemic side-effects and the significant toxicity, especially when in combination with other drugs, the dose has been re-evaluated, and more recent therapeutic regimens recommend low doses of prednisone or prednisolone (0.5 mg$\cdot$kg$^{-1}\cdot$day^{-1} for 4 weeks, followed by 0.25 mg$\cdot$kg$^{-1}\cdot$day^{-1} for 8 weeks, then 0.125 mg$\cdot$kg$^{-1}\cdot$day^{-1}). The rate of taper depends on the patient's individual characteristics. In the case of responders with clinical and radiological improvement, prolonged maintenance therapy with low dose alternate-day prednisone may be prescribed to reduce the chance of recrudescent disease.

In case of exacerbation, 2 mg$\cdot$kg$^{-1}\cdot$day^{-1} of methylprednisolone for ∼14 days should be administered, depending on individual clinical response. The rapid decline of pulmonary function may lead to important respiratory failure; accordingly, patients require supplemental oxygen and noninvasive positive pressure mechanical ventilation. In the most severe cases, intubation may be necessary.

Azathioprine and cyclophosphamide are the most frequently used second-line drugs, alone or in combination with corticosteroids. Azathioprine is the most frequently used cytotoxic agent and usually is well tolerated. Its metabolism leads to the production of mercaptopurine, similar to purine, which inhibits DNA synthesis. Azathioprine is administered *per os*, usually in combination with low-dose corticosteroids; initial dose is 25–50 mg·day^{-1} (2–3 mg·kg^{-1}·day^{-1}). If adverse effects do not appear, an increase of 25 mg every 7–14 days is recommended, until a maximum dose of 150 mg·day^{-1} is reached. There are no clinical trials which confirm a certain benefit of combination (corticosteroids+azathioprine) therapy. Given the minor toxicity compared to cyclophosphamide, azathioprine should be administered in patients with symptomatic or progressive disease for 6 months unless adverse effects which suggest interruption or modification of the treatment appear.

Cyclophosphamide is usually used as a second-line drug for patients who have presented adverse effects to high-dose corticosteroid therapy. The route of administration is usually oral or intravenous, but it can also be administered by intramuscular injection. Generally, cyclophosphamide is used in combination with low-dose corticosteroids. Scientific evidence confirming the efficacy of cyclophosphamide in the treatment of IPFs is lacking; no clinical benefit regarding survival and progression of the disease has been reported.

Cyclosporine is a fungus-derived peptide which exerts potent immunosuppressive effects; it inhibits lymphocyte T proliferation by inhibiting the release of IL-2. Cyclosporine is rarely used for IIP treatment and its use is limited for selected patients awaiting a lung transplant. There are no clinical trials showing that cyclosporine therapy is beneficial.

Novel therapeutic strategies Interferon (IFN)-γ-1b is a novel biological antifibrotic drug with a number of inhibitory effects on fibroblasts. In the literature there are only few studies relative to the real efficacy of IFN-γ, either alone or in combination therapy with low dose corticosteroids.

Colchicine inhibits the synthesis of collagen and suppresses growth factors that are necessary for fibroblast proliferation. On the basis of these properties, the use of this drug is being tested. Data are limited, although there is no evidence that colchicine improves the progression of the disease and survival.

D-Penicillamine is a thiolic compound which interferes with collagen turnover. Indeed, it inhibits collagen synthesis and deposition by interrupting cross-linking of collagen molecules. There are no controlled clinical trials showing any benefit of D-penicillamine therapy. Given the frequent adverse effects, D-penicillamine does not appear to be a treatment choice in IIPs.

Pirfenidone (5-methyl-1-phenyl-2[1H]-pyridone) attenuates pulmonary fibrosis in animal models. It reduces synthesis of collagen (I and III) and TNF-α, and inhibits TGF-β-stimulated collagen synthesis. Moreover, it decreases synthesis of the extracellular matrix and blocks the mitogenic effect of profibrotic cytokines.

Experimental models *in vitro* and *in vivo* showed that angiotensin-converting enzyme inhibitors (ACEI) and statins possess antifibrotic properties. However, there is no evidence of improved survival in treated patients.

There is evidence that the production of oxidative agents increases in IIP. In particular, neutrophils, macrophages and fibroblasts release oxidative agents, such as reactive oxygen species (ROS), hydrogen peroxide (H_2O_2) and superoxide anion. These factors, in addition to the reduction of antioxidants, facilitate fibroblast deregulation and deposition of extracellular matrix. *N*-acetylcysteine (NAC) is derived from the amino acid cysteine. It is considered a precursor of glutathione (GSH) and it stimulates GSH synthesis. GSH has strong antioxidative properties, as it removes free oxygen radicals and decreases H_2O_2. The route of administration is oral at a dose of 1,800 mg·die^{-1} and only in association with conventional therapy with corticosteroids and azathioprine. A significant difference in the rate of decline of FVC and $T_{L,CO}$ has been described in patients treated with NAC, even if no difference was observed in mortality.

Endothelin (ET)-1 is a potent mitogen for endothelial and smooth muscle cells. ET-1 is strongly upregulated in patients with IPF and is mainly expressed in epithelial cells. Some studies have suggested that inhibition of ET-1 could have antifibrotic effects. Bosentan is a non-selective ET(A) and ET(B) receptor antagonist which is used in patients with pulmonary hypertension and it could delay the progression of IPF. However, in the treatment of IPF, clinical trials have been disappointing.

TNF-α antagonist – etanercept has been found to be significantly elevated in bleomycin-induced pulmonary fibrosis (BIPF). TNF-α stimulates a series of cytokines, such as TGF-β, IL-5 and modifies eosinophil recruitment in the parenchyma. Both antibodies anti-TNF-α and TNF-α soluble receptor antagonists have been found to reduce fibrotic processes in animals.

The typical fibroproliferative process in IPF seems to be related to inflammation and vascular injury. Indeed, endothelium damage causes exposition of the intimale tissue to circulation, thereby inducing thrombotic events. Pulmonary embolism is one of the most common causes of death in IPF patients and D-dimer levels often increase during exacerbation of the disease. Recently, the role of thrombotic events in the natural history of the disease and survival in IPF patients has been evaluated. Patients treated with warfarin added to corticosteroids had significantly higher survival after exacerbation when compared to patients treated with corticosteroids alone. D-dimer levels and number of days free of exacerbation did not differ between the two groups. The mechanisms underlying increased survival are unclear. Certainly extravascular deposition of fibrin and thrombotic events play main roles in the fibroproliferative process and acute lung injury. Hence, anticoagulant therapy may be considered as an important additional therapeutic support in IIP treatment.

Lung transplantation Lung transplantation is the only option which definitely improves survival in IPF patients and the only option for patients refractory to medical therapy. IIPs represent the second most frequent disease which requires lung transplantation. It is extremely important to decide when to list a patient for transplantation. Given the legal complexity of

Table 3. International Society for Heart and Lung Transplantation guidelines

For referral
Radiographic or histological evidence of UIP irrespective of vital capacity
Histological evidence of fibrotic NSIP
For listing
Radiographic or histological evidence of UIP and any of the following: $T_{L,CO}$ <39% predicted; >10% reduction in FVC in the last 6 months; oxygen saturation <88% during 6MWT; honeycombing on HRCT (fibrosis score >2)
Histological evidence of NSIP and any of the following: $T_{L,CO}$ < 35% predicted; >10% reduction in FVC or >15% in $T_{L,CO}$ in the last 6 months
$D_{L,CO}$: transfer factor of the lung for carbon dioxide; FVC: forced vital capacity; 6MWT: 6-min walk test.

the process, early listing is urged. Recently, the International Society for Heart and Lung Transplantation published guidelines for establishing the characteristics and the criteria for transplantation and listing (table 3).

Unfortunately, many patients die while awaiting a transplant because of the poor availability of donor organs. Post-operative mortality in transplanted patients is high, because of rejection, infections and other complications. Two- and 5-yr survival rates following single lung transplants are approximately 70% and 50%, respectively.

References

- American Thoracic Society, Idiopathic pulmonary fibrosis: diagnosis and treatment. International consensus statement. *Am J Respir Crit Care Med* 2000; 161: 646-664.
- American Thoracic Society/European Respiratory Society International Multidisciplinary Consensus Classification of the Idiopathic Interstitial Pneumonias. *Am J Respir Crit Care Med* 2002; 165: 277-304.
- Bouros D, Antoniou KM. Current and future therapeutic approaches in idiopathic pulmonary fibrosis. *Eur Respir J* 2005; 26: 693-703.
- Chetta A, *et al.* Pulmonary function testing in interstitial lung diseases. *Respiration* 2004; 71: 209-213.
- Coultas DB, *et al.* The epidemiology of interstitial lung diseases. *Am J Respir Crit Care Med* 1994; 150: 967-972.
- Demedts M, *et al.* High-dose acetylcysteine in idiopathic pulmonary fibrosis. *N Engl J Med* 2005; 353: 2229-2242.
- Hospenthal MA. Diagnosis and management of idiopathic pulmonary fibrosis: implications for respiratory care. *Respir Care* 2006; 51: 382-391.
- Hyzy R, *et al.* Acute exacerbation of idiopathic pulmonary fibrosis. *Chest* 2007; 132: 1652-1658.
- Kubo H, *et al.* Anticoagulant therapy for idiopathic pulmonary fibrosis. *Chest* 2005; 128: 1475-1482.
- Noble PW, Hormer RJ. Idiopathic pulmonary fibrosis: new insights into pathogenesis. *Clin Chest Med* 2005; 25: 749-758.
- Noth I, Martinez FJ. Recent advances in idiopathic pulmonary fibrosis. *Chest* 2007; 132: 637-650.
- O'Callaghan D, Gaine SP. Bosentan: a novel agent for the treatment of pulmonary arterial hypertension. *Int J Clin Pract* 2004; 58: 69-73.
- Orens JB, *et al.* Pulmonary Scientific Council of the International Society for Heart and Lung Transplantation. International guidelines for the selection of lung transplant candidates: 2006 update a consensus report from the Pulmonary Scientific Council of the International Society for Heart and Lung Transplantation. *J Heart Lung Transplant* 2006; 25: 745-755.
- Raghu G, *et al.* A placebo-controlled trial of interferon gamma-1b in patients with idiopathic pulmonary fibrosis. *J Clin Invest* 2004; 114: 438-446.
- Raghu G, *et al.* Azathioprine combined with prednisone in the treatment of idiopathic pulmonary fibrosis: a prospective, double-blind randomized, placebo-controlled clinical trial. *Am Rev Respir Dis* 1991; 144: 291-296.
- Richeldi L, *et al.* Costicosteroids for idiopathic pulmonary fibrosis. *Cochrane Database Syst Rev* 2003; 3.

EOSINOPHILIC DISEASES

A. Menzies-Gow
Royal Brompton and Harefield NHS Foundation Trust, London, UK
E-mail: a.menzies-gow@rbht.nhs.uk

The exact role of the eosinophil has yet to be determined. It is believed to play a role in combating helminthic parasitic infections and, in health, eosinophils primarily reside within the gastrointestinal mucosa. Eosinophilic lung diseases cover a wide spectrum of pathology ranging from airways disease, such as eosinophilic bronchitis, to parenchymal disease, such as eosinophilic pneumonia, and also systemic diseases, such as the hypereosinophilic syndrome.

Nonasthmatic eosinophilic bronchitis

Eosinophilic bronchitis is a common and treatable form of chronic cough that was first identified in 1989. Nonasthmatic eosinophilic bronchitis is a condition that presents with a corticosteroid-responsive chronic cough in nonsmokers. These patients have evidence of eosinophilic airways inflammation without the variable airflow obstruction or airways hyperresponsiveness characteristic of asthma.

Eosinophilic bronchitis accounts for 10–30% of cases of chronic cough referred for specialist investigation. Eosinophilic bronchitis is defined as a chronic cough in patients with no symptoms or objective evidence of airflow obstruction, a histamine/methacholine provocative concentration causing a 20% fall in forced expiratory volume in 1 s of >16 mg·mL^{-1} and >3% sputum eosinophilia.

It is unclear why eosinophilic inflammation leads to asthma in some individuals and eosinophilic bronchitis in others. Studies by BRIGHTLING (2006) suggest that the key may be mast cell localisation. In asthmatics, mast cells infiltrate airways smooth muscle, resulting in airflow obstruction and hyperresponsiveness. In eosinophilic bronchitis, mast cells infiltrate the airway epithelium leading to bronchitis and cough.

Anti-inflammatory therapy with inhaled corticosteroids is the mainstay for the treatment of eosinophilic bronchitis. Inhaled corticosteroids produce a significant improvement in symptoms as well as a fall in sputum eosinophilia. There is no evidence to suggest that any one inhaled corticosteroid is more effective. Data is also not available to guide the dose or duration of inhaled corticosteroid therapy. Logically, antileukotrienes may be of benefit, but this hypothesis has not been tested in clinical trials. In very resistant cases, oral corticosteroids may be required for symptom control.

Little is known about the natural history of the condition, but it can be transient, episodic or persistent unless treated.

Key points

- Eosinophilic lung disease covers a wide spectrum of pathology from airways to parachymal lung disease.

- Always exclude secondary causes of eosinophilia before diagnosing acute or chronic eosinophilic pneumonia.

- Novel therapies are being introduced for eosinophilia including tyrosine kinase inhibitors and monoclonal antibodies against interleukin 5.

Acute and chronic eosinophilic pneumonia

Acute eosinophilic pneumonia presents as an acute febrile illness of <5 days' duration. The average age at presentation is 30 yrs with symptoms of dyspnoea, cough, myalgia and fevers. Patients often present with severe type I respiratory failure requiring ventilation. Unlike other pulmonary eosinophilic syndromes, the blood eosinophil count is usually normal. The chest radiograph demonstrates diffuse alveolar and interstitial infiltrates. The diagnosis is confirmed by the presence of a bronchoalveolar lavage eosinophilia of >25% in the absence of parasitic, fungal or other infections and no history of drug hypersensitivity. Acute eosinophilic pneumonia responds quickly to oral corticosteroids with no relapse after stopping therapy.

Chronic eosinophilic pneumonia typically presents in middle-aged asthmatic women, but it can also develop in nonasthmatic individuals. The symptoms are gradually progressive and include shortness of breath, cough, fever and weight loss. Clinical examination demonstrates wheezing and hypoxia. Patients usually have a raised blood eosinophil count at the time of an acute exacerbation along with elevated inflammatory markers. The majority of patients have infiltrates visible on chest radiograph, and they are peripherally distributed in about two-thirds of cases (fig. 1).

High-resolution computed tomography is more sensitive at demonstrating infiltrates and ~50% of patients also have mediastinal adenopathy. Patients respond well to oral corticosteroids, but tend to relapse on discontinuation of therapy. Many patients require long-term, low-dose oral corticosteroids to control the condition; in a small minority, alternative steroid-sparing agents have been used. This condition is frequently misdiagnosed as asthma. Blood eosinophilia and pulmonary infiltrates respond to corticosteroids within 24–48 h, making it easy to miss this condition if the relevant investigations are not performed prior to starting steroids.

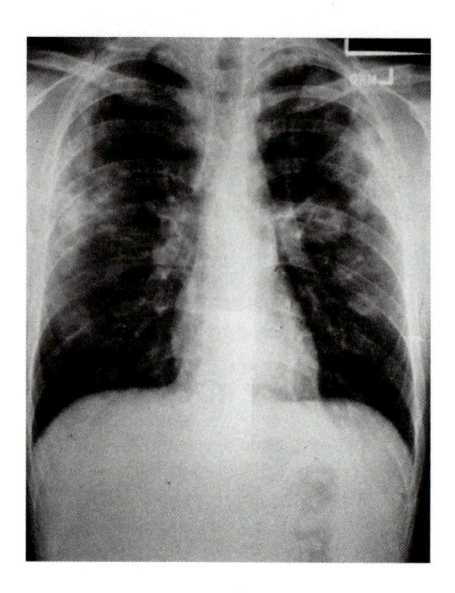

Figure 1. Chest radiograph of patient presenting with chronic eosinophilic pneumonia demonstrating the characteristic peripheral infiltrates.

Both acute and chronic eosinophilic pneumonia are idiopathic conditions. It is important to exclude secondary causes of eosinophilia before diagnosing either condition. In clinical practice, this requires a careful travel history asking about residence in areas of endemic parasitic infection and a careful drug history including illicit substances. The other main causes of a pulmonary eosinophilic syndrome are as follows: allergic bronchopulmonary aspergillosis, the hypereosinophilic syndrome, and Churg–Strauss syndrome, which should also be excluded at the time of diagnosis.

Hypereosinophilic syndrome

The hypereosinophilic syndrome (HES) is a heterogeneous group of disorders characterised by the presence of marked blood and tissue eosinophilia resulting in a variety of clinical manifestations. The following criteria are used to define idiopathic HES: 1) blood eosinophilia $>1,500 \cdot mm^{-3}$ for $\geqslant 6$ months; 2) absence of an underlying cause for the eosinophilia; and 3) end-organ damage due to the eosinophilia.

Idiopathic HES can occur at any age, but tends to develop in the fourth or fifth decade of life, with a male predominance. Nonspecific systemic symptoms are common. More specific symptoms will depend upon which organs are affected. The lungs are involved in ~40% of patients, leading to cough and airflow limitation. Pulmonary function tests demonstrate an obstructive pattern in patients with cough. In patients with cardiac involvement, concomitant pulmonary fibrosis can occur leading to a restrictive or mixed pattern. The chest radiograph can be normal or demonstrate spontaneously clearing airspace shadowing in early disease. At a later stage with multi-organ involvement, up to one-third of cases will have diffuse, nonsegmental interstitial infiltrates.

The most important cause of morbidity and mortality in idiopathic HES is cardiovascular involvement. Thromboembolic disease and involvement of the nervous system are also common presentations.

Until recently, oral corticosteroids have been the mainstay of treatment. Better understanding of eosinophil biology has led to the use of more logical targeted therapies. Distinct HES subtypes are now recognised. The myeloproliferative variant is associated with the presence of a fusion tyrosine kinase, FIP1L1/PDGFRA. These patients historically had a poor prognosis with poor steroid responsiveness. The use of the tyrosine kinase inhibitor, imatinib, in this group of patients has significantly improved their outcome.

The lymphoproliferative variant is a consequence of increased production of eosinophilopoietic cytokines by clonal populations of phenotypically abnormal, activated T-lymphocytes. Identification of interleukin-5 (IL-5) as a key mediator of eosinophilopoiesis led to the use in clinical trials of an anti-IL-5 monoclonal antibody (mepolizumab) for HES. Mepolizumab is an effective corticosteroid sparing agent in patients with HES negative for FIP1L1/PDGFRA.

References

- Allen J. Acute eosinophilic pneumonia. *Semin Respir Crit Care Me*d 2006; 27: 142-147.
- Brightling CE. Chronic cough due to nonasthmatic eosinophilic bronchitis: ACCP evidence based clinical practice guidelines. *Chest* 2006; 129: 116S-121S.
- Klion AD, *et al.* Approaches to the treatment of hypereosinophilic syndromes: a workshop summary report. *J Allergy Clin Immunol* 2006; 117: 1292-1302.
- Marchand E, Cordier JF. Idiopathic chronic eosinophilic pneumonia. *Semin Respir Crit Care Med* 2006; 27: 134-141.
- Rothenberg ME, *et al.* Treatment of patients with the hypereosinophilic syndrome with mepolizumab. *N Engl J Med* 2008; 358: 1215-1228.

DRUG-INDUCED RESPIRATORY DISEASE

Ph. Camus
Dept of Pulmonary & Intensive Care, UMC Dijon Bocage, Dijon, France
E-mail: ph.camus@chu-dijon.fr

Key points

- DIRD is not uncommon and is multifaceted, with involvement of the airways, lung, pleura, pulmonary circulation and neuromuscular system.

- Chemotherapy agents, amiodarone, ACE inhibitors, NSAIDs and β-blockers in particular pose the risk of adverse respiratory effects.

- The clinical and imaging expression of DIRD closely resembles that of illnesses of other causes or that occur idiopathically. Pathology is rarely specific for the drug aetiology.

- Diagnosing DIRD requires a high degree of awareness, up-to-date knowledge and ruling out of other causes, particularly infection.

- Stopping the drug is often followed by improvement in symptoms and imaging. However, this should be done carefully to avoid relapse of the underlying condition for which the drug was given.

- Corticosteroid therapy is reserved for severe cases and where dechallenge does not produce measurable improvement. Duration of corticosteroid therapy varies with drug and pattern of involvement.

- Generally, rechallenge with the drug is discouraged as severe relapse of DIRD can occur.

Drug-induced and iatrogenic respiratory disease (DIRD) is a classic, not uncommon and often unpredictable complication of exposure to therapy drugs, including the novel biological kinase inhibitors gefitinib, erlotinib, imatinib, dasatinib and monoclonal antibody therapy, irradiation, abused substances, herbal therapy and vaccines. The diagnosis of DIRD is one of exclusion (table 1), and aetiologies other than the drug or drugs must be ruled out, particularly an infection due to *Pneumocystis jiroveci* or other opportunistic pathogens. Patients exposed to methotrexate, anti-tumour necrosis factor (TNF) agents, immunosuppressive drugs, chemotherapy agents and rituximab are at risk of developing opportunistic infections, and further tests are required to rule out an infection in such patients.

DIRD is probably under-reported. Incidence is greater with chemotherapy agents (up to 40% depending on which drug regimen is used and which test is used to diagnose the condition) or amiodarone or methotrexate (1–2% per year) compared with other drugs. With most of the other 400 or so drugs known to cause respiratory injury, DIRD is uncommon.

The respiratory system includes the lung, airways, pulmonary circulation, pleura, haemoglobin and neuromuscular system. Each of these can be the target of drug-induced injury, causing varied imaging patterns of involvement (table 2).

Accordingly, DIRD can occur in the form of interstitial lung disease (ILD), where drugs may account for 3% of ILD cases, upper airway obstruction (UAO), bronchospasm or bronchiolitis obliterans, pulmonary hypertension, pleural effusion or thickening, impaired oxygen carrying capacity of haemoglobin and reduced inspiratory muscle force. Potentially severe DIRD includes acute angioedema from angiotensin-converting enzyme (ACE) inhibitors, catastrophic bronchospasm from nonsteroidal antiinflammatory drugs (NSAIDs), β-blockers or aspirin, acute methotrexate pneumonitis or minocycline-induced eosinophilic pneumonia, pulmonary oedema from tocolytic agents or chemotherapy drugs, anticoagulant-induced diffuse alveolar haemorrhage, large-volume pleural effusion and acute methaemoglobinemia and drug-induced neuromuscular acute respiratory failure. These drug-induced complications portend immediate severity and may have fatal consequences. In such cases, prompt recognition of the drug aetiology, emergent management of the airway and of respiratory failure and early drug withdrawal are warranted. A maintained list of drugs and patterns of drug-induced respiratory involvement is available on the Pneumotox website at www.pneumotox.com.

Pathophysiology: mechanisms

Drug-induced ILD is characterised by homing, proliferation and persistence of immune-effector cells including eosinophils in lung tissue. This causes pulmonary shadowing, increases in bronchoalveolar lavage (BAL) cells and hindrance to gas exchange. Corticosteroid therapy usually quenches drug-induced pulmonary inflammation and is followed by improvement in symptoms and imaging. Rechallenge with the causal drug often but not always produces relapse of DIRD. The mechanisms for drug-induced cell influx are generally unknown.

Table 1. Checklist for diagnosing drug-induced respiratory disease

1. Maintain a high degree of awareness of drug-induced disease *vis à vis* any new respiratory sign and symptom if not explained otherwise. Use Pneumotox website as needed[#]
2. Record medical history including history of exposure to drugs, radiation and substances of abuse
3. Evaluate the possibility or likelihood of pulmonary involvement from an underlying condition if present
4. Retrieve pre-therapy imaging and pulmonary function data. Compare with present tests
5. Review timing of exposure to drug *versus* onset of symptoms (minutes to years, depending on drug and pattern)
6. Try to define pattern of injury in the most conservative way (lung biopsy can be risky; pathology may show nonspecific findings)
7. Evaluate drug causality, taking into account each drug taken in isolation. Correlate with pattern of involvement[#]
8. Evaluate the likelihood of disease caused by drug *versus* underlying condition, (an opportunistic infection, other drugs, or incidental disease) using the above and BAL
9. *In vitro* tests of mononuclear cell migration are cumbersome and none has yet proved useful
10. Evaluate literature pertaining to the specific drug or pattern of involvement[#]
11. Dicontinue drug, patient condition permitting. This may not be followed by improvement in patients with acute disease. Check whether the underlying illness needs a substitute drug
12. Evaluate whether corticosteroid therapy is indicated (depending on drug, severity, pattern and effect of drug discontinuance)
13. Organise appropriate follow-up including imaging and pulmonary physiology
14. Discuss rechallenge only if no other drug available to treat the patient's condition. Otherwise avoid

BAL: bronchoalveolar lavage; [#]: match drug and pattern using Pneumotox website.

Table 2. Main imaging pathological patterns of drug-induced infiltrative lung disease

Pattern on chest radiograph or CT	Causal drugs	Pathology correlate
Diffuse haze or ground-glass opacity	Drugs that cause interstitial pneumonia[#]	Interstitial inflammation, cellular interstitial pneumonia
	Chemotherapy agents	Early/mild pulmonary oedema, alveolar haemorrhage or DAD
Localised ground-glass opacity	Radiation therapy[#]	Early or mild radiation lung injury (interstitial oedema, cell sloughing, cell debris)
Diffuse white-out – white lungs	Drugs that produce acute ILD, pulmonary oedema, DAD, eosinophilic pneumonia or DAH[#]	Dense cellular interstitial pneumonia with or without tissue eosinophilia. Acute pulmonary oedema. DAH
Disseminated areas of ground-glass with a mosaic pattern of distribution	Drugs that cause interstitial pneumonia[#]	Cellular interstitial pneumonia. DIP
Bilateral perihilar alveolar opacities with a batwing pattern of distribution	Drugs causing pulmonary oedema, DAD or DAH[#]	Pulmonary oedema, DAD, DAH
Multiple subpleural areas of condensation	Drugs causing pumonary eosinophilia or BOOP. Statins[#]	Eosinophilic pneumonia, BOOP
Opacities with a recognisable segmental or lobar pattern of distribution	Amiodarone[#]	Phosphoilipidosis, organising pneumonia
	Statins[#]	BOOP
	Paraffin[#]	Exogenous lipoid pneumonia
Diffuse miliary pattern	BCG therapy, methotrexate, sirolimus[#]	Granulomatous reaction[¶]
Area of condensation. A mass	Drugs causing BOOP or eosinophilic pneumonia[#]	BOOP, eosinophilic pneumonia
	Amiodarone	Phospholipidosis, APT features, amiodaronoma
	Paraffin	Paraffinoma
Wandering opacities	Drugs which cause organising or eosinophilic pneumonia[#]	BOOP, eosinophilic pneumonia
	Irradiation for breast carcinoma[#]	BOOP
Multiple nodular opacities	Amiodarone[#]	APT features
	Bleomycin[#]	BOOP
		Areas of nodular fibrosis
Pulmonary fibrosis. Low lung volumes	Chemotherapy agents. Amiodarone. Nitrofurantoin. Irradiation	Pulmonary fibrosis. UIP pattern

CT: computed tomography; DAD: diffuse alveolar damage; ILD: interstitial lung disease; DAH: diffuse alveolar haemorrhage; DIP: desquamative interstitial pneumonia pattern; BOOP : bronchiolitis obliterans organising pneumonia; APT: amiodarone pulmonary toxicity; UIP: usual interstitial pneumonia; [#]: see appropriate pattern on Pneumotox website; [¶]: interferons and anti-tumour necrosis factor agents may produce a mimic of sarcoidosis.

With some drugs (chemotherapy agents, and drugs that cause pulmonary oedema or bronchospasm), the respiratory reaction is dose dependent. Above a certain drug dosage, most patients exhibit some form of adverse reaction, suggesting a dose-related cytopathic mechanism. Patients on chemotherapy for haematological malignancies or solid tumours may exhibit a time- or dose-related decrease in the diffusing capacity for carbon monoxide, thought to reflect subclinical dose-related pulmonary toxicity, without necessarily exhibiting clinically detectable disease.

However, most drug reactions are idiosyncratic and occur unpredictably in only a few individuals, regardless of dose or time on the drug.

Several drugs in a pharmacological class may cause the same pattern of injury. Examples include the association: of β-blockers or NSAIDs and acute bronchospasm; of chemotherapy agents and pulmonary oedema, acute lung injury (ALI), diffuse alveolar damage (DAD) or pulmonary fibrosis; and of ergots with pleural thickening. This also suggests that a common pathogenetic mechanism caused the injury.

Experimental and clinical evidence suggests that drug disposition in lung is a critical factor for toxicity. For instance, amiodarone and its main metabolite sequester in lung, reaching tissue concentrations that are above the threshold for toxicity to lung cells. This may cause cell toxicity despite serum concentrations being within the therapeutic range. The slow efflux of amiodarone and metabolite from the lung are consistent with for the slow resolution of amiodarone pulmonary toxicity (APT) in the clinic, except when corticosteroid therapy is added.

A few drugs are known to undergo metabolic activation in designated lung cells, leading to the formation of reactive drug species that bind avidly and covalently to cell macromolecules, causing injury or cell loss. Metabolism of nitrofurantoin, cyclophosphamide, mitomycin, bleomycin and the herbicide paraquat can generate reactive oxygen species, which attack cell constituents and deplete reducing equivalents. This may lead to cell death and consequent pulmonary inflammation and/or fibrosis. Of note, the heterogenous distribution of activating enzymes in the lung may account for the selective alveolar or bronchial injury seen with a specific agent. The delicate and/or unstable architecture of the lung may expose it to potentially severe consequences of even small amounts of tissue damage.

An immunological reaction is thought to cause the adverse reaction to some drugs. For instance, transfusion-related ALI is caused by the binding of human leukocyte antigen antibodies of donor origin to circulating blood cells in the recipient, causing cell activation, endothelial cell injury and an increase in vascular permeability with consequent alveolar oedema. The drug-induced lupus syndrome is characterised by a positive anti-nuclear and sometimes anti-DNA antibody test. The antibody may be at the origin of the adverse pleural reaction that is a hallmark of the drug-induced lupus. Drug-induced asthma is largely non-immunoglobulin E-dependent. Nevertheless, small incremental doses of NSAIDs or aspirin can be given to asthmatics who are intolerant to these drugs and thus a state of tolerance can be induced, should such patients need to be treated with this class of medications.

Alveolar haemorrhage can complicate treatments with variegated anticoagulant drugs, and overdose is thought to account for this complication although not all cases exhibit abnormal coagulation studies. Only a few drugs produce pulmonary capillaritis with consequent alveolar haemorrhage.

Rare cases of drug-induced injury result from deposition of the drug excipient in lung tissue, notably the pulmonary circulation, causing reactive foreign body granulomas around pulmonary arterioles.

Clinical presentation

A high degree of suspicion must be maintained at all times, and drugs should be a diagnostic consideration in any patient with otherwise unexplained respiratory symptoms, abnormal pulmonary physiology or new radiographic findings while being treated with therapy or other drugs. Some adverse reactions to drugs exhibit a short time to onset (e.g. β-blocker-induced bronchospasm, chemotherapy-induced pulmonary oedema), and this readily suggests causality. For most drugs, however, there is a long time delay for DIRD to present and thus, consideration of the drug aetiology is not always raised in due time. Drugs can cause lung injury when administered by the oral, intravenous or intramuscular, inhaled, pleural or intrathecal route or following delivery in a distant organ that is situated upstream of the lung (e.g. bone, brain or liver).

Symptoms of DIRD at presentation may include a nonproductive cough, dyspnoea, wheezing, cyanosis and rigors. Acute bronchospasm, angio-oedema and shock characterise those cases with drug-induced anaphylaxis. Occasional patients present with stridor, hoarseness, wheezing, haemoptysis or acute chest pain. Extrarespiratory signs, symptoms and laboratory features include a cutaneous rash, lymph-node enlargement and hepatitis. Rare patients present with full-blown systemic reactions resembling lupus erythematosus, Churg–Strauss syndrome, Wegener's granulomatosis or polymyositis.

The severity of DIRD relates to the acuteness, extent, location and reversibility of the adverse reaction. Life-threatening presentations are in patients with acute dense ILD, upper airway oedema, massive pleural effusion or drug-induced systemic involvement.

Drug withdrawal followed by abatement of signs and symptoms is a simple and straightforward test to confirm the drug aetiology. The risk of rechallenge should be balanced against the merit of securing the diagnosis, as fatal reactions may follow rechallenge with the causal agent.

However, many clinical situations are complex. It is possible that patients are exposed to several causal drugs with each drug having differing delay times for DIRD to present, or they have received chest irradiation, or DIRD cannot be confidently separated from pulmonary involvement of the underlying disease for which the drug was given. Examples include patients with thoracic malignancies or rheumatoid arthritis, when they are exposed to corticosteroids and/or novel biological drugs including tyrosine kinase inhibitors or anti-TNF antibody therapy. Similarly, diagnosing DIRD is difficult in patients with autoimmune conditions or recipients of solid organ or bone marrow transplant who are receiving long-term treatments with immunosuppressive drugs, corticosteroids or sirolimus.

Imaging

Imaging features of DIRD are diverse, as are their clinical presentations.

Drug-induced bronchospasm may present with hyperinflation concomitant with bronchospasm on imaging.

On CT, airway narrowing can be documented in patients with drug-induced angio-oedema or haematoma and UAO.

Patients with ILD generally present with bilateral lung shadowing (table 2) that may localise in the bases, mid-lung regions or apices or can be diffuse. Both the density and extent of pulmonary involvement correlate with the degree of respiratory impairment. On computed tomography, there is inter- or intralobular septal thickening and lobular or more widespread alveolar filling, depending on patient, drug and pattern of involvement. Pleural effusions may be present in severe ILD presentation. APT may cause electron-dense areas of condensation with, often, pleural effusion. Chemotherapy lung is in the form of basilar opacities or a more diffuse haze or consolidation. In eosinophilic pneumonia, the pulmonary opacities tend to predominate in the lung periphery. Acute nitrofurantoin lung is in the form of diffuse haze. Chronic nitrofurantoin lung is with scattered peribronchovascular areas of consolidation.

Bronchiolitis obliterans organising pneumonia (BOOP) typically presents with migratory alveolar opacities on serial chest films. Mediastinal or hilar lymph node enlargement characterises those cases with a granulomatous pattern of reaction. The pulmonary opacities in exogenous lipoid pneumonia typically have low attenuation numbers. Radiation pneumonia generally develops in the area of the radiation beam. Only in severe cases does the shadowing extend outside the radiation beam. It is very difficult if not impossible to infer pathology from the pattern on imaging.

Drug-induced pleural effusion is undistinguishable from an effusion of other causes, except when APT is present in association. An air–fluid level can be present when the pleural pathology occurs as a complication of chemotherapy in patients with pulmonary metastases adjacent to the pleural surface.

Pathology and other diagnostic tests

BAL is used to rule out an infection, and to evaluate alveolitis by enumerating cell numbers and percentages. Inflammatory cells decrease upon drug withdrawal.

On pathology, drugs can cause virtually any pattern of ILD, including cellular or fibrotic interstitial pneumonia, eosinophilic pneumonia, acute lung injury or diffuse alveolar damage, pulmonary granulomas, DAD, BOOP, desquamative or lymphocytic interstitial pneumonia, a usual interstitial pneumonia pattern or rarely, pulmonary alveolar proteinosis. These patterns are not specific to the drug aetiology and cannot be separated reliably from the idiopathic variant. Thus, while pathology may help eliminate conditions other than drugs, lung biopsy is rarely used to document drug-induced ILD. Notable exceptions include APT and exogenous lipoid pneumonia, which may display characteristic features on pathology.

No *in vitro* test of monocyte cell migration in the presence of the drug has demonstrated diagnostic utility in DIRD.

Specific reactions

Airways Angio-oedema is a well-demarcated oedema that is classically caused by ACE inhibitors. The condition develops shortly after first exposure to the drug or it occurs later after uneventful weeks or months of treatment in the form of rapidly developing breathing difficulty or asphyxia due to airway narrowing. The condition is more common in elderly African-American women. About 40% of the cases require admission to intensive care. This complication requires emergent identification of the airway, and orotracheal intubation or tracheostomy are indicated in severe cases to stabilise the airway. Even though patients tend to improve quickly upon drug discontinuance, close patient follow-up is required since a rebound can occur after a few hours. Patients should not be rechallenged with any ACE inhibitor, as severe relapse may occur in patients so tested.

Catastrophic bronchospasm may closely follow exposure to as little as one tablet of NSAID, aspirin or a nonselective β-blocker in aspirin-sensitive individuals, atopics, asthmatics or in a patient known to react adversely to these classes of medications. About 15% of acute asthma attack cases admitted to intensive care are thought to be triggered by exposure to drugs. Rechallenge is hazardous and leads to severe relapse with consequent anoxic brain damage and death.

An annoying cough is a frequent complication of treatments with ACE inhibitors. Incidence varies according to the drug used and ethnicity. The condition remits within days or a few weeks with cessation of exposure to the drug.

Parenchymal lung disease Methotrexate pneumonitis is a form of acute, severe and reversible ILD. The condition develops unexpectedly in patients on methotrexate long term – typically rheumatoid arthritis patients. A background of previous ILD is a risk factor for developing methotrexate lung. The disease typically manifests dense diffuse pulmonary shadowing and respiratory failure. Lymphocytes are the predominant cell type in the BAL. The main differential diagnosis is *Pneumocystis jiroveci* pneumonia or pneumonia due to other opportunistic microorganisms. These need be ruled out confidently using the BAL and molecular diagnostic tools. Mild cases of methotrexate lung exist. In rare cases, pulmonary fibrosis follows an episode of otherwise classic methotrexate pneumonia.

Eosinophilic pneumonia is a common pattern of reaction to drugs. Other causes of pulmonary infiltrates and eosinophilia must be ruled out. The condition shows bilateral shadowing in the context of peripheral and BAL eosinophilia. Acute eosinophilic pneumonia is a severe form of ILD with acute respiratory failure and sometimes, pleural effusion is present. Characteristic causal agents include NSAIDs, antibiotics (*e.g.* minocycline), abused drugs and exposure to tobacco smoke of recent onset. Rechallenge is contraindicated, as relapse will almost inevitably occur. Severe systemic presentations can occur and are characterised by a cutaneous rash and deep-seated organ involvement. This is called the drug rash with eosinophilia and systemic symptoms (DRESS).

APT is a distinctive condition that develops insidiously after months or years on the drug, in the form of asymmetrical consolidation that may be electron-dense. Pulmonary function is restrictive in nature. Foam cells are present in the BAL and are an aid to diagnosis of APT, although this does not prove toxicity and is a routine finding on the drug. The clinical–imaging–pathological expression of APT is multifaceted and includes ground-glass shadowing, lung nodules, pulmonary fibrosis or, rarely, pleural effusion in isolation. Amiodarone withdrawal may not suffice for APT to clear, due to the high affinity and peristence of amiodarone in lung tissue. Corticosteroid therapy often is required to accelerate recovery. Severe APT may occur in the setting of thoracic surgery and can be in the form of an ARDS picture.

Several drugs can acutely produce lung permeability changes. Pulmonary oedema is mainly observed following exposure to chemotherapy agents including taxanes, gemcitabine, mitomycin and rituximab, blood and blood products. There is a spectrum of severity ranging from transient pulmonary infiltrates following each exposure to the drug to acute pulmonary edema or an acute respiratory distress syndrome (ARDS) picture. Severe cases may develop at once, or after several bouts of pulmonary infiltrates, indicating impending toxicity. Outcome is good in early or mild cases. Severe cases may evolve to refractory respiratory failure.

Chemotherapy agents may cause a peculiar form of acute ILD called chemotherapy lung. The condition is in the form of pulmonary infiltrates during or shortly after completion of treatment with the drug. Bleomycin, cyclophosphamide, gemcitabine, nitrosoureas and taxanes are classic causal drugs, with recent evidence implicating targeted therapies (gefitinib, erlotinib, pemetrexed). On pathology, there is moderate interstitial interstitial inflammation and oedema, along with a reactive epithelium and widespread areas of acute lung injury or alveolar damage. The condition may or may not improve upon drug discontinuance and corticosteroid therapy. In more severe cases an ARDS picture or an accelerated form of pulmonary fibrosis develop.

Drug-induced BOOP resembles BOOP of other causes or which occurs idiopathically. It takes the form of migratory opacities, fixed opacities or masses or diffuse shadowing with respiratory failure. Main causal agents include amiodarone, interferon, methotrexate, minocycline, rituximab, statins and radiation therapy to the breast. Drug withdrawal is indicated in all cases and it is followed by disappearance of signs and symptoms of the condition. Otherwise, sequential relapses may occur. Costicosteroid therapy is reserved for severe cases and in those with equivocal effect of drug withdrawal.

Interferons, anti-TNF agents and a few other drugs may occasion a granulomatous pattern of pulmonary and lymph node reaction that may closely mimic sarcoidosis. Pulmonary infiltrates and lymph node enlargement are present on imaging. A confirmatory transbronchial lung biopsy may be required, except if granulomas are present on a readily-accessible tissue such as the dermis.

Drug-induced diffuse alveolar haemorrhage is diagnosed by BAL, which shows a hemorrhagic return. Oral or parenteral anticoagulants, fibrinolytic agents, abciximab, ticlopidine and clopidogrel can cause the syndrome. Rarely, alveolar haemorrhage is a manifestation of drug (mainly propylthiouracil)-induced anti-neutrophil cytoplasmic antibody vasculitis.

Drug-induced pulmonary fibrosis can occur as a complication of treatments with chemotherapy agents, amiodarone and irradiation (fibrosis is localised in the latter). Patients present with dyspnoea. On imaging there are diffuse linear or streaky opacities and volume loss. The condition may stabilise with drug discontinuance. In most patients, however, the disease is progressive and response to corticosteroid therapy is limited.

When drug aetiology is considered likely, corticosteroid therapy is indicated in severe ILD cases and wherever drug withdrawal is not followed by improvement in a few days or weeks.

Pleura Many drugs can injure the pleura, including the novel targeted agent dasatinib. Involvement is in the form of a pleural exudate with or without pleural eosinophilia or a serosanguineous effusion. Lupus-inducing drugs may cause drug lupus with pleural or pleuropericardial effusion in the context of positive antinuclear antibodies (ANA). The novel anti-TNF agents infliximab, etanercept and adalimumab may cause a form of lupus syndrome with anti-double-strand DNA in addition to the ANA antibodies, an unusual finding in classic drug-induced lupus.

Ergots are notable for the insidious development of diffuse pleural thickening with or without an effusion causing dyspnoea, chest pain and restrictive lung dysfunction. There is slow improvement with discontinuance of the ergot.

Pulmonary vasculopathy This condition mainly is in the form of pulmonary hypertension similar to primary pulmonary hypertension. Anorectic agents, benfluorex and crushed tablets injected intravenously as a form of drug abuse can effectuate the condition.

Methaemoglobinaemia

Methaemoglobinaemia is a drug-induced state of oxidation of the iron in haemoglobin, and methaemoglobin is a poor oxygen carrier. The condition is diagnosed by slate-grey cyanosis, a low pulse oxygen saturation, normal arterial oxygen tension and calculated arterial oxygen saturation, and measurement of methaemoglobin in a patient receiving an eligible drug.

References

- Babu KS, Marshall BG. Drug-induced airways diseases. *Clin Chest Med* 2004; 25: 113-122.
- Briasoulis E, Pavlidis N. Noncardiogenic pulmonary edema: an unusual and serious complication of anticancer therapy. *The Oncologist* 2001; 6: 153-161.
- Goldblatt M, et al. Dasatinib-induced pleural effusions: A lymphatic network disorder? *Am J Med Sci* 2009; 338: 414-417.
- Khasnis AA, Calabrese LH. Tumor necrosis factor inhibitors and lung disease: A paradox of efficacy and risk. *Semin Arthritis Rheum* 2010 [Epub ahead of print. DOI: 10.1016/j.semarthrit.2009.09.001].
- Lara AR, Schwarz MI. Diffuse alveolar hemorrhage. *Chest* 2010; 137: 1164-1171.
- Rubin RL. Drug-induced lupus. *Toxicology* 2005; 209: 135-147.
- Sondhi D, et al. Airway compromise due to angiotensin-converting enzyme inhibitor-induced angioedema: clinical experience at a large community teaching hospital. *Chest* 2004; 126: 400-404.
- Vahid B, Marik PE. Pulmonary complications of novel antineoplastic agents for solid tumors. *Chest* 2008; 133: 528-538.
- Foucher P, Camus P. Pneumotox® Website, 1997. www.pneumotox.com Date last updated: June 4, 2010.

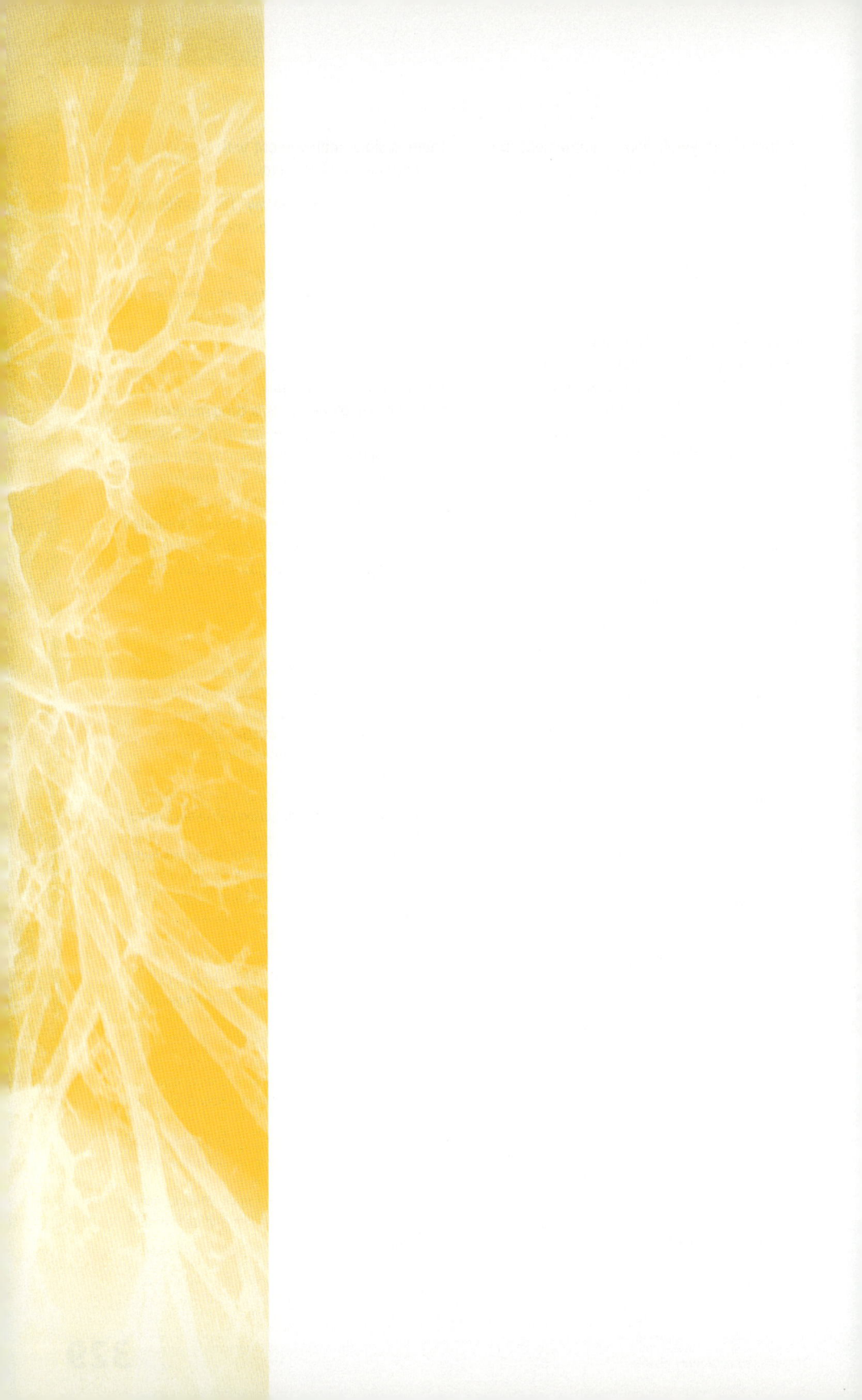

CHAPTER 12:

PULMONARY VASCULAR DISEASES

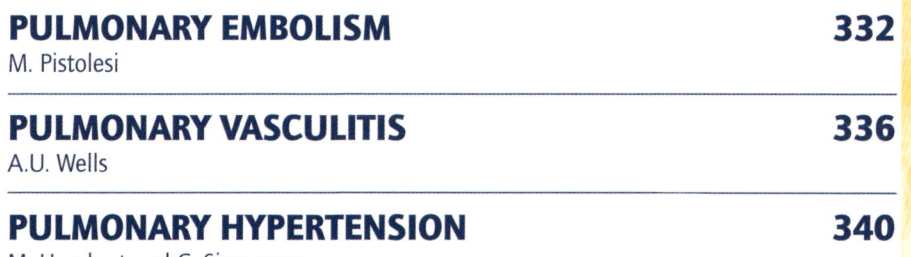

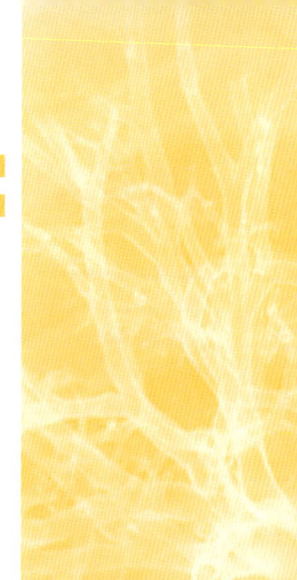

PULMONARY EMBOLISM   332
M. Pistolesi

PULMONARY VASCULITIS   336
A.U. Wells

PULMONARY HYPERTENSION   340
M. Humbert and G. Simonneau

PULMONARY EMBOLISM

M. Pistolesi
Section of Respiratory Medicine, Department of Internal Medicine,
University of Florence, Florence, Italy
E-mail: massimo.pistolesi@unifi.it

Despite the recent advances in prevention and diagnostic imaging, pulmonary embolism (PE) remains a major health problem. The incidence of this pathological condition is as high as one in 1,000 per year in the general population. Early diagnosis is fundamental since early treatment is highly effective. However, due to the low specificity of its clinical presentation, this common disease is still underdiagnosed and it is estimated that in the USA ~50,000 people die each year of PE.

Several points are summarised below concerning the diagnostic strategies to be adopted in patients with clinical suspicion of PE that have been highlighted and brought to the attention of the scientific community by recent scientific publications, expert reviews, and international guidelines.

General rules for the diagnostic work-up of patients clinically suspected of PE

- Pre-test clinical probability of PE should be objectively assessed in each patient.
- D-Dimer should be determined if pre-test probability of PE is low or intermediate.
- Diagnostic imaging of the chest should be used to assess post-test probability of PE in most patients. Further testing is necessary when post-test probability of PE is neither sufficiently low nor sufficiently high to permit therapeutic decisions.
- Diagnostic strategies of PE could differ significantly in different clinical contexts and special conditions.

Key points

- Although early treatment is highly effective, PE is underdiagnosed and therefore it remains a major health problem.
- Diagnostic strategy should be based on clinical evaluation of the probablility of PE.

Pre-test clinical probability of PE

A thorough clinical evaluation is the key step in raising the suspicion of the disease and setting-up appropriate diagnostic strategies. Although the diagnostic yield of individual clinical symptoms, signs and common laboratory tests is limited, the combination of these variables, either by empirical assessment or by a prediction rule, can be used to stratify patients into an increased risk of PE (low, intermediate or high). The results of two broad prospective studies in the 1990s (Prospective Investigation of Pulmonary Embolism Diagnosis (PIOPED) and Prospective Investigative Study of Acute Pulmonary Embolism Diagnosis (PISA-PED)) indicate that physicians' estimates of the clinical likelihood of PE, even if based on empirical assessment, do have predictive value.

Three objective scoring systems have been tested prospectively and validated in large-scale clinical trials: Wells score, Geneva score and Pisa score. The three scoring systems perform reasonably well to assess objectively the clinical probability of PE in outpatients or emergency room patients. The Pisa score seems to perform better than other scoring systems in hospitalised patients. It appears that fully standardised scoring systems, such as Wells and Geneva scores, with no implicit evaluation of symptoms (*e.g.* dyspnoea, chest pain) and simple instrumental findings (ECG, chest radiograph) could not perform better than subjective clinical judgment of experienced physicians, as it was obtained in the PIOPED and the PISA-PED studies. Conversely, interpretation of ECG and chest radiograph in these patients, as requested by the Pisa score, necessitates a certain level of clinical experience and is hard to be standardised.

Nevertheless, several prospective studies have shown that, whatever scoring method is used, pre-test clinical probability categorises patients into subgroups with a different prevalence for PE and that the positive and negative predictive value of various objective tests is strongly conditioned by the independently assessed pre-test clinical probability. Accordingly, recent international guidelines recommend that the clinical probability of the disease should be assessed in each patient with suspected PE before any further objective testing occurs. Future research is needed to develop standardised models, of varying degree of complexity, which may find application in different clinical settings to predict the probability of PE.

D-Dimer

D-Dimer plasma levels are elevated in the presence of simultaneous activation of coagulation and fibrinolysis. A normal D-dimer level has, consequently, a high negative predictive value for PE or deep vein thrombosis (DVT). However, fibrin endogenous production may be increased in a wide variety of conditions including, among others, cancer, inflammation, infection, pregnancy and chronic illnesses. Elevated plasma D-dimer levels have, for this reason, a low positive predictive value for PE and DVT.

The value of D-dimer measurement in the diagnostic work-up of each patient must be considered according to the determined PE clinical probability and the sensitivity of the particular D-dimer method of measurement employed. A negative D-dimer test result, measured by any method, in combination with a low probability clinical assessment, excludes PE with accuracy. An intermediate clinical probability also would exclude PE with reasonable certainty if D-dimer was measured by a high sensitivity ELISA method. It has been shown that the 3-month risk of PE or DVT in untreated patients with a negative D-dimer and a low or intermediate clinical probability is <1%. Conversely, if clinical assessment results in high probability for PE, a concomitant negative D-dimer test does not exclude PE.

The number of patients with suspected PE in whom D-Dimer must be measured to exclude one PE episode ranges between three in the emergency dept and ≥10 in hospitalised patients. It then appears recommendable to consider D-Dimer measurement in the diagnostic work-up of PE only in outpatients or in patients of the emergency dept with low or intermediate levels of clinical probability.

The sensitivity of D-Dimer testing for pulmonary embolism increases with the extent of PE. D-Dimer concentrations are the highest in patients with PE involving the pulmonary trunk and lobar arteries and with perfusion scan defects involving >50% of the pulmonary circulation.

Diagnostic imaging of the chest (post-test probability of PE)

The contribution of computed tomography angiography (CTA) in the diagnosis of PE has in recent years greatly increased as a consequence of the extraordinary advancement in CTA technology. Multidetector CTA has become the most widely used technique for the diagnosis or exclusion of PE and has almost replaced lung scanning as a screening test and conventional pulmonary angiography as the reference standard for the diagnosis of acute pulmonary embolism. CTA, however, does not escape the simple rule that the combined use of the estimated clinical probability and the results of one noninvasive test substantially increases the accuracy in confirming or ruling out a disease, as compared with either assessment alone. As shown by the PIOPED II trial, the predictive value of CTA is high with a concordant clinical assessment, but additional testing is necessary when clinical probability is inconsistent with the imaging results.

Perfusion (Q') lung scan was introduced 40 yrs ago as the first chest imaging method for the diagnosis of PE. A normal Q' scan excludes PE (high sensitivity and high negative predictive value), whatever the pre-test clinical probability. However, Q' scanning was thought to be poorly specific (low positive predictive value) for PE because all common pulmonary diseases (infections, neoplasms, chronic obstructive pulmonary disease) can produce decreased blood flow to the affected regions. Ventilation (V') scan was added to Q' scan to increase the specificity of scintigraphy. This diagnostic approach is based on the flawed expectation that regions of the lung excluded from perfusion by emboli maintain normal ventilation, thus giving rise to V'/Q' mismatch. This criterion to diagnose PE is at variance with the notion that ventilation is shifted away from embolised lung regions. The concept that dead space ventilation is not significantly increased in the course of PE was widely held in respiratory pathophysiology before the V'/Q' scanning approach was developed as it was asserted by COMROE (1966), who foresaw that "decrease in wasted ventilation (ventilation to unperfused or poorly perfused lung) helps the patient but hinders the physician in diagnosis.". This is in keeping with the results of the PIOPED trial, in which it was shown that the high probability V'/Q' scan (Q' defects without matching V' abnormalities) lacks sensitivity in diagnosing PE since it fails to identify 59% of PE patients (sensitivity 41%, specificity 97%). The combination of clinical probability and V'/Q' scan results either confirms or excludes PE in <30% of patients. The diagnostic value of the Q' scan (without V' imaging) was reappraised in the PISA-PED study, in which Q' scans were read either as compatible with PE when featuring wedge-shaped (segmental) perfusion defects or not compatible with PE when featuring defects other than wedge-shaped or normal perfusion. When compared with the original PIOPED protocol, the PISA-PED approach has several advantages, as follows: 1) Q' scan either confirms or excludes the clinical suspicion of PE (thus virtually eliminating nondiagnostic examinations); 2) the sensitivity of lung scintigraphy is greatly increased (86% versus 41%), yet with minor reduction of specificity (from 97% to 93%); 3) the combination of clinical probability and Q' scan results confirms or excludes PE in ~80% of patients. More recently the diagnostic performance of Q' scan for PE was confirmed by examining 889 scans from the PIOPED II. PIOPED II data were used to test the hypothesis that reading Q' scans without V scans, and categorising the Q' scan as "PE present", "PE absent", or "nondiagnostic" can result in clinically useful sensitivity and specificity in a high proportion of patients. The study has confirmed that Q' scan and CTA have comparable positive and negative predictive values, with no nondiagnostic readings for the Q' scan (table 1).

Diagnostic strategies in different clinical contexts and special conditions

Most clinicians and diagnostic radiologists feel, however, more comfortable with an anatomical demonstration of whether a clot is present or not as compared to assess a PE probability by looking at V'/Q' mismatches (PIOPED) or to evaluate the shape of a perfusion defect (PISA-PED). Furthermore, contrary to scintigraphy, in most hospitals, CTA is available 24 h/7 days a week. However, CTA cannot be performed in the whole population of patients suspected of PE. As shown in the PIOPED II trial, ~50% of the recruited patients did not undergo CTA for documented contraindications, such as renal failure, abnormal creatinine levels, allergy to contrast agent, possible pregnancy, critical illness, requirement of ventilator support, or recent myocardial infarction. In all these conditions, Q' scan could be the preferred alternative approach to the diagnosis of PE.

Table 1. Predictive value of multidetector computed tomography angiography (CTA) and perfusion scintigraphy (Q') scan from retrospective evaluation of PIOPED II data

Imaging test	Positive predictive value %	Negative predictive value %	Nondiagnostic %
Q' scan	85	96	0
CTA	86	95	6

This approach is particularly important for reproductive-age female patients in whom the breast irradiation dose from CT angiography can be minimised by using the Q' scan as the first imaging test.

Under circumstances in which clinical probability and imaging test (CTA or scintigraphy) results are discordant and further testing, such as lower limb compression ultrasonography, is required to either confirm or exclude the diagnosis. Another practical approach could be to image the pulmonary circulation with CTA if Q' scan was the first imaging test used or *vice versa*.

Summary and conclusions

The choice of a diagnostic strategy for pulmonary embolism depends on the pre-test clinical probability of PE, the condition of the patient, the availability of the necessary test, the risks of testing, the risk of an inaccurate positive or negative diagnosis, and the cost. Clinical evaluation makes it possible to classify patients into probability categories corresponding to an increasing prevalence of PE, whether assessed by implicit clinical judgment or by a validated prediction rule. Structured models to assess clinical probability so far developed have different performances in patients of the emergency department and those who are hospitalised. Exclusion of PE by clinical probability assessment and D-dimer spares the cost and radiation of an imaging evaluation. CTA has become the method of choice for imaging the pulmonary vasculature when PE is suspected in routine clinical practice. Scintigraphy can be considered as the preferred alternative chest imaging technique for patients with contraindication to CTA. If scintigraphy is used, eliminating the ventilation scan can reduce cost and radiation load with gain in diagnostic yield.

References

- Comroe JH Jr. The main function of the pulmonary circulation. *Circulation* 1966; 33: 146-158.
- Eisner MD. Before diagnostic testing for pulmonary embolism: estimating the prior probability of disease. *Am J Med* 2003; 114: 232-234.
- Miniati M, et al. Value of perfusion lung scan in the diagnosis of pulmonary embolism: results of the Prospective Investigative Study of Acute Pulmonary Embolism Diagnosis (PISA-PED). *Am J Respir Crit Care Med* 1996; 154: 1387-1393.
- Lucignani G, Pistolesi M. Diagnosing pulmonary embolism: clinical problem or methodological issue? *Eur J Nucl Med Mol Med* 2009; 36: 522-528.
- PIOPED Investigators. Value of the ventilation-perfusion scan in acute pulmonary embolism: results of the Prospective Investigation of Pulmonary Embolism Diagnosis (PIOPED). *JAMA* 1990; 263: 2753-2759.
- Remy-Jardin M, et al. Management of suspected acute pulmonary embolism in the era of CT angiography. A statement from the Fleischner Society. *Radiology* 2007; 245: 315-329.
- Sostman HD, et al. Sensitivity and specificity of perfusion scintigraphy for acute pulmonary embolism in PIOPED II. *J Nucl Med* 2008; 49: 1741-1748.
- Stein PD, et al. Challenges in the diagnosis of acute pulmonary embolism. *Am J Med* 2008; 121: 565-571.
- Stein PD, et al. Multidetector computed tomography for acute pulmonary embolism. *N Engl J Med* 2006; 354: 2317-2327.
- The Task Force for the Diagnosis and Management of Acute Pulmonary Embolism of the European Society of Cardiology, Guidelines on the diagnosis and management of acute pulmonary embolism. *Eur Heart J* 2008; 29: 2276-2315.

PULMONARY VASCULITIS

A.U. Wells
Interstitial Lung Disease Unit, Royal Brompton Hospital, London, UK
E-mail: a.wells@rbh.nthames.nhs.uk

The principles of diagnosis and management are broadly similar across the individual pulmonary vasculitides, sub-divided into primary systemic and secondary disorders (table 1). The main challenges for the clinician are to recognise that vasculitis is a possible diagnosis, to make the diagnosis in nonclassical disease and to select a level of treatment appropriate to disease severity. Wegener's granulomatosis (WG) and Churg–Strauss syndrome (CSS) are the most frequent examples of life-threatening disease.

Epidemiology and pathogenesis

WG is the third most prevalent systemic vasculitis (after giant cell arteritis and vasculitis in rheumatoid arthritis), with an annual incidence of 3–11 per million, largely affecting adults aged 30–50 yrs. CSS has an annual incidence of ~3 per million and mainly affects adults aged 30–50 yrs. In neither disorder is there a strong sex predilection.

Key points

- Haemoptysis is often scanty or absent in disffuse alveolar haemorrhage.
- Vasculitis must often be treated empirically, in the absence of full diagnostic clinical criteria or a histological diagnosis.
- Initial treatment should be definitive, even when the diagnosis is tentative.
- Chronic infection and malignancy are the most frequent differential diagnosis.

Antineutrophil cytoplasmic antibodies (ANCA) are often present in systemic vasculitides involving the small- and medium-sized vessels, including CSS, WG and microscopic polyangiitis. ANCA are subcategorised as cytoplasmic, perinuclear or atypical and are directed primarily against proteinase 3 in WG (cytoplasmic) and against myeloperoxidase in CSS (perinuclear), although all ANCA patterns have been reported in both disorders. *In vitro* and animal data suggest that ANCA interact with primed neutrophils, leading to endothelial damage and further neutrophil recruitment. Both diseases are generally considered to be triggered by foreign agents, including drugs and infections, with the most suggestive data relating to chronic nasal carriage of *Staphylococcus aureus* in WG.

Clinical presentation

Vasculitis should be suspected in diffuse alveolar haemorrhage, which may be difficult to diagnose as haemoptysis is often absent or scanty. Diffuse alveolar haemorrhage should be suspected when unexplained infiltrates on chest imaging are associated with a fall in haemoglobin over a day or two or, in chronic low-grade haemorrhage, with an iron-deficiency anaemia. Bronchoalveolar lavage is usually diagnostic of haemorrhage. Vasculitis should also be suspected: 1) in patients presenting with breathlessness on exertion and an unexplained isolated or disproportionate reduction in carbon monoxide diffusing capacity; and 2) in patients with features of an underlying systemic vasculitis, such as WG, CSS or a pulmonary–renal syndrome (of which Goodpasture's disease is the best-known example).

Investigations that tend to be useful in suspected vasculitis are shown in table 2.

Table 1. Classification of pulmonary vasculitis

Primary vasculitides (Chapel Hill International Consensus nomenclature)	**Frequency of lung involvement**
Large vessel	
Giant-cell arteritis	Rare
Takayasu's arteritis	Frequent
Medium-sized vessel	
Polyarteritis nodosa	Rare
Kawasaki disease	No
Small vessel (with variable medium-sized vessel involvement)	
Wegener's granulomatosis	Frequent
Churg–Strauss syndrome	Frequent
Microscopic polyangiitis	Frequent
Henoch–Schönlein purpura	No
Essential cryoglobulinaemia	No
Secondary vasculitides	
Rheumatological	
Pulmonary–renal (*e.g.* Goodpastures' syndrome)	
Relapsing polychronditis	
Behćet's syndrome	
Chronic infection	
Lymphoma	
Drugs	

Churg–Strauss Syndrome

The American College of Rheumatology definition of CSS requires the satisfaction of at least four of six criteria (table 3). There is typically a prodrome of rhinitis with nasal polyps and the eventual development of late-onset asthma, followed by eosinophilia in tissue or peripheral blood and, ultimately, systemic vasculitis. Other frequent sites of involvement include the central nervous system (especially mononeuritis multiplex in 75%), skin (60%), heart (50%), joints and, less frequently, the kidneys and gastrointestinal tract. The classical triad at lung biopsy is necrotising angiitis, granulomas and tissue eosinophilia. Pulmonary infiltrates on chest imaging are more common than pulmonary nodules (which very seldom cavitate). Pleural disease is present in 50% of cases. The diagnostic role of ANCA continues to be debated. ANCA, usually p-ANCA, are present in up to two-thirds of patients, but also occur in many other nonvasculitic autoimmune and infectious conditions. Thus, neither the presence nor the absence of p-ANCA is diagnostically definitive, and is no more than a useful ancillary finding, increasing or decreasing the diagnostic likelihood.

Wegener's granulomatosis

The classic historical WG triad consists of renal, lower respiratory tract and upper respiratory tract involvement. Most often, chronic rhinitis, sinusitis or mastoiditis progresses to generalised disease over months to years with lower respiratory tract involvement in 65–85%, including diffuse alveolar haemorrhage, which may be life-threatening. Fever and weight loss are frequent. There is a wide range of extrapulmonary organ involvement. Lung involvement is asymptomatic in a third of cases. The cardinal histological features are granulomatous inflammation and necrotising vasculitis, affecting small- to medium-sized vessels. Chest imaging may show one or more nodules which can cavitate, localised or diffuse infiltrates (which may represent alveolar haemorrhage), or evidence of large and small airway disease. As in CSS, the diagnosis should never be dependent upon ANCA positivity:

Table 2. Useful investigations for suspected pulmonary vasculitis

Imaging
Chest radiography, high-resolution computed tomography

Lung function tests
Pulmonary function tests, arterial gases

Renal function
Urine dipstick testing and microscopy for proteinuria, haematuria and cellular casts; estimation of renal function; consider renal biopsy (if evidence of nephritis)

Immunology
Antineutrophil cytoplasmic antibodies (ANCA), antiglomerular basement membrane (anti-GBM), immune complexes, rheumatoid factor, antinuclear antibodies (ANA), antiphospholipid antibodies

Bronchoalveolar lavage
Iron-laden macrophages

Biopsy
Renal
Skin
Lung (surgical)

c-ANCA are not present in all cases and are also found in other vasculitides, chronic bacterial infections and cryoglobulinaemia.

Among vasculitides, microscopic polyangiitis, a necrotising vasculitis affecting small to medium-sized vessels, is the main clinical mimic of WG. This disorder also often presents with diffuse alveolar haemorrhage, which can have a poor prognosis. Necrotising glomerulonephritis, mononeuritis multiplex, and skin lesions are variably present. The cardinal histological distinction is the absence of granulomas, which are characteristically present in WG.

Diagnosis of vasculitis

A confident diagnosis requires histological confirmation or satisfaction of the requisite

Table 3. ACR diagnostic criteria for CSS (four out of six are required)

1. Presence of asthma
2. Peripheral blood eosinophilia (>10%)
3. Evidence of a neuropathy in a vasculitic pattern (*e.g.* mononeuritis multiplex)
4. Transient pulmonary infiltrates
5. A history of sinus disease
6. Evidence of extra-vascular eosinophilia on biopsy

number of clinical criteria. However, many patients with vasculitis have features overlapping between diagnostic entities with transient or nonfulfilment of diagnostic criteria. Thus, a versatile diagnostic approach is required. When vasculitis is suspected but full clinical criteria are not satisfied, a histological diagnosis should be made, if possible. However, a negative biopsy does not exclude vasculitis, which may be patchy or give rise to nonspecific inflammatory change (as in upper airway biopsies in WG patients).

Thus, the diagnosis of a vasculitic syndrome is sometimes necessarily empirical, with chronic infection and malignancy the most frequent differential diagnoses. In such cases, initial treatment and monitoring should be as for the vasculitic syndrome most closely corresponding to the clinical presentation in that patient. Initial treatment should be definitive, as a clear response provides important support for the diagnosis, whereas a tentative therapeutic approach often prolongs diagnostic uncertainty.

Prognosis

The poor historical outcome of the vasculitic syndromes has been transformed by more aggressive therapy, but also by the increasing detection of milder disease, including patients with limited involvement. In localised pulmonary WG and CSS alike, the outcome is much better than with multi-organ involvement. In CSS, the prognosis worsens strikingly with two or more extrapulmonary complications (5-yr survival 54%). Mortality is largely ascribable to sepsis (as a complication of treatment) or disease progression. Death from progressive disease is most commonly due to renal failure or lung involvement in WG, and to renal failure, cerebrovascular involvement and gastrointestinal disease in CSS (with 10% of deaths accounted for by lung disease).

Treatment

In most patients with WG, and in severe vasculitis in general, intense immunosuppression to induce remission is usual. In WG, oral cyclophosphamide (2.0 mg·kg^{-1}·day^{-1}) and intravenous cyclophosphamide (600 mg·m^{-2} at 3-4 weekly intervals, depending on disease severity) are equally successful in inducing remission. Intravenous therapy is associated with a slightly higher relapse rate, but is much less toxic in the short-term and is much less likely to provoke haemorrhagic cystitis and subsequent malignancy, based on long-term systemic lupus erythematosus data. In life-threatening disease, cyclophosphamide and intravenous methyl prednisolone should be administered concurrently. Prophylactic co-trimoxazole (trimethoprim 160 mg/ sulfamethoxazole 800 mg three times a week) is often used with prolonged intense immunosuppression, to reduce the risk of *Pneumocystis carinii* opportunistic infection.

In less severe vasculitis, a less aggressive initial approach is justified. In isolated pulmonary CSS, a good response is usual with oral prednisolone (1 mg·kg^{-1}·day^{-1}, up to 60 mg·day^{-1}) or, in more severe disease, intravenous methylprednisolone (up to 1 g daily on three successive days). In WG without major organ involvement, methotrexate (0.3 mg·kg^{-1}·week^{-1}) is as effective as daily oral cyclophosphamide in the induction of remission, although relapse is more likely with cessation of treatment at 12 months.

Following initial treatment, less intense long-term therapy is almost invariably required. In WG, standard maintenance treatment has consisted of azathioprine (2.0 mg·kg^{-1}·day^{-1}), usually with low-dose corticosteroid therapy, although no comparison with other agents (such as methotrexate and mycophenolate mofetil) has been undertaken, either in WG or other vasculitides. In WG, co-trimoxazole therapy has been efficacious in localised respiratory tract disease and may have an ancillary role in maintaining remission.

Intravenous immunoglobulin and anti-thymocyte globulin have been variably efficacious in resistant WG. Rituximab therapy is more promising, based on striking responses recently reported in patients refractory to standard treatments.

References

- Conron M, Beynon HLC. Churg-Strauss syndrome. Thorax Rare Disease Series. *Thorax* 2000; 55: 870-877.
- Guillevin L, *et al*. Prognostic factors in polyarteritis nodosa and Churg-Strauss syndrome. A prospective study in 342 patients. *Medicine* 1996; 75: 17-28.
- Jayne D, *et al*. A randomized trial of maintenance therapy for vasculitis associated with antineutrophil cytoplasmic autoantibodies. *New Engl J Med* 2003; 349: 36-44.
- Jennette JC, *et al*. Nomenclature of systemic vasculitides. Proposal of an international consensus conference. *Arthritis Rheumatism* 1994; 37: 187-192.
- Keogh KA, *et al*. Rituximab for refractory Wegener's Granulomatosis: report of a prospective, open-label pilot trial. *Am J Respir Crit Care Med* 2006; 173: 180-187.
- Lanham JG, *et al*. Systemic vasculitis with asthma and eosinophilia: the clinical approach to the Churg-Strauss syndrome. *Medicine (Baltimore)* 1984; 63: 65-681.
- Lhote F, Guillevin L. Polyarteritis nodosa, microscopic polyangiitis and Churg-Strauss syndrome. Semin Respir Crit Care Med 1998; 19: 27-46.
- Specks U. Pulmonary vasculitis. In: Schwarz MI, King TE Jr, eds. Interstitial lung disease. Hamilton, Canada, BC Dekker, 1998; pp. 507-534.

PULMONARY HYPERTENSION

M. Humbert and G. Simonneau
Univ Paris-Sud, Orsay, Centre National de Référence de l'Hypertension Pulmonaire Sévère, Service de Pneumologie et Réanimation Respiratoire, Hôpital Antoine Béclère, AP-HP, Clamart, and INSERM U999, Hypertension Artérielle Pulmonaire, Physiopathologie et Innovation Thérapeutique, Centre Chirurgical Marie Lannelongue, Le Plessis Robinson, France
E-mail: gerald.simonneau@abc.aphp.fr

Pulmonary hypertension (PH) is defined as an increase in mean pulmonary arterial pressure $\bar{P}_{pa} \geqslant 25$ mmHg at rest as assessed by right heart catheterisation.

Classification

According to values of pulmonary wedge pressure (P_{pw}), PH can be pre-capillary ($P_{pw} \leqslant 15$ mmHg) or post-capillary ($P_{pw} > 15$ mmHg).

PH can be classified into five groups according to pathological, pathophysiological and therapeutic characteristics. Despite comparable elevations of $\bar{P}_{pa}$ in the different clinical groups, the underlying mechanisms, diagnostic approaches, and prognostic and therapeutic implications are completely different.

The new clinical classification is shown in Table 1. Group 1 relates to pulmonary arterial hypertension (PAH), corresponding to idiopathic, heritable and associated pre-capillary pulmonary hypertension. The term familial PAH has been replaced by heritable PAH because specific gene mutations have been identified in sporadic cases with no family history. Heritable forms of PAH include clinically sporadic idiopathic PAH with germline mutations (mainly bone morphogenetic protein receptor 2 gene as well as activin receptor-like kinase type-1 gene or endoglin gene) and clinical familial cases with or without identified mutation. Associated PAH includes conditions that can have a similar clinical presentation to that seen in idiopathic PAH with comparable histological findings. Associated PAH account for approximately half of the patients followed at specialised centres. Pulmonary veno-occlusive disease (PVOD) and pulmonary capillary haemangiomatosis remain difficult disorders to classify since they share some

Key points

- PAH is a rare condition characterised by elevated pulmonary arterial resistance leading to right heart failure and death.

- PAH can be sporadic (idiopathic PAH), heritable, induced by drugs or toxins, or associated with other conditions such as connective tissue diseases.

- Doppler echocardiography is the investigation of choice for noninvasive screening but measurement of haemodynamic parameters during right heart catheterisation is mandatory to confirm the diagnosis (mean pulmonary artery pressure $\geqslant 25$ mmHg and pulmonary artery wedge pressure $\leqslant 15$ mmHg).

- Recent advances in the management of PAH include prostaglandins, endothelin receptor antagonists and type 5 phosphodiesterase inhibitors.

- Lung transplantation is an option for severe patients deteriorating despite medical treatment.

Table 1. Updated clinical classification of pulmonary hypertension (PH)

1 PAH
1.1 Idiopathic PAH
1.2 Heritable
1.2.1 BMPR2
1.2.2 ALK1, endoglin (with or without hereditary haemorrhagic telangiectasia)
1.2.3 Unknown.
1.3 Drugs and toxins induced
1.4 APAH:
1.4.1 Connective tissue diseases
1.4.2 HIV infection
1.4.3 Portal hypertension
1.4.4 Congenital heart disease
1.4.5 Schistosomiasis
1.4.6 Chronic haemolytic anaemia
1.5 Persistent PH of the newborn
1' Pulmonary veno-occlusive disease and/or pulmonary capillary haemangiomatosis
2 PH due to left heart disease
2.1 Systolic dysfunction
2.2 Diastolic dysfunction
2.3 Valvular disease
3 PH due to lung diseases and/or hypoxia
3.1 Chronic obstructive pulmonary disease
3.2 Interstitial lung disease
3.3 Other pulmonary diseases with mixed restrictive and obstructive pattern
3.4 Sleep-disordered breathing
3.5 Alveolar hypoventilation disorders
3.6 Chronic exposure to high altitude
3.7 Developmental abnormalities
4 Chronic thromboembolic PH
5 PH with unclear and/or multifactorial mechanisms
5.1 Haematological disorders: myeloproliferative disorders, splenectomy.
5.2 Systemic disorders, sarcoidosis, pulmonary Langerhans' cell histiocytosis, lymphangioleiomyomatosis, neurofibromatosis, vasculitis
5.3 Metabolic disorders: glycogen storage disease, Gaucher disease, thyroid disorders
5.4 Others: tumoral obstruction, fibrosing mediastinitis, chronic renal failure on dialysis

PAH: pulmonary arterial hypertension; BMPR2: Bone morphogenetic protein receptor, type II; ALK-1: Activin receptor-like kinase 1 gene; APAH: associated PAH. Reproduced from SIMONNEAU et al. (2009), with permission from the publisher.

characteristics with PAH but also demonstrate a number of differences. Given the current evidence, these conditions have been individualised as a distinct category but not completely separated from PAH and have been designated as clinical group 1'. Chronic thromboembolic pulmonary hypertension (CTEPH) is an important subcategory of PH, which may be cured by surgical pulmonary endarterectomy. It was decided to maintain only a single category of CTEPH without attempting to distinguish between proximal and distal forms. The most frequent causes of PH are those complicating left heart diseases (group 2) and pulmonary diseases (group 3).

All forms of PH have some common pathologic features regardless of their aetiology: medial hypertrophy of muscular and elastic arteries; dilation and intimal atheromas of elastic pulmonary arteries; and right ventricular hypertrophy. In addition to the aforementioned pathologic changes common to all forms of PH, PAH is characterised by constrictive and complex arterial lesions involving to varying degrees the pre- and intra-acinar pulmonary arteries The plexiform lesion is a focal proliferation of endothelial channels lined by myofibroblasts, smooth muscle cells, and connective tissue matrix. The lesion is located within pre- and intra-acinar pulmonary arteries, and is associated with expansion and partial destruction of the arterial wall with extension of the plexiform lesion into the perivascular connective tissue. The plexiform lesion is often located at an arterial branching point (fig. 1).

Epidemiology and survival

PAH is a rare condition with a prevalence ranging 15–50 per million in western Europe. The prevalence of idiopathic PAH was about 6 per million in the French Registry and its incidence was 2 per million per yr. Median survival of idiopathic PAH was 2.8 yrs in the National Institutes of Health Registry before the recent development of PAH-specific therapies. Despite improvements in recent years, idiopathic, familial, and anorexigen-associated PAH remains a progressive, fatal disease in the modern management era. Mortality is most closely associated with male sex, right ventricular haemodynamic function and exercise limitation.

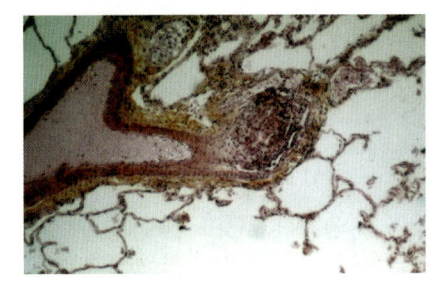

Figure 1. A typical plexiform lesion in a patient with idiopathic PAH. The lesion is located at an arterial branching point.

Diagnosis

The diagnostic process starts with the identification of the more common clinical groups of PH (group 2 – left heart diseases and group 3 – pulmonary diseases), to distinguish group 4 – CTEPH and finally to make the diagnosis and recognise the different types of group 1 – PAH and the rarer conditions of group 5.

PAH should be considered in the differential diagnosis of exertional dyspnoea, syncope, angina and/or progressive limitation of exercise capacity, particularly in patients without apparent risk factors, symptoms or signs of common cardiovascular and respiratory disorders. Special awareness should be directed towards patients with associated conditions and/or risk factors for development of PAH such as family history, connective tissue diseases, congenital heart diseases, HIV infection, portal hypertension, haemolytic anaemia, or a history of drug and toxin intake known to induce PAH. In everyday clinical practice, such awareness may be low. More often, PH is found unexpectedly on transthoracic echocardiography requested for another indication.

If noninvasive assessment is compatible with PH, clinical history, symptoms, signs, ECG, chest radiograph, transthoracic echocardiogram, pulmonary function tests (including nocturnal oximetry if required) and high-resolution computed tomography (HRCT) of the chest are requested to identify the presence of group 2 – left heart diseases or group 3 – pulmonary diseases. If these are not found or if PH seems "out of proportion" to their severity, less common causes of PH should be sought. Ventilation/perfusion lung scan should be considered. If ventilation/perfusion scan shows multiple segmental perfusion defects, a diagnosis of group 4 – CTEPH should be suspected. The final diagnosis of CTEPH (and the assessment of suitability for pulmonary endarterectomy) will require helical computed tomography of the chest, right heart catheterisation and selective pulmonary angiography. HRCT of the chest may also show signs suggestive of

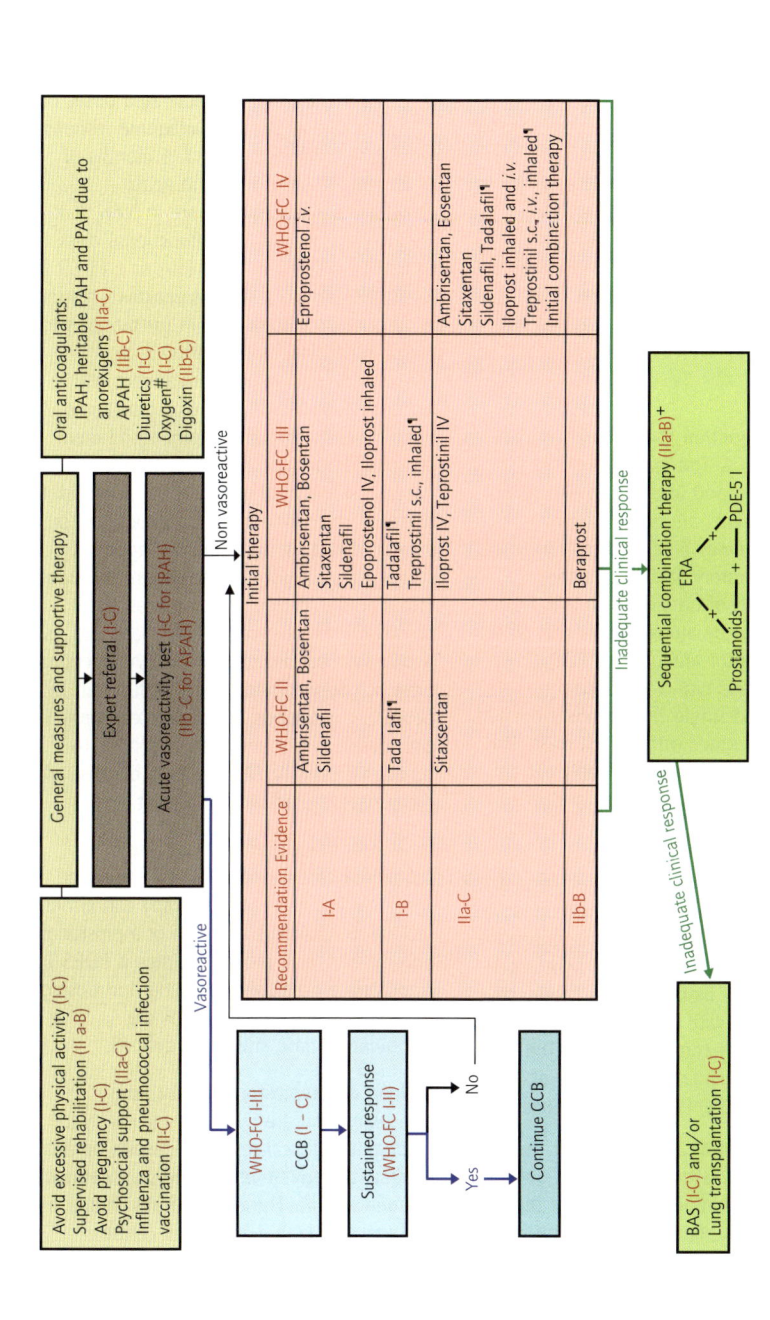

Figure 2. Evidence-based treatment algorithm for pulmonary arterial hypertension (PAH) patients (for group 1 patients only). Level of recommendation and evidence have been evaluated in the ESC/ERS European Guidelines. IPAH: idiopathic pulmonary arterial hypertension; APAH: associated pulmonary arterial hypertension; WHO-FC: World Health Organization functional class; CCB: calcium channel blockers; *i.v.*: intravenous; s.c.: subcutaneous; BAS: balloon atrial septostomy; ERA: endothelin receptor antagonist; PDE5 I: phosphodiesterase type-5 inhibitor. #: to maintain arterial blood O_2 pressure ≥ 8 kPa (60 mmHg); ¶: under regulatory review; +: IIa-C for W-O-FC II.

Pulmonary hypertension

343

group 1' – PVOD. If a ventilation/perfusion scan is normal or shows only subsegmental "patchy" perfusion defects, a tentative diagnosis of group 1 - PAH or the rarer conditions of group 5 is made. Performing a right heart catheterisation will be necessary to confirm the diagnosis and assess hemodynamic severity. Additional specific diagnostic tests, including haematology, biochemistry, immunology, serology and ultrasonography, will allow the final diagnosis to be refined. 6-min walk distance is an important marker of exercise limitation with prognostic value in PAH.

Treatment

A treatment algorithm for PAH patients is shown in figure 2. The grades of recommendation and levels of evidence for the PAH treatments are derived from European Guidelines published jointly by the European Respiratory Society and the European Society of Cardiology in 2010. Drug classes are listed by alphabetical order (ERA: endothelin receptor antagonists; PDE5 I: phosphodiesterase type-5 inhibitors; prostanoids) and single compounds are listed by alphabetical order within each class. The treatment algorithm does not apply to patients in other clinical groups, and in particular not to patients with PH associated with group 2 – left heart disease or with group 3 – pulmonary diseases. In addition, the different treatments have been evaluated by randomised control trials mainly in idiopathic PAH, heritable PAH, PAH due to anorexigen drugs and in PAH associated with connective tissue diseases or with congenital heart diseases (surgically corrected or not). The grades of recommendation and levels of evidence for the other PAH subgroups are lower.

The suggested initial approach, after the diagnosis of PAH, is the adoption of general measures, the initiation of supportive therapy and referral to an expert centre. Acute vasoreactivity testing with inhaled nitric oxide or intravenous prostacyclin or adenosine should be performed in all patients with group 1 - PAH, although patients with idiopathic PAH, heritable PAH, and PAH associated with anorexigen use are the most likely to exhibit an acute positive response and to profit from high-dose calcium-channel blocker therapy. Vasoreactive patients should be treated with optimally tolerated doses of calcium channel blockers; adequate response should be confirmed after 3–4 months of treatment. Nonresponders to acute vasoreactivity testing who are in New York Heart Association (NYHA) functional class II should be treated with an ERA or a PDE5 I. Nonresponders to acute vasoreactivity testing, or responders who remain in (or progress to) NYHA functional class III should be considered candidates for treatment with either an ERA or a PDE5 I or a prostanoid. As head-to-head comparisons among different compounds are not available, no evidence-based first-line treatment can be proposed. In this case, the choice of drug is dependent on a variety of factors, including the approval status, the route of administration, the side-effect profile, patients' preferences and physicians' experience. Some experts still use first-line *i.v.* epoprostenol in NYHA functional class III patients, because of its survival benefits. Continuous *i.v.* epoprostenol may be considered as first-line therapy for NYHA functional class IV PAH patients because of the survival benefit in this subset.

In case of inadequate clinical response, sequential combination therapy should be considered. Combination therapy can either include an ERA plus a PDE5 I or a prostanoid plus an ERA or a prostanoid plus a PDE5 I. Appropriate protocols for timing and dosing to limit possible side-effects of the combination have still to be defined.

Balloon atrioseptostomy and/or lung transplantation are indicated for PAH with inadequate clinical response despite optimal medical therapy or where medical treatments are unavailable. These procedures should be performed only in experienced centres.

References

- D'Alonzo GE, *et al*. Survival in patients with primary pulmonary hypertension. *Ann Int Med* 1991; 115: 343–349.

- Galiè N, et al. Guidelines for the diagnosis and treatment of pulmonary hypertension. The task force for the diagnosis and treatment of pulmonary hypertension of the European Society of Cardiology (ESC) and the European Respiratory Society (ERS), endorsed by the International Society of Heart and Lung Transplantation (ISHLT). *Eur Respir J* 2009; 34: 1219-1263.
- Humbert M, et al. Pulmonary arterial hypertension in France: results from a national registry. *Am J Respir Crit Care Med* 2006; 173: 1023-1030.
- Humbert M, et al. Survival in patients with idiopathic, familial, and anorexigen-associated pulmonary arterial hypertension in the modern management era. *Circulation* 2010; 122: 156-163.
- Rich S, et al. Primary pulmonary hypertension: a national prospective study. *Ann Int Med* 1987; 107: 216-223.
- Simonneau G, et al. Updated clinical classification of pulmonary hypertension. *J Am Coll Cardiol* 2009; 54: Suppl. 1, S43-S54.

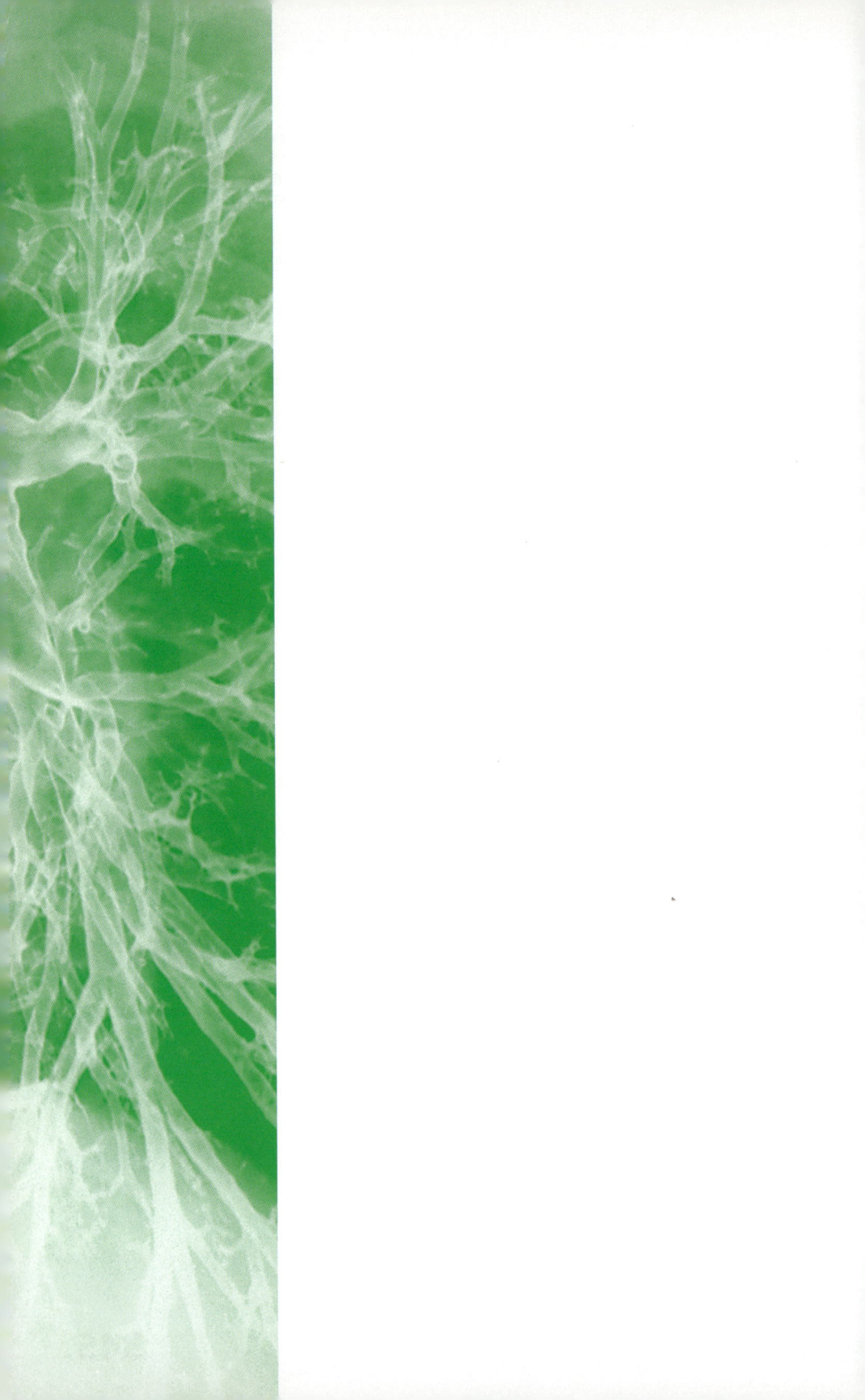

CHAPTER 13:

PLEURAL, MEDIASTINAL AND CHEST WALL DISEASES

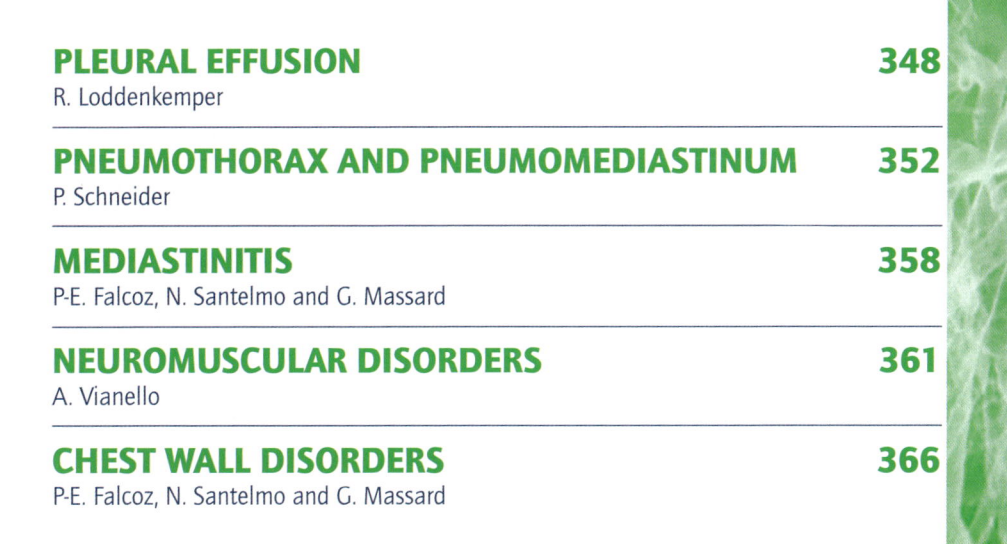

PLEURAL EFFUSION — 348
R. Loddenkemper

PNEUMOTHORAX AND PNEUMOMEDIASTINUM — 352
P. Schneider

MEDIASTINITIS — 358
P-E. Falcoz, N. Santelmo and G. Massard

NEUROMUSCULAR DISORDERS — 361
A. Vianello

CHEST WALL DISORDERS — 366
P-E. Falcoz, N. Santelmo and G. Massard

PLEURAL EFFUSION

R. Loddenkemper
Former Chief of Department of Pneumology II, Lungenklinik Heckeshorn,
HELIOS Klinikum Emil von Behring, Berlin, Germany
E-mail: rloddenkemper@dzk-tuberkulose.de

Key points

- Pleural effusions may present as primary manifestations of many diseases. However, most often they are observed as secondary manifestations or complications of other diseases.
- Cardiac failure is the main cause of pleural effusions.
- Of noncardiac causes, parapneumonic effusions are commonest, followed by malignant pleural effusions.
- Small pleural effusions can be detected best by ultrasound (or CT).
- Pleural effusion can in the majority of cases be diagnosed by case history, clinical presentation, imaging techniques and examination of pleural fluid.
- The most important laboratory parameter of pleural fluid is total protein, distinguishing trans- and exudates.
- Biopsy procedures such as closed-needle biopsy or medical thoracoscopy/ pleuroscopy may be necessary to confirm or exclude malignant or tuberculous causes.
- Treatment depends upon the underlying disease.
- Local treatment options include therapeutic thoracentesis, chest-tube drainage, chemical pleurodesis and, rarely, surgical interventions.

Pleural effusion is defined as accumulation of fluid in the pleural space that exceeds the physiological amounts of 10–20 mL. Pleural effusion develops either when the formation of pleural fluid is excessive or when fluid resorption is disturbed. Pleural effusions may represent a primary manifestation of many diseases, but most often they are observed as secondary manifestations or complications of other diseases.

Pleural effusion is found in almost 10% of patients who have internal diseases and the main cause in 30–40% of these is cardiac failure. Among the noncardiac effusions, parapneumonic effusions are the most common at 48%, of which ~75% are of bacterial and 25% of viral origin. Malignant pleural effusions follow in 24% of cases, half of which are caused by lung or breast cancer. Pleural effusion is secondary to pulmonary embolism in 18% of cases, to liver cirrhosis in 6%, and to gastrointestinal diseases, mainly pancreatitis, in 3% of cases. Many other possible causes, albeit extremely rare, play an important role in differential diagnosis.

Pleural effusion may result from a number of pathophysiological mechanisms, all of which disturb the physiological balance between the formation and removal of pleural fluid (normal production estimated at 15 mL·day^{-1} in a 60-kg person). Most effusions develop from both an increase in the entry rate of liquid into the pleural space and a decrease in the maximal exit rate of liquid from the pleural space. Transudative effusions are caused either by increased hydrostatic pressure (*e.g.* in cardiac failure), or by reduced plasma oncotic pressure because of protein deficiency (*e.g.* liver cirrhosis, nephrotic syndrome). The pleura itself remains intact. Rarely, transudates may arise from the entry of liquids with low protein concentrations (*e.g.* urine, cerebrospinal fluid or iatrogenic intrapleural infusion of fluids). In contrast, pathological changes in the pleura result in exudation caused by diffuse increase of capillary permeability, due to localised ruptures (*e.g.* blood vessels, lymphatic vessels, lung abscess, oesophagus) or to disturbed absorption (*e.g.* lymphatic blockage).

Pleural effusion may present at all ages, but is mainly found in adults. Malignant pleural effusions are observed mainly in patients aged >60 yrs; the most common presentations are dyspnoea and chest pain, and those of the individual underlying diseases. Physical examination reveals dullness on percussion, usually at the base of the thorax, and decreased breath sounds.

Pleural effusion may be demonstrated by a number of techniques with different sensitivities. The demonstration by percussion requires at least 300-400 mL of fluid, whereas at least 200-300 mL is necessary for standard chest radiography. Smaller amounts can be recognised by lateral decubitus radiography, which also demonstrates whether the fluid is moving freely. Ultrasound is able to demonstrate small effusions, and the sensitivity is almost 100% for volumes of ≥100 mL. Computed tomography and magnetic resonance imaging have very similar sensitivities, but require a more advanced technology and are therefore much more expensive.

In the majority of cases, the aetiology is based on the case history, clinical presentation, imaging techniques and examination of the pleural fluid.

The presence of a pleural effusion is established only by thoracentesis. The site should be selected according to the results of the diagnostic procedures. If the effusion is small, thoracentesis can be performed under ultrasound guidance. Thoracentesis is indicated in all cases of pleural effusion of unknown origin and in effusions that do not resolve after appropriate treatment. Additional biopsy procedures, such as closed needle biopsy or medical thoracoscopy/pleuroscopy, may be necessary to confirm or exclude malignant or tuberculous causes. These are performed in a stepwise diagnostic approach (fig. 1).

In many cases, evaluation of the pleural fluid yields valuable diagnostic information or even permits a clear diagnosis. The most important criteria are appearance, protein content and cellular components. In case of more specific diagnostic questions, routine measurement of the glucose content is supplemented by determination of further laboratory

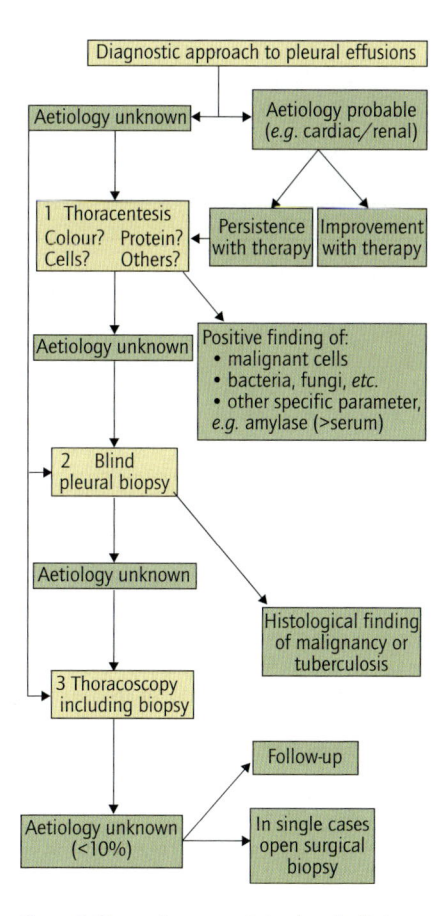

Figure 1. Diagnostic approach to pleural effusions.

Table 1. Investigative parameters of pleural effusion

Obligatory
Appearance
Total protein
Cell differentiation (cytology)
Optional
Glucose (pH)
Lactate dehydrogenase
Cholesterol
NT-proBNP
Triglycerides
Amylase
Bilirubin
Creatinine
Haematocrit
Immunocytology
Tumour markers
Adenosine deaminase
Interferon-γ release assay
Antinuclear factor, rheumatoid factors, *etc.*
Search for infecting organisms
Tubercle bacilli
Gram staining
Anaerobic, aerobic bacteria
Fungi, parasites
NT-proBNP: N-terminal pro-B-type natriuretic peptide.

parameters and search for infecting organisms (table 1).

The most important laboratory parameter is total protein content in the effusion, for which a threshold value of 30 g·L^{-1} separates a transudate from an exudate. However, this value is not exclusive, and additional parameters such as lactate dehydrogenase (LDH >200 U·L^{-1}) or cholesterol (>0.55 mmol·L^{-1} (60 mg·dL^{-1})) may be helpful (table 2). The simultaneous determination of serum values is important, because these may strongly influence the values in the pleura. Low glucose values may indicate rheumatoid pleuritis, lupus pleuritis, empyema, tuberculous or malignant effusion or oesophageal perforation.

Markedly elevated amylase values are observed in acute pancreatitis and pancreatic pseudocysts, oesophageal perforation and occasionally in malignant effusions.

Haemothorax is characterised by purely bloody effusions and haematocrit values that exceed those in peripheral blood by >50%. Increased triglycerides distinguish chylous from pseudochylous effusions. Although nonspecific, adenosine deaminase and T-cell-based interferon-γ release assays may allow the diagnosis of tuberculosis as cause of pleural effusion with high sensitivity and specificity.

Diagnostic testing for the infecting organisms that cause pleural effusion is indicated in empyemas with aerobic and anaerobic cultures and in suspected tuberculous, fungal or parasitic effusions.

Therapeutic aims in patients with pleural effusion are palliation of symptoms (pain, dyspnoea), treatment of underlying diseases, prevention of pleural fibrosis with reduction of pulmonary function, and prevention of recurrences. The therapeutic approach depends on the availability of options for causal or only symptomatic treatments.

Empyema usually requires, besides antibiotic treatment, additional pleural drainage. Resolution may be further facilitated by instillation of a fibrinolytic agent. In malignant pleural effusions, therapeutic thoracentesis or chest-tube drainage combined with chemical pleurodesis or medical thoracoscopy with talc poudrage are the preferred options for local treatment. In those resulting from tumours likely to respond to chemotherapy or hormonal treatment, systemic treatment should be started and may be combined with therapeutic thoracentesis or pleurodesis.

Table 2. Light's criteria for exudates

TP >3 g·dL^{-1}	TP - pleura/TP - serum >0.5
LDH >200 U·L^{-1}	LDH – pleura/LDH – serum >0.6
TP: total protein; LDH: lactate dehydrogenase. Sensitivity of ratios 89.5/91.4, accuracy 95.4/94.7.	

References

- Antony VB, et al. Management of malignant pleural effusions. (ATS/ERS Statement). *Eur Respir J* 2001; 18: 402–419.
- Antunes G. BTS guidelines for the management of malignant pleural effusions. *Thorax* 2003; 58: Suppl. 2, ii29–ii38.
- Chegou NN, et al. Evaluation of adapted whole-blood interferon-gamma release assays for the diagnosis of pleural tuberculosis. *Respiration* 2008; 76: 131–138.
- Colice GL, et al. Medical and surgical treatment of parapneumonic effusions: an evidence-based guideline. *Chest* 2000; 118: 1158–1171.
- Heffner JE, et al. Diagnostic value of tests that discriminate between exudative and transudative pleural effusions. *Chest* 1997; 111: 970–979.
- Koegelenberg CF, et al. Parapneumonic pleural effusions and empyema. *Respiration* 2008; 75: 241–250.
- Kolditz M, et al. High diagnostic accuracy of NT-proBNP for cardiac origin of pleural effusions. *Eur Respir J* 2006; 28: 114–150.
- Light RW. Diagnostic approach in a patient with pleural effusion. *Eur Respir Mon* 2002; 22: 131–145.
- Light RW, ed, Pleural Diseases. 5th Edn. Philadelphia, Lippincott Williams & Wilkins, 2007.
- Maskell NA, et al. BTS guidelines for the investigation of a unilateral pleural effusion in adults. *Thorax* 2003; 58: Suppl. 2, ii8–ii17.
- Rodriguez-Panadero F, et al. Thoracoscopy: general overview and place in the diagnosis and management of pleural effusion. *Eur Respir J* 2006; 28: 409–422.
- Trajman A, et al. Novel tests for diagnosing tuberculous pleural effusion: what works and what does not? *Eur Respir J* 2008; 31: 1098–1106.

PNEUMOTHORAX AND PNEUMOMEDIASTINUM

P. Schneider
DRK Kliniken Berlin, Thoracic Surgery, Berlin, Germany
E-mail: p.schneider@drk-kliniken-berlin.de

Introduction and classification

Pneumothorax is defined as an accumulation of air in the pleural space with secondary lung collapse. This accumulation is of diverse derivation, but visceral pleural rupture with air leakage is the most common cause. An original possible ruptured oesophagus with diminished chest wall integrity can cause free air in the pleural space, and more rarely a gas-forming organism.

Key points

- The most likely cause of a primary spontaneous pneumothorax is the rupture of small subpleural bulla.

- Pneumothorax usually present with acute chest pain and dyspnoea.

- Pneumothorax can be complicated by persistent air leak >3 days, pneumomediastinum and haemopneumothorax.

- Recurrence is the most common indication for surgery in patients with a primary spontaneous pneumothorax.

- Surgery is accomplished by a video-assisted thoracoscopy mechanical abrasion, or by parietal apical pleurectomy in association with resection of the lung.

- In secondary pneumothorax the mortality rate for surgery may reach 10 percent and the morbidity is significant.

In most instances the pneumothorax presents with minor symptoms without any physiological changes. Rarely, a simple pneumothorax progresses and develops with significant haemodynamic and respiratory instability, hypoxia and shock. This clinical presentation is accompanied by a tension pneumothorax and demands emergency treatment.

The pneumothorax can be classified according to cause or clinical presentation; or of spontaneous, traumatic or iatrogenic aetiology (table 1). The first category includes primary and secondary causes. A primary spontaneous pneumothorax occurs in individuals with no known pulmonary disease. A secondary pneumothorax occurs in patients with clinical or radiographic evidence of underlying lung disease. Traumatic pneumothorax occurs as a result of penetrating or blunt trauma with disruption of the bronchus, the lung, or the oesophagus. A traumatic pneumothorax is defined as "open" with an associated disruption of the chest wall. Iatrogenic pneumothorax includes the diagnostic and therapeutic pneumothorax, which are relatively common in the hospital environment but will not be considered in this discussion.

Primary spontaneous pneumothorax

Clinical features The most likely cause of a primary spontaneous pneumothorax is the rupture of small subpleural bulla (fig. 1), occuring at rest or during exercise. It is seen most often in young, tall male patients with admitted cigarette or cannabis smoking habits. Hereditary aspects have been described.

Table 1. Classification of pneumothorax

Spontaneous
  Primary (healthy individuals)
  Secondary (underlying pulmonary disease)
    Chronic obstructive pulmonary disease
    Infection
    Neoplasm
    Catamenial
    Miscellaneous
Traumatic
  Blunt
  Penetrating
Iatrogenic
  Inadvertent
  Diagnostic
  Therapeutic

In the North American population, incidence varies from 6-7 per 100,000 men to 1-2 per 100,000 women. Bilateral pneumothoraces occur in <10% of patients. Recurrences are observed in 42% of patients, usually within 2 yrs. After the second pneumothorax, the chances of having a third episode increase to >50%.

The clinical presentation usually relates to the degree of pulmonary collapse. Although some patients have an asymptomatic pneumothorax, more often they present with acute chest pain and dyspnoea.

Physical findings may be totally absent if the collapse is minimal, while substantial collapse is defined in decreased chest wall movement on the affected side. Percussion of the chest cavity is hyperresonant and tympanic, and on auscultation breath sounds are decreased or absent. A pleural friction rub can sometimes be heard. Tachycardia is found in most patients.

Diagnosis The clinical diagnosis of a pneumothorax is best confirmed by erect posteroanterior and lateral chest radiographs. Expiration posteroanterior chest radiography may be useful to demonstrate a small pneumothorax not seen on standard film.

Computed tomography scanning is generally not necessary unless abnormalities are noted on the plain chest radiograph or for further evaluation (*e.g.* suspected secondary pneumothorax), or if an aberrant chest drain emplacement is suspected.

Complications Air leakage may persist for >48 h after the treatment of a pneumothorax. Often the air leak is seen in patients with a secondary pneumothorax, but occasionally patients with a primary spontaneous pneumothorax develop this complication. In this instance, surgery must be considered.

Pneumomediastinum (fig. 2) is secondary to the dissection of air along the bronchial and pulmonary vessel sheets or as a complication of a spontaneous pneumothorax. It is generally of no clinical consequence, but other causes of pneumomediastinum, such as injury to major airways or oesophagus perforation, may be needed to be excluded! Pneumoperitoneum secondary to a pneumothorax is rare, and it must be differentiated from a pneumoperitoneum associated with a perforated abdominal organ. Interstitial and subcutaneous emphysema are usually of no consequence.

Haemothorax (fig. 3) is a rare complication of a pneumothorax and results more often from the rupture of a small vessel located in adhesions between the visceral and the parietal pleura. Often re-expansion of the lung with a chest drain helps to tamponade the bleeding point.

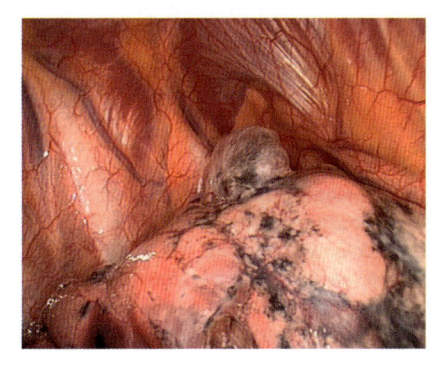

Figure 1. Bulla on the apex.

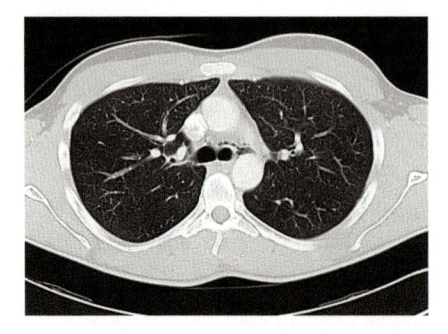

Figure 2. Pneumomediastinum.

Occasionally the patient becomes hypotensive and requires emergency surgery.

Bilateral pneumothorax happens in <1% of cases and can be simultaneous or, more commonly, sequential.

Management The different clinical situations in spontaneous pneumothorax require different therapeutic approaches. The nonoperative approach includes observation, simple aspiration, and thoracostomy with ambulatory chest drainage. Chemical pleurodesis with tetracycline or talc are options that can be used to reduce the risk of recurrence. Surgical intervention entails apical bullectomy with or without pleurodesis by pleurectomy or gauze abrasion.

Observation Asymptomatic patients in good health (<20%) with a small pneumothorax and no evidence of radiographic progression may be treated per observation. To ensure no complications develop, it is recommended that these patients be observed in hospital for 24–48 h. Before discharge, patients must be warned of a potential tension pneumothorax development. A weekly follow-up with clinical examination and chest radiograph is to be carried out until the pneumothorax has been completely resolved. The main inconvenience in this form of therapy is the duration, which far exceeds what is seen with conventional pleural drainage plus the added risk of a tension pneumothorax development. Therefore observation only is inappropriate in most cases.

Aspiration and small chest tube drainage Simple aspiration of air with a 16-gauge intravenous cannula connected to a three-way stopcock and a 60-mL syringe is an option.

Small 9-Fr. chest tubes with or without flutter valves have also been used as an alternative to larger and more conventional thoracostomy tubes. The success rate is high, but problems associated with kinking and occlusion of the drains have been described. Treatment is still controversial. Simple aspiration is recommended by the British Thoracic Society – but not by the American College of Chest Physicians – as first-line treatment for the primary pneumothorax requiring intervention. Acceptance by medical staff is seemingly modest.

Conventional tube thoracostomy Conventional tube thoracostomy remains the procedure of choice for the management of moderate-to-large pneumothoraces. The drain allows for rapid and complete evacuation of air from the pleural space. Although underwater-seal drainage is sufficient for most cases of

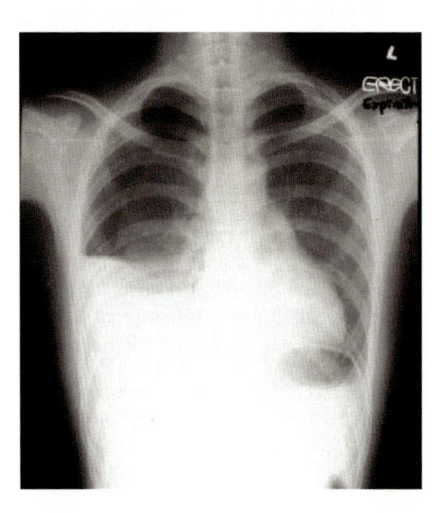

Figure 3. Haemopneumothorax on the right side.

pneumothorax, the current author prefers the use of negative intrapleural pressure to maintain lung re-expansion over a period of 5 days.

Nonsurgical therapy of recurrences Most surgeons are concerned about the routine use of chemopleurodesis in the treatment of spontaneous pneumothorax. Being a benign disease occurring in young people who may require surgery in later life (for other disease development) the important symphysis which follows chemopleurodesis complicates and multiplies the risk in association with high morbidity rates, especially if lung resection or transplantation is considered. Chemical pleurodesis should therefore be used only in selected cases.

Indications for surgery Surgery may be indicated in the first instance, if the pneumothorax is complicated by a persisting air leak over 3 days. Furthermore, haemothorax development, failure to re-expand the lung, bilateral involvement and tension hazard are indications. Patients with an occupational risk hazard are a classic indication. Some authors have proposed that all young patients with a diagnosed spontaneous pneumothorax should be spared a drain thoracostomy and proceed directly to surgical intervention. This approach is not standard treatment, though many patients are operated on as a result of complication or disease recurrence. See table 2 for indications for surgery in primary spontaneous pneumothorax.

Surgical therapy The principles of surgical intervention for spontaneous pneumothorax consist of bulla or bleb resection (fig. 4) and obliteration of the pleural space to prevent recurrence.

Recurrence is the most common indication for surgery in patients with a primary spontaneous pneumothorax.

Multiple wedge resections may also be required when the disease is present at several sites. Segmentectomy and lobectomy are usually unnecessary and are contraindicated.

Obliteration of the pleural space is thought to be necessary to prevent recurrences. It is accomplished by mechanical abrasion, or by parietal apical pleurectomy (fig. 5), which is performed in association with resection of the lung during a video-assisted thoracoscopy.

This operation is carried out under general anaesthesia with a dual-lumen endotracheal tube. Only two thoracic incisions are made for the thoracoscope and dissecting or stapling instruments.

Apical parietal pleurectomy can be performed easily using this technique with modern endo-scissors and forceps.

Video-assisted surgery is recommended as the first-line surgical treatment for patients with recurrent primary spontaneous pneumothorax. This recommendation is based on its favourable early postoperative course without major complication and the long-term outcome with 3% recurrence and patient satisfaction.

Secondary pneumothorax

Spontaneous pneumothorax can be secondary to a variety of pulmonary and nonpulmonary disorders.

Table 2. Indications for surgery in primary spontaneous pneumothorax

First episode
Prolonged air leak
Non re-expansion of the lung
Bilateral pneumothoraces
Haemopneumothorax
Occupational hazard (flight personnel, divers)
Absence of medical facilities in isolated area
Tension pneumothorax
Associated single large bulla
Individual indication
Second episode
Ipsilateral recurrence
Contralateral recurrence after a first pneumothorax

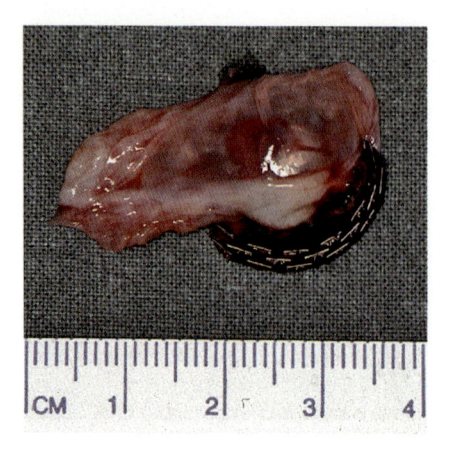

Figure 4. Specimen of an apical bulla resected by stapler.

Chronic obstructive pulmonary disease (COPD) is the most common cause of secondary pneumothorax (fig. 6, table 3). It occurs typically in patients aged >50 yrs and is the result of a bulla rupture into the pleural space.

Most patients with COPD and pneumothorax present with chest pain and acute sudden respiratory distress. These patients show little tolerance to even a small pneumothorax because of their limited pulmonary function. The diagnosis is difficult due to physical findings associated with COPD

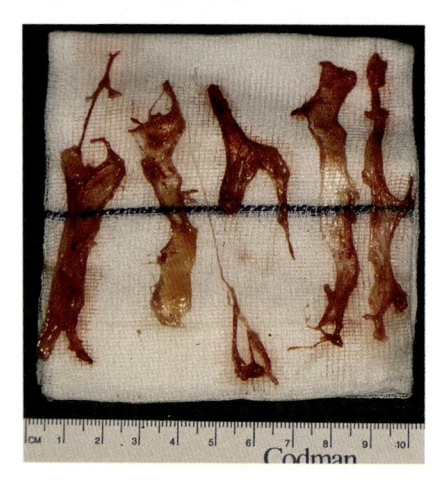

Figure 5. Specimen of apical parietal pleurectomy.

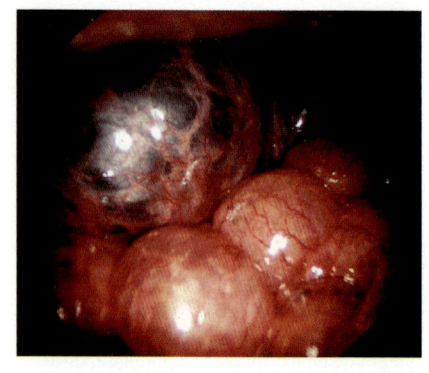

Figure 6. Thoracoscopic view of bullous emphysema with pneumothorax.

(*e.g.* hyperresonance on percussion and diminished breath sounds at auscultation). In most cases, the diagnosis is made by chest radiographs, which are also difficult to interpret because of the increased radiolucency of the diseased lung. For these difficult cases, computed tomography may be necessary to confirm the diagnosis, localise the pneumothorax and facilitate distinction between a large bulla and a pneumothorax.

The emergency treatment of patients with a secondary pneumothorax is similar to that described for primary spontaneous pneumothorax, except that observation alone is seldom justified. If the pleural space is adequately drained and the lung maintains a re-expanded state, the air leak eventually closes. In some patients, however, a bronchopleural fistula persists for 10–15 days, and surgical repair must be considered.

When surgery is required, the procedure must be individualised and based on the extent and disease infiltration, as well as the air leak location.

Staple resection of the bullae should be carried out, followed by a subtotal parietal pleurectomy or pleural abrasion.

The mortality rate for this surgery may reach 10% and morbidity is significant in those individuals with a poor overall physical condition. Other options, such as chemical

Table 3. Causes of secondary pneumothorax

Airway and pulmonary disease
Chronic obstructive pulmonary disease (bullous or diffuse emphysema)
Asthma
Cystic fibrosis
Intersitial lung disease
Pulmonary fibrosis (fig. 7)
Sarcoidosis
Infectious disease
Tubercular and other mycobacterial
Bacterial
Pneumocystis carinii
Parasitic
Mycotic
AIDS
Neoplasic
Bronchogenic carcinoma
Metastatic (lymphoma or sarcoma)
Catamenial
Endometriosis
Miscellaneous
Marfan's syndrome
Ehlers-Danlos syndrome
Histiocytosis X
Scleroderma
Lymphangiomyomatosis
Collagen disease

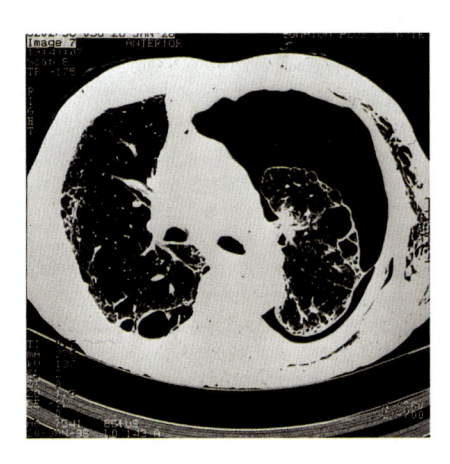

Figure 7. Severe pulmonary fibrosis with pneumothorax on the left side.

pleurodesis, autologous blood injection and permanent fistula drainage can be considered in individual cases.

Summary

Primary spontaneous pneumothorax occurs in young patients with no evidence of coexisting lung disease while secondary pneumothorax is mostly seen in emphysema patients. Unless there is a complication, most surgeons will manage the first episode by conventional tube drainage. Recurrences are treated by bulla or bleb resection with apical parietal pleurectomy. Video-assisted surgery is the safest approach with excellent long-term results.

References

- Abolnik IZ, et al. On the inheritance of primary spontaneous pneumothorax. *Am J Med Genet* 1991; 40: 155-158.
- Aguinagalde B, et al. Percutaneous aspiration versus tube drainage for spontaneous pneumothorax: systematic review and meta-analysis. *Eur J Cardiothorac Surg* 2010; 37: 1129-1135.
- Baumann MH, et al. Management of spontaneous pneumothorax: an American College of Chest Physicians Delphi consensus statement. *Chest* 2001; 119: 590-602.
- Ben-Nun A, et al. Video-assisted thoracoscopic surgery for recurrent spontaneous pneumothorax: the long-term benefit. *World J Surg* 2006; 30: 285-290.
- Beshay M, et al. Emphysema and secondary pneumothorax in young adults smoking cannabis. *Eur J Cardiothorac Surg* 2007; 32: 834-838.
- Chambers A, Scarci M. In patients with first-episode primary spontaneous pneumothorax is video-assisted thoracoscopic surgery superior to tube thoracostomy alone in terms of time to resolution of pneumothorax and incidence of recurrence? *Interact Cardiovasc Thorac Surg* 2009; 9: 1003-1008.
- Chen JS, et al. Management of recurrent primary spontaneous pneumothorax after thoracoscopic surgery: should observation, drainage, redo thoracoscopy, or thoracotomy be used? *Surg Endosc* 2009; 23: 2438-2444.
- Henry M, et al. BTS guidelines for the management of spontaneous pneumothorax. *Thorax* 2003; 58: Suppl. 2, ii39-ii52.

MEDIASTINITIS

P-E. Falcoz, N. Santelmo and G. Massard
Université Louis Pasteur and Hôpitaux Universitaires de Strasbourg, Strasbourg, France
E-mail: pierre-emmanuel.falcoz@wanadoo.fr

The majority of acute mediastinal infections results from oesophageal perforation or infection following a trans-sternal cardiac procedure. Occasionally, acute mediastinitis results from oropharyngeal abscesses with severe cervical infection spreading along the fascial planes into the mediastinum. This particularly virulent form of mediastinal infection is described as descending necrotising mediastinitis (DNM).

DNM is a potentially lethal condition especially if diagnosis or treatment is delayed or inappropriate. Despite the introduction of modern antimicrobial therapy and computed tomographic (CT) imaging, DNM has continued to produce high mortality rates (reported between 25% and 40%).

Criteria for diagnosis of DNM

Criteria for diagnosis of DNM have been accurately defined as follows:

- Clinical manifestations of a severe infection.
- Establishment of a relationship between an oropharyngeal or cervical infection and subsequent mediastinitis.
- Demonstration of radiographic features characteristic of DNM.
- Documentation of a necrotising mediastinal infection at the time of operative debridement or necropsy.

Epidemiology

Primary sites of infection are peridontal abscess, retropharyngeal abscess, and peritonsillar abscess. According to

Key points

- DNM is a particularly virulent and potentially lethal mediastinal infection.
- Initial presentation is toxic shock and respiratory difficulty, sometimes with other signs such as erythema and oedema of the neck and upper chest.
- DNM is an emergency, and should be treated with broad-spectrum *i.v.* antibiotics as well as early and aggressive surgical drainage.

WHEATLEY *et al.* (1990), the most common primary oropharyngeal infection is odontogenic (25 of 43 cases) with mandibular second or third molar abscess.

Route of diffusion

Familiarity with the cervical fascial planes is essential in understanding the propagation pathways, symptoms and thoracic complications of cervical infections. The infection from neck to mediastinum spreads along three primary routes: *via* the retropharyngeal space, the perivascular space and the pretracheal space. The retropharyngeal space has been thought to be the most important route by which a cervical infectious disease spreads to the mediastinum (70% of cases in the series of MONCADA *et al.* (1978)). Rapid spread of infection is facilitated by tissue necrosis (loose of anatomical structure), gravity and negative intrathoracic pressure.

Pathogens involved

DNM is a polymicrobial process with anaerobic organisms being the most predominant. FREEMAN et al. (2000) reviewed the English literature and found 96 patients with DNM between 1990 and 1999. All but four (4%) had mixed aerobic and anaerobic infection, with those pathogens acting often synergistically; in the four exceptions, the sole pathogen was β-haemolytic *Streptococcus*. CHOW et al. (1978) reported that anaerobes had been recovered from 94% of patients with DNM; 52% had mixed infections and 88% had polymicrobial infections.

Clinical and radiological signs

Anamnesis:

- *Phase I*: periodontal or peritonsillar abscess treated by simple antibiotherapy.
- *Phase II*: erythema and oedema of the neck ± associated with subcutaneous emphysema.
- *Phase III*: acute aggravation of the infectious syndrome; onset of cough, dyspnoea, sternal pain and painful dysphagia.

Patients with DNM usually present with toxic shock and respiratory difficulty. Other presenting signs may include erythema and oedema of the neck and upper chest. In severe infections, frank necrosis of skin, fascia and muscle may be present. In the chest, DNM may produce abscesses and empyemas, pleural and pericardial effusions, intrathoracic haemorrhage and cardiac tamponade, and frequently results in the death of the patient.

Delay of diagnosis is one of the primary reasons for high mortality in DNM. Diagnosis of DNM from conventional radiographic studies may be difficult, principally because the signs appear late in the course of the disease. Cervicothoracic CT imaging is currently considered as the diagnostic study of choice for patients in whom DNM is suspected. Indeed, CT scan findings have been proven to confirmed the diagnosis of DNM with high accuracy in these patients who often have a nonspecific constellation of symptoms. Various CT imaging findings are increased attenuation of mediastinal fat, air fluid levels, pleural and pericardial effusions, oesophageal thickening and enlarged lymph nodes. BRUNELLI et al. (1996) found cervicothoracic CT imaging to be immediately diagnostic in all patients in whom it was used.

Treatment

Principles of treatment are:

- Emergency.
- Intravenous broad-spectrum antibiotic therapy: probabilistic and secondarily adapted to the pathogen(s).
- Early and aggressive surgical drainage: extensive debridement, excision of necrotic tissue, bacteriological sampling, mediastinal and pleural irrigation, feeding jejunostomy.

The decision on the type of surgical drainage to be employed is a crucial one. Four approaches have been classically reported: transcervical, standard posterolateral thoracotomy, median sternotomy and transthoracic *via* subyphoid or clamshell incision. Thoracoscopic approach and video-assisted mediastinoscopic drainage can also be found. Although each of these techniques offers potential advantages and disadvantages, the posterolateral thoracotomy incision (sometimes bilateral) remains the standard by which other transthoracic approaches should be measured.

The optimal surgical approach for mediastinal drainage is theoritically dependent on the level of diffusion of necrotising process. Several studies have reported that mediastinal drainage is best accomplished through a transthoracic approach when the necrotising process extends below the level of the fourth thoracic vertebra posteriorly or the tracheal bifurcation anteriorly. However, because of the rapid spread of this type of infection, other investigators have advocated mandatory transthoracic mediastinal exploration regardless of the level of infection. This latter point was confirmed in a meta-analysis, where a statistically significant difference ($p<0.05$) in survival was found between patients undergoing transcervical mediastinal drainage (53%) *versus* those receiving transthoracic mediastinal drainage (81%).

Close-watch care Recurrent abscesses and collections are common after first operative drainage (50%) and they should be drained promptly. CT scan (at best) or ultrasound-guided percutaneous drainage (for lack) of recurrent abscesses and collections may decrease the need for recurrent surgical procedures in these critically ill patients. Surveillance should be continued until no evidence of progressive infection is found on CT imaging and the patient displays no clinical signs of infection. Hyperbaric oxygen therapy has not shown any real proof of effectiveness in this particular framework, when looking at evidence-based medicine. It should not take the place or delay surgical treatment.

Mediastinal fibrosis Fibrosing mediastinitis is an uncommon chronic sequela of prior infectious mediastinal involvement. A chronic, noninfectious inflammatory process results in progressive mediastinal fibrosis. The fibrosis may constrict or obstruct virtually any of the mediastinal organs (in particular, superior vena cava, oesophagus, pulmonary vein or artery). CT scans demonstrate a localised (or less frequently diffuse) mass infiltrating the mediastinum and constricting the structure; extensive calcification is associated with the fibrotic mass in a vast majority of the cases. This appearance is pathognomonic of the disorder.

Conclusions

DNM is caused by downward spread of neck infections and constitutes a highly fatal complication of oropharyngeal lesions. CT imaging should be performed in all patients with persistent symptoms of septicaemia after being treated for oropharyngeal infections. Prompt surgical drainage of the mediastinum should be performed. Optimal mediastinal drainage method should be tailored to each patient's condition and extension of the mediastinitis (posterolateral thoracotomy is frequently required). In the postoperative period, progression of the disease and effectiveness of surgical therapy should be monitered by CT scanning. Further drainage should be carried out if necessary either surgically or by percutaneous drainage.

References

- Brunelli A, *et al.* Descending necrotizing mediastinitis: cervicotomy or thoracotomy? *J Thorac Cardiovasc Surg* 1996; 111: 485-486.
- Chow AW, *et al.* Orofacial odontogenic infections. *Ann Intern Med* 1978; 88: 392-402.
- Corsten MJ, *et al.* Optimal treatment of descending necrotizing mediastinitis. *Thorax* 1997; 52: 702-708.
- Devaraj A, *et al.* Computed tomography findings in fibrosing mediastinitis. *Clin Radiol* 2007; 62: 781-786.
- Estera AS, *et al.* Descending necrotizing mediastinitis. *Surg Gynecol Obstet* 1983; 157: 545-552.
- Freeman RK, *et al.* Descending necrotizing mediastinitis: an analysis of the effects of serial surgical debridement on patient mortality. *J Thorac Cardiovasc Surg* 2000; 119: 260-267.
- Marty-Ané CH, *et al.* Management of descending necrotizing mediastinitis: an aggressive treatment for an aggressive disease. *Ann Thorac Surg* 1999; 68: 212-217.
- Moncada R, *et al.* Mediastinitis from odontogenic and deep cervical infection: anatomic pathways of propagation. *Chest* 1978; 73: 497-500.
- Shimizu K, *et al.* Successful video-assisted mediastinoscopic drainage of descending necrotizing mediastinitis. *Ann Thorac Surg* 2006; 81: 2279-2281.
- Wheatley MJ, *et al.* Descending necrotizing mediastinitis: transcervical drainage is not enough. *Ann Thorac Surg* 1990; 49: 780-784.

NEUROMUSCULAR DISORDERS

A. Vianello
Respiratory Physiology Division, University-City Hospital of Padova, Padova, Italy
E-mail: avianello@qubisoft.it

Various neuromuscular diseases (NMD) can progress to the point where they cause pulmonary complications (table 1); a careful respiratory follow-up adapted to the variable time course of each disease is therefore mandatory. Although the diseases have different causes and clinical courses, common principles apply in their management.

Key points

- NMD have a range of causes, but common principles apply to their treatment.
- Treatment focuses on ventilatory assistance and assisted coughing techniques.

Evaluation of patients with suspected respiratory impairment

Clinical evaluation As the first step, a systematic clinical evaluation is essential to detect the subtle respiratory symptoms and signs related to respiratory muscle failure. Symptoms are frequently nonspecific, including fatigue, lethargy, or difficulty in concentrating. Dyspnoea and orthopnoea are often late findings in patients with usually severe functional impairment due to peripheral muscle weakness. Patients with sleep-disordered breathing (SDB) often seem to have symptoms such as an unrefreshed feeling upon awakening, morning headaches, disappearance of snoring, daytime tiredness, and irritability as a result of repeated arousals and carbon dioxide retention. Physical evaluation is essential and may reveal an increase in respiratory rate, followed by alternating abdominal and rib cage breathing (respiratory alternans), the absence of outward excursion of the abdomen during inspiration or even paradoxical inward inspiratory movement due to diaphragm weakness (abdominal paradox), accessory muscle recruitment, and mucous encumbrance of upper or lower airways.

Indicators of bulbar muscle involvement include dysarthria, trouble swallowing liquids, aspiration manifesting as a new-onset cough, or frank choking.

Pulmonary function testing Pulmonary function tests (PFT) should be routinely performed during the evaluation of patients with NMD. Because of the inadequacy of inspiratory muscle function, PFT generally reveals a pattern of restrictive ventilatory defect, with the following characteristics:

- preserved total lung capacity until a far-advanced stage of the disease
- elevated residual volume
- reduced vital capacity (VC)
- preserved functional residual capacity

When VC falls below 55% of predicted values, the onset of insidiously progressive hypercapnia is likely. A significant difference between upright and recumbent lung volumes has been reported frequently for patients with

Table 1. NMD affecting respiratory function

Site of lesion	Specific disorders
Anterior horn cell	Amyotrophic lateral sclerosis Poliomyelitis Type I SMA, intermediate SMA
Peripheral nerve and/or nerve roots	Guillain–Barrè Syndrome Charcot–Marie–Tooth disease
Neuromuscular junction	Congenital myasthenia
Muscle	Duchenne/Becker muscular dystrophy Limb-girdle muscular dystrophy (especially types 2C-2F-2I) Facio-scapolo-humeral muscular dystrophy Congenital muscular dystrophy Congenital myotonic dystrophy Acid maltase deficiency Congenital myopathy Mitochondrial myopathy Bethlem myopathy

SMA: spinal muscular atrophy.

NMD; in particular, a fall in VC of ⩾25% has been considered a sensitive indicator of diaphragmatic weakness. A specific evaluation of respiratory muscle strength is mandatory as these tests are both sensitive and highly prognostic. A high-negative maximal inspiratory pressure (MIP) result (<-80 cm H_2O) or a high positive maximal expiratory pressure result (>+90 cmH_2O) excludes clinically relevant inspiratory or expiratory muscle weakness. Cough peak expiratory flow (CPEF) is the single most important factor in determining whether the ability to eliminate bronchial secretions is well preserved. Patients who either alone or with assistance are able to generate a CPEF >260 $L·min^{-1}$ can effectively remove bronchial secretions, whereas those with a CPEF <160 $L·min^{-1}$ usually require tracheal suctioning at the onset of respiratory infections. The frequency of pulmonary function monitoring depends on the rapidity of progression of the neuromuscular syndrome and may range from every 1–2 months to yearly. Once the VC drops below 40–50% predicted, or MIP below 30% predicted, daytime arterial blood gases should be performed.

Sleep study All patients with NMD should be monitored carefully for the presence of SDB. Nocturnal oximetry alone is inadequate at detecting sleep apnoea and hypoventilation. In addition, criteria defining significant desaturations remain controversial. Overnight polysomnography (PLSG) or respiratory polygraphy (RP) is advisable for patients who develop symptoms and signs of

Examinations required in the assessment of respiratory function in patients with NMD are:

- Checklist of symptoms and signs.
- Vital capacity sitting or standing, and lying.
- Maximal inspiratory and expiratory pressures.
- Cough-peak expiratory flow.
- Arterial blood gases, if symptoms present.
- PLSG or RP, if symptoms or nocturnal RF present.

sleep-wake abnormality or nocturnal respiratory failure (RF). It has been suggested that PLSG or RP should be performed in all NMD patients as early as possible to take a baseline recording. It should be repeated according to the course of the disease to detect abnormalities during sleep and subsequent indication to long-term ventilatory treatment.

Management

Noninvasive positive pressure ventilation (NPPV) In recent years, the approach of care in neuromuscular RF has been revised, due to two new critical developments: 1) technology has advanced and several new types of ventilatory aids have been introduced, which deliver effective mechanical ventilation (MV), even noninvasively. 2) the majority of severely disabled ventilator users have expressed satisfaction with their lives, even though they are usually unable to achieve some of the goals associated with acceptable quality of life in the "normal" population.

As a consequence, increasing numbers of NMD patients with advanced respiratory impairment are now being successfully treated by long-term NPPV usually in the home setting. The non-invasive administration of positive pressure ventilation requires a positive pressure ventilator delivering pressurised gas to the lungs through an interface with the nose or mouth, or both. In recent years, manufacturers have developed a new generation of microprocessor-controlled ventilators that supply both volume- and pressure-limited modes. Also, special features have been incorporated that are designed to facilitate the application of noninvasive techniques and are simple, reliable and easy for the patient to use.

Long-term NPPV is required when spontaneous respiratory muscle efforts are unable to sustain adequate alveolar ventilation, causing chronic-stable, or slowly progressive RF.

Indications for NPPV therapy in chronic NMD are:

1. Symptoms (such as fatigue, dyspnoea, morning headache) and one of the following:

2. Physiological criteria:

- Significant daytime CO_2 retention (arterial CO_2 tension > 50 mmHg).

- Nocturnal oxygen desaturation (arterial oxygen saturation $<88\%$ for at least five consecutive minutes).

- Forced VC $<50\%$ predicted or MIP <60 cmH_2O, only for rapidly progressive disease.

The following complications are considered to be contraindications for the noninvasive ventilatory approach:

- Severely impaired swallowing, leading to chronic aspiration and repeated pneumonia.

- Ineffective clearing of tracheobronchial secretions, despite the use of noninvasive manual or mechanical expiratory aids.

- The need for around-the-clock (>20 h) ventilatory support.

These conditions usually require an invasive application of MV *via* tracheostomy. There is no consensus on the optimal interface to use in delivering NPPV: nasal masks are usually preferable for nocturnal ventilation, due to the fact that they are more comfortable and permit better speech; conversely, oronasal interfaces may be a suitable alternative for subjects who have excessive air leaking through the mouth or nose. Mouthpiece interfaces have also been successfully used to deliver NPPV for up to 24 h·day[-1]. Finally, the choice of ventilator and interface in most cases is individualised according to patients' preference and physicians' intuition and experience, rather than based on standardised evidence-based guidelines. Administration of NPPV to NMD patients with chronic RF may be expected to allow some individuals with nonprogressive pathology to live to nearly normal life expectancy, extend survival by many years in patients with other conditions, improve physiological lung function and quality of life (QoL), as well as decrease the frequency of exacerbations requiring acute care facilities. Although ineffective for prolonging survival in patients with rapidly progressive conditions and advanced bulbar muscle involvement, such as amyotrophic lateral sclerosis/motor neurone disease, NPPV may be added with the aim of improving some aspects of the QoL, in particular energy, vitality and symptoms related to SDB, being considered as an important part of the total palliative care plan for terminally ill cases.

Assisted coughing techniques The onset of acute RF in patients with advanced stage NMD may be caused by airway encumbrance with mucous as a result of weakened respiratory muscles and an inability to cough effectively. A noninvasive approach to the management of tracheobronchial secretions, based on the combination of expiratory muscle aid and NPPV, has been proposed. This treatment strategy may result in a reduced need for nasal suctioning and conventional intubation, and/or tracheostomy. Among noninvasive expiratory aids, manually assisted coughing (MAC) techniques have been demonstrated to be effective in facilitating the elimination of airway secretions. Additionally, mechanical insufflation-exsufflation (MI-E) has been shown to effectively mobilise mucous secretions and has been proposed as a complement to MAC techniques in the prevention of pulmonary morbidity during respiratory tract infections (fig. 1). MI-E can be administered by a device consisting of a two-stage axial compressor that provides positive pressure to the airway, then rapidly shifts to negative pressure, thereby generating a forced expiration.

Conclusion

It is now clear that life can be greatly prolonged for most individuals with NMD by the availability of noninvasive aids and that the great majority of severely disabled patients submitted to ventilatory assistance are satisfied with their lives. Clinicians with a special competence in the management of such patients have the responsibility of offering these treatment options, encouraging the patients to decide in advance whether or not these measures would be acceptable.

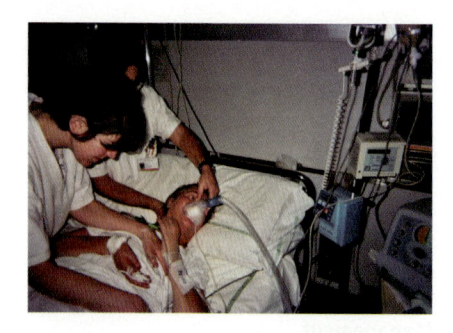

Figure 1. Application of mechanical insufflation-exsufflation combined with manually assisted coughing during respiratory tract infection.

References

- Bach JR, et al. Prevention of pulmonary morbidity for patients with Duchenne muscular dystrophy. Chest 1997; 112: 1024-1028.
- Bourke SC, et al. Effects of non-invasive ventilation on survival and quality of life in patients with amyotrophiclateral sclerosis: a randomised controlled trial. Lancet Neurol 2006; 5: 140-147.
- Braun NM, et al. Respiratory muscle and pulmonary function in polymyositis and other proximal myopathies. Thorax 1983; 38: 616-623.
- Clinical indications for noninvasive positive pressure ventilation in chronic respiratory failure due to restrictive lung disease, COPD, and nocturnal hypoventilation – a consensus conference report. Chest 1999; 116: 521-534.
- Gomez-Merino E, Bach JR. Duchenne muscular dystrophy: prolongation of life by noninvasive ventilation and mechanically assisted coughing. Am J Phys Med Rehabil 2002; 81: 411-415.
- Hill NS. Ventilator management for neuromuscular disease. Semin Respir Crit Care Med 2002; 23: 293-305.
- Kohler M, et al. Quality of life, physical disability, and respiratory impairment in Duchenne muscular dystrophy. Am J Respir Crit Care Med 2005; 172: 1032-1036.
- Lofaso F, Quera-Salva MA. Polysomnography for the management of progressive neuromuscular disorders. Eur Respir J 2002; 19: 989-990.

- Mellies U, *et al.* Daytime predictors of sleep disordered breathing in children and adolescents with neuromuscular disorders. *Neuromusc Disord* 2003; 13: 123-128.
- Polkey MI, *et al.* Respiratory aspects of neurological disease. *J Neurol Neurosurg Psychiatry* 1999; 66: 5-15.
- Simonds A, *et al.* Impact of nasal ventilation on survival in hypercapnic Duchenne muscular dystrophy. *Thorax* 1998; 53: 949-952.
- Simonds AK. Recent advances in respiratory care for neuromuscular disease. *Chest* 2006; 130: 1879-1886.
- Vianello A, *et al.* Long-term nasal intermittent positive pressure ventilation in advanced Duchenne's muscular dystrophy. *Chest* 1994; 105: 445-448.
- Vianello A, *et al.* Mechanical insufflation-exsufflation improves outcomes for neuromuscular disease patients with respiratory tract infections. *Am J Phys Med Rehabil* 2005; 84: 83-88.
- Vianello A, *et al.* Non-invasive ventilatory approach to treatment of acute respiratory failure in neuromuscular disorders. A comparison with endotracheal intubation. *Int Care Med* 2000; 26: 384-390.

CHEST WALL DISORDERS

P-E. Falcoz, N. Santelmo and G. Massard
Université de Strasbourg and Hôpitaux Universitaires de Strasbourg, Strasbourg, France
E-mail: pierre-emmanuel.falcoz@chru-strasbourg.fr

There is a large and diverse group of congenital abnormalities of the thorax that manifest as deformities and/or defect of the anterior chest wall. Depending on the severity of the case, the cardiopulmonary sphere (tolerance to exercise) as well as the psychological area may be implicated.

This diverse group includes pectus excavatum (PE), pectus carinatum (PC), Poland syndrome and cleft sternum. Among them, the two most common chest wall abnormalities are PE ("funnel chest") and PC ("keel chest").

Pathogenesis

Over the years, the theories concerning the pathogenesis of pectus deformities evolved from substernal ligament traction to overgrowth of the rib cartilage and later to a stress–strain imbalance. The genetic aspects of pectus deformities have just started to emerge and hopefully will answer many questions unanswered so far.

PE

PE is a recessively inherited chest wall deformities with an occurrence of 0.3% of all births (9:1 predominance in males). In patients with PE, the normal moderately convex contour of the anterior chest wall is replaced by precordial depression. Depending on the severity of the anomaly, the sterno-vertebral space is narrowed, there is a shift of the heart into the left hemithorax and pulmonary expansion is confined.

The PE indications for surgery may be summarised as follows:

- Aesthetic (psychological repercussion)
- Symptom
- Exercise intolerance; decreased endurance; exercise-induced asthma
- Body images issues (computed tomography (CT) scan)
- Pain
- Abnormal/low forced vital capacity, forced expiratory volume in 1 s, maximum voluntary ventilation
- Decreased oxygen pulse, oxygen uptake, minute ventilation
- Echocardiogram: compression of right atrium/right ventricle (rare)
- CT Haller index >3.0
- Calliper measurement depth > 2.5

Key points

- The two most common chest wall abnormalities are pectus excavatum and pectus carinatum.
- The two most common surgical procedures for pectus excavatum repair are the modified Ravitch technique and the Nuss technique.
- Careful pre-operative evaluation on the basis of clinical but also psychological symptoms is required to select potential candidates for surgical remodelling.
- The optimal timing of surgical repair would be after the main growth has stopped (late teens or early 20s).

PC

In PC, the clinical aspect includes a variety of protrusion deformities of the anterior chest wall. The most common variety consists of anterior displacement of the sternal gladiolus with the appropriate cartilages in tow. In severe forms, there is also a narrowing of the transverse diameter of the chest, which seems to further exaggerate the anomaly.

The PC indications for surgery may be summarised as follows:

- Aesthetic (psychological repercussion)
- Pain
- Frequent injury
- Body image issues
- Abnormal pulmonary function testing

Surgical treatment

PE Although there are a number of different techniques utilised by surgeons, most repairs performed today will be either the modified Ravitch technique or the Nuss procedure (note that the "Wada" procedure of sternal turnover is no longer realised).

The *Ravitch technique* requires the exposition of the thorax's anterior region (horizontal inframammary fold incision preferred) with resection of costal cartilages affected bilaterally, the performance of a cross-sternal osteotomy with the placing of a temporary stabiliser (support bar anterior to the sternum), and the development of a muscular flap.

The *Nuss technique* is an alternative and new technique done by means of minimally invasive surgery and based on the skeleton's malleability and the remodelling capacity of the thorax. The techique consists in the implantation of a retrosternal steel bar that would modify the concavity of the sternum while maintaining the contour of the reformed thorax, all done by means of two small incisions on each side of the thorax.

PC The repair of PC, including exposure, detachment of the pectoralis muscles, transverse osteotomy and resection of the deformed cartilages, is largely identical to that described in PE. Operative correction required double bilateral chondrotomy parasternally and at points of transition to normal ribs, followed by detorsion of the sternum, retrosternal mobilisation and correction of the everted sternum, as well as of the everted and inverted ribs. After incomplete wedge osteotomy the mobilised sternum is finally stabilised by a temporary support bar anterior to the sternum and cartilages (in place for at least 6 months).

Controversies

Some controversies do need to be mentioned:

First, concerning PE, there has never been a randomised controlled trial comparing the results of the two most common surgical procedures (there is currently an ongoing evaluation from a multi-centre study). Secondly, concerning the optimal timing of surgical repair, it seems that the best time for repair would be after the main growth has stopped (*i.e.* after adolescence in the late teens or early 20s), as opposed to an early repair. Although the operation is more traumatic after adolescence, the results are far better with minimal recurrence. Thirdly, the goal of such an approach remains elusive. Not only are we unable to reach an agreement on such simple issues as how to measure the clinical or even the anatomical severity of pectues deformities, but we are still engaged in a seemingly endless debate with the insurance companies as to whether these often physiologically and psychologically crippling abnormalities should be even considered a "disease" at all.

Conclusions

Chest wall abnormalities, PE and PC, are a relatively rare problem, but are commonly seen in the practice of general thoracic surgery. Careful pre-operative evaluation on the basis of clinical but also psychological symptoms is required to select potential candidates for surgical remodelling. Surgical procedures, based on the surgeon's personal expertise, are currently relatively well codified and provide satisfactory results with a low rate of complications.

References

- Colombani PM. Preoperative assessment of chest wall deformities. *Semin Thorac Cardiovasc Surg* 2009; 21: 58-63.
- Feng J, *et al.* The biomechanical, morphologic, and histochemical properties of the costal cartilages in children with pectus excavatum. *J Pediatr Surg* 2001; 36: 1770-1776.
- Fonkalsrud EW, Anselmo DM. Less extensive techniques for repair of pectus carinatum: the undertreated chest deformity. *J Am Coll Surg* 2004; 198: 898-905.
- Gurnett CA, *et al.* Genetic linkage localizes an adolescent idiopathic scoliosis and pectus excavatum gene to chromosome 18 q. *Spine (Phila Pa 1976)* 2009; 34: E94-E100.
- Haller JA, *et al.* Evolving management of pectus excavatum based on a single institutional experience of 664 patients. *Ann Surg* 1989; 209: 578-583.
- Huddelston CB. Pectus excavatum. *Semin Thorac Cardiovasc Surg* 2004; 16: 225-232.
- Nuss D, *et al.* A ten-year review of minimally invasive technique for the correction of pectus excavatum. *J Pediatr Surg* 1998; 33: 545-552.
- Ravitch MM. The operative treatment of pectus excavatum. *Ann Surg* 1949; 129: 429-444.
- Robicsek F, Fokin AA. Surgical repair of anterior chest wall deformities: the past, the present, the future. Introduction. *Semin Thorac Cardiovasc Surg* 2009; 21: 43.
- Robiscek F, *et al.* Surgical repair of pectus excavatum and carinatum. *Semin Thorac Cardiovasc Surg* 2009; 21: 64-75.
- Saxena AK, Willital GH. Surgical repair of pectus carinatum. *Int Surg* 1999; 84: 326-330.
- Shamberger SC, Hardy Hendren W III. Congenital deformities. *In*: Pearson FG, et al., eds. Thoracic Surgery. New York, Churchill Livingstone, 1995; pp. 1189-1209.

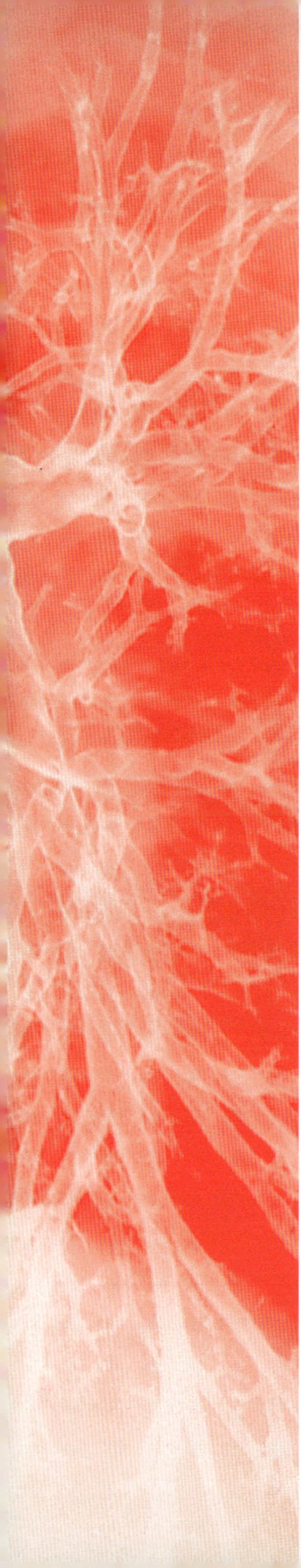

CHAPTER 14:

THORACIC TUMOURS

LUNG CANCER   372
J. Vansteenkiste and S. Derijcke

CHEMOTHERAPY AND OTHER ANTI-TUMOUR   377
THERAPY FOR THORACIC MALIGNANCIES
A. Tufman and R.M. Huber

PRINCIPLES OF SURGICAL TREATMENT FOR   382
EARLY-STAGE NONSMALL CELL LUNG CANCER
G. Massard, N. Santelmo and P-E. Falcoz

METASTATIC TUMOURS   388
E. Quoix

PLEURAL AND CHEST WALL TUMOURS   392
A. Scherpereel

MEDIASTINAL TUMOURS   399
P.E. Van Schil, P. Lauwers and J.M. Hendriks

LUNG CANCER

J. Vansteenkiste and S. Derijcke
Respiratory Oncology Unit/Pulmonology, University Hospital Leuven, Belgium
E-mail: johan.vansteenkiste@uz.kuleuven.ac.be

Lung cancer is the most common cause of cancer-related mortality worldwide for both males and females, with an incidence of about 1.3 million cases per year. The term lung cancer, or bronchogenic carcinoma, refers to malignancies that originate in the airways or pulmonary parenchyma.

Epidemiology

Lung cancer occurs through a complex multistage process that results from the combination of carcinogen exposure and genetic susceptibility (fig. 1).

A number of lifestyle and environmental factors have been associated with the development of lung cancer, of which cigarette smoking is the most important. Cigarette smoking accounts for ~80–90% of all lung cancers. Compared with nonsmokers, smokers have an ~20-fold increase in lung cancer risk, depending on the duration of smoking and the number of cigarettes smoked per day. Cigarette smokers can benefit at any age from smoking cessation: as the period of abstinence from smoking increases, the risk of lung cancer decreases, although it remains elevated compared with never-smokers. In recent years, an increasing number of never-smoker patients present with a lung cancer, often of adenocarcinoma histology. A number of other factors may also affect the risk of developing lung cancer, such as underlying acquired lung diseases (chronic obstructive pulmonary disease and pulmonary fibrosis) and environmental exposures, often synergistically with smoking (asbestos, radon, metals, ionising radiation including previous radiotherapy and polycyclic aromatic hydrocarbons).

Several molecular genetic abnormalities have been described in lung cancer, including chromosomal aberrations (*e.g.* chromosome 3p or 8p deletions), overexpression of oncogenes (K-ras, c-MET, Bcl-2, *etc.*), deletions and/or mutations in tumour suppressor genes (p53, retinoblastoma gene, genes on chromosome 3p) or altered telomerase activity.

Classification of malignant lung tumours

The World Health Organization (WHO) classification of lung tumours is based on histological characteristics in surgical samples or biopsies and is primarily based on light-optic microscopy. The following major subcategories can be distinguished:

Pre-invasive lesions: mild, moderate, severe squamous dysplasia and carcinoma *in situ* are precursors of squamous cell carcinoma, atypical adenomatous hyperplasia of adenocarcinoma; and diffuse idiopathic pulmonary neuroendocrine cell hyperplasia of neuroendocrine tumours.

Small cell lung cancer (SCLC): carcinoma with typical small cells, closely linked to smoking. A

Key points

- Combined modality treatment has improved cure rates for nonmetastatic patients.
- Systemic therapy has improved quantity and quality of life for metastatic patients.

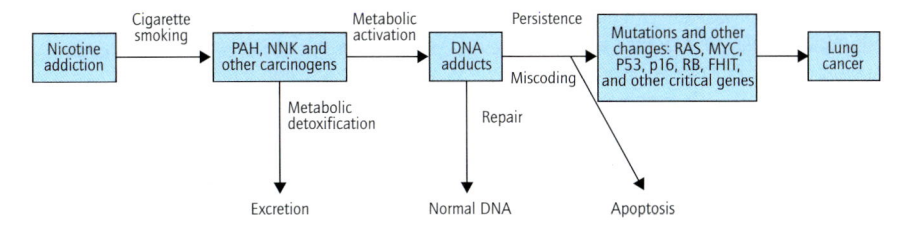

Figure 1. The multistep process leading from nicotine addiction to lung cancer. PAH: polyaromatic hydrocarbons; NHK: nicotine-derived nitrosamine ketone. Reproduced from HECHT (1999), with permission from the publisher.

variant 'combined' type harbours >10% nonsmall cell components.

Nonsmall cell lung cancer (NSCLC): carcinoma with larger cells and a varying degree of squamous epithelial or glandular differentiation. *Squamous cell carcinoma* is a typically centrally located tumour in smokers. *Adenocarcinoma* is the predominant histological subtype and the most prevalent form of lung cancer in younger males (<50 yrs old) and in females of all ages, in never- and former-smokers. *Large cell carcinoma* and large cell neuroendocrine carcinoma (LCNEC); the latter is also described in the spectrum of neuroendocrine tumours extending from the low-grade typical carcinoid over the intermediate-grade atypical carcinoid to high-grade neuroendocrine tumours (LCNEC and SCLC).

Immunohistochemistry (and electron microscopy) are valuable adjuncts for differential diagnosis, *e.g.* the subclassification of NSCLC, the distinction between pleural metastatic adenocarcinoma and mesothelioma (calretinin and cytokeratin). They are required for diagnosis of LCNEC (chromogranin, synaptophysin, neural cell adhesion molecule).

Clinical manifestations

The majority of patients with lung cancer have advanced disease at clinical presentation, which reflects the frequent asymptomatic course of early stage lung cancer.

Symptoms due to the intrathoracic effects of the tumour are cough (central airway or pleural involvement), haemoptysis, chest pain, dyspnoea, hoarseness (laryngeal nerve involvement), superior vena cava syndrome (dilated neck veins, facial oedema), Pancoast's syndrome (pain, Horner sign, hand muscle atrophy).

In addition, paraneoplastic effects of lung cancer are common: hypercalcaemia (nausea, lethargy, dehydration), syndrome of inappropriate antidiuretic hormone (hyponatraemia), hypertrophic osteo-arthropathy (clubbing, periostal proliferation of tubular bones), dermatomyositis, haematological manifestations (anaemia, leukocytosis, thrombocytosis), hypercoagulability, Cushing's syndrome, neurological syndromes (Lambert–Eaton). It is important to distinguish paraneoplastic effects from symptoms due to metastasis, as only the latter impede a radical approach.

As for extrathoracic disease, the most frequent sites of distant metastasis are the liver (pain, constitutional symptoms), adrenal glands, bones (pain) and brain (headache, paresis, seizures). General symptoms such as anorexia, weight loss and asthenia are often also present.

Diagnosis

Bronchoscopy is the appropriate test for centrally located tumours, where a pathological diagnosis will be obtained in ~90% of cases, by means of forceps biopsy, bronchial brushing or washing.

Peripheral lesions, especially solitary pulmonary nodules, can be a diagnostic challenge. Noninvasive techniques are positron emission tomography with ^{18}F-2-fluoro-2-deoxy-D-glucose positron emission tomography (FDG-PET: enhanced uptake of FDG in tumours) or contrast enhanced computed tomography (CT). For most lesions, pathological documentation is needed: peripheral sampling of tissue by bronchoscopy (nowadays with help of endobronchial ultrasound), fine needle aspiration by CT guidance, sometimes surgical sampling by video-assisted thoracoscopy.

Staging

A proposal for revision of the Tumour-Node-Metastasis (TNM) classification of lung tumours was officially adopted for NSCLC, SCLC and carcinoid tumours in 2010. The combination of T, N, and M descriptors determines the overall disease stage: stage I (localised tumour, no lymph node spread), stage II (spread to hilar nodes), stage III (more advanced tumour and/or mediastinal lymph node spread) and stage IV (distant metastasis). The stage defines the prognosis and guides management.

A detailed medical history, physical examination, blood testing and contrast-enhanced CT from the adrenal gland to the lung apex should be performed. According to symptoms and locoregional spread, a CT or magnetic resonnance image of the brain, a bone scintigraphy or other tests may be appropriate. Patients without evident metastatic disease benefit from FDG-PET or fusion FDG-PET-CT, which improve staging of locoregional lymph node and distant spread. The role of PET for SCLC is less well defined.

Functional assessment

In patients scheduled for radical treatment (surgical or nonsurgical combined modality treatment), an appropriate functional evaluation is needed. This can be simple (ECG and basic pulmonary function tests) in fit individuals, but is often more complex because of co-existing smoking-related cardiopulmonary disease. Diffusion capacity, cardiopulmonary exercise testing, measurement of left/right distribution of pulmonary function by, for example, scintigraphy, echocardiography, and other tests may be appropriate.

Performance status (PS), measured by, for example, the Karnofsky or WHO scale, is very important in patients with advanced disease, where it is strongly related to prognosis and treatment choices.

Treatment of NSCLC (table 1)

For fit patients with stage I and II, upfront surgical resection is indicated, followed by adjuvant cisplatin-based chemotherapy in case of lymph node spread or larger-sized (>4–5 cm) primary tumour. Curative conformal radiotherapy is to be considered in medically inoperable patients.

Stage III is subdivided into stage IIIA (ipsilateral mediastinal lymph node spread) or stage IIIB (contralateral). In stage IIIA patients, assessment of resectability in a multidisciplinary group is essential. Patients with resectable stage IIIA benefit from surgical combined modality treatment (induction therapy followed by complete resection), as this approach improves local control, progression-free survival and overall survival if pneumonectomy can be avoided. For patients with unresectable stage IIIA or stage IIIB, nonsurgical combined modality treatment is preferred (chemotherapy plus radiotherapy). For fit patients, concurrent administration is preferred; for others, a sequential approach.

In patients with advanced NSCLC and good PS (Karnofsky >80%), two-drug platinum-based chemotherapy is indicated because of modest gain in survival and improved symptom control and quality-of-life. Recent data point at the importance of histology for treatment: patients with adenocarcinoma have a superior outcome with cisplatin-pemetrexed chemotherapy, while the opposite is true for squamous cell carcinoma, where gemcitabine, vinorelbine, or a taxane can be added to platinum. Moreover, some

Table 1. Major staging groups, preferred treatment patterns, and expected 5-yr survival rates for nonsmall cell lung cancer

Group	Stage	Treatment	5-year survival
Early stages	Stage I	Surgical resection (adjuvant chemotherapy for large tumours) Radiotherapy if medically inoperable	58-73%
	Stage II	Surgical resection + adjuvant chemotherapy Radiotherapy if medically inoperable	36-46%
Locally advanced stages	Stage IIIA	Surgical or nonsurgical combined modality treatment	24%
	Stage IIIB	Nonsurgical combined modality treatment	9%
Advanced stage	Stage IV	Chemotherapy and/or targeted agents	<5%

Data from GOLDSTRAW et al. (2007).

adenocarcinomas harbour activating mutations in the epidermal growth factor receptor (EGFR) gene, which predicts a sustained tumour control in case of therapy with EGFR tyrosine kinase inhibitors. Second-line systemic treatment (docetaxel, pemetrexed, erlotinib) also improves disease-related symptoms and survival. Nevertheless, quite some patients have a lower PS. They may be treated with single-agent chemotherapy or best supportive care.

Treatment of SCLC

Patients with stages I–III should be treated with four to six cycles of cisplatin-etoposide chemotherapy in combination with thoracic radiotherapy. Concurrent administration is preferred if the patient is fit enough and if the tumour volume is not too bulky. Prophylactic cranial irradiation (PCI) should be offered to patients with response following chemoradiotherapy, as it reduces the risk of cerebral metastases and improves survival. Patients with stage IV should be treated with platinum (cisplatin or carboplatin) in combination with etoposide for four to six cycles. PCI is added in case of major response after chemotherapy. Patients with good performance status relapsing after response to first-line chemotherapy should be considered for re-treatment, either with repeat platinum-etoposide or with topotecan.

General treatment measures

Radiotherapy plays an important role in palliation of local problems such as vena cava superior syndrome, haemoptysis, postobstructive pneumonia, bone pain and brain metastasis. Endobronchial treatment (cryotherapy, laser resection, endobronchial stenting) may relieve symptoms in patients with major airway obstruction. Overall supportive measures, such as analgesics, corticosteroids, biphosphonates in the case of bone disease, *etc.*, should accompany the primary tumour treatment, or may be the only option in patients with very poor performance status. A multidisciplinary team including doctors, nurses, psychologists, social workers and others will have a major role in the latter situation. Smoking cessation should be advised to all patients in remission after treatment.

References

- Albain KS, *et al.* Radiotherapy plus chemotherapy with or without surgical resection for stage III non-small-cell lung cancer: a phase III randomised controlled trial. *Lancet* 2009; 374: 379–386.
- Alberg AJ, *et al.* Epidemiology of lung cancer: ACCP evidence-based clinical practice guidelines (2nd edition). *Chest* 2007; 132: Suppl. 3, 29S–55S.
- Brambilla E, *et al.* The new World Health Organization classification of lung tumours. *Eur Respir J* 2001; 18: 1059–1068.

- Brunelli A, *et al.* ERS/ESTS clinical guidelines on fitness for radical therapy in lung cancer patients (surgery and chemo-radiotherapy). *Eur Respir J* 2009; 34: 17–41.
- D'Addario G, Felip E. Non-small cell lung cancer: ESMO clinical recommendations for diagnosis, treatment and follow-up. *Ann Oncol* 2009; 20: Suppl. 4, 68–70.
- Goldstraw P, *et al.* The IASLC Lung Cancer Staging Project: proposals for the revision of the TNM stage groupings in the forthcoming (seventh) edition of the TNM Classification of malignant tumours. *J Thorac Oncol* 2007; 2: 706–714.
- Hecht SS. Tobacco smoke carcinogens and lung cancer. *J Natl Cancer Inst* 1999; 91: 1194–1210.
- The International Adjuvant Lung Cancer Trial Collaborative Group, et al, Cisplatin-based adjuvant chemotherapy in patients with completely resected non-small cell lung cancer. *N Engl J Med* 2004; 350: 351–360.
- Mok TS, *et al.* Gefitinib or carboplatin-paclitaxel in pulmonary adenocarcinoma. *N Engl J Med* 2009; 361: 947–957.
- Scagliotti G, *et al.* Phase III study comparing cisplatin plus gemcitabine with cisplatin plus pemetrexed in chemotherapy-naive patients with advanced stage non-small cell lung cancer. *J Clin Oncol* 2008; 26: 3543–3551.
- Sorensen M, Felip E. Small cell lung cancer: ESMO clinical recommendations for diagnosis, treatment and follow-up. *Ann Oncol* 2009; 20: Suppl. 4, 71–72.
- Toh CK, *et al.* Never-smokers with lung cancer: epidemiologic evidence of a distinct disease entity. *J Clin Oncol* 2006; 24: 2245–51.
- Vansteenkiste JF, *et al.* Lymph node staging in non-small cell lung cancer with FDG-PET scan: a prospective study on 690 lymph node stations from 68 patients. *J Clin Oncol* 1998; 16: 2142–2149.

CHEMOTHERAPY AND OTHER ANTI-TUMOUR THERAPY FOR THORACIC MALIGNANCIES

A. Tufman and R.M. Huber
Division of Respiratory Medicine, Medizinische Klinik-Innenstadt,
Ludwig-Maximilians-University, Munich, Germany
E-mail: huber@med.uni-muenchen.de

Key points

- Due to the interdisciplinary nature of lung cancer treatment, decision-making should take place in structured tumour boards.
- SCLC generally responds well to initial chemotherapy.
- Prophylactic cranial irradiation has an important role in the treatment of SCLC.
- First-line treatment of NSCLC is generally a platinum-based doublet.
- Performance status is an important parameter in treatment decision-making.
- The individualisation of treatment based on histology and molecular biology is of increasing importance in NSCLC.
- The side-effects of chemotherapy vary between agents and should be taken into account during treatment planning.
- Endobronchial techniques are an important tool in the palliation of lung cancer patients.

In oncology, chemotherapy involves the use of substances with nonspecific cytotoxic and anti-proliferative properties to control tumour spread and symptoms, improve quality of life and lengthen survival.

Depending on the clinical situation, either a single chemotherapeutic agent or a doublet may be given. In metastatic lung cancer, chemotherapy is palliative; however, in earlier stages of disease it can be curative when combined with local irradiation (radiochemotherapy) or surgery. Chemotherapy given after surgery is known as adjuvant chemotherapy; that administered before surgery is neoadjuvant or induction chemotherapy. Generally, chemotherapy is administered intravenously, although some agents may be given orally. There are also circumstances in which chemotherapeutic agents may be administered locally (intrathecally or in the pleural space). Although most modern chemotherapeutic agents have milder side-effects than the older agents, side-effects remain problematic and include neutropenia, neuropathy, nephropathy, fatigue, hair loss and nausea and vomiting (table 1).

The decision how to treat a patient is dependant not only on the diagnosis itself, but on the patient's comorbidities and overall medical condition, as well as on the overall prognosis and goal of treatment (table 2). Performance status scales attempt to standardise the assessment of a patient's

Table 1. The major side-effects of chemotherapeutic agents

Nausea and vomiting	Cisplatin is highly emetogenic
	Prophylactic anti-emetics should be given to all patients receiving chemotherapy
	Delayed nausea and vomiting may occur days after administration
	Commonly used anti-emetics include dexamethasone, serotonin antagonists and neurokinin-1 inhibition
Neutropenia	Severe neutropenia refers to peripheral neutrophil counts <500 cells·μL^{-1}
	Reverse isolation in hospitalised patients with severe neutropenia may reduce the risk of nosocomial infections
	Febrile neutropenia refers to elevated oral or axillary temperature (>38°C for >1 h, or >38.2°C one-time measurement) in the setting of severe neutropenia, and should be treated with intravenous antibiotics
	The prophylactic use of granulocyte colony-stimulating factors can be considered in those at increased risk of developing febrile neutropenia
Anaemia	Consider transfusion in symptomatic patients or those with very low haemoglobin
	The use of erythrocyte-stimulating factors (*e.g.* erythropoietin) is generally not recommended; however, it can reduce the number of transfusions and improves fatigue
Neuropathy	Most commonly caused by the taxanes and vinorelbine
Fatigue	Multifactorial
	Malnutrition, anaemia and depression commonly play a role

general state of health; the Karnofsky scale and the World Health Organization/Eastern Cooperative Oncology Group (WHO/ECOG) scale are commonly used (table 3).

In most cases the overall management of lung cancer involves a combination of chemotherapy, radiation, bronchoscopic intervention and surgery. For this reason, interdisciplinary tumour boards are an important forum for discussion and decision making in the care of lung cancer patients.

Chemotherapy in small cell lung cancer

First line Small cell lung cancer (SCLC) is almost always a systemic disease and in most cases the initial response to chemotherapy is quite good.

Cisplatin plus etoposide is a frequently used first-line combination, although carboplatin can be used instead of cisplatin in patients with poor prognosis/performance status or contraindications to cisplatin. Another commonly used but less effective regimen is adriamycin, cyclophosphamid, vincristin. In small cell lung cancer, chemotherapy offers a clear survival benefit, from 4–6-week survival in untreated patients with extensive disease, to 12-month survival in extensive disease with chemotherapy.

Second line The second-line treatment of SCLC has been shown to increase survival and quality of life compared with best supportive care alone. Here the choice of medications depends on the length of time since the initial remission. For patients whose tumours initially respond well to chemotherapy and then go on to recur or progress >3–6 months later, the medications used in first-line treatment can be given again. Tumours that progress <3 months after the end of first-line therapy should be treated with different agents: in this setting, topotecan monotherapy is a common choice and can be given intravenously or orally. If the tumour does not respond to first-line therapies or progresses quickly after chemotherapy, second-line treatment is

Table 2. Considerations for individual chemotherapeutic agents

Cisplatin	Highly emetogenic (appropriate use of anti-emetics is essential)
	Nephrotoxic. Avoid in patients with reduced GFR
	Prehydration ($\geq$500 mL NaCl 0.9% per 50 mg cisplatin) reduces the risk of nephrotoxicity
Carboplatin	Consider as alternative to cisplatin in elderly patients or those with contraindications to cisplatin, dosed at AUC
Vinorelbine	May cause neuropathy or neutropenia
	Available in pill form for oral administration
Gemcitabine	30-min infusion time (more toxicity with slower infusion), avoid combination with radiotherapy due to increased side-effects
Pemetrexed	Short (10-min) infusion time
	Effective in patients with nonsquamous cell NSCLC and mesothelioma
	The risk of myelosuppression can be significantly reduced by vitamin B12 (1,000 IU *i.m.* every 9 weeks) and folate (0.35–1 mg·day^{-1})
Paclitaxel	Premedication to prevent allergic reaction is required (dexamethasone and antihistamine)
Docetaxel	Premedication to prevent allergic reaction is required (dexamethasone)

GFR: glomerular filtration rate; AUC: area under the curve; NSCLC: nonsmall cell lung cancer; *i.m.*: intramuscular.

usually recommended. Inclusion in clinical trials or best supportive care alone also are also reasonable options.

Multimodal therapy Studies have shown that adjuvant chemotherapy improves survival in SCLC patients with completely resected very limited disease. In patients with limited disease, local radiation is generally combined with chemotherapy. Concurrent chemoradiation regimens including cisplatin are the most effective. In extensive disease SCLC, thoracic radiation may be considered in patients who have responded well to chemotherapy.

Prophylactic cranial irradiation has been shown to improve survival in SCLC patients who reach good remission after chemotherapy, including those with extensive disease at the time of diagnosis.

Nonsmall cell lung cancer

Chemotherapy is the treatment of choice for nonsmall cell lung cancer (NSCLC) patients with distant metastases or malignant pleural

Table 3. The World Health Organization/Eastern Cooperative Oncology Group (WHO/ECOG) scale

WHO/ECOG Performance status	Description
0	Patient is fully active and unrestricted in daily activities
1	Patient cannot carry out physically strenuous activities, but is able to care for self and carry out light work
2	Patient is ambulatory and can care for self but is unable to work. Up and about for >50% of waking hours
3	Patient is limited in self care activities and confined to bed or chair for >50% of waking hours
4	Completely disabled. Cannot care for self. Totally confined to bed or chair

effusion, although its efficacy is limited. In fit patients, first-line treatment should consist of cisplatin or carboplatin paired with one of gemcitabine, docetaxel, paclitaxel, pemetrexed or vinorelbine, administered over 4–6 cycles. The increase in survival offered by platinum-based chemotherapy is in the range of several months, although some patients experience durable remissions, and there is evidence that chemotherapy improves patients' quality of life and performance status. Unfortunately, ~40% of NSCLC tumours do not respond to chemotherapy and only 20% of NSCLC patients experience significant regression of their tumours. In earlier randomised trials with platinum-based chemotherapy doublets (cisplatin/paclitaxel, cisplatin/gemcitabine, cisplatin/docetaxel, vinorelbin/cisplatin or carboplatin/paclitaxel), there were no significant differences in response rate or overall survival. More recent studies show that histology plays a role in the response of NSCLC to various chemotherapeutic medications. In particular, nonsquamous histology (adenocarcinomas and large cell NSCLC) is predictive for better activity of pemetrexed.

Patients with poor performance status may not tolerate platinum-based doublet chemothrapy, but can often be treated with a single chemotherapeutic agent, for instance gemcitabine or paclitaxel, or in some cases with a carboplatin-based doublet.

Second-/third-line chemotherapy Second/third-line chemotherapy in NSCLC generally involves monotherapy with a chemotherapeutic agent (docetaxel and pemetrexed are licensed in this setting) or, in selected patients, erlotinib. Participation in phase II or III clinical trials with newer targeted agents may offer patients the option of treatment with medications not yet available on the market. There is some recent evidence that early second-line or maintenance therapy may be beneficial, especially for patients who did not respond particularly well to first-line chemotherapy (stable disease patients compared to partial/complete responders).

Targeted therapies The role of targeted therapies in NSCLC is growing rapidly. Unlike traditional chemotherapeutics, which interfere with cell division in all rapidly dividing cells, targeted therapies attempt to inhibit cell activity more selectively at the level of growth factor receptors and intracellular signalling cascades.

The epidermal growth factor receptor (EGFR) is involved in signalling cascades leading to cell division and proliferation. In tumour cells, mutations and overexpression in EGFR or in downstream components of the EGFR pathway increase proliferation, survival and metastasis. Several targeted therapies attempt to interfere with this abnormal EGFR activity: erlotinib and gefitinib are both tyrosine kinase inhibitors (TKIs) which inactivate the intracellular portion or EGFR, whereas cetuximab, as an antibody, binds to the extracellular domain of the receptor. EGFR inhibitors do not cause typical chemotherapy side-effects, but commonly cause clinically significant rash, diarrhoea and liver enzyme elevation.

There is evidence that EGFR mutations in exon 19 and 21 ("activating mutations") predict a good response to EGFR TKIs, whereas other mutations such as T790M predict resistance. Response to EGFR inhibitors is also associated with certain clinical characteristics (female patients, nonsmokers, adenocarcinoma, Asian ethnicity). Erlotinib is approved as a second- or third-line therapy in NSCLC. Gefitinib is only approved for use in patients with a documented activating mutation in EGFR.

Because tumours are dependent on the growth of new blood vessels, inhibition of angiogenesis is of major therapeutic interest. Bevacizumab is a monoclonal antibody against the vascular endothelial growth factor. In stage IIIB and IV NSCLC patients, there is evidence that the addition of bevacizumab to platinum-based doublets is beneficial. The combination of bevacizumab with carboplatin + paclitaxel was shown to provide a survival benefit, whereas the combination of bevacizumab with cisplatin + gemcitabine only showed a benefit in progression-free survival.

Bevacizumab can cause severe haemoptysis, seen in the randomised phase II trial mostly in patients with squamous cell histology. Thereafter, most studies have excluded patients with brain metastases, previous haemoptysis, cavitary lung lesions or concurrent anticoagulation.

Malignant mesothelioma

If systemic treatment is applied, usually cisplatin plus pemetrexed are given. Often more than 6 cycles are used. In patients with contraindications to cisplatin, the off-label use of carboplatin can be considered. There is evidence supporting off-label second-line treatment with vinorelbin, gemcitabine or in some cases with pemetrexed.

Palliative treatments

In advanced lung cancer, progressive tumour growth in the central airways can produce haemoptysis, cough, and airway obstruction leading to shortness of breath or pneumonia. In these situations quality of life may primarily be improved through the palliative use of endoscopic tumour debulking techniques or prosthetic measures. Brachytherapy is also an effective option for the local treatment of tumour growth in or around the central airways, and stents may be used to maintain airway patency in patients with compression due to tumour.

Palliative radiation provides symptomatic relief in patients with brain and bone metastases. Pleurodesis is an option for patients with recurrent malignant pleural effusions.

References

- D'Addario G, Felip E Non-small-cell lung cancer. ESMO Clinical Recommendations for diagnosis, treatment and follow-up. Ann Oncol 2009; 20: Suppl. 4, iv68–iv70.
- Sørensen M, Felip E. Small-cell lung cancer: ESMO Clinical Recommendations for diagnosis, treatment and follow-up. Ann Oncol 2009; 20: Suppl. 4, iv71–iv72.
- Spiro SG, Huber RM, Janes SM. Thoracic Malignancies. *Eur Respir Mon* 2009; 44.
- Stahel RA, Weder W, Felip E. Malignant pleural mesothelioma: ESMO Clinical Recommendations for diagnosis, treatment and follow-up. Ann Oncol 2009; 20: Suppl. 4, iv73–iv75.

Weblinks

- American Society of Clinical Oncology. www.ASCO.org.
- American College of Chest Physicians. www.chestnet.org.

PRINCIPLES OF SURGICAL TREATMENT FOR EARLY-STAGE NONSMALL CELL LUNG CANCER

G. Massard, N. Santelmo and P-E. Falcoz
Department of Thoracic Surgery, Hôpitaux Universitaires de Strasbourg, Strasbourg, France
E-mail: Gilbert.Massard@chru-strasbourg.fr

Despite the progress made in thoracic oncology over the past 30 yrs, surgical resection remains the mainstay of curative treatment for nonsmall cell lung cancer (NSCLC). Although combined modality treatments based on neoadjuvant or adjuvant chemotherapy are credited with a slight advantage in survival, the area under the survival curve proves that the most substantial part of cure is owed to surgery. Contemporary alternatives to surgery for small tumours are stereotaxic radiotherapy and radiofrequency ablation; these treatments are not yet scientifically validated and ignore lymphatic spread (see below). In the N2 category, surgery has been challenged by exclusive radiochemotherapy in a recent multicentre trial by VAN MEERBEECK *et al.* (2007), whose conclusions are not acceptable: the surgical arm comprised an incomplete resection rate of nearly 50%. Most patients nowadays are subjected to combined treatments, but the scientific evidence remains ambiguous and controversial. It is unclear whether neoadjuvant therapies are more beneficial to the N2 population, or to those with incipient disease. Meta-analysis demonstrated a benefit for patients undergoing adjuvant therapy; the latter is of weak clinical relevance for the individual patient, knowing that treatment of 20 patients is needed to save one at 2 yrs. The result deteriorates in the long term, and long-term complications of chemotherapy appear in survivors.

Work-up of the patient should include a check-up of fitness according to European Respiratory Society/European Society of Thoracic Surgeons guidelines.

> **Key points**
>
> The following recommendations are evidence-based:
>
> - Optimal results are obtained by specialised surgeons working in large-volume units.
> - Anatomical resection combined with a complete lymph node dissection is the gold standard.
> - Bronchoplastic and angioplastic lobectomies are viable alternatives to pneumonectomy, provided that a complete resection may be achieved.
> - Segmentectomies could be applied to high-risk patients with tumours <2 cm in diameter; wedge excisions may be recommended for very small bronchoalveolar carcinoma (ground-glass opacity).

The aim of this article is to describe the quality requirements of contemporary oncologic thoracic surgery, based on recommendations issued by a working group of the French Society for Thoracic and Cardiovascular Surgery.

How can we define early-stage lung cancer?

Although there is no clear definition, it seems adequate to restrict this label to patients with reasonable chances for survival. Since lymph node invasion at the N2 level is a marker of poor prognosis, the medical oncologist would certainly restrict the definition to stages N0 and N1.

For the surgeon, resectable disease offers an advantage over nonresectable disease. Minimal N2, defined as microscopic metastasis to a single N2 node, is credited with a survival rate of 30–35% at 5 yrs, which is comparable to the worst N1. Further, resectable T4N0 disease, such as selected cases of Pancoast tumors or main carinal invasion, may achieve a 5-yr survival of >40%.

Any marginal situation needs to be discussed with a qualified thoracic surgeon, and any decision not to operate should be validated by a qualified thoracic surgeon in a multidisciplinary discussion.

What are the usual survival figures?

The following figures drawn from the classic surgical literature apply to surgical treatment, regardless of any neoadjuvant or adjuvant treatment.

For stage I, the usual figures vary from 55–75% with a substantial difference between T1 and T2. Survival is further influenced by the type of resection (lobectomy *versus* pneumonectomy) and the comorbidity, which accounts for half of late deaths (table 1).

For stage II, reported 5-yr survival rates vary between 35–50%. Besides a difference between T1N1 and T2N1, there is a very dissimilar survival pattern according to the intralobar or extralobar location of the N1 node. Intralobar N1 is credited with 5-yr survival close to 55%, whereas in extralobar N1 it reaches only 35% (table 2).

For stage IIIA-N2, survival rates at 5 yrs are considerably lower and range from 15–25%. However, minimal N2 is a subgroup with a possible survival rate of 35% at 5 yrs. There is a small subset of completely resectable IIIA - T4N0 disease (Pancoast tumors, main carina involvement) that can achieve a survival of close to 50% at 5 yrs.

The large majority of patients with stage IIIB are inoperable, and global survival at 5 yrs is <5%.

Quality requirements: what depends on the surgeon and his institution!

Thoracic oncologic surgery is a specialised medical activity. The best results are obtained by well-trained specialised thoracic surgeons, working in high-volume units.

1. Qualification of the individual surgeon

A comparison of the results of lung resections performed by either general or well-trained thoracic surgeons in a cohort of 1,583 cases of resection for lung cancer performed between 1991 and 1995 showed that operative mortality was twice as high when resection was performed by general surgeons. It is remarkable that 75% of general surgeons performed fewer than 10 resections during the observation period.

2. Hospital volume and its impact on post-operative mortality

A review of data from the Medicare registry between 1994 and 1999 revealed that operative mortality following lobectomy varied from 6.4% in a low-activity centre (<9 cases per year) to 4.2% in a high-activity centre (>46 cases per year); following pneumonectomy, the range extended from 17% to 10.6%.

We may conclude that a high hospital volume warrants the necessary routine not only of the operating surgeon, but also of the surrounding team.

Table 1. Survival following stage I disease: independent factors of prognosis

	Yes %	No %	p-value	Relative risk
Pneumonectomy	53	62.7	0.031	1.55
Angio-invasion	54.5	61.9	0.029	1.85
Atherosclerosis	46.3	64.3	0.017	1.55
Adapted from THOMAS et al. (2002).				

3. Hospital volume and its impact on long-term survival It has been confirmed that hospital volume affects not only early outcome, but also long-term survival, in a study that included 2,118 patients operated upon in one of 76 hospitals over a 10-yr period, divided into quintiles according to hospital volume. Operative mortality ranged from 3% at high-volume units to 6% at low-volume units; operative morbidity ranged 20–44%. The 5-yr survival decreased from 44% at high-volume units to 33% at low-volume centres.

This study suggests that appropriate decision making is enhanced by routine.

Basic principles of surgical treatment: complete anatomic resection and complete lymph node dissection.

The basic principles described here are based on recommendations issued by a working group of the French Society for Thoracic and Cardiovascular Surgery. A complete cancer operation requires anatomic resection of the primary lesion and complete homolateral lymph-node dissection.

1. Complete anatomic resection Anatomic resection means either lobectomy or pneumonectomy with precise hilar dissection, according to the loco-regional extent of the tumour. The rule is to privilege lobectomy whenever it enables a complete resection. Standard lobectomy is not possible if the tumour extends across the fissure, invades the main pulmonary artery or involves the bronchial tree proximal to the lobar take-off; a double location in different lobes is also an indication for pneumonectomy.

Lobectomy is preferred to pneumonectomy because of a substantially lower operative risk. Operative mortality is ~2% following lobectomy, and ranges from 6–10 % following pneumonectomy. Mortality after pneumonectomy may be >10% in patients aged >70 yrs, or in case of extended resection. There is an ongoing debate whether mortality of pneumonectomy is increased after induction chemotherapy, especially on the right side. We have recently demonstrated a similar risk when compared to standard operations, and a survival advantage even if the patient remains stage N2. Other disadvantages of pneumonectomy are decreased quality of life owing to loss of respiratory function, and decreased possibilities of repeated curative resection, should a metachronous primary cancer occur (~10% of stages I and II).

To resect less than a pulmonary lobe is not recommended as a routine. The Lung Cancer

Table 2. Comparison of 5-yr survival for intralobar and extralobar N1

First author	Patients n	5-yr survival %	
		Intralobar N1	Extralobar N1
YANO	78	64	39
VAN VELZEN	391	57	30
RIQUET	256	53	38

Study Group (GINSBERG et al. (1995)) compared lobectomy and segmentectomy (or wedge excision) for T1N0 cancer in a randomised trial. There was a drop of 20% in 5-yr survival for patients subjected to segmentectomy, and a 3-fold increase of local recurrence following segmentectomy or wedge excision. More recent investigations from Japan conclude that wedge excisions are valuable in small bronchoalveolar carcinoma; similarly, segmentectomies could be applied to stage I tumours <2 cm.

When the tumour is invading surrounding anatomical structures, an enlarged en bloc R-0 resection may achieve satisfactory long-term results; this should be carried out in specialised institutions so that an excessive operative mortality does not erase the survival benefit of resection.

2. Complete homolateral lymph node dissection
The goals of lymph node dissection are: 1) to ascertain staging; and 2) to ensure complete resection of the disease.

Staging is important on the individual level to set prognosis and to define the most appropriate treatment strategy. On the collective level, adequate staging facilitates comparison of different treatment modalities, or results from different institutions.

Leaving unrecognised lymph node metastases obviously leads to "local recurrence". Medical imaging has serious pitfalls. Computed tomography underestimates N2 stage in one patient out of five, and overestimates in one patient out of two. A negative positron emission tomography (PET) scan matches with mediastinoscopy, but the latter is subject to 10–15% failures; a positive PET requires histologic assessment because the false-positive rate is >40%. Furthermore, >30% of patients with N2 disease have no apparent disease at the N1 level (so called skip metastases). Even among patients with T1 disease, 22% have mediastinal lymph node involvement.

As such, intraoperative exploration of the mediastinum is mandatory, and can be achieved by two different procedures: either random sampling of nodes, or complete node dissection. Obviously, only complete dissection appears to be serious and reliable. The arguments are as follows.

In patients with pathological stage I-N0 disease, survival increases with the number of dissected nodes. This demonstrates that the more lymph nodes are harvested, the lower the risk of ignoring an invaded node, and the more reliable the staging.

In a cross-sectional analysis, we have compared sampling and dissection in each single case of 248 resections. Sampling identified 52% of N2; multilevel N2 was identified in 42% of events only. Resection based on sampling alone would have been complete in only 12%.

The standard lymph node dissection is defined as an en bloc dissection of all lymphatic tissue along its anatomical borders (tracheobronchial tree, sheets of major vessels, oesophagus). On the right side, it includes lower oesophageal nodes within the

Table 3. Lymph node dissection increases survival! Results of a randomised study

	5-yr survival %	
	268 dissections	**264 samplings**
Stage I	82.2	57.5
Stage II	50.4	34.0
Stage III	27.0	6.2
Global	**48.4**	**36.9**

Reproduced from WU et al. (2002), with permission from the publisher.

Table 4. Survival following bronchoplastic lobectomy

First author	Stage I %	Stage II %	Stage III %
TEDDER	63	37	21
MEHRAN	57	46	0
VAN SCHIL	62	31	31
MASSARD	70	37	8
ICARD,	60	30	27
TRONC	63	48	8

pulmonary ligament, subcarinal space and paratracheal space. On the left side, it includes pulmonary ligament, subcarinal space, aorto–pulmonary window, phrenic nodes and subaortic nodes up to the left tracheo-bronchial angle.

Formal lymph node dissection does not increase the postoperative complication rate. There is increasing evidence for a positive effect on survival. A first, nonrandomised study compared sampling to dissection in stage II and III and concluded that there is a survival advantage following dissection.

A randomised study including >500 patients demonstrated a survival advantage of node dissection without relation to a stage migration effect: it was observed not only stage by stage, but also when comparing the two investigated groups as a whole (table 3).

A meta-analysis concluded that 4-yr survival was increased in patients having undergone node dissection, with a hazard ratio of 0.78.

Are there alternatives to pneumonectomy?

Given the high operative mortality rate of pneumonectomy, it is meaningful to look for alternatives. Bronchoplastic operations (sleeve lobectomy) are indicated: 1) when the tumour involves the lobar take-off on the endobronchial side; and 2) when positive N1 nodes with capsular disruption are identified at the origin of the lobar bronchus. Angioplastic lobectomies are indicated when the lobar branches destined to the upper lobe cannot be divided safely with tumour-free margins; this situation is much more frequent on the left side for anatomical reasons.

The operative risk of bronchoplastic lobectomy is comparable to standard lobectomy, with a mortality of ⩽2%. Long-term survival and rate of local recurrence match with reported data per stage (table 4). A meta-analysis published by MA et al. (2007) showed that mortality was almost half that after pneumonectomy in experienced teams; 1-year survival was improved after bronchoplastic resection.

References

- Allen MS, et al. Mortality and morbidity of major pulmonary resections in patients with early stage lung cancer: initial results of the randomized prospective ACOSOG Z0030 trial. Ann Thorac Surg 2006; 81: 1013–1019.
- Berghmans T, et al. Survival improvement in respectable non-small cell lung cancer with (neo)adjuvant chemotherapy: results of a meta-analysis of the literature. Lung Cancer 2005; 49: 13–23.
- Brunelli A, et al. ERS/ESTS guidelines on fitness for radical therapy in lung cancer patients (surgery and chemo-radiotherapy). Eur Respir J 2009; 34: 17–41.
- Cerfolio RJ, et al. The role of FDG-PET scan in staging poatients with nonsmall cell carcinoma. Ann Thorac Surg 2003; 76: 861–866.
- Ginsberg RJ, et al. Randomized trial of lobectomy versus limited resection for T1N0 non-small cell lung cancer. Ann Thorac Surg 1995; 60: 615–623.
- Mansour Z, et al. Induction chemotherapy does not increase the operative risk of pneumonectomy! Eur J Cardiothorac Surg 2007; 31: 181–185.

- Martinod E, et al. Management of superior sulcus tumors : experience with 139 cases treated by surgical resection. *Ann Thorac Surg* 2002; 73: 1534-1540.
- Massard G. Local control of disease and survival following bronchoplastic lobectomy for non-small cell lung cancer. *Eur J Cardiothorac Surg* 1999; 16: 276-282.
- Riquet M, et al. Prognostic value of T and N in non small cell lung cancer three centimeters or less in diameter. *Eur J Cardiothorac Surg* 1997; 11: 440-444.
- Thomas P, Doddoli C, Thirion X, et al. Stage I non-small cell lung cancer : a pragmatic approach to prognosis after complete resection. *Ann Thorac Surg* 2002; 73: 1065-70.
- Van Meerbeeck JP, et al. Randomized controlled trial of resection versus radiotherapy after induction chemotherapy in stage IIIA-N2 non-small cell lung cancer. *J Natl Cancer Instit* 2007; 99: 442-450.
- Wright G, et al. Surgery for non-small cell lung cancer : systematic review and meta-analysis of randomized trials. *Thorax* 2006; 61: 597-603.
- Wu YL, et al. A randomized trial of systematic nodal dissection in respectable non-small cell lung cancer. *Lung Cancer* 2002; 36: 1-6.

METASTATIC TUMOURS

E. Quoix
University of Strasbourg, University Hospital, Pneumology, Strasbourg, France
E-mail: elisabeth.quoix@chru-strasbourg.fr

The thorax is a common site of metastasis from various cancers, which may affect the hilar or mediastinal lymph nodes, bone (chest wall and vertebrae), lung, pleura, muscle or heart, and pericardium. These metastases may induce mediastinal compression syndromes (Pancoast, superior vena cava syndrome, dysphagia *etc*., just like locoregional extension of a primary lung cancer).

Pleural metastases

Pleural metastasis occur commonly in patients with haematological or solid tumours. In an already old series of 133 patients, the most common primary sites appear to be breast carcinoma (35 patients), lung cancer (32), lymphomas (20), Hodgkin's disease (12), ovary carcinoma (9), adenocarcinoma of unknown primary tumour (6) and melanoma (4). In women specifically, 37% of malignant pleural effusions were due to breast cancer, 20% to gynaecological cancers and 15% to lung cancer. Probably, with the increase of the frequency of lung cancer in women, there will be a higher percentage of malignant pleural effusions secondary to lung cancer in the forthcoming years.

Key points

- The thorax is a common site of metastasis from several cancers.
- It is sometimes difficult to distinguish between primary lung cancer and metastases from other primaries.
- Prognosis is linked to the underlying primitive.

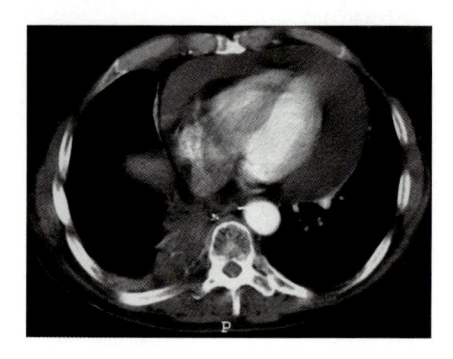

Figure 1. Neoplasic pericardial effusion in a patient with lung cancer.

Pericardial effusions

Out of 55 patients admitted to an intensive care unit with malignant pericardial effusion, 30 had a lung carcinoma as a primary tumour, nine breast cancer, five haematological malignancies and 11 other solid tumours. Figure 1 shows a neoplastic pericardial effusion in a patient with lung cancer.

Pulmonary metastases

Endothoracic metastases of breast cancer are essentially pleuropulmonary (figs 2a and b, and 3). In a review of 660 cases of breast cancers followed during a period of 5 yrs between 1975 and 1979, 119 endothoracic metastases were recorded. Among them, 79 were pleural or pleuroparietal, 80 were pulmonary (lymphangitis 41, multiple nodules 34, solitary nodules nine, endobronchial seven, tumoral emboli two, alveolar metastasis one), 46 hilar or mediastinal, and two myocardial metastases CHATKIN *et al*. (2007).

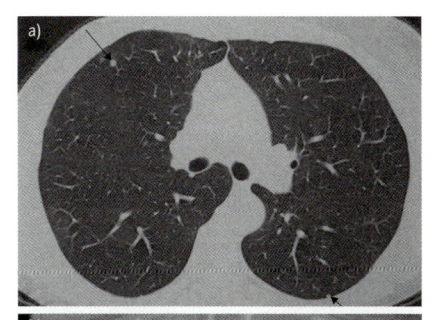

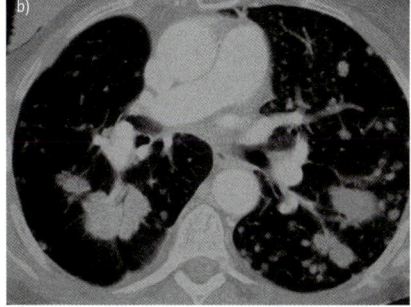

Figure 2. a) Multiple micronodules in a woman who developed chronic cough 2 yrs after a breast cancer. b) Same patient 6 yrs later with multiple nodules, some displaying a pneumonic pattern.

Pulmonary metastases were also frequent in lung cancer and their prognosis appeared to be of intermediate value if there is no other site involved. In fact, they will be classified as M1a in the new staging classification. Sometimes, pulmonary metastases may be excavated (fig. 4).

Endobronchial metastasis is an infrequent feature (table 1), the most frequent primary site being head and neck (although, it might be difficult to distinguish them from a primary lung cancer) followed by breast and kidney.

It may be quite difficult, if not impossible, to distinguish a primary lung cancer from endobronchial metastasis on a computed tomography (CT) scan. Endobronchial metastases from melanoma are often black. Endobronchial metastases of a kidney cancer display strong enhancement on the contrast-enhanced CT images. Whenever a bronchofibroscopy is performed, there may be

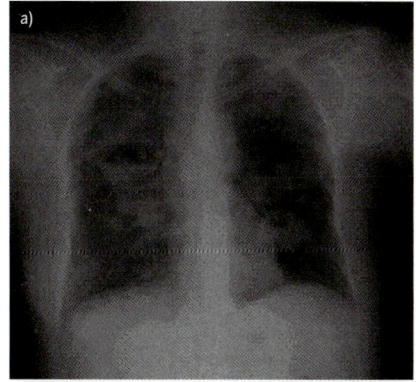

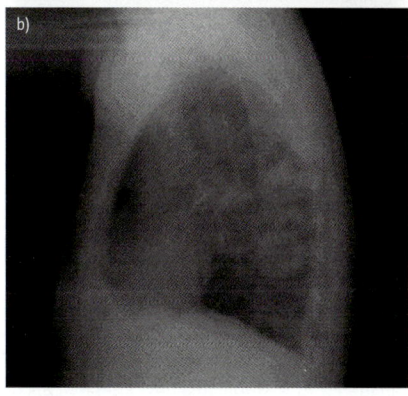

Figure 3. Multiple excavated pulmonary metastases.

quite severe bleeding at biopsy attempt. In fact, cough with haempoptysis is the most frequent symptom.

Tumoral emboli may provide similar clinical and radiological features as cruoric emboli; however, peripheral tumoral micro-emboli are characterised by respiratory failure despite normal imaging. Diagnosis may be obtained by transbronchial biopsy or by video-thoracoscopy with, at histology, multiple carcinomatous emboli in distal pulmonary arteries, veins and lymphatics.

Hilar and mediastinal metastatic lymph nodes

Of course, metastatic hilar and mediastinal lymph nodes are usually linked to an intrathoracic carcinoma. Among 565 patients, only 37 had a history of extrathoracic

Table 1. Endobronchial metastases: frequency by primary site

Primary tumour	n (%)
Head and neck	71 (31)
Breast	32 (14)
Kidney	31 (13)
Colon/rectum	25 (11)
Melanoma	18 (8)
Sarcoma	10 (4)
Thyroid	9 (4)
Bladder	6 (3)
Ovarian	5 (2)
Prostate	4 (2)
Oesophagus	3 (1)
Testis	3 (1)
Pancreas	3 (1)
Adrenal gland	2 (1)
Stomach	2 (1)
Other	3 (1)
Modified from SORENSEN (2004).	

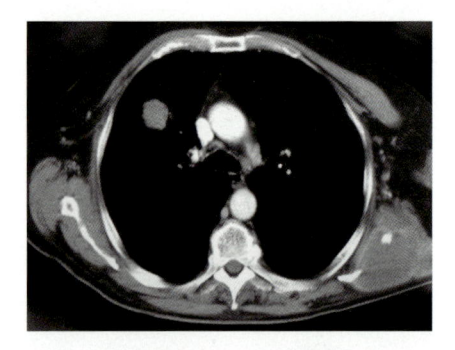

Figure 4. Left scapula osteolytic metastasis of a right upperlobe adenocarcinoma.

carcinoma in a surgical series. Primary cancer was most frequently breast but also kidney, testis, prostate, thyroid and other. Metastasis of breast cancer to intrathoracic nodes seems to occur quite frequently. In an autopsy series of women who had died of disseminated breast cancer, metastatic involvement of intrathoracic lymph nodes was found in 71% of cases. Lymph node involvement was more extensive in the mediastinum ipsilateral to the primary breast cancer than in the contralateral mediastinum.

Bone metastases in the chest

Bone metastases in the chest are common sites of secondary lesions of lung, prostate and breast cancer in which bone is the most common metastatic site. Bone metastases affect 8% of patients with breast cancer. Bone scans remain the primary means for detection of bone metastases. In a meta-analysis of six studies comparing bone scan and positron-emission tomography (PET) scan without CT, a pooled lesion-based sensitivity of 88% and specificity of 87% in breast cancer was found for bone scan and a pooled lesion-based sensitivity of 69% and a specificity of 98% was found for PET scan. With regard to lung cancer, bone is also a frequent metastatic site (fig. 4). In a recent study of 1,000 patients, 105 (10.5%) had bone metastases at diagnosis. Sensitivity of PET-scan and CT was 94.3% compared with 78.1% with bone scan and specificity was 98.8% and 97.4%, respectively. Among the 346 bone metastases detected by PET scan and CT, 55 were in the thoracic spine, 28 in the scapula or clavicles (fig. 4), 12 in the sternum and 56 in the ribs (fig. 5); *i.e.* 44% of the foci were in the chest. The main problem of PET scan is poor anatomical resolution (fig. 6).

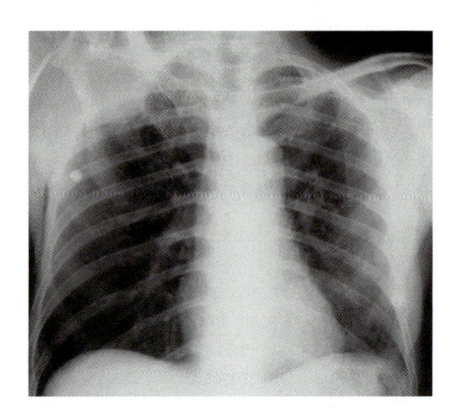

Figure 5. Osteolytic metastasis of the second right rib.

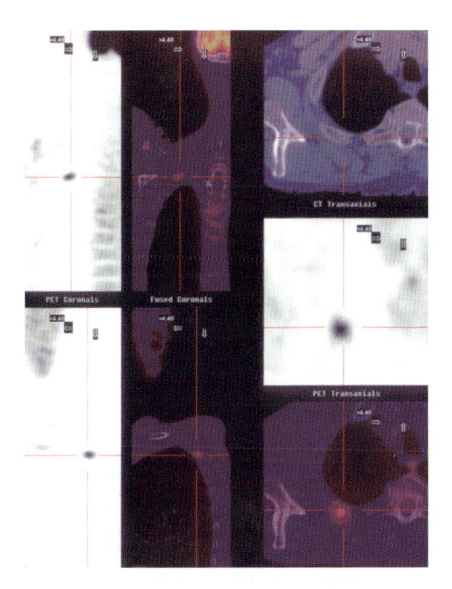

Figure 6. Rib metastasis in a patient with a left hilar relapse of a lung adenocarcinoma.

Magnetic resonance imaging is the best imaging procedure whenever spinal cord compression is suspected.

Conclusions

The chest is a frequent site of metastasis especially for lung, breast, kidney, prostate, colon and ovary carcinomas. The prognosis of these metastases is more related to the possibilities of control of the underlying neoplasm than to their possible immediate complications, such as tamponade. However, some of the metastases may especially alter quality of life, such as bone metastases with a special attention to be paid to the spine because of the risk of cord compression.

References

- Anderson CB, et al. The treatment of malignant pleural effusion. *Cancer* 1974; 33: 916-922.
- Chatkin JM, et al. Microscopic pulmonary neoplastic emboli : report of a case with respiratory failure but normal imaging. *Prim Care Respir* 2007; 16: 115-117.
- Costelloe CM, et al. Imaging bone metastases in breast cancer : techniques and recommendations for diagnosis. *Lancet Oncol* 2009; 10: 606-614.
- Dequanter D, et al. Severe pericardial effusion in patients with concurrent malignancy : a retrospective analysis of prognostic factors influencing survival. *Ann Surg Oncol* 2008; 15: 3268-3271.
- Dizon DS, et al. The differential diagnosis of dyspnea in a woman with metastatic breast cancer – consideration beyond pulmonary embolism. *The Breast Journal* 2008; 14: 90-91.
- Milleron B, et al. Endobronchial metastases of cancer. A propos of 29 cases. *Rev Pneumol Clin* 1986; 42: 231-234.
- Ou SH, Zell JA. Validation study of the proposed IASLC staging revisions of the T4 and M non-small cell lung cancer descriptors using data from 23583 patients in the California Cancer registry. *J Thorac Oncol* 2008; 3: 216-227.
- Park CM, et al. Endobronchial metastasis from renal cell carcinoma: CT findings in four patients. *Eur J Radiol* 2004; 51: 155-159.
- Riquet M, et al. Intrathoracic lymph node metastases from extrathoracic carcinoma : the place of surgery. *Ann Thorac Surg* 2009; 88: 200-205.
- Shie P, et al. Meta-analysis: comparison of F-18 fluorodeoxyglucose-positron emission tomography and bone scintigraphy in the detection of bone metastases in patients with breast cancer. *Clin Nucl Med* 2008; 33: 97-101.
- Song JW, et al. Efficacy comparison between 18-FDG PET/CT and bone scintigrapgy in detecting bony metastases of non-small cell lung cancer. *Lung Cancer* 2009; 65: 333-338.
- Sorensen B. Endobronchial metastases from extrapulmonary solid tumors. *Acta Oncologica* 2004; 43: 73-79.
- Thomas JM, et al. The spread of breast cancer: importance of the intrathoracic lymphatic route and its relevance to treatment. *Br J Cancer* 1979; 40: 540-547.

PLEURAL AND CHEST WALL TUMOURS

A. Scherpereel[1,2]
[1] Pulmonary and Thoracic Oncology Dept, Hospital of the University of Lille II, Hôpital Calmette
[2] INSERM Unit 1019, Pasteur Institute of Lille, Lille, France
E-mail: arnaud.scherpereel@chru-lille.fr

Pleural and chest wall malignancies are quite common diseases in our practice. Malignant pleural effusions (MPEs) and pleural metastases are much more frequent than primary tumours of these tissues (mesothelioma, sarcoma, lymphoma, *etc.*). Primary chest wall tumours are a heterogeneous group of rare tumours (<2% of all primary tumours; 60% of them are malignant) developing in the bones and soft tissues of the thoracic cage, but have similar diagnostic and therapeutic issues.

Epidemiology and pathogenesis

Malignant pleural mesothelioma (MPM)
Malignant mesothelioma, a highly aggressive tumour involving the pleura in 90% of cases, is a rare tumour but with increasing incidence. MPM may occur in subjects up to 40 yrs after occupational asbestos exposure (found in >80% of male cases but <40% in female), the main factor involved in MPM pathogenesis.

Pleural metastases and MPEs
Pleural tumour involvement may result from a direct invasion from adjacent structures (lung, chest wall, *etc.*), blood dissemination or more often from tumour emboli to the visceral pleura with secondary seeding to the parietal pleura (lung cancer). Effusion may be due to the pleural tumour lesions or to a lymphatic blockade at the mediastinal level. MPEs also depend on interactions between tumour cells and mesothelial cells through growth factors such as vascular endothelial growth factor

Key points

- MPEs are much more frequent than primary pleural or chest wall tumours.
- Diagnostic strategy includes pleural cytology, but a firm and reliable diagnosis of cancer is based on histology usually best obtained by biopsies during thoracoscopy.
- Talc pleurodesis by thoracoscopy is the best local treatment of recurrent or massive MPE, but indwelling pleural catheter represents an interesting alternative.
- Figures 1 and 2 summarise a proposal for MPE and MPM management.

that increase vascular permeability and angiogenesis.

An MPE is found in up to 6% of patients with malignancy. In half of these cases, MPE may reveal the cancer. Neoplasias responsible for pleural metastases and/or MPE are mostly lung cancer (approximately one-third of cases) or breast cancer (10–15%), but other cancers include carcinomas (ovary, stomach, *etc.*) or noncarcinoma proliferations such as lymphoma, sarcoma, melanoma, seminoma or thymoma.

Pleural effusion is the main clinical element but it is not found in all pleural malignancies. Moreover, pleurisy is not systematically synonymous with MPE in cancer patients because it may be induced by other mechanisms such as pneumonia and/or atelectasia due to bronchial obstruction, transudate induced by severe denutrition or cardiac failure, or even drug- or radiotherapy-induced effusion. Therefore the diagnostic strategy may differ whether the patient has a cancer background or not, but should always rely on cytology or, better still, on histology.

Lymphoma and chest wall sarcoma Initial thoracic involvement of lymphoma is common but mostly involves the mediastinum. Lung parenchyma and/or pleural localisations are less frequent and need to be histologically proven because they modify the staging and prognosis of the tumour. Primary soft-tissue sarcoma of the chest wall is a rare disease (<10% of the 8,000 new cases per year of soft-tissue sarcomas in the USA).

Prognosis

The prognosis of patients with pleural metastases or MPM is poor (median 1-yr survival 13%, and median survival <12 months, respectively). However survival may vary according to the primary cancer: from a few months usually for lung cancer to a potential much longer survival in breast cancer or lymphoma. In fact, lymphoma is characterised by a good outcome (cure rate >80%). Sarcomas have a variable prognosis, with a reported 5-yr survival from 15% up to 90%, depending mostly of the localisation, the grade and the differentiation the tumour and the possibility to achieve an early wide resection of the sarcoma.

Diagnosis

Clinical signs Dyspnoea on exertion and dry cough are the most common signs of MPE. Dyspnoea is usually progressive and more marked as the effusion becomes larger, but it may be also modulated by other factors: bronchus obstruction, carcinomatous lymphangitis or associated (pulmonary, cardiac) comorbidities. Chest pain suggests chest wall involvement. Other signs may include weight loss, anorexia, asthenia, haemoptysis (lung cancer), adenopathy, peritoneal effusion, *etc*. However, MPE or MPM may be diagnosed in asymptomatic patients by routine chest imaging. A diagnosis of MPM should not be based on unspecific and usually late clinical signs. However, the association of chest pain, thoracic "shrinkage", and/or a unilateral pleural effusion or thoracic mass in asbestos-exposed patients may suggest this diagnosis.

There are no reliable clinical features for distinguishing benign from malignant chest wall tumours. A palpable mass and pain are common in both groups of tumours. The final diagnosis is often obtained only after surgery.

Imaging Pleural metastases usually exhibit a moderate-to-large, nonloculated and unilateral pleural effusion. MPE may be associated with an irregular pleural thickening. Typically this large pleural effusion induces a contralateral mediastinal shift. If not, one should suspect an obstruction of a main bronchus by lung cancer or metastasis, a fixed mediastinum caused by the cancer and/or lymph nodes, an extensive tumour infiltration of the ipsilatary lung mimicking a large effusion, or MPM.

Chest radiograph or, better, computed tomography (CT) scan shows typically an unspecific, unilateral (95% of cases) pleural effusion ± mediastinal shift in MPM patients. More rarely, pleural thickening or mass, without pleuresy, may be observed. Pleural plugs are very common (70% of cases); about 20% of patients exhibit the association of asbestos-induced pulmonary interstitial fibrosis. Definitive diagnosis of MPM is not possible by CT scan, but is recommended for diagnosis and staging (after removal of pleural effusion if applicable). Magnetic resonance imaging is mostly useful to assess the tumour extent into the diaphragm and chest wall.

18-Fluorodeoxyglucose-positron emission tomography (^{18}FDG-PET) usually shows

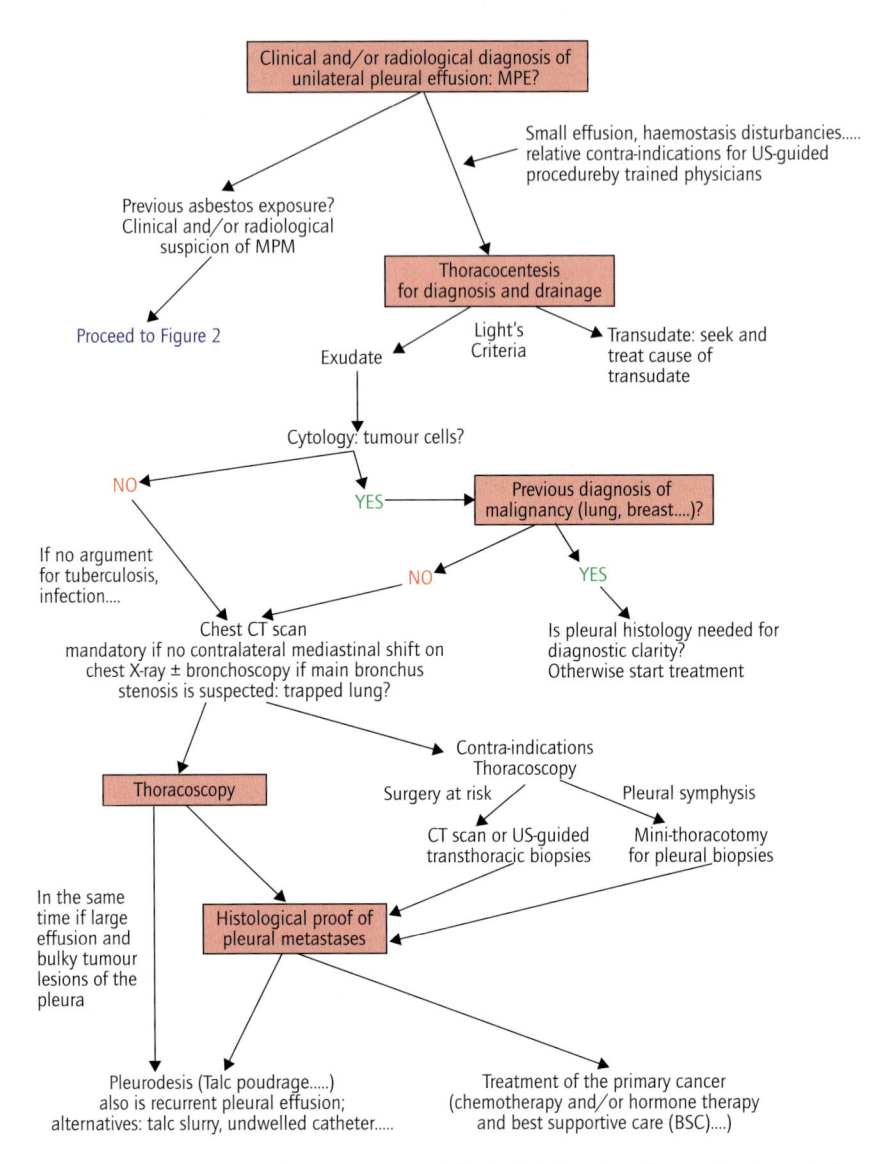

Figure 1. Proposed management for malignant pleural effusion (MPE). MPM: malignant pleural mesothelioma; US: ultrasound; CT: computed tomography; BSC: best supportive care.

hypermetabolism of pleural mesothelioma, metastatic adenopathy and metastasis, but should not be currently performed for the diagnosis of MPM. Pleural hypermetabolism is also found after talc pleurodesis. PET may be helpful for the staging of pleural malignancies, or in the search of primary cancer.

Pathology and diagnostic procedures In patients suspected of malignancy with pleural effusion, a thoracocentesis is the first diagnostic step (American Thoracic Society/ European Respiratory Society (ERS) guidelines). Pleural fluid analysis finds usually an exudate according to Light's criteria, but a

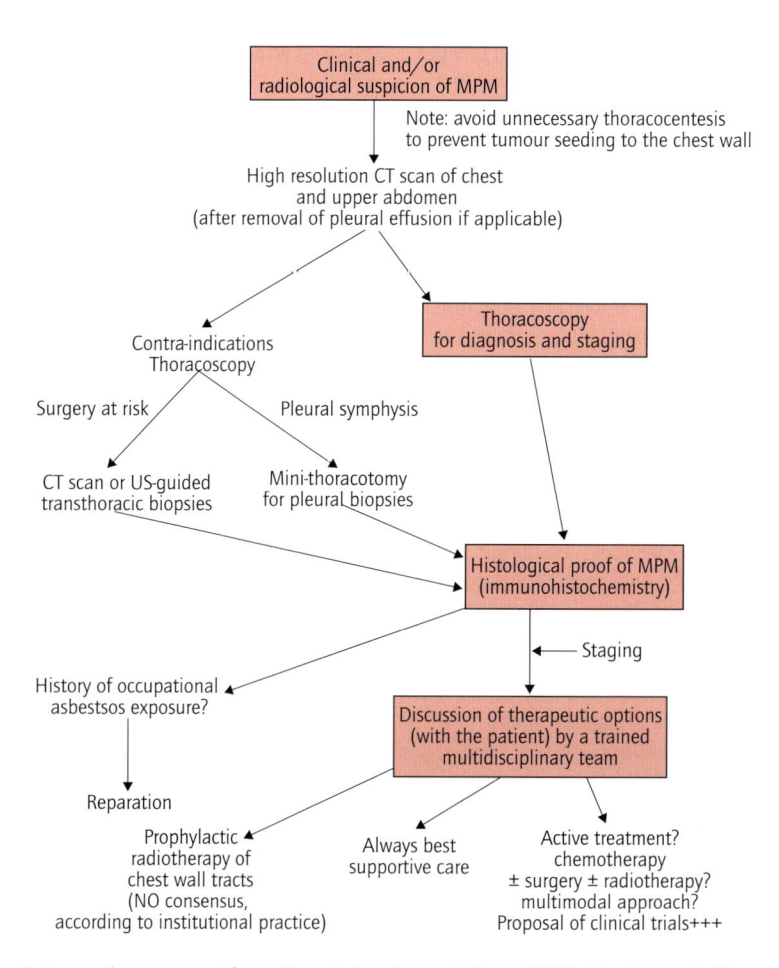

Figure 2. Proposed management for malignant pleural mesothelioma (MPM). US: ultrasound; CT: computed tomography.

transudate due to major hypoprotidaemia with cachexia or to malignant pericardial effusion does not eliminate the diagnosis of MPE. Assessment of the adenosine deaminase (ADA) pleural level can bring false-positive results in some cases of MPM or lymphoma, but may be helpful in countries with medium-to-high prevalence of tuberculosis. The diagnostic sensitivity of pleural cytology in MPE may vary, depending of the extension of the pleural lesions and the primary cancer, from 62–90% in series. Thus in a patient with a history of cancer, cytology may be enough for the diagnosis of pleural metastases. A diagnosis of MPM should not be based on cytology alone because of its poor sensitivity (30%) and specificity (potential confusion with reactive mesothelial cells or adenocarcinoma cells).

Closed, percutaneous needle (*e.g.* Abrams) pleural biopsies are quite easy to perform with local anaesthesia on an outpatient basis. However, due to the potentially scarce and irregular distribution of the tumour lesions in the pleural cavity, a positive yield of blind biopsies is low (30–40%), adding little to a negative cytology.

Guided biopsies did better than blind biopsies in series of MPEs (70–80% sensitivity), but did worse than thoracoscopy, and are not recommended for the diagnosis of MPM except in patients for whom thoracoscopy (or mini-thoracotomy if pleural symphysis) is contra-indicated or rejected by the patient. If MPM is not clearly suspected, closed needle biopsies may be first proposed in young patients with pleural lesions and exudative, cytology-negative pleural effusion from countries with a relatively high prevalence of tuberculosis.

Medical (pleuroscopy) or surgical (video-assisted thoracoscopic surgery (VATS)) thoracoscopy with multiple pleural biopsies is the "gold standard" to obtain the diagnosis of MPM or pleural metastasis. Diagnostic accuracy is >90% and complications occur in <10% of cases. MPM or pleural metastasis will usually appear as nodules or masses of various diameters. Thoracoscopy is also useful for the staging of MPM and may permit talc pleurodesis in case of massive and/or recurrent pleural effusion.

Immunohistochemistry is helpful in the search of primary cancer for pleural metastases or to obtain an accurate diagnosis of mesothelioma, referring to the international classification of pleural tumours (World Health Organization (WHO) 2004). Epithelioid subtype is the most frequent mesothelioma subtype.

Soluble biomarkers have been searched to obtain an early and reliable diagnosis of pleural malignancies but none was considered as valuable in routine. Soluble mesothelin (or soluble mesothelin-related peptides (SMRPs)) levels were increased in serum and pleural fluid of patients with MPM compared with healthy asbestos-exposed subjects or patients with benign pleural lesions or pleural metastasis. SMRPs showed interesting sensitivity (70–80%) and specificity (80–100%) as diagnostic markers for MPM. However, SMRPs do not capture sarcomatoid (and some mixed) mesothelioma subtypes, and should not be used for MPM screening.

Staging and pre-therapeutic assessment of MPM

It is recommended to use the Union Internationale Contre le Cancer/International Mesothelioma Interest Group 1995 TNM staging system, even if it is inaccurate in describing T and N extent by current imaging procedures. Only a patient's performance status (PS) and histological subtype are recognised as prognostic factors for the management of MPM in routine.

To identify candidates for proper treatment, the 2008 ERS/European Society of Thoracic Surgeons (ESTS) experts on MPM proposed a simple and sequential three-step pre-treatment assessment (see references for full details).

Treatment

It includes palliative local therapies, mostly to improve the patient's symptoms, and a treatment of primary cancer depending of the nature of the malignancy, the clinical status and the wishes of the patient.

Treatment of primary cancer MPM treatment relies mostly on best supportive care (BSC: oxygen, pain relief, nutrition, *etc.*) associated with chemotherapy, and has been summarised by the 2008 ERS/ESTS guidelines, as follows.

Surgery has very little indication in MPM. Debulking surgery (pleurectomy/decortication) should not be proposed with a curative intent, but can be considered to obtain symptom control, especially in symptomatic patients with entrapped lung syndrome who cannot benefit from chemical pleurodesis. There is limited evidence for the efficacy of radical surgery for mesothelioma, except parietal pleurectomy in very early and rare stage Ia disease. Extrapleural pneumonectomy (EPP), as well as post-operative irradiation, should be performed only in clinical trials, in specialised centres, as a part of multimodal treatment.

Palliative radiotherapy aimed at pain relief may be considered in case of painful chest wall infiltration or nodules. The value of prophylactic radiotherapy to prevent subcutaneous metastasis developing along drainage channels or thoracocentesis tracts is questionable after recent studies and did not permit any recommendation.

When a decision is made to treat patients with chemotherapy, subjects with a good PS should be treated with first-line chemotherapy combining of platinum and anti-metabolite (pemetrexed), or could be included in clinical trials. No drug has been validated in second-line chemotherapy, and patients with a good PS should rather be proposed to enter into clinical trials. Patients demonstrating prolonged symptomatic and objective response with first-line chemotherapy may be treated again with the same regimen in the event of recurrence or relapse. For assessment and follow-up of MPM, only chest CT scan is recommended. PET scan and biological markers are still under investigation. The modified Response Evaluation Criteria In Solid Tumors (RECIST) criteria are the preferred method of measuring response to treatment.

Pleural metastases Because of the systemic dissemination of the cancer, it relies on chemotherapy and/or hormone therapy, associated with BSC. The choice of cytotoxic drugs depends on the nature of the primary cancer. Mediastinal and/or abdominal radiotherapy may be combined with chemotherapy for lymphoma.

Chest wall sarcomas The treatment of choice is an early adequate and wide resection of the sarcoma. Adjuvant radio- and/or chemotherapy are considered for high/grade sarcomas.

Local treatment Pleurodesis is useful in treating a patient's symptoms and in preventing recurrent effusions. Sterile talc is preferred to other agents and may be administered in the pleural space through a chest drain ("talc slurry", TS) or better during medical (pleuroscopy) or surgical thoracoscopy (VATS) ("talc poudrage", TP). Pleurodesis is most effective when performed early in the disease process before effusions have become loculated and/or the lung has become fixed and is unable to expand fully, but it should not be performed before sufficient tissue for diagnosis has been obtained. Criteria for talc pleurodesis are a sufficient WHO PS <2, an estimated survival >3 months, an established diagnosis of the tumour, and no arguments for either a trapped lung (suspected if a pneumothorax persists after thoracocentesis) or an endobronchial tumour (massive pleural effusion without a contralateral mediastinal shift). This may justify a bronchoscopy or a pleural manometry before the pleurodesis. To decrease the risk of pleurodesis failure in MPE, it is recommended to use 4 g of talc after complete aspiration of pleural effusion. In a phase III multicentric randomised study, success rates in TP *versus* TS in patients with MPE were respectively 67% *versus* 56% (p=0.045), and 82% *versus* 67% in the subgroup of lung or breast cancers (p=0.022). Benign usual side-effects of talc (fever, chest pain) were observed with both methods, but no acute respiratory distress syndrome and death.

Alternatives to talc pleurodesis are repeated pleural punctures or indwelling pleural catheters. This last ambulatory procedure has to be proposed rather than a second talc pleurodesis in the case of trapped lung, a pleuro-peritoneal shunt with a high risk of complications, or a parietal pleurectomy in frail patients. Spontaneous pleurodesis may be obtained by indwelling pleural catheter without mortality or major morbidity in nearly half of the cases when pleural drainage is done *via* the catheter every other day, or even up to 70% in MPE patients fit for pleurodesis.

References

- Scherpereel A, *et al*. Guidelines of the European Respiratory Society and the European Society of Thoracic Surgeons for management of malignant pleural mesothelioma. *Eur Respir J* 2010; 35: 479–495.
- Rodriguez-Panadero F. Effusions from malignancy. *In*: Light RW, Gary Lee YC, eds. Textbook of Pleural Diseases, 2nd Edn. Hodder Arnold, London, 2008; pp. 323–337.

- Sahn SA. Malignant pleural effusions. *In*: Bouros D, ed. Pleural disease, Vol. 186. Marcel Dekker, New York, 2004: pp. 411-438.
- Antony VB, *et al.* Management of malignant pleural effusions. ERS/ATS statement. *Eur Respir J* 2001; 18: 402-419.
- Maskell NA, *et al.* Standard pleural biopsy versus CT-guided cutting-needle biopsy for diagnosis of malignant disease in pleural effusions: a randomised controlled trial. *Lancet* 2003; 361: 1326-1330.
- Janssen JP, *et al.* Safety of pleurodesis with talc poudrage in malignant pleural effusion: a prospective cohort study. *Lancet* 2007; 369: 1535-1539.
- Tremblay A, *et al.* Use of tunnelled catheters for malignant pleural effusions in patients fit for pleurodesis. *Eur Respir J* 2007; 30: 759-762.
- Grigoriu B, *et al.* Utility of osteopontin and serum mesothelin in MPM diagnosis and prognosis assessment. *Clin Can Res* 2007; 13: 2928-2935.
- Travis WD, *et al.*, eds. World Health Organization Classification of tumors. Tumors of the lung, pleura, thymus and heart. Lyon, France, IARC; 2004.
- Gross JL, *et al.* Soft-tissue sarcomas of the chest wall: prognostic factors. *Chest* 2005; 127: 902-908.

MEDIASTINAL TUMOURS

P.E. Van Schil, P. Lauwers and J.M. Hendriks
Department of Thoracic and Vascular Surgery, Antwerp University Hospital, Belgium
E-mail: paul.van.schil@uza.be

The mediastinum, which is defined as the anatomical compartment between both lungs, is a fascinating region due to its surprising complexity and variety.

Variety of compartments and organs

Although no universal agreement exists, the mediastinum is commonly divided into a superior compartment above a straight line from the sternal angle of Louis to the vertebral column, and an inferior part below this imaginary line. The latter is composed of an anterior compartment in front of the heart, a middle compartment at the level of the heart, and a posterior part lying behind the heart. Each compartment contains different organs and structures, varying from heart and great vessels to lymphatic tissue and pluripotent cells.

Variety of histological types and tumours

In both young and old patients, a range of primary tumours and cysts is encountered in the mediastinum; these are summarised in table 1. Metastases may also occur in the mediastinum.

Variety of symptoms

Mediastinal tumours can grow to a large size before symptoms appear. Pressure on surrounding structures may result in hoarseness, dyspnoea, dysphagia and superior vena cava syndrome. Various paraneoplastic syndromes have been described, such as myasthenia gravis and pure red cell aplasia in case of thymoma (fig. 1).

Variety of diagnostic means

Chest computed tomography (CT), magnetic resonance imaging and positron emission tomography provide exact anatomical delineation of a tumour and may suggest a specific entity. To obtain a precise histological diagnosis, CT-guided puncture, endoscopic or endobronchial ultrasound, mediastinoscopy, mediastinotomy and video-assisted thoracic surgery are utilised. In the case of suspicion of lymphoma, germ cell tumour or thymoma,

---

Key points

- Mediastinal tumours are characterised by a wide variation in clinical presentation, histological features and treatment options.
- A multidisciplinary approach is necessary to determine optimal treatment.
- Surgical treatment should aim at complete resection.

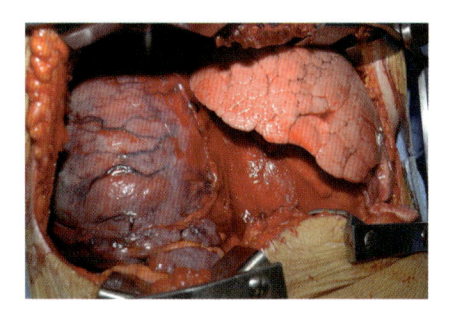

Figure 1. A large thymoma in the right hemithorax presenting with myasthenia gravis. The tumour was resected by a bilateral anterior thoracotomy (clam-shell incision).

Table 1. Primary tumours and cysts encountered in the mediastinum

Superior mediastinum		Substernal goitre
		Ectopic thyroid
Inferior mediastinum	Anterior	Thymoma
		Thymic cyst
		Germ cell tumours
		Pleuropericardial cysts
	Middle	Lymphoma
		Bronchogenic cyst
	Posterior	Neurogenic tumours
		Enterogenic cysts

large biopsies are required. Well-circumscribed tumours in young patients should be excised at once so as not to breach the surrounding capsule.

Variety of therapeutic strategies

Operable lesions are treated by surgical excision. Minimally invasive and even robotic techniques can be applied if a complete resection can be obtained by this approach. In the case of incomplete resection or capsular invasion, adjuvant radio- or chemotherapy may be indicated. Inoperable lesions and lymphomas are treated by a combination of chemo- and radiotherapy. In selected cases, induction therapy may be a valid approach to downstage a locally aggressive tumour. Salvage surgery may be attempted in tumours that are no longer responsive to chemo- or radiotherapy. Long-term survival depends on histological type and completeness of resection.

References

- Date H. Diagnostic strategies for mediastinal tumors and cysts. *Thorac Surg Clin* 2009; 19: 29–35.
- Hoffman R, et al., eds. Hematology: Basic Principles and Practice, 5th Edn. Philadelphia, Churchill Livingstone Elsevier, 2009.

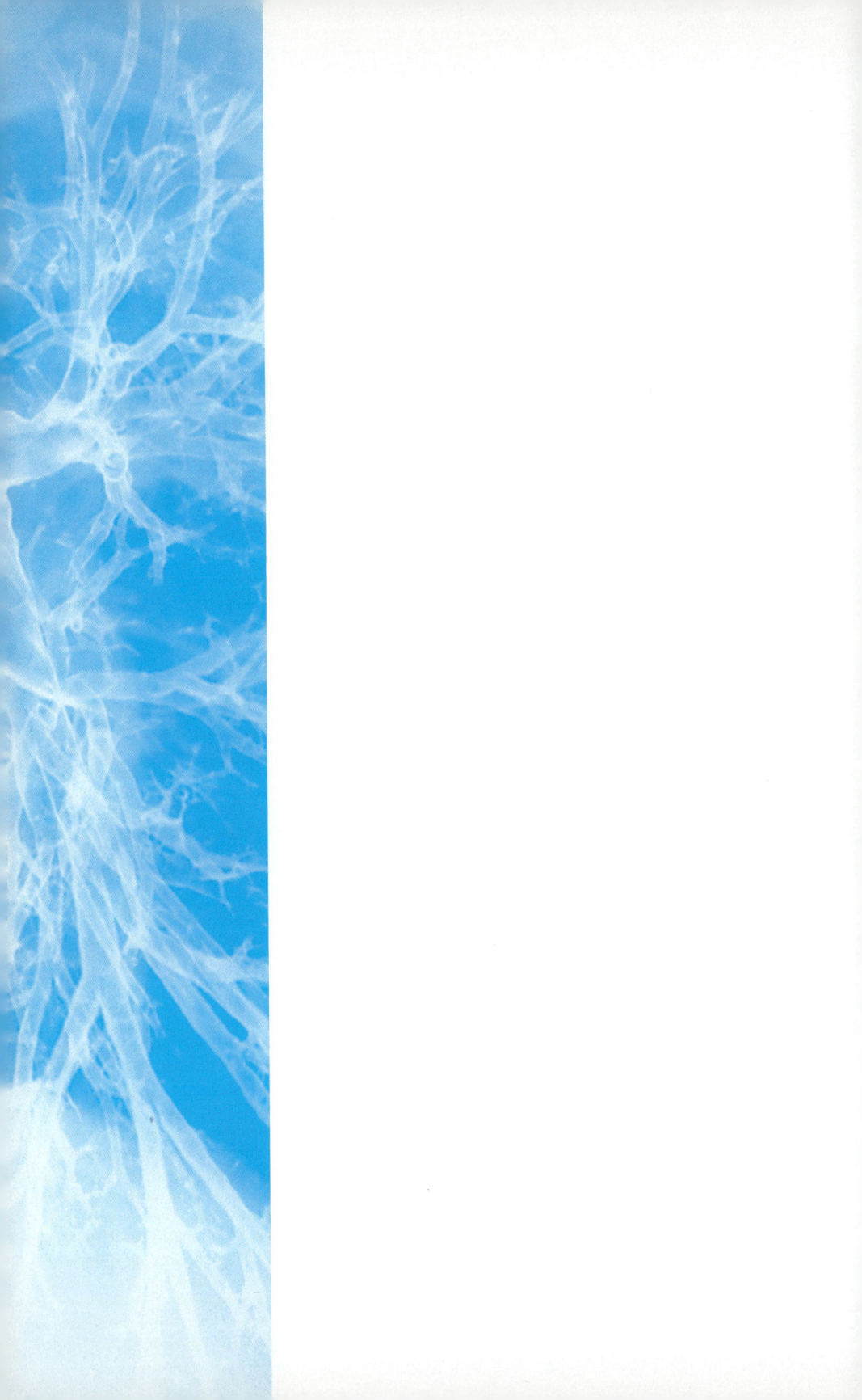

CHAPTER 15:

SLEEP-RELATED DISORDERS

OBSTRUCTIVE SLEEP APNOEA/ HYPOPNOEA SYNDROME 404
W. De Backer

CENTRAL SLEEP APNOEA 410
K.E. Bloch and T. Brack

HYPOVENTILATION SYNDROMES 414
J-F. Muir

OBSTRUCTIVE SLEEP APNOEA/HYPOPNOEA SYNDROME

W. De Backer
Dept of Pulmonary Medicine, University of Antwerp, Antwerp, Belgium
E-mail: wilfried.debacker@ua.ac.be

Obstructive sleep apnoea/hypopnoea syndrome (OSAHS) is characterised by recurrent episodes of partial or complete upper airway collapse during sleep. The collapse is highlighted by a reduction in, or complete cessation of, airflow despite ongoing inspiratory efforts. Due to the lack of adequate alveolar ventilation that results from the upper airway narrowing, oxygen saturation may drop and partial pressure of CO_2 may occasionally increase. The events are mostly terminated by arousals. Clinical consequences are excessive daytime sleepiness related to the sleep disruption. Minimal diagnostic criteria have been defined for OSAHS. Patients should have excessive daytime sleepiness that can not be better explained by other factors, or experience two or more of the following symptoms, again that are not better explained by other factors: choking or gasping during sleep; recurrent awakenings from sleep; unrefreshing sleep; daytime fatigue; and impaired concentration.

Key points

- OSAHS is characterised by recurrent episodes or partial or complete upper airway collapse during sleep.
- Minimal diagnostic criteria exist for OSAHS.
- Overnight polysomnography is the gold standard for OSAHS diagnosis.

All patients should have more than five obstructed breathing events per hour during sleep. An obstructive apnoea or hypopnoea can be defined as an event that lasts for $\geqslant 10$ s and is characterised by an absence or a decrease from baseline in the amplitude of a valid measure of breathing during sleep that either reaches >50% with an oxygen desaturation of 3% or an arousal (alternatively a 30% reduction with 4% desaturation). These definitions are recommended by the American Academy of Sleep Medicine (AASM). The Task Force of the AASM also states that there are common pathogenic mechanisms for obstructive apnoea syndrome, central apnoea syndrome, sleep hypoventilation syndrome and Cheyne–Stokes breathing. It was more preferable to discuss each of these separately; although, they could be placed under the common denominator of "sleep-disordered breathing syndrome". The definition of OSAHS using two components, daytime symptoms and breathing pattern disturbances during sleep, may suggest that there is a tight correlation between the two. However, unfortunately this is not the case. The breathing pattern abnormalities, mostly described by an apnoea/hypopnoea index (AHI), only weakly correlate with quantified measures of sleepiness, such as the Epworth Sleepiness Scale (ESS). This probably means that inter-individual sensitivity, with some individuals coping better with sleep fragmentation than others, does compromise the relationship between the AHI and daytime sleepiness scores. In addition, epidemiological studies show a broad range of sleepiness in the general population. Obviously, epidemiological studies investigating the prevalence of OSAHS are all biased by the lack of a uniform definition. The prevalence of an AHI of >5 events·h^{-1} in a general population (without taking into account symptoms of sleepiness) has previously been estimated to be 24% in a male population. When symptoms of sleepiness were also taken into account, the prevalence decreased to 4% in males and 2% in females.

Assessment of OSAHS

The most widely used gold standard for diagnosis is overnight polysomnography including nasal and/or oral airflow, thoraco-abdominal movement, snoring, EEG, EOG, EMG and oxygen saturation. Cardiorespiratory monitoring alone can be considered as highly sensitive (78–100%) and specific (67–100%). Sleepiness is often evaluated using the ESS, which assesses global level of sleepiness and is independent of short-term variations in sleepiness. The ESS discriminates between normal and pathological sleepiness.

Pathophysiology

Structural narrowing of the upper airway at one specific location is unlikely to be a major cause. Studies have shown that the upper airway collapse is not restricted to one place but is rather a dynamic phenomenon starting at a certain level and spreading caudally. Upper airway obstruction involves more than one specific site of the upper airway in the majority of sleep apnoea patients. The upper airway can collapse when insufficient load compensation is generated when an imbalance between the activation of the upper airway dilator muscles and the diaphragm occurs. When this occurs, the airway will collapse during inspiration or at least narrow with the development of flow limitation. However, there is increasing evidence that the collapse of the upper airway occurs during expiration. Furthermore, it has been convincingly shown that the upper airway behaves like a Starling resistor, making the collapse independent of the suction force brought about by the diaphragm, but rather dependent on the balance between the upper airway pressure and the tissue pressure at the collapsible site. The airway remains patent, regardless of the excessive pressure applied as long as the critical pressure of positive end-expiratory pressure (P_{crit}) remains low relative to P_u (pressure upstream to the collapsible segment). Closure of the upper airway occurs when P_u falls below the surrounding tissue pressure (P_{crit}). In the model of the Starling resistor, maximal flow (V'_{max}) becomes a function of the pressure gradient and the resistance in the segment upstream to the collapsible segment R_u: $V'_{max}=(P_u-P_{crit})/R_u$. The collapse of the upper airway then finally occurs during expiration when, due to the absence of dilator muscle, P_{crit} exceeds the upstream pressures. Prolonged expiratory time, as occurs during central apnoeas, therefore predisposes to collapse, but other factors may contribute and can be considered as risk factors (table 1).

Central and obstructive events are closely linked. Sometimes a central event with already partially collapsed upper airway can transit towards an obstructive event with ongoing occlusion of the upper airway despite the resumption of effort. Often, however, with resumption of effort at the end of the central apnoea, the obstruction of the upper airway disappears, presumably due to reactivation of the upper airway dilator muscles. However, the mechanisms remain unclear and more research is needed to understand why central apnoeas are sometimes followed by obstructive apnoeas and in some cases followed by reopening of the airways. In any case, since central apnoeas can trigger classical obstructive apnoeas, the mechanisms leading to unstable breathing (and thus central apnoeas) are also important in the genesis of obstructive apnoeas.

Consequences

Cardiovascular consequences Obstructed airways may generate negative intrathoracic pressure that increases left ventricular

Table 1. Risk factors for obstructive sleep apnoea: factors promoting upper airway collapse

Abnormal anatomy of the upper airway
Skeletal factors
Maxillary and/or mandibular hypoplasia or retroposition
Hyoid position (inferior displacement)
Soft tissue factors
Increased volume of soft tissues
Adenotonsillar hypertrophy
Macroglossia
Thickened lateral pharyngeal walls
Increased fat deposition
Pharyngeal inflammation and/or oedema
Increased vascular volume
Increased muscle volume
Pharyngeal muscle factors
Insufficient reflex activation of upper airway dilator muscles
Impaired strength and endurance of pharyngeal dilators
Pharyngeal compliance
Increased upper airway collapsibility
Sensory function
Impaired pharyngeal dilator reflexes
Impaired mechanoreceptor sensitivity
Lung volume dependence of upper airway cross-sectional area
Increased below functional residual capacity
Ventilatory control system factors
Unstable ventilatory control
Increased ventilatory responses and loop gains
Sex factors
Male influences
Centripetal pattern of obesity
Absence of progesterone
Presence of testosterone
Weight
Obesity causing peripharyngeal fat accumulation

Reproduced from VERBRAECKEN *et al.* (2009), with permission from the publisher.

transmural pressure and left ventricular afterload. The negative pressure also draws more blood into the thorax and increases right ventricular preload. Intermittent hypoxia related to obstructive sleep apnoea (OSA) will also impair cardiac contractility and diastolic relaxation (fig. 1).

OSA patients also have attenuated endothelium-dependent vasodilation and decreased circulating markers of nitric oxide. These effects, together with increased sympathetic vasoconstrictor activity and inflammation, will predispose to hypertension and atherosclerosis. In addition, platelet activation and aggregability are increased and predispose to thrombotic disease. Epidemiological studies indicate that OSA can initiate or promote cardiovascular disease, such as hypertension, coronary heart disease, heart failure, cardiac arrhythmias (bradyarrhythmias, atrial fibrillation and ventricular ectopy) and cerebrovascular disease.

Metabolic consequences OSA is associated with several components of the metabolic syndrome (MetS), mainly insulin resistance (IR) and abnormal lipid metabolism. Sleep restriction causes IR by inducing a pro-inflammatory state (increased release of interleukin-6 and tumour necrosis factor-α). Epidemiological studies have shown that sleep-related hypoxaemia is associated with glucose intolerance independent of age, sex, body mass index and waist circumference. MetS can be triggered by both intermittent hypoxia and sleep fragmentation/deprivation. The mechanisms are shown in figure 2.

MetS can be due to the release of free fatty acids, agiotensin II and adipokines by adipose tissue, which may damage the pancreas, leading to insufficient insulin release and apparent IR.

Mean and nadir arterial oxygen saturation during sleep is an independent predictor of MetS in overweight children and adolescents.

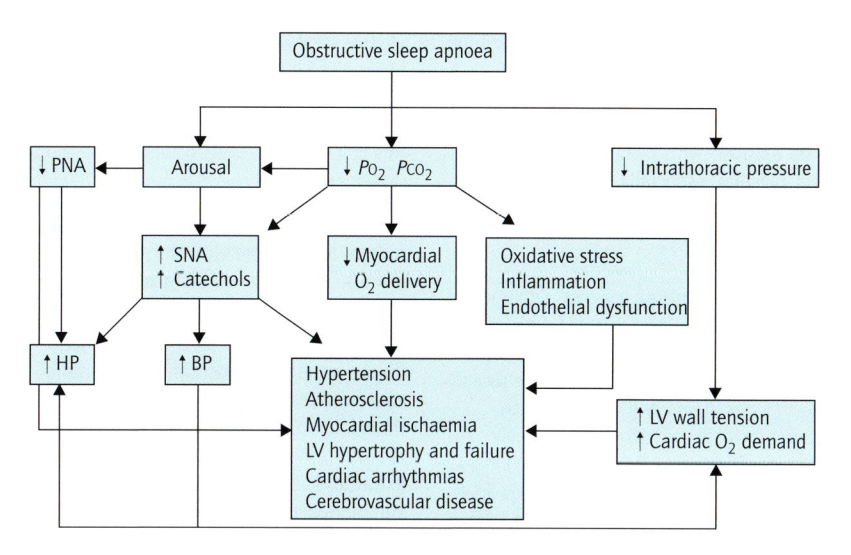

Figure 1. Cardiovascular consequences of obstructive sleep apnoea. PNA: parasympathetic nerve activity; P_{O_2}: oxygen tension; P_{CO_2}: carbon dioxide tension; SNA: sympathetic nerve activity; HR: heart rate; BP: blood pressure; LV: left ventricle. Modified from Bradley et al. (2009).

CPAP treatment

Therapy with nasal continuous positive pressure: mode of action Treatment with nasal continuous positive pressure (nCPAP) is perceived by most physicians as a very effective treatment for sleep apnoea and has been shown to be effective in controlled studies. nCPAP results in better sleep quality with lower arousal index: less stage 1 and more stage 3 and 4 sleep in a placebo-controlled (using placebo capsules) study. In addition, in milder forms of sleep apnoea nCPAP improved self-reported symptoms of

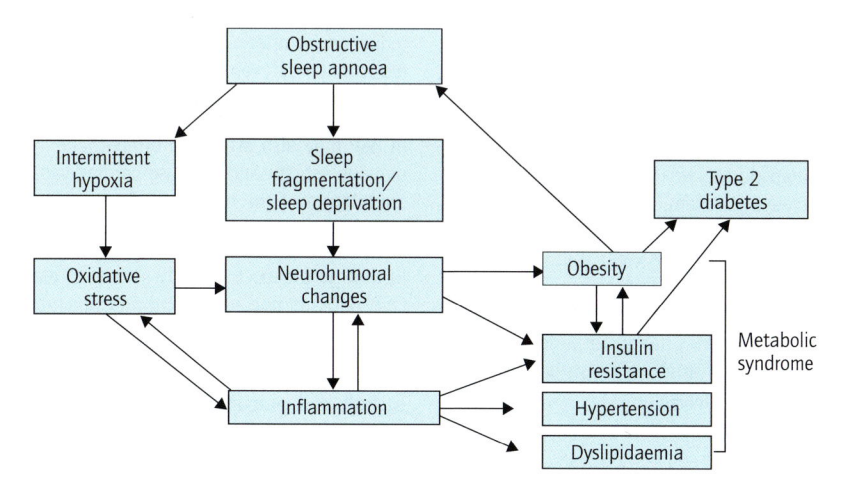

Figure 2. Mechanisms linking obstructive sleep apnoea and the metabolic syndrome. Modified from Tasali et al. (2008).

OSA, including snoring, restless sleep, daytime sleepiness and irritability. Neuropsychological tests also improved after nCPAP compared with ineffective nCPAP. Blood pressure can also be reduced with nCPAP when compared to oral placebo, especially in patients using nCPAP for $\geqslant 3.5$ h·night^{-1} and in those with >20 desaturations of 4% per hour.

nCPAP and the upper airway Occlusion of the upper airway can be prevented when either the resistance of the upper airway upstream, R_u or P_{crit} can be lowered. Regardless of the severity of the changes in P_{crit} and P_u, nCPAP can effectively increase (or restore) flow, largely through its effect on P_u ($V'_{max}=(P_u-P_{crit})/R_u$). Appropriate titration of the CPAP restores flow. nCPAP can increase P_u much more than local interventions, such as uvulopalatopharyngoplasty, can. Therefore, it also explains that overall nCPAP is much more clinically effective than was shown in previous controlled studies.

nCPAP and control of breathing As mentioned previously, some clinical observations initially indicated that unstable breathing is part of OSA syndrome, while more recent systematic analysis confirmed the increased loop gain and instability in the breathing pattern in OSA patients. It can be questioned, therefore, whether nCPAP can influence control of breathing in (obstructive) sleep apnoea patients. One could demonstrate that prolonged treatment with nCPAP significantly decreases the slope of the hypercapnic ventilatory response curve when measured during wakefulness, together with an increase in arterial oxygen tension and a decrease in the arterial–alveolar oxygen tension difference. It is clear that all of these changes may contribute to lowering of the gain in the system and promote a more stable breathing pattern. Changes in lung volume, although mostly small, can also be observed during nCPAP therapy.

nCPAP has also been demonstrated to be effective in central sleep apnoea. nCPAP can increase carbon dioxide tension above the apnoeic threshold and, therefore, eliminate central apnoeas. However, central apnoeas are often also characterised by (near) occlusion of the upper airway; as highlighted earlier, nCPAP can also presumably be effective in preventing this collapse and its associated local reflexes.

nCPAP and the heart nCPAP can effectively be used to treat acute cardiogenic pulmonary oedema with shifting volume from intra- to extrathoracic compartments.

nCPAP may relieve CSA in chronic heart failure patients by increasing the arterial carbon dioxide tension above the apnoeic threshold. nCPAP may reduce ventilation by redistributing excess lung water to extrathoracic compartments thereby reducing stimulation of pulmonary vagal irritant receptors. nCPAP may also unload the inspiratory muscles by increasing lung compliance, again due to extrathoracic redistribution of lung water.

nCPAP may significantly reduce left ventricular afterload by lowering the transmural pressure in patients with compromised cardiac function. In the normal heart, where cardiac output is largely preload dependent, CPAP decreases cardiac output by reducing left ventricular preload. In contrast, the failing heart is relatively insensitive to changes in preload but very sensitive to reductions in afterload. CPAP induced reductions in left ventricular transmural pressure (and afterload) can augment cardiac output.

nCPAP may also attenuate sympathetic nervous activity and increase cardiac vagal modulation of the heart with favourable effects on blood pressure regulation.

In a large prospective study severe untreated OSA patients had more fatal and non-fatal cardiovascular events, this difference disappeared with nCPAP treatment.

nCPAP and metabolic/systemic effects of OSA nCPAP may improve MetS although it is not always certain that nCPAP has an independent effect. nCPAP also lowers tumour necrosis factor-α, interleukin-6 and C-reactive protein.

Non-CPAP treatment

Mandibular advancement device

Mandibular advancement devices (MAD) are the most common oral appliances used for the treatment of OSA and/or snoring. They have either a one-piece (monobloc) or two-piece (duobloc) configuration while customised devices have a better retention, tolerance and efficacy. MAD are effective if they increase the volume of the upper airway, which may enlarge at some sites and also narrow at other sites. Therefore, the overall efficacy is sometimes suboptimal; 65% of patients achieve a 50% reduction in AHI. Also snoring, excessive daytime sleepiness, neuropsychological function and cardiovascular risk may decrease. It is important to try to predict the outcome. Imaging and modelling studies can be of help for this purpose.

Surgical treatment

Several techniques have been performed, all with the aim of enlarging the volume of the upper airway and reducing the closing pressure. Uvulopalatopharyngoplasty reduces upper airway obstruction by shortening the uvula, trimming the soft plate and suturing back the anterior and posterior pharyngeal pillars. Tonsillectomy is performed at the same time if tonsils are found to be enlarged. Maxillomandibular advancement osteotomy advances the maxilla and mandible to enlarge the retrolingual and retropalatal spaces. Adenotonsillectomy is first-line treatment in children. Electrical stimulation of the genioglossus with an implanted pacemaker has recently been tested and found to be efficient in selected patients, although more clinical studies are needed in order to learn which patients will benefit most.

References

- Bradley TD, Floras JS. Obstructive sleep apnoea and its cardiovascular consequences. *Lancet* 2009; 373: 82-93.
- Chan AS, *et al*. Non-positive airway pressure modalities: mandibular advancement devices/positional therapy. *Proc Am Thorac Soc* 2008; 5: 179-184.
- De Backer WJ, *et al*. Novel imaging techniques using computer methods for the evaluation of the upper airway in patients with sleep-disordered breathing: a comprehensive review. *Sleep Med Rev* 2008; 12: 437-447.
- Jennum P, Riha RL. Epidemiology of sleep apnoea/hypopnoea syndrome and sleep-disordered breathing. *Eur Respir J* 2009; 33: 907-914.
- Levy, P., et al, Sleep, sleep-disordered breathing and metabolic consequences. *Eur Respir J* 2009; 34: 243-260.
- Marin JM, *et al*. Long-term cardiovascular outcomes in men with obstructive sleep apnoea-hypopnoea with or without treatment with continuous positive airway pressure: an observational study. *Lancet* 2005; 365: 1046-1053.
- McArdle, N., Douglas NJ, Effect of continuous positive airway pressure on sleep architecture in the sleep apnea-hypopnea syndrome: a randomized controlled trial. *Am J Respir Crit Care Med* 2001; 164: 1459-1463.
- Sleep-related breathing disorders in adults: recommendations for syndrome definition and measurement techniques in clinical research. The Report of an American Academy of Sleep Medicine Task Force. *Sleep* 1999; 22: 667-689.
- Tasali E, Ip MS. Obstructive sleep apnea and metabolic syndrome: alterations in glucose metabolism and inflammation. *Proc Am Thorac Soc* 2008; 5: 207-217.
- Verbraecken JA, De Backer WA. Upper airway mechanics. *Respiration* 2009; 78: 121-133.
- Verhulst SL, *et al*. Sleep-disordered breathing and the metabolic syndrome in overweight and obese children and adolescents. *J Pediatr* 2007; 150: 608-612.
- Won CH, *et al*. Surgical treatment of obstructive sleep apnea: upper airway and maxillomandibular surgery. *Proc Am Thorac Soc* 2008; 5: 193-199.
- Young TM, *et al*. The occurrence of sleep-disordered breathing among middle-aged adults. *N Engl J Med* 1993; 328: 1230-1235.
- Younes M, *et al*. Mechanisms of breathing instability in patients with obstructive sleep apnea. *J Appl Physiol* 2007; 103: 1929-1941.

CENTRAL SLEEP APNOEA

K.E. Bloch[1] and T. Brack[2]
[1] Pulmonary Division, University Hospital of Zurich, Zurich
[2] Cantonal Hospital Glarus, Glarus, Switzerland
E-mail: konrad.bloch@usz.ch

Central sleep apnoea/hypopnoea (CSA) refers to the cessation or reduction of ventilation lasting for $\geqslant 10$ s (in adults) due to transient loss of neural output to the respiratory muscles. Many patients with CSA have mild hypocapnia or normocapnia, but rarely are hypercapnia and hypoventilation also observed. A periodic pattern of waxing and waning of ventilation with periods of hyperventilation alternating with central apnoea/hypopnoea is termed Cheyne-Stokes respiration (CSR).

Prevalence, aetiology and pathophsiology

The prevalence of CSA in the general population is not known. However, it seems to be significantly less common than obstructive sleep apnoea (OSA), as <5% of patients referred to a sleep laboratory revealed predominant CSA. In contrast, a relatively high prevalence of CSA is observed in association with various conditions including congestive heart failure, pulmonary hypertension, ischaemic stroke, neuromuscular disease, obesity hypoventilation syndrome and narcotic use, or during initiation of continuous positive airway pressure (CPAP) therapy in patients with OSA. In healthy subjects, CSA may occur during hypoxia at altitude. In addition, idiopathic CSA is not associated with any comorbid condition.

Pathophysiological mechanisms underlying CSA include: respiratory control instability, due to an increased chemical drive that moves the prevailing arterial carbon dioxide tension closer to the apnoea threshold; a prolonged circulation time; and altered respiratory mechanics. Subsequently, different forms of CSA will be discussed.

CSR/CSA syndrome in heart failure patients

The prevalence of CSR/CSA with an apnoea/hypopnoea index of >15 events·h^{-1} has been found to be very high (15-37%) and OSA is even common (10-26%) among patients with severe heart failure (left ventricular ejection fraction $\leqslant 45\%$) irrespective of a suspicion of sleep apnoea. In some patients CSR/CSA and OSA may coexist and alternate over the course of a night. Symptoms attributable to CSR/CSA are not well defined and may

Key points

- CSA is the loss or reduction in ventilation due to transient loss of neural output to the respiratory muscles.
- A high prevalence of CSA is observed in association with other conditions, such as congestive heart failure, pulmonary hypertension, ischaemic stroke, neuromuscular disease, obesity hypoventilation syndrome and narcotic use.
- Risk factors for CSA/CSR are age >60 yrs, male sex, severe heart failure, hypocapnia and atrial fibrillation.
- Treatment includes oxygen, acetazolamide and positive pressure ventilation, in particular adaptive servo-ventilation.

include paroxysmal nocturnal dyspnoea, poor sleep quality, excessive daytime sleepiness, fatigue and poor exercise tolerance.

CSR/CSA in heart failure patients is associated with poor prognosis. Several studies have found an increased mortality in patients with CSR/CSA even after controlling for the severity of heart failure, age, sex and other potential confounders. Mortality was particularly high in patients presenting with CSR during physical activity during the day (fig. 1).

Sleep-related breathing disturbances should be suspected in all patients with heart failure who suffer from nocturnal dyspnoea, unrefreshing sleep or daytime sleepiness. Particular risk factors for CSA/CSR include: severe heart failure, older age ($\geqslant 60$ yrs), male sex, hypocapnia, atrial fibrillation and CSR observed during the day. The diagnosis should be evaluated by polysomnography or a cardiorespiratory sleep study, since pulse oximetry can not make the important distinction between CSA and OSA.

Optimised medical therapy of heart failure is the first step in the treatment of CSR/CSA. Cardiac resynchronisation by biventricular pacing and heart transplantation may also alleviate CSR/CSA. If medical therapy is ineffective, noninvasive ventilation may additionally be required. Nocturnal CPAP has been shown to improve nocturnal CSR/CSA, oxygen saturation, left ventricular ejection fraction, sympathetic nervous system activity and the 6 min walking distance. However, CPAP did not prolong survival without heart transplantation during a 2-yr follow-up in a large trial (CANPAP), although a *post hoc* analysis suggested a survival benefit if CPAP sufficiently suppressed CSR/CSA. Adaptive servo-ventilation is a mode of bi-level positive airway pressure ventilation that continuously adjusts pressure support according to the breathing pattern of the patient in order to stabilise periodic breathing. It is a promising treatment option for CSR/CSA as it has been shown to improve nocturnal breathing pattern, daytime vigilance and quality of life after treatment for several weeks. Studies in larger patient cohorts over longer time periods are needed to confirm these effects and to evaluate a potentially improved

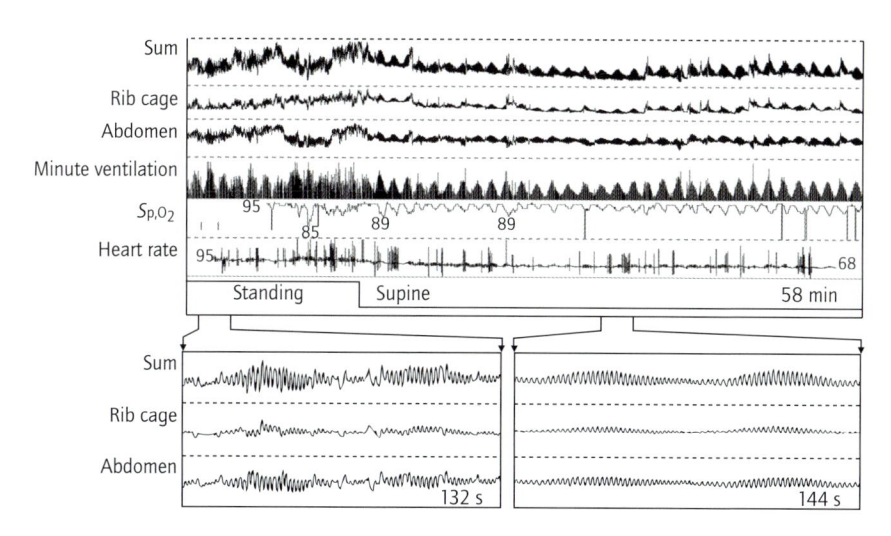

Figure 1. Cheyne–Stokes breathing in a patient with congestive heart failure. Inductive plethysmographic signals from rib cage and abdominal sensors showing regular waxing and waning of ventilation with central hypopnoea and corresponding oscillations of oxygen saturation. The upper panel represents a 58-min daytime recording, the lower panels show enlarged portions obtained while standing (left) and in the supine position (right). S_{p,O_2}: arterial oxygen saturation measured by pulse oximetry. Modified from Brack *et al.* (2007).

Central sleep apnoea

survival. Supplemental oxygen and acetazolamide have also been shown to alleviate CSR/CSA. Further studies are required to better define the role of these adjuncts for the treatment of heart failure in patients with CSR/CSA.

Complex sleep apnoea syndrome

In some patients diagnosed with OSA a CSR/CSA breathing pattern may emerge during initial CPAP therapy. The clinical relevance of this phenomenon, referred to as complex sleep apnoea, is still a matter of debate since studies suggest that CSA disappears in the majority of OSA patients during prolonged CPAP therapy. However, persistent residual CSA may disturb sleep quality, prevent complete symptomatic improvement and may lead to CPAP intolerance in OSA patients. In this setting adaptive servo-ventilation has been successfully used to normalise the breathing pattern and improve sleep quality.

Idiopathic CSA apnoea syndrome

Idiopathic CSA syndrome (fig. 2) is, by definition, not associated with any underlying disease. CSA causes sleep fragmentation which may be perceived as unrefreshing sleep and may result in daytime sleepiness. Idiopathic CSA is thought to be much less common than OSA, although no systematic epidemiological studies have been performed. Treatment options include acetazolamide, theophylline, CPAP and adaptive servo-ventilation.

CSA in various conditions

CSA and ataxic breathing have been observed in patients on chronic opioid medication and can be successfully treated with adaptive servo-ventilation, although the relevance of the breathing disturbances requires further study. Patients with stroke and neuromuscular disease, such as post-polio syndrome, motor neuron disease, multiple system atrophy or with idiopathic central hypoventilation, may

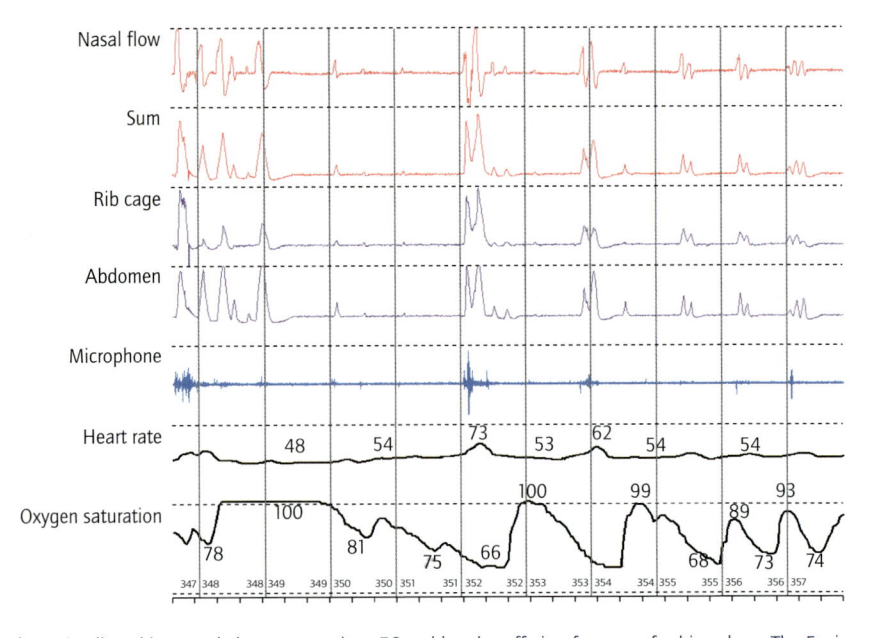

Figure 2. Idiopathic central sleep apnoea in a 56-yr-old male suffering from unrefreshing sleep. The 5-min recording shows repetitive central apnoeas of variable duration (20–90 s) associated with severe oxygen desaturation (minimal value of 66%). The absence of excursions in the inductive plethysmographic rib cage and abdominal signals during cessation of airflow indicates that apnoeas are due to intermittent loss of neuromuscular drive.

exhibit CSA with or without associated OSA and/or hypoventilation. Depending on the prevailing breathing disturbance, bi-level positive pressure ventilation, CPAP or adaptive servo-ventilation may improve breathing and alleviate symptoms.

High-altitude periodic breathing

In healthy subjects, hypobaric hypoxia at altitudes of >2,000 m may induce periodic breathing with central apnoea/hypopnoea. Breathing instability is related to an enhanced chemosensitivity (high controller gain) causing a tendency for a ventilatory overshoot and hyperventilation with a reduced CO_2 reserve, *i.e.* the eupneic carbon dioxide tension approaches the apnoeic threshold which promotes apnoea during minor ventilatory alterations. Symptoms may include paroxysmal dyspnoea and poor sleep quality. In some subjects, high-altitude periodic breathing is associated with acute mountain sickness; a syndrome characterised by headaches, insomnia, poor appetite, fatigue and, in more severe forms, ataxia and altered consciousness. The diagnosis of high-altitude periodic breathing is based on clinical observations in the appropriate context combined with pulse oximetry or more sophisticated sleep studies if feasible. Treatment is often not required but can be performed by altitude descent or the administration of supplemental oxygen or acetazolamide, which is also effective against acute mountain sickness.

Conclusions

In conclusion, CSA/CSR is less common than OSA. However, in certain conditions, including congestive heart failure, neuromuscular disorders, during opioid use and at high altitude, the prevalence of CSA is high. Treatment for CSA is not as well established as that for OSA, and may include oxygen, acetazolamide and positive pressure ventilation, in particular adaptive servo-ventilation.

References

- Brack T, *et al.* Daytime Cheyne–Stokes respiration in ambulatory patients with severe congestive heart failure is associated with increased mortality. *Chest* 2007; 132: 1463–1471.
- Dai Y, Bradley DT. Central sleep apnea and Cheyne-Stokes respiration. *Proc Am Thorac Soc* 2008; 5: 226–236.
- Eckert DJ, *et al.* Central sleep apnea. *Chest* 2007; 131: 595–607.
- Javaheri S, *et al.* The prevalence and natural history of complex sleep apnea. *J Clin Sleep Med* 2009; 5: 205–211.
- Walker JM, *et al.* Chronic opioid use is a risk factor for the development of central sleep apnea and ataxic breathing. *J Clin Sleep Med* 2007; 3: 455–461.
- Bradley DT, *et al.* Continuous positive airway pressure for central sleep apnea and heart failure. *N Engl J Med* 2005; 353: 2025–2033.
- UpToDate for Patients. Central sleep apnea syndrome. www.uptodate.com/patients/content/search.do?search=central+sleep+apnea.

HYPOVENTILATION SYNDROMES

J-F. Muir
Respiratory Dept and Respiratory Intensive Care Unit, Rouen Hospital, Rouen, France
E-mail: Jean-Francois.Muir@chu-rouen.fr

Sleep-related hypoventilation syndromes, together with central and obstructive sleep apnoea syndromes, are sleep-related breathing disorders (table 1).

Sleep-induced hypoventilation is characterised by elevated levels of arterial carbon dioxide tension (Pa,CO_2) of >45 mmHg while asleep or disproportionately increased relative to levels during wakefulness.

Pathophysiology

Nocturnal hypoventilation can be attributed to decreased ventilatory drive (won't breathe), which may be due to respiratory dysfunction (polio sequelae, central hypoventilation, amyotrophic lateral sclerosis or Arnold–Chiari malformation), or the following: depression (hypnotics); alteration of respiratory nerve conduction (Guillain–Barré syndrome), transmission to the respiratory muscles (myasthenia) or worsening mechanics (can't breathe) with respiratory muscle alteration (muscular dystrophy); chest wall deformities; or severe obesity. In the latter situations, lungs are normal and associated hypoxaemia is due to the displacement of oxygen in the alveoli from increasing CO_2 levels, as predicted by the alveolar air equation. If the lungs are abnormal (chronic obstructive pulmonary disease (COPD), tuberculous sequelae, cystic fibrosis or diffuse bronchiectasis), hypercapnia is mainly due to worsening mechanics and ventilation–perfusion inequalities.

During the night, ventilatory response to hypoxaemia and hypercapnia is largely reduced during rapid eye movement (REM) sleep with dysrythmic breathing and less reduced during non-REM sleep. The result is a reduction of alveolar hypoventilation by altering minute ventilation and/or dead space volume/tidal volume.

Respiratory mechanics change during sleep and thereby worsen gas exchange, particularly in neuromuscular diseases and obstructive airways diseases. REM sleep induces skeletal muscle hypotonia sparing the diaphragm and not the accessory respiratory muscles, with

Key points

- Sleep-induced hypoventilation is characterised by increased Pa,CO_2 levels of >45 mmHg

- Nocturnal hypoventilation is associated with decreased ventilatory drive, respiratory iatrogenic depression, alteration of respiratory nerve conductance, chest wall deformities or severe obesity

- OHS is the association of obesity and sleep-disordered breathing with daytime hypersomnolence and hypercapnia in the absence of other respiratory diseases

- Polysomnographic evaluation is needed in order to diagnose OHS

- NIV is used as the first-line treatment with supplementary oxygen

Table 1. Sleep related hypoventilation/hypoxaemic syndromes[#]

Sleep-related hypoventilation/hypoxaemic syndromes
Sleep-related non-obstructive alveolar hypoventilation, idiopathic congenital central alveolar hypoventilation syndrome
Sleep-related hypoventilation/hypoxaemia due to a medical condition
Sleep-related hypoventilation/hypoxaemia due to pulmonary parenchymal or vascular pathology
Sleep-related hypoventilation/hypoxaemia due to lower airways obstruction
Sleep-related hypoventilation/hypoxaemia due to neuromuscular or chest wall disorders

[#]: according to the International Classification of Sleep Disorders-2 classification.

deleterious effects in conditions where these muscles are necessary to maintain normal ventilation. REM sleep also alters upper airways patency and reduces chronic respiratory failure.

Clinical features

Hypoventilation *per se* generates a clinical syndrome associated with, in typical cases, dyspnoea during activities of daily living in the absence of paralysis, poor sleep quality, excessive daytime fatigue and sleepiness, nocturnal or early morning headache, cyanosis and evidence of right heart failure.

Diagnosis

The presence of such symptoms highlights the need to perform a physical examination, pulmonary function tests, a chest radiograph as well as measure arterial blood gases and recordings of sleep, *i.e.* arterial oxygen saturation and transcutaneous carbon dioxide tension. The results of this initial investigation will be concluded by full night ventilatory polygraphy (respiratory signals only) or polysomnography (respiratory and neurological signals; EEG, EOG, EMG). Chronic daytime hypercapnia is associated with and preceded by sleep-related hypoventilation.

Aetiology

Presence of an extrapulmonary restrictive disorder
If obesity is present the most frequent diagnosis is obesity hypoventilation syndrome. Previously called the "Pickwickian syndrome", obesity hypoventilation syndrome (OHS) is defined as the association of obesity (body mass index (BMI) >30 kg·m^{-2}) and sleep-disordered breathing with daytime hypersomnolence and hypercapnia (Pa,CO_2 >45 mmHg) in the absence of any other respiratory disease. The prevalence of OHS is 36% in patients with a BMI of 35–40 kg·m^{-2} and 48% if BMI is ⩾50 kg·m^{-2}.

The pathogenesis of OHS involves abnormal pulmonary mechanics with an excessive work of breathing and altered hypoxic and hypercapnic ventilatory responses, linked, in part, to chronic hypoxaemia and poor sleep quality, upper airway obstruction and, possibly, the influence of leptin.

Without adequate treatment, patients with OHS develop cor pulmonale, recurrent episodes of hypercapnic respiratory failure and loss of survival. OHS is one of the many aetiologies of chronic respiratory failure and has become a growing indication to initiate acute and/or long-term noninvasive mechanical ventilation (NIV). Mechanisms of action include resting of the respiratory muscles, an increase in thoracic compliance and resetting of the respiratory centres. In OHS, nocturnal NIV has been shown to be clinically effective because of a rapid and sustained improvement of daytime arterial blood gas levels and a net reduction of daytime sleepiness.

In order to establish a diagnosis of OHS polysomnographic evaluation is needed and the ventilatory treatment needs to be adapted. The sleep respiratory pattern can present as obstructive apnoeas and hypopnoeas (90% of cases), obstructive hypoventilation due to increased upper airway resistance and/or central hypoventilation (10%) (fig. 1).

Recent data from a large cohort of OHS patients who had been treated with NIV and pressure-cycled ventilators showed a very significant decrease in the number of hospital stays for cardiac and/or respiratory illness for the 3 yrs following the initiation of NIV, compared with the year prior to the start of treatment. A dramatic improvement in arterial blood gases was observed and a good compliance suggests that this treatment is cost-effective and improves morbidity and mortality in such patients. NIV is used as first-line treatment with supplemental oxygen; expiratory airway pressure is titrated to control hypopnoeas and apnoeas and inspiratory airway pressure is added to control Pa,CO_2. If pressure pre-set NIV fails, nasal volume pre-set ventilation may be used. In patients with OHS and predominant OSA, once hypercapnia has improved using NIV (which may take several weeks), NIV may be changed to nasal continuous positive airway pressure (fig. 2). NIV has also largely

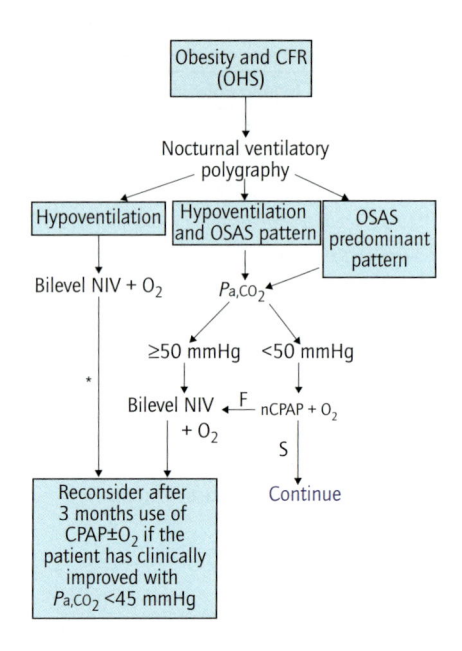

Figure 2. A ventilator management algorithm in a patient with severe obesity hypoventilation (OHS) presenting with chronic respiratory failure (CRF). OSAS: obstructive sleep apnoea syndrome; NIV: noninvasive ventilation; Pa,CO_2: arterial carbon dioxide tension; CPAP: continuous positive airway pressure; F: failure; S: success. [#]: an alternative is assisted control ventilation.

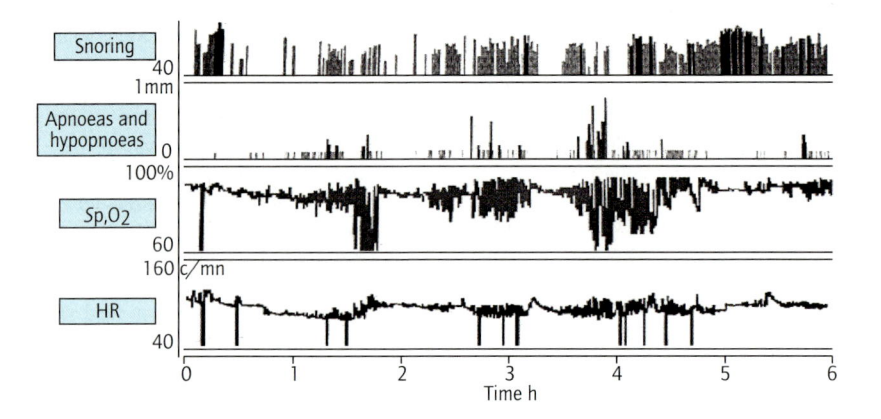

Figure 1. A ventilator polygraphy from a patient with severe obesity hypoventilation syndrome. Apnoea/hypopnoea index: 26 events·h[-1]; arterial oxygen tension: 9.6 kPa; arterial carbon dioxide tension: 8.5 kPa. Sp,O_2: arterial oxygen saturation measured by pulse oximetry; HR: heart rate.

improved the immediate vital prognosis of OHS and acute respiratory failure.

The medical management is mainly orientated towards weight loss. A reduction of 5-10% of body weight can result in a significant decrease in Pa,CO_2. Unfortunately, weight loss by diet alone is difficult to achieve and sustain; thus, bariatric surgery has been advocated. After significant weight reduction surgery patients with OHS experience long-term improvement of arterial blood gases and dyspnoea.

If obesity is absent or not predominant, the most frequent conditions are: neuromuscular diseases with Duchenne muscular dystrophy; Steiner myotony; polio sequelae; amyotrophic lateral sclerosis; and high spinal injuries with tetraplegia and respiratory paralysis. Less frequent are acid maltase deficiency and spinal muscular atrophy.

Chest wall diseases with kyphoscoliosis and tuberculosis sequelae are a category of diseases that represent the best indication for the application of acute and chronic mechanical ventilation mainly with NIV, and in some severe situations or after failure of NIV with invasive mechanical ventilation with tracheostomy.

Presence of an obstructive disorder

COPD, diffuse bronchiectasis and cystic fibrosis are the most frequent conditions. During sleep there is a worsening of awake hypoxaemia and hypercapnia, especially during REM sleep. NIV is generally proposed after failure of long-term oxygen therapy in hypercapnic COPD when frequent episodes of acute respiratory decompensation occur and/or when baseline Pa,CO_2 progressively worsens. COPD patients with obesity must be investigated for possible overlap syndrome, which is associated with obstructive sleep apnoea and COPD.

Congenital central hypoventilation syndrome

Congenital central hypoventilation syndrome is a rare disorder of ventilatory control that typically presents in newborns and mainly results from a polyalanin repeat expansion mutation in the PHOX2B gene. It results in the failure of automatic central control of breathing in infants who do not breathe spontaneously or who breathe shallowly and erratically. Sufferers are generally treated by mechanical ventilation with tracheostomy and, in less severe situations, by NIV. Electrostimulation of the phrenic nerves and or the diaphragm is currently being tested as a new therapeutic option.

References

- Bannerjee D, Yee BJ, et al. Obesity hypoventilation syndrome: hypoxemia during CPAP. Chest 2007; 131: 1678-1684.
- Casey KR, Contillo KO, et al. Sleep related hypoxemic/hypoventilation syndromes. Chest 2007; 131: 1936-1948.
- Cuvelier A, Muir JF. Obesity hypoventilation syndrome: new insights in the Pickwick papers. Chest 2007; 131: 7-8.
- de Lucas-Ramos P, de Miguel-Diez J, et al. Benefits at 1 year of nocturnal intermittent positive pressure ventilation in patients with obesity-hypoventilation syndrome. Respir Med 2004; 98: 961-967.
- Guo YF, Sforza E, et al. Respiratory patterns during sleep in OHS patients treated with nocturnal pressure support. Chest 2007; 131: 1090-1099.
- Hill NS. Noninvasive ventilation. Does it work, for whom, and how? Am Rev Respir Dis 1993; 147: 1050-1055.
- Janssens JP, Derivaz S, et al. Changing patterns in long-term noninvasive ventilation: a 7-year pro-spective study in the Geneva Lake area. Chest 2003; 123: 67-79.
- Kessler, R, Chaouat, A, et al, The obesity-hypoventilation syndrome revisited: a prospective study of 34 consecutive cases. Chest 2001; 120: 369-376.
- Mokhlesi B, Tulaimat A, et al. Impact of adherence with positive airway pressure therapy on hypercapnia in OSA. J Clin Sleep Med 2006; 2: 57-62.
- Muir JF, Cuvelier A. Management of chronic respiratory failure and obesity. In: Ambrosino N, Goldstein R, eds. Ventilatory Support for Chronic Respiratory Failure. Vol. 1. New York, Informa Healthcare, 2008; pp. 433-444.
- Nowbar R, Burkart KM, et al. Obesity associated hypoventilation in hospitalized patients: prevalence, effects and outcome. Am J Med 2004; 116: 1-7.

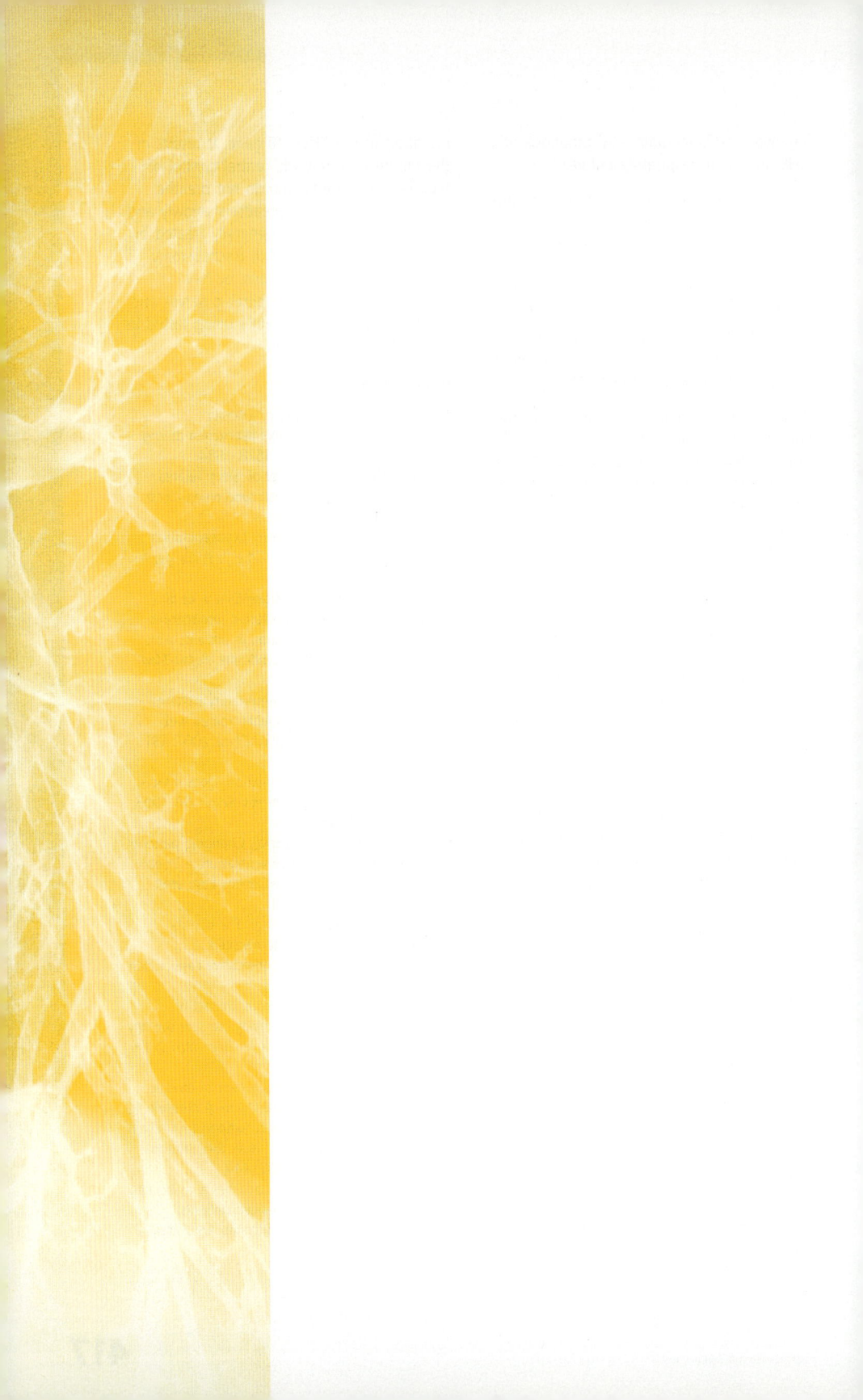

CHAPTER 16:

IMMUNODEFICIENCY DISORDERS AND ORPHAN LUNG DISEASE

PULMONARY DISEASES IN PRIMARY IMMUNODEFICIENCY SYNDROMES I. Quinti, C. Milito, L. Bonanni and F. La Marra	**420**
HIV-RELATED DISEASE M.C.I. Lipman and R.F. Miller	**423**
GRAFT *VERSUS* HOST DISEASE I. Quinti, C. Milito, L. Bonanni and F. La Marra	**430**
AMYLOIDOSIS H.J. Lachmann	**433**
PULMONARY ALVEOLAR PROTEINOSIS M. Luisetti	**435**
ADULT PULMONARY LANGERHANS' CELL HISTIOCYTOSIS J-F. Cordier and V. Cottin	**438**
LYMPHANGIOLEIOMYOMATOSIS J-F. Cordier and V. Cottin	**441**

PULMONARY DISEASES IN PRIMARY IMMUNODEFICIENCY SYNDROMES

I. Quinti, C. Milito, L. Bonanni and F. La Marra
Dept of Clinical Medicine, Reference Centre for Primary Immunodeficiencies, Sapienza University of Rome, Rome, Italy
E-mail: isabella.quinti@uniroma1.it

The definition of primary immunodeficiencies (PID) includes multiple genetic defects that belong to the group of rare diseases. The World Health Organization recognises more than 70 diseases classified as PID. The risk and type of infections change according to the main defects of the immune system, and are classified as antibody deficiencies, combined immunodeficiencies and phagocytic disorders (table 1). In some cases there are unique features of lung abnormalities in specific defects.

Severe and recurrent infections with capsulated bacteria, asthma and bronchiectasis represent the most important morbidity and mortality factors of the patients affected by primary antibody deficiencies. The common pathogens isolated from the sputum are *Haemophilus influenzae*, *Streptococcus pneumoniae* and *Streptococcus pyogenes*, with *Pseudomonas aeruginosa* and *Moraxella catarrhalis* occurring less frequently. Chronic lung disease (CLD) represents the principal morbidity factor. In primary antibody deficiencies where the defect is an inability to produce an effective antibody response to pathogens, only immunoglobin (Ig)G antibodies might be replaced. The substitutive therapy with Ig reduces the risk of acute respiratory infections, particularly pneumonia, but has low efficacy in reduction of chronic lung complications, infective exacerbations and asthma, which are promoted by vicious circle infection–inflammation. Despite *i.v.* Ig treatment, the number of patients with CLD and bronchiectasis increases with time for almost all age groups (prevalence of CLD >50% in adults, 30–40% in children). The overall probability of developing CLD reached ~80% after 17 yrs of follow-up. As already

> **Key points**
>
> - Primary immunodeficiencies (PID) include multiple genetic defects that belong to the group of rare diseases.
> - More than 70 diseases are classified as PID.
> - The risk and type of infections change according to the main defects of the immune system, and are classified as antibody deficiencies, combined immunodeficiencies and phagocytic disorders.
> - A PID diagnosis should be considered in patients presenting with severe and recurrent respiratory infections, with granulomatous diseases or with life-threatening invasive pulmonary infections.

Table 1. Microorganisms in primary immunodeficiencies

	Antibody deficiencies	**Combined immunodeficiencies**	**Phagocytic defects**
Viruses	Enteroviruses	CMV, respiratory syncytial virus, EBV, parainfluenza type 3	No
Bacteria	Streptococcus pneumoniae, Haemophilus influenzae, Moraxella catarrhalis, Pseudomonas aeruginosa, Staphylococcus aureus, Neisseria meningitidis, Mycoplasma pneumoniae, Campylobacter	As for antibody deficiencies, also: Salmonella typhi, Listeria monocytogenes, Candida, Pneumocysitis carinii	S. aureus, P. aeruginosa, Nocardia asteroides, S. typhi, Aspergillus
Mycobacteria	No	Nontuberculous, including BCG	Nontuberculous, BCG

CMV: cytomegalovirus; EBV: Epstein-Barr virus; BCG: bacille Calmette-Guerin. Adapted from Notarangelo (2010).

demonstrated in patients with cystic fibrosis, dyspnoea and sputum production are conditioning factors of increased morbidity. Accumulated mucus in the airways is the prominent feature of bronchiectasis, leading to airway obstruction, bacterial colonisation and recurrent infections. The events that define the pathogenesis of an infection depend on a large range of variables, including the specific infecting organism and its virulence and the overall immunological state of the host. IgG antibodies are only one player in the complex network of cells and mediators required to protect the respiratory tract against various insults, including infections. In support of this evidence, data indicate the role of a very low IgA level as a major independent risk factor for all the main PID-associated clinical conditions (pneumonia, chronic lung disease, acute and chronic sinusitis), underlining the well known role of IgA antibodies on immune defence against a variety of potentially pathogenic organisms when they are encountered in the respiratory or the intestinal tracts. The generation of secretory IgA has a basic impact on the epithelial barrier, a function lacking in the majority of PID patients. Moreover, low IgA levels reflect a severely impaired isotype-switching process. Thus, the loss of function of memory B-cells seems to represent the major cause of PID-associated clinical conditions as already demonstrated in common variable immunodeficiency patients with bronchiectasis. Aside from Ig replacement, a strategy to reduce lung damage should then be approached. Prophylactic antibiotics, macrolides as anti-inflammatory agents, inhaled corticosteroids, bronchodilators, mucolytics, or mechanical or rehabilitative respiratory methods need to be considered.

In patients with cellular and combined immunodeficiencies and in patients with PID who require bone marrow transplantation, respiratory viral infections are major causes of morbidity and mortality. All viruses might be detected, all worsening the clinical outcome (table 1). Herpes viruses, paramyxoviruses and adenoviruses are common, significant pathogens in these patients. Aggressive treatments may reduce viral replication and damage. Fungal infections are less frequent compared with bacterial or viral infections among patients with PID. However, fungal infections can result in significant morbidity and potentially fatal outcome if misdiagnosed or not treated correctly. In this context, the knowledge of fungal pathogens likely to cause disease as well as of the expected clinical presentation of the infection is important.

Noninfectious associated respiratory diseases might also occur in PID patients and should be taken into consideration in the differential diagnosis. Medical imaging, especially computed tomography, plays a crucial role in the initial detection and characterisation of changes and in monitoring the response to therapy. The spectrum of abnormalities seen at thoracic imaging includes noninfectious airway disorders, infections, CLD, chronic inflammatory conditions, and benign and malignant neoplasms.

In conclusion, a PID diagnosis should be considered in patients presenting with severe and recurrent respiratory infections, with granulomatous diseases or with life-threatening invasive pulmonary infections.

References

- Alachkar H, et al. Memory switched B cell percentage and not serum immunoglobulin concentration is associated with clinical complications in children and adults with specific antibody deficiency and common variable immunodeficiency. Clin Immunol 2006; 120: 310-318.
- Carsetti R, et al. The loss of IgM memory B cells correlates with clinical disease in common variable immunodeficiency. J Allergy Clin Immunol 2005; 115: 412-417.
- Crooks BN, et al. Respiratory viral infections in primary immune deficiencies: significance and relevance to clinical outcome in a single BMT unit. Bone Marrow Transplant 2000; 26: 1097-1102.
- Notarangelo LD. Primary immunodeficiencies. J Allergy Clin Immunol 2010; 125: Suppl. 2, S182-S194.
- Pilette C, et al. Lung mucosal immunity: immunoglobulin-A revisited. Eur Respir J 2001; 18: 571-588.
- Plebani A, et al. Clinical, immunological, and molecular analysis in a large cohort of patients with X-linked agammaglobulinemia: an Italian multicenter study. Clin Immunol 2002; 104: 221-230.
- Primary immunodeficiency diseases. Report of an IUIS Scientific Committee. International Union of Immunological Societies. Clin Exp Immunol 1999; 118: Suppl. 1, 1-28.
- Quinti I, et al. Long-term follow-up and outcome of a large cohort of patients with common variable immunodeficiency. J Clin Immunol 2007; 27: 308-316.
- Sanchez-Ramon S, et al. Memory B cells in common variable immunodeficiency: clinical associations and sex differences. Clin Immunol 2008; 128: 314-321.
- Thickett KM, et al. Common variable immune deficiency: respiratory manifestations, pulmonary function and high-resolution CT scan findings. QJM 2002; 95: 655-662.
- Wood P, et al. Recognition, clinical diagnosis and management of patients with primary antibody deficiencies: a systematic review. Clin Exp Immunol 2007; 149: 410-423.

Weblink

- Associazione Italiana Ematologia Oncologia Pediatrica. www.aieop.org.

HIV-RELATED DISEASE

M.C.I. Lipman[1,2] and R.F. Miller[1,3]
[1] University College Medical School
[2] Royal Free Hospital, and
[3] London School of Hygiene and Tropical Medicine, London, UK
E-mail: marclipman@nhs.net

Most HIV-infected patients experience at least one significant episode of respiratory disease during their lifetime. A very wide variety of illnesses and pathogens can be encountered, and systematic investigation is vital. This chapter will focus upon common causes of HIV-related disease (table 1). It uses blood absolute CD4 counts to categorise the stages of HIV infection. This is a reasonably accurate measure of systemic and local immunity (in HIV-uninfected individuals, the CD4 count is typically >500 cells·μL^{-1}). In HIV-infected subjects with reasonably preserved immunity, typical community-acquired infections occur but at greater frequency than in the general population. With advancing HIV-induced immunosuppression (CD4 counts <200 cells·μL^{-1}), the risk of opportunistic infections and malignancy increases.

Use of effective combination antiretroviral therapy (CART) leads to 50–90% reductions in the incidence of HIV-associated opportunistic infections and malignancies. However, respiratory problems remain a major cause of disease. This results from the worldwide limited availability of CART (particularly in resource-poor settings), the failure of sustained HIV suppression in almost half of patients using it, the failure of prophylaxis for specific opportunistic infections, the continuing late presentation of patients with previously undiagnosed HIV infection and ongoing cofactors such as smoking, which are common in many HIV-infected populations.

Infections

Bacterial infection Upper respiratory tract infections, acute bronchitis and acute and symptomatic chronic sinusitis occur more frequently in HIV-infected patients than in the general population.

Key points

- More than 50% of HIV-infected patients suffer a respiratory episode during the course of their HIV disease.

- In populations with access to antiretroviral therapy, use of combination antiretroviral therapy (CART) has led to a marked reduction in the incidence of many HIV-associated opportunistic infections.

- *Pneumocystis jirovecii* is the new name for *Pneumocystis carinii*, the cause of *Pneumocystis* pneumonia in humans. The acronym PCP still applies.

- Bacterial infections are more common in HIV-infected patients than in the HIV-negative general population.

- In response to starting CART, there may be an overexuberant and uncontrolled immune response to exogenous antigen. This phenomenon is called immune reconstitution inflammatory syndrome.

- Tuberculosis may occur at any stage of HIV infection, is common, and is a public, as well as personal, health issue.

Table 1. Common causes of HIV-associated respiratory disease

Infectious disease	Non-infectious disease

Upper respiratory tract infection
Acute bronchitis
Acute sinusitis
Chronic sinusitis
	Malignancy
	  Kaposi sarcoma
	  Lymphoma
	  Bronchial carcinoma

Bronchiectasis
Bacterial pneumonia
  Streptococcus pneumoniae
  Haemophilus influenzae
Tuberculosis
Fungal infections
  Pneumocystis pneumonia
  Histoplasma capsulatum
  Cryptococcus neoformans
	Nonmalignant conditions
	  Chronic obstructive pulmonary disease
	  HIV-associated pneumonitis *e.g.* NSIP & LIP
	  Pulmonary arterial hypertension
	  Pneumothorax
	  HIV therapy causing respiratory symptoms *e.g.* IRIS

NSIP: nonspecific interstitial pneumonitis; LIP: lymphocytic interstitial pneumonitis; IRIS: immune reconstitution inflammatory syndrome.

Bronchiectasis is increasingly recognised in patients with advanced HIV disease. It probably arises as a consequence of recurrent *Pneumocystis jirovecii* pneumonia or bacterial infection.

Compared with HIV-negative populations, bacterial pneumonia is six to ten times more frequent in HIV-infected subjects not using highly active antiretroviral therapy. Injecting drug users are particularly vulnerable (approximately double that of other HIV risk groups). The presentation of community-acquired bacterial pneumonia in HIV-infected individuals is similar to HIV-negative subjects. However, the chest radiograph may be atypical, and mimic *P. jirovecii* pneumonia in up to half of cases. The usual pathogens isolated are *Streptococcus pneumoniae* and *Haemophilus influenzae*. Infection with *Staphylococcus aureus* and Gram-negative organisms may occur in advanced HIV disease. *Mycoplasma*, *Legionella* and *Chlamyida* species do not appear to be more frequent.

Bacteraemia is up to 100 times more common in HIV-infected patients with bacterial pneumonia, irrespective of CD4 count. Complications include intrapulmonary cavitation, abscess formation and empyema. There is a high relapse rate, despite appropriate antibiotic therapy.

Immunisation with pneumococcal vaccine is recommended in all adults and adolescents (at diagnosis of HIV infection and after 5 yrs); although humoral responses and clinical efficacy are probably impaired in those with CD4 counts <200 cells·μL^{-1}.

Fungal infection *P. jirovecii*, formerly called *P. carinii*, is the cause of *Pneumocystis* pneumonia (the acronym PCP still applies: *PneumoCystis P*neumonia). It remains a common problem in individuals unaware of their HIV serostatus and also among HIV-infected patients intolerant of, or nonadherent to, PCP prophylaxis and/or CART.

Patients present with nonproductive cough and progressive exertional breathlessness of several days' to weeks' duration, with or without fever. On auscultation the chest is usually clear; occasionally, end-inspiratory crackles are audible. In early PCP the chest radiograph may be normal (~10% cases). The most common abnormality is bilateral, perihilar interstitial infiltrates, which may progress to diffuse alveolar shadowing over a period of a few days. Atypical radiographic appearances include upper zone infiltrates resembling tuberculosis (TB), hilar/mediastinal lymphadenopathy, intrapulmonary nodules and lobar consolidation (present in up to 20%).

Treatment is usually started empirically in patients with typical clinical and radiological features and a CD4 count of <200 cells·μL^{-1}, pending diagnosis by cytological analysis of bronchoalveolar lavage (BAL) fluid or induced sputum samples.

Several factors present at or soon after hospitalisation predict poor outcome from PCP. These include increasing patient age, a second or third episode of PCP, hypoxaemia, low haemoglobin, co-existent pulmonary Kaposi sarcoma and medical comorbidity. Once hospitalised, development of pneumothorax, admission to the intensive care unit and need for mechanical ventilation are associated with worse outcome.

PCP can be stratified clinically as mild (arterial oxygen tension (P_{a,O_2}) >11.0 kPa, arterial oxygen saturation (S_{a,O_2}) >96% (breathing air at rest)), moderate (P_{a,O_2} 8.0–11.0 kPa, S_{a,O_2} 91–96%) or severe (P_{a,O_2} <8.0 kPa, S_{a,O_2} <91%). This categorisation is helpful, as oral therapy may be given to those with mild disease. First-choice treatment for PCP of all severity is high-dose co-trimoxazole (sulphamethoxazole 100 mg·kg^{-1}·day^{-1} with trimethoprim 20 mg·kg^{-1}·day^{-1}) in two to four divided doses orally or intravenously for 21 days. Approximately two-thirds of patients will successfully complete this regimen. Treatment-limiting drug toxicity is common and <10% will not respond to treatment (defined by deterioration after ≥5 days of therapy).

In patients who develop toxicity or do not respond to co-trimoxazole, alternative therapy in mild/moderate disease includes clindamycin (450–600 mg *q.i.d.* orally or *i.v.*) plus oral primaquine (15 mg daily), oral dapsone (100 mg daily) with trimethoprim (20 mg·kg^{-1}·day^{-1}), or oral atovaquone suspension (750 mg *b.i.d.*). In severe disease, alternative therapy is clindamycin with primaquine or intravenous pentamidine (4 mg·kg^{-1} daily).

Patients with an admission P_{a,O_2} ≤9.3 kPa should also receive adjuvant glucocorticoids within 72 h of starting specific anti-PCP treatment. A frequently used regimen is prednisolone, 40 mg *b.i.d.* for 5 days then 40 mg daily on days 6–10 and 20 mg daily on days 11–21. This has been shown to reduce mortality.

Co-trimoxazole, dapsone and primaquine should be avoided in patients with glucose-6-phosphate dehydrogenase deficiency.

Patients are at increased risk of PCP as their CD4 count decreases. Recommended regimens for PCP prophylaxis are listed in table 2.

Indications for primary prophylaxis are:

- blood absolute CD4 count <200 cells·μL^{-1}
- blood CD4 count <14% of total lymphocyte count
- unexplained fever (>3 weeks' duration)
- persistent or recurrent oral/pharyngeal *Candida*
- history of another AIDS-defining diagnosis *e.g.* Kaposi sarcoma

Indications for secondary prophylaxis are:

- all patients after an episode of *Pneumocystis* pneumonia

Indications for discontinuing secondary prophylaxis are:

- patients on combination antiretroviral therapy with sustained increase in blood CD4 count (>200 cells·μL^{-1}) and undetectable plasma HIV RNA for ≥3 months (note that if CD4 count subsequently falls <200 cells·μL^{-1} and/or the HIV RNA load increases, prophylaxis should be re-instituted)

Tuberculosis All patients with TB and unknown HIV status should be offered an HIV test. Active TB is estimated to occur between 20 and 40 times more frequently in HIV-infected subjects. Approximately 15% of all new TB cases globally occur in HIV-infected subjects, and it accounts for ~25% of all HIV-related deaths. TB is also covered in other chapters, so here the focus is on issues of particular relevance to HIV-infected subjects.

More than two-thirds of patients with TB and HIV co-infection present with pulmonary disease. When blood CD4 counts are normal or only slightly reduced, clinical features are similar to adult post-primary disease. Chest radiography often shows upper lobe infiltrates and cavitary changes. Sputum and BAL fluid are often smear positive.

In advanced HIV disease, and with a low blood CD4 count (<200 cells·μL^{-1}), the presentation is often with nonspecific malaise, fatigue, weight loss and fever. Chest radiographic abnormalities may not be obvious although they can include diffuse or miliary shadowing, mediastinal/hilar lymphadenopathy and pleural effusions; cavitation is uncommon. Sputum or BAL fluid is often smear negative but culture positive. Extrapulmonary TB is common in patients with CD4 counts <100 cells·μL^{-1}. Local or disseminated infection may involve lymph nodes and bone marrow; blood cultures may be positive; and it is worth obtaining specimens from several body sites or fluids if possible, as there is a reasonable yield *e.g.* from early morning urine cultures.

If smears or unspeciated mycobacterial cultures are positive, treatment should initially include a four-drug anti-TB regimen with rifamycin plus isoniazid, pyrazinamide and ethambutol, until mycobacterial identification and drug sensitivities are known. TB diagnosis using nucleic acid amplification tests is limited by poor sensitivity, although it can distinguish *Mycobacterium tuberculosis* from opportunistic mycobacteria and identify common mutations in the *rpoB* gene associated with rifampicin resistance, as well as isoniazid (*katG* and *inhA* genes).

Response to treatment with a 6-month four-drug regimen is generally good, although patients with disseminated disease are often treated for 9–12 months. Given the reported increased risk of developing drug-resistant disease, it is recommended that HIV patients with high mycobacterial loads (*e.g.* disseminated disease, as seen in patients with low blood CD4 counts) receive daily and not

Table 2. Recommended *Pneumocystis* pneumonia prophylaxis regimens

	Drug	Dosage	Notes
First choice	Co-trimoxazole (sulphamethoxazole + trimethoprim 5:1)	960 mg *q.d.*[#] 480 mg *q.d.* 960 mg thrice weekly	Protects against certain bacterial infections and reactivation of toxoplasmosis; adverse effects include nausea (40%), rash (up to 20%), bone marrow suppression (20%)
Second choice	Aerosolised pentamidine	300 mg once per month *via* jet nebuliser	Use once per fortnight if CD4 count <50 cells·μL^{-1}
	Dapsone	100 mg *q.d.*	Plus oral pyrimethamine 25 mg once per week against reactivation of toxoplasmosis
Third choice	Atovaquone	Suspension 750 mg *b.i.d.*	
	Azithromycin	1250 mg once per week	

[#]: the use of lower doses of co-trimoxazole may be associated with fewer adverse effects.

higher-dose (twice- or thrice-weekly) intermittent therapy. Compared with non-HIV-infected individuals, there is a possible greater incidence of adverse reactions to anti-TB drugs, and an increased risk of death.

CART reduces short- and long-term mortality in co-infected patients and should be started as soon as possible in subjects receiving treatment for active TB. However, there are issues with its early use in patients on anti-TB therapy. Generally, the lower the blood CD4 count, the more pressing is the clinical need to start CART (i.e. 2-4 weeks).

Issues with early use of combination antiretroviral therapy (CART) in tuberculosis patients:

- high pill burden
- overlapping toxicities, e.g. neuropathy
- drug–drug interactions, e.g. CART and rifamycins
- poor adherence to complex regimen
- immune reconstitution inflammatory disease more likely

Multidrug- and extensively drug-resistant TB has been associated epidemiologically with HIV infection. This is probably due to the rapid development of active (and hence infectious) TB in the HIV co-infected population exposed to drug-resistant cases, and hence reflects general susceptibility to developing mycobacterial disease, rather than to infection with specific drug-resistant strains.

Given the high risk of latent TB infection (LTBI) progressing to active disease, the World Health Organization recommends that HIV-infected patients with LTBI should receive prophylactic treatment. As, by definition, LTBI diagnosis requires a positive immune response (e.g. tuberculin skin test or blood interferon-γ release assay) in an asymptomatic individual, these assessments are hampered by the immune dysregulation present in HIV co-infected subjects.

Malignant conditions

Kaposi sarcoma Kaposi sarcoma is the commonest HIV-associated malignancy. Before the advent of CART, 15–20% of AIDS diagnoses were due to Kaposi sarcoma. It is associated with human herpes virus-8 (also called Kaposi sarcoma-associated virus) co-infection. Pulmonary Kaposi sarcoma is almost always accompanied by cutaneous or lymphadenopathic Kaposi sarcoma (palatal disease strongly predicts the presence of pulmonary lesions). Presentation is with nonspecific cough and progressive dyspnoea; haemoptysis is less common.

As Kaposi sarcoma may involve both the airways and lung parenchyma, radiological findings include interstitial or nodular infiltrates and alveolar consolidation. Hilar/mediastinal lymphadenopathy occurs in ~25% of patients and up to 40% have a pleural effusion.

Diagnosis is confirmed at bronchoscopy in >50% cases by the appearance of multiple, raised or flat, red or purple endotracheal and endobronchial lesions. Biopsy is rarely performed since cutaneous Kaposi sarcoma is usually present and diagnostic yield from biopsy is <20%. CART may induce remission of lesions, and is used in addition to chemotherapy.

Lymphoma High-grade B-cell non-Hodgkin lymphoma is the commonest HIV-associated thoracic lymphoma, and is usually found in association with disease elsewhere. Presenting symptoms are nonspecific. Chest radiographic abnormalities include mediastinal lymphadenopathy, pleural masses or effusions. The prognosis is better if patients treated with chemotherapy also receive CART.

Bronchial carcinoma Lung cancer appears to be two to four times more common in HIV-infected smokers. It is now more frequently diagnosed than in the pre-CART era. Whether this reflects the impact of CART protecting patients from other conditions, or some other mechanism, is uncertain. Presentation is usually with disseminated disease, and the prognosis is therefore poor.

Nonmalignant, noninfectious conditions

Chronic obstructive pulmonary disease

HIV-infected smokers appear to be at increased risk (~60%) of developing chronic obstructive pulmonary disease. The synergistic effects of smoking, recurrent bacterial and opportunistic infections, injecting drug use and possibly direct effect of HIV in the lung, argue strongly for scaling up smoking cessation services. This will also impact on other smoking-related illnesses such as cardiovascular disease, which are increasingly prevalent in HIV-infected communities.

HIV-associated pneumonitis
Nonspecific pneumonitis mimics PCP but often occurs at higher blood CD4 counts. Diagnosis requires transbronchial, video-assisted thoracoscopic or open-lung biopsy. Most episodes are self limiting, but prednisolone may be beneficial.

Lymphocytic interstitial pneumonitis is generally seen in HIV-infected children and clinically resembles idiopathic pulmonary fibrosis. Diagnosis requires biopsy. Treatment with CART is often effective.

Pulmonary arterial hypertension
Pulmonary arterial hypertension is reported to be six to 12 times more common in HIV-infected populations. The presentation and management are similar to nonimmunocompromised individuals, although CART is associated with improved haemodynamics and survival.

Pneumothorax
Pneumothorax occurs more frequently in HIV-infected patients than in the age-matched general medical population. Cigarette smoking and receipt of nebulised pentamidine are risk factors. PCP should be excluded in any patient presenting with a pneumothorax.

HIV therapy causing respiratory symptoms
In response to starting CART there may be an overexuberant immune response to exogenous antigen (from a current or previous opportunistic infection). This is well described for many conditions, although in particular for mycobacterial disease, and has been given several names including immune reconstitution inflammatory syndrome and immune reconstitution disease (IRD). Using TB as an example, subjects with known TB responding to treatment start CART and within a median of 2 weeks develop new clinical manifestations, *e.g.* peripheral lymphadenopathy, pleural or pericardial effusions or cerebral disease. There is no specific diagnostic test and drug resistance, patient nonadherence and other disease processes must be actively excluded. It is more likely in subjects with low baseline CD4 counts (<100 cells·μL^{-1}), more rapid suppression of HIV viral load and shorter time between starting anti-TB therapy and CART. It is reported in up to 30% subjects and, while often severe, is rarely fatal. Treatment is largely symptomatic, and may involve oral glucocorticoid therapy.

A second form of IRD is the "unmasking" of TB. Here, a patient with latent, asymptomatic infection will rapidly develop highly inflammatory active TB at a median of 40 days after starting CART. Treatment is generally directed at the underlying mycobacterial infection.

Lactic acidosis, typically due to the (nucleoside analogue) reverse transcriptase inhibitors didanosine and stavudine, may present with progressive breathlessness. Also, the nucleoside analogue abacavir can cause a hypersensitivity reaction (in up to 3% of subjects) with fever, rash and pulmonary symptoms. In these cases, recovery occurs if the drug is withdrawn.

References

- Benfield T, *et al.* Second-line salvage treatment of AIDS-associated *Pneumocystis jirovecii* pneumonia: a case series and systematic review. *J Acquir Immune Defic Syndr* 2008; 48: 63–67.

- Benfield T. Non-infectious conditions (AIDS). *In*: Albert R, Spiro S, Jett J, eds. Comprehensive Respiratory Medicine. 3rd Edn. Philadelphia, Mosby Elsevier, 2008.
- Davis JL, Huang L. Pneumocystis pneumonia. *In*: Volberding PA, Sande MA, Lange J, Greene WC, eds. Global HIV/AIDS Medicine. Philadelphia, Saunders Elsevier, 2008.
- Grogg KL, *et al*. HIV infection and lymphoma. *J Clin Pathol* 2007; 60: 1365–1372.
- Kaplan JE, *et al*. Guidelines for prevention and treatment of opportunistic infections in HIV-infected adults and adolescents: recommendations from CDC, the National Institutes of Health, and the HIV Medicine Association of the Infectious Diseases Society of America. *MMWR Recomm Rep* 2009; 58: 1–207.
- Lipman MCI, *et al*. An Atlas of Differential Diagnosis in HIV Disease. 2nd Edn. London, Parthenon Publishing, 2004.
- Miller RF, Lipman MCI. Pulmonary infections (AIDS). *In*: Albert R, Spiro S, Jett J, eds. Comprehensive Respiratory Medicine. 3rd Edn. Philadelphia, Mosby Elsevier, 2008.
- Pozniak AL, *et al*. BHIVA treatment guidelines for TB/HIV infection 2010. *HIV Med* 2010; in press.
- Stringer JR, *et al*. A new name (*Pneumocystis jirovecii*) for *Pneumocystis* from humans. *Emerg Infect Dis* 2002; 8: 891–896.
- Walzer PD, *et al*. Early predictors of mortality from *Pneumocystis jirovecii* pneumonia in HIV-infected patients: 1985–2006. *Clin Infect Dis* 2008; 46: 625–633.

GRAFT *VERSUS* HOST DISEASE

I. Quinti, C. Milito, L. Bonanni and F. La Marra
Dept of Clinical Medicine, Reference Centre for Primary Immunodeficiencies, Sapienza University of Rome, Rome, Italy
E-mail: isabella.quinti@uniroma1.it

Pathogenesis

Graft *versus* host disease (GVHD) is the principal complication of allogeneic bone marrow transplantation (BMT). The number of patients at high risk for GVHD is increasing, as more BMTs are performed from unrelated donors and older patients. Vascular endothelial damage and increased secretion of pro-inflammatory cytokines are involved in systemic disorders post-BMT, including GVHD and cytomegalovirus (CMV) infection. The pathology of acute GVHD can be considered in a framework of sequential phases. Initially, the recipient-conditioning regimen damages host tissues and causes release of pro-inflammatory cytokines; host antigen-presenting cells mature, acquire adhesion and co-stimulatory molecules that activate mature donor T-cells; these cells proliferate and produce additional cytokines inducing inflammatory and cellular effectors that amplify the inflammatory responses that cause tissue damage. Obstacles to the improvement of BMT include the linkage between GVHD toxicity and the beneficial graft-*versus*-leukaemia effect, as well as the impairment of immune reconstitution leading to life-threatening infections.

Key points

- GVHD is the principal complication of allogeneic BMT.
- Vascular endothelial damage and increased secretion of pro-inflammatory cytokines are involved in the pathogenesis of lung disorders.
- Acute and subacute patterns of lung injury include: idiopathic interstitial pneumonitis, bronchiolitis obliterans syndrome, organising pneumonia, alveolar haemorrhage, capillaritis, post-transplant lymphoproliferative disorders.
- CMV infection is the most frequent viral complication in patients undergoing BMT and acute GVHD significantly affects active CMV infection recurrence.

Treatment

Novel approaches to prevent or treat GVHD are linked to the generation of new monoclonal antibodies, immunomodulatory therapy, innovative strategies that target both soluble and cellular effectors. Among such agents are sirolimus, anti-tumour necrosis factor and antilymphocyte function-associated (LFA)-3 antibodies, extracorporeal photopheresis, mesenchymal stem cells and regulatory T-cells.

Noninfectious pulmonary-associated complications

Common pulmonary complications occur in 25–50% of BMT recipients and are responsible for 50% of transplant related deaths (table 1). Acute and subacute patterns of lung injury have been recognised. The idiopathic pneumonia syndrome occurs within the first 120 days after BMT with a rapidly

Table 1. Frequency and mortality due to pulmonary complications after bone marrow transplantation

	Frequency %	**Mortality %**
Infectious aetiology	34.3	50
CMV pneumonitis		71.4
Tuberculosis		33.4
PCP		0
Aspergillosis		0
Noninfectious aetiology	65.7	30.4
Idiopathic interstitial pneumonitis		14.3
Organising pneumonia		20
Alveolar haemorrhage		100
Capillaritis		100
Post-transplant lymphoproliferative disorders		100

CMV: cytomegalovirus; PCP: *Pneumocystis carinii* pneumonia. Adapted from WANG *et al.* (2004)

progressing fulminant course resulting in death in 60–80% of patients. By contrast, subacute noninfectious lung injury (alloimmune lung syndromes), including idiopathic pneumonia syndrome, bronchiolitis obliterans syndrome and bronchiolitis obliterans with organising pneumonia, can occur in the early post-transplant period or in the months post-BMT. Although long-term disease-free survival after BMT could exceed 60%, pulmonary infiltrates, due to either inflammatory or infectious pneumonitis, occur in 40–60% of BMT recipients causing 80% of transplant-related deaths. In children undergoing BMT, the incidence of pulmonary complications varies from 10–25%. Open lung biopsy has been recommended to make a definitive diagnosis and the appropriate treatment. Idiopathic interstitial pneumonitis and CMV pneumonitis are the most common causes and should be suspected in patients with diffuse interstitial infiltrates.

Epidemiological data suggest that, although GVHD reactions may play an aetiological role, the major contributing factor is conditioning-related toxicity. Moreover, engraftment syndrome, diffuse alveolar haemorrhage and pulmonary veno-occlusive disease are also possible complications.

Infectious pulmonary-associated complications

Respiratory virus infections in BMT patients are seen in 1–56%. CMV infection is the most frequent viral complication in patients undergoing BMT. Despite advanced diagnostic methods and pre-emptive antiviral therapy, CMV disease continues to be a life-threatening complication. Clinical manifestations could vary from an asymptomatic infection, defined as active CMV replication in the blood in the absence of clinical manifestations, or organ failure abnormalities characterised by CMV infection with clinical symptoms or organ function abnormalities. Active CMV infection interacts significantly in several ways with GVHD. Acute GVHD increases the chances of a poor outcome. CMV prophylaxis or pre-emptive therapy adopted during the last few years in allogeneic BMT recipients has changed the natural history of the disease. In prophylaxis, antiviral drugs are administered before any evidence of the virus, and in pre-emptive therapy, antiviral drugs are administered when there is laboratory evidence of an active but asymptomatic infection. Acute GVHD significantly affects active CMV infection recurrence. CMV infection recurrence is more frequent with short courses of antiviral therapy. The poor bioavailability of oral ganciclovir may account for this; drug resistance may also be a supplementary factor. Knowledge of these complications is now a part of the contemporary practice of pulmonary medicine, no longer isolated to the transplant pulmonologist.

References

- Takatsuka H, et al. Complications after bone marrow transplantation are manifestations of systemic inflammatory response syndrome. *Bone Marrow Transplant* 2000; 26: 419–426.
- Paczesny S, et al. Acute graft-*versus*-host disease: new treatment strategies. *Curr Opin Hematol* 2009; 16: 427–436.
- Versluys AB, et al. Strong association between respiratory viral infection early after hematopoietic stem cell transplantation and the development of life-threatening acute and chronic alloimmune lung syndromes. *Biol Blood Marrow Transplant* 2010; 16: 782–791.
- Yoshihara S, et al. Bronchiolitis obliterans syndrome (BOS), bronchiolitis obliterans organizing pneumonia (BOOP) and other late-onset noninfectious pulmonary complications following allogeneic hematopoietic stem cell transplantation. *Biol Blood Marrow Transplant* 2007; 13: 749–759.
- Castagnola E, et al. Cytomegalovirus infection after bone marrow transplantation in children. *Human Immunol* 2004; 65: 416–422.
- Wang JY, et al. Diffuse pulmonary infiltrates after bone marrow transplantation: the role of open lung biopsy. *Ann Thorac Surg* 2004; 78: 267–272.

AMYLOIDOSIS

H.J. Lachmann
UK National Amyloidosis Centre, Dept of Medicine, University College London Medical School, Royal Free Campus, London, UK
E-mail: h.lachmann@medsch.ucl.ac.uk

Amyloidosis is a group of diseases caused by accumulation of protein as insoluble fibrillar deposits in the extracellular space. These progressively disrupt the structure and function of affected tissues. Diagnosis is made by biopsy and Congo red staining, and classification is by the fibril precursor protein. Untreated amyloidosis progresses relentlessly, but deposits can regress if the supply of fibril precursors is reduced.

Amyloidosis can present to respiratory physicians in a number of ways: chronic lung conditions can give rise to systemic amyloidosis; systemic amyloidosis may present with respiratory symptoms; and localised pulmonary and respiratory tract amyloid deposits may present symptomatically or incidentally.

Key points

- Amyloidosis is a protein deposition disease.
- Diagnosis is by biopsy and Congo red staining.
- Systemic amyloidoiss usually affects serveral organs.
- Localised amyloidosis can present with obstructive symptoms, haemoptysis or as an incidental finding on imaging.
- Treatment depends on the type and distribution of amyloid deposits.

Systemic amyloidosis complicating respiratory diseases

Amyloid A (AA) amyloidosis This causes proteinuric renal failure and is a potential complication of any sustained inflammation. The amyloid fibrils are derived from the acute phase reactant, serum amyloid A protein (SAA). The major respiratory disease underlying AA amyloidosis in the industrialised world is bronchiectasis. Previously tuberculosis was common and other associations include cystic fibrosis, sarcoidosis, lung neoplasia and Kartagener's syndrome. The prognosis of AA amyloidosis depends on the degree of renal damage and whether the underlying inflammatory disease can be completely controlled. Treatment depends on the underlying disease and may involve surgery, antimicrobials or immunosuppression.

Systemic, amyloid light chain (AL) amyloidosis This may occur in association with any B-cell dyscrasia as it is derived from monoclonal immunoglobulin light chains. A number of chest-localised conditions can underlie systemic AL amyloidosis including Sjögren's syndrome, plasmacytomas and Castleman's tumours.

Respiratory system symptoms arising from systemic AL amyloidosis

Although lung deposits are universal at *post mortem*, symptoms are rare and dyspnoea generally reflects amyloid cardiomyopathy. Chest radiographs are usually normal. Lung function tests may be restrictive and extensive alveolar deposits can reduce gas transfer. Persistent pleural effusions are usually due to cardiac infiltration by amyloid but can rarely be caused by amyloidotic disruption of the pleura and may require recurrent drainage or pleurodesis. Treatment of systemic AL amyloidosis is chemotherapy directed against the underlying B-cell clone.

Amyloidosis localised to the respiratory tract

This results either from local production of fibril precursors, or from a microenvironment that favours fibril formation from a widely distributed protein. The majority of deposits are AL type associated with monoclonal B-cells confined to the affected site. Apparently localised amyloid deposits can be manifestations of systemic disease and should always be fully investigated to exclude systemic amyloidosis.

Laryngeal amyloidosis

Amyloid represents 0.5-1% of benign laryngeal disease and the incidence increases with age. It usually presents as hoarseness and is relatively benign but can be progressive or recur after treatment. Fatal haemorrhage has been reported. Endoscopic or laser excision is the treatment of choice, aiming to preserve voice quality and airway patency. Very rarely apparently localised laryngeal amyloid deposits can be a feature of hereditary apolipoprotein AL amyloidosis.

Tracheobronchial amyloidosis

This typically presents in the fifth or sixth decades with dyspnoea, cough and haemoptysis. Airway narrowing may cause pneumonia or lobar collapse and solitary nodules can mimic endobronchial neoplasia. There is no proven therapy although chemotherapy has been tried in patients with progressive disease. Management is dictated by symptoms and includes resection, stenting or laser ablation. Survival is <45% at 6 yrs.

Parenchymal pulmonary amyloidosis

This is typically an incidental finding on chest radiography of solitary/multiple nodules or a diffuse alveolar-septal pattern. Although the lesions must be differentiated from neoplasia the prognosis is usually excellent and no treatment is required.

Mediastinal and hilar amyloid lymphadenopathy

The lymphadenopathy may be massive and typically complicates a low-grade lymphoma. Disease progression is slow and calcification frequent. Tracheal compression or superior vena caval obstruction occasionally result.

Conclusion

Amyloidosis can both complicate long-standing pulmonary disease and be deposited within the respiratory system. The presentation and prognosis of amyloid deposits depend on their aetiology and distribution and can be benign or life threatening. In most cases of localised disease, management is essentially supportive or involves resection of symptomatic deposits. In contrast, systemic treatment can be extremely effective in patients with generalised AA and AL amyloidosis.

References

- Berk JL, *et al.* Pulmonary and tracheobronchial amyloidosis. *Semin Respir Crit Care Med* 2002; 23: 155-165.
- Lachmann HJ, Hawkins PN. Amyloidosis and the lung. *Chron Respir Dis* 2006; 3: 203-214.
- Lachmann HJ, *et al.* Natural history and outcome in systemic AA amyloidosis. *N Engl J Med* 2007; 356: 2361-2371.
- Linder J, *et al.* Amyloidosis complicating hairy cell leukaemia. *Am J Clin Pathol* 1982; 78: 864-867.
- Osserman EF, *et al.* The pathogenesis of "amyloidosis". Studies on the role of abnormal gammaglobulins and gammaglobulin fragments of the Bence Jones (L-polypeptide) types in the pathogenesis of "primary" and "secondary" amyloidosis associated with plasma cell myeloma. *Semin Hematol* 1964; 1: 3.
- Pepys MB. Amyloidosis. *Annu Rev Med* 2006; 57: 223-241.
- Shah PL, *et al.* The importance of complete screening for amyloid fibril type and systemic disease in patients with amyloidosis in the respiratory tract. *Sarcoidosis Vasc Diffuse Lung Dis* 2002; 19: 134-142.
- Travis WD, et al. Non-neoplastic disorders of the lower respiratory tract. In: Atlas of Nontumor Pathology. Washington DC, American Registry of Pathology, 2002; pp. 873-881.

PULMONARY ALVEOLAR PROTEINOSIS

M. Luisetti
University of Pavia, Clinica Malattie Apparato Respiratorio, IRCCS
Policlinico San Matteo, Pavia, Italy
E-mail: m.luisetti@smatteo.pv.it

Pulmonary alveolar proteinosis (PAP) is a rare syndrome occurring worldwide with an estimated prevalence of 0.1 per 100,000 individuals. PAP is characterised by accumulation of surfactant within alveolar macrophages in the alveoli and terminal airspaces, with impairment of gas transfer, and by a variable clinical course, ranging from spontaneous resolution to progressive respiratory failure.

A surfactant clearance impairment is the likely common pathophysiology of PAP, which can be classified as follows.

Primary PAP is due to disruption of granulocyte macrophage-colony stimulating factor (GM-CSF) signalling, either by the presence in plasma and lungs of high levels of neutralising anti-GM-CSF autoantibodies (GMAb) (autoimmune PAP, formerly known as idiopathic PAP), or to mutations in the GM-CSF receptor α or β chains.

Secondary PAP occurs as a consequence of the presence of several underlying diseases associated with PAP, such as haematologic disorders (mostly myelodysplatic syndrome), immunodeficiency status, dust inhalation, or lysinuric protein intolerance.

A third group (PAP-like diseases) is characterised by surfactant production impairment and includes genetic disorders due to mutations in the SP-B and SP-C genes, as well as in the ABCA3 gene.

According to a recently published meta-analysis and large cohort report, >90% of immune PAP patients are middle-aged adults,

> **Key points**
>
> - Pulmonary alveolar proteinosis (PAP) is a rare syndrome caused by surfactant clearance impairment.
>
> - More than 90% of PAP cases are associated with the presence of neutralising autoantibodies anti GM-CSF (GMAb; primary autoimmune PAP).
>
> - Diagnosis of primary autoimmune PAP is based of the following triad : 1) crazy paving pattern at HR CT scan; 2) milky appearance and cytology of BALF; 3) elevated serum level of GMAb.
>
> - Whole lung lavage is the current standard of care of PAP, but alternative therapy (especially GM-CSF administration) are under active investigation.

complaining about progressive exertional dyspnoea and cough; interestingly, about one-third of a large Japanese PAP series was asymptomatic. Physical examination of PAP patients is often unremarkable. Pulmonary function tests may be normal, but usually the first abnormality is represented by a decrease in lung diffusing capacity, and exertional increased alveolar–arterial oxygen tension gradient. The classic chest radiographic presentation is a diffuse bilateral infiltrate, with a distribution sometimes similar to pulmonary oedema (fig. 1a). More typical is the high-resolution computed tomography

(HRCT) presentation defined as "crazy paving" (thickening of interlobular and intralobular septa, and ground-glass opacities, with patchy distribution) (fig. 1b). Although surgical biopsy is traditionally considered mandatory to establish the diagnosis of PAP, more recently the triad represented by: 1) typical radiological findings on HRCT; 2) macroscopic appearance of milky fluid and cytology of bronchoalveolar lavage (BAL) fluid; and 3) elevated serum level of GMAb (whose sensitivity and specificity for diagnosing PAP is approximately 100%) is now considered sufficient to establish the diagnosis of autoimmune PAP. Lung biopsy should be considered when one or more of the previous findings are unclear. Histopathology usually shows well preserved alveolar wall architecture, and alveolar spaces filled with lipoproteinaceous, eosinophilic, Periodic Acid–Schiff-positive material and foamy macrophages.

The natural history of the PAP has been greatly influenced by the treatment. In the pre-whole-lung lavage (WLL) era, progressive deterioration occurred in ~30% of PAP patients. Death occurred mostly because of irreversible respiratory failure and, to a lesser extent, respiratory infection. The latter is a typical complication of the clinical course of PAP: pulmonary and systemic infections due to opportunistic organisms such as *Nocardia*, mycobacteria and *Cryptococcus* are often reported. Increased susceptibility to lung infections is traditionally attributed to the impairment of alveolar macrophages engulfed by surfactant, but systemic infections have been ascribed more recently to GM-CSF signalling impairment.

The adoption of WLL, first described in the mid-1960s has changed the natural history of PAP, by dramatically reducing the death rate. It is considered the standard care of PAP, and 95% of PAP patients respond positively to the procedure, although a considerable fraction of patients may show relapses or incomplete resolution. GM-CSF administration, based on the pathophysiology of the disorder, is considered an attractive alternative to WLL. Unfortunately, limited experience and, more importantly, difficult access to the drug have so far precluded diffusion of this therapeutic option. Possible alternatives are plasmapheresis or immunosuppressive agents such as rituximab, but data are so far insufficient. Lung transplantation is considered in end-stage disease, but PAP may recur.

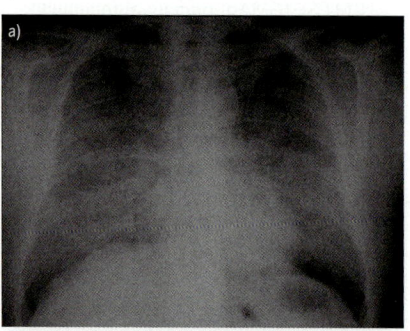

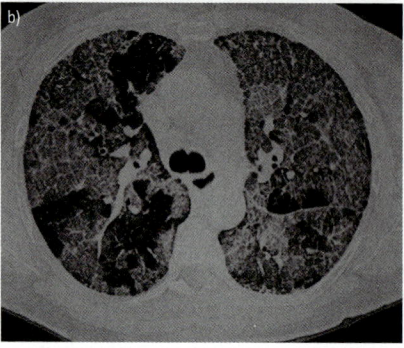

Figure 1. a) Radiographic and b) high-resolution computed tomography 'crazy paving' presentation of pulmonary alveolar proteinosis.

References

- Beccaria M, et al. Long-term durable benefit after whole lung lavage in pulmonary alveolar proteinosis. *Eur Respir J* 2004; 23: 526–531.
- Inoue Y, et al. Characteristics of a large cohort of patients with autoimmune pulmonary alveolar proteinosis in Japan. *Am J Respir Crit Care Med* 2008; 177: 752–762.
- Luisetti M, Trapnell BC. Pulmonary alveolar proteinosis. *In:* Schwarz MI, King TE, eds. Interstitial Lung Disease, 5th Edn. Maidenhead, McGraw-Hill, 2010.
- Orphanet Series. November 2009, no.1. www.orpha.net/consor/cgi-bin/Education_Home.php?lng=EN Date last accessed: March 8, 2010.

- Presneill JJ, *et al*. Pulmonary alveolar proteinosis. *Clin Chest Med* 2004; 25: 593-613.
- Ramirez-R J, *et al*. Pulmonary alveolar proteinosis: a new technique and rationale for treatment. *Arch Int Med* 1963; 112: 419-431.
- Seymour JF, *et al*. Efficacy of granulocyte-macrophage colony stimulating factor in acquired pulmonary alveolar proteinosis. *N Engl J Med* 1996; 335: 1924-1925.
- Seymour JF, Presneill JJ. Pulmonary alveolar proteinosis: progress in the first 44 years. *Am J Respir Crit Care Med* 2002; 166: 215-235.
- Trapnell BC, *et al*. Pulmonary alveolar proteinosis. *N Engl J Med* 2003; 349: 2527-2539.
- Uchida K, *et al*. GM-CSF autoantibodies and neutrophil dysfunction in pulmonary alveolar proteinosis. *N Engl J Med* 2007; 356: 567-579.

ADULT PULMONARY LANGERHANS' CELL HISTIOCYTOSIS

J-F. Cordier and V. Cottin
Department of Respiratory Diseases, Hôpital Louis Pradel, Lyon, France
E-mail: jean-francois.cordier@chu-lyon.fr

Langerhans' cell (LC) histiocytosis (LCH) in adults may involve especially the lungs, bone, the skin, and the pituitary gland. The disease presentation in childhood is different, with acute disseminated disease with a poor prognosis, and in older children and adolescents with multifocal involvement including bone. Single-system involvement by LCH is possible.

Epidemiology

Pulmonary LCH in adults is a rare disease with an estimated prevalence <1 in 200,000. It occurs almost exclusively in smokers, with no gender predominance, between the ages of 20–40 yrs, and is more common in the white population.

Pathologic features

Pulmonary LCH is characterised by the granulomatous bronchiolocentric organisation of LCs associated with inflammatory cells including eosinophils. The LCs do not differ from their counterparts in other tissues, exhibiting convoluted irregular nuclei with characteristic Birbeck granules on electron microscopy. These cells stain positive with anti-CD1a and anti-CD207 antibodies. Some features of alveolar macrophage pneumonitis (desquamative interstitial pneumonia) or respiratory bronchiolitis with interstitial lung disease are often associated. The progression of the bronchiole-centered granulomatous lesions results in fibrosis with end-stage stellar fibrotic scars and adjacent cystic cavities.

Clinical features

The respiratory manifestations are not specific, with cough (often overlooked since patients are smokers), and dyspnoea on exercise. Spontaneous pneumothorax is the first manifestation leading to diagnosis in ~10-20 % of patients. A number of patients have almost no reported symptoms and diagnosis is made by routine chest radiography.

Pulmonary LCH is solitary in a large majority of patients; however, involvement of other systems may be the first manifestation of the disease. These include bone lesions (which are often characteristic, well demarcated and osteolytic on imaging; rib involvement with chest pain is possible), hypothalamic–pituitary involvement resulting in diabetes insipidus (polyuria, polydipsia) and skin lesions.

> **Key points**
>
> - Pulmonary LCH is characterised by cough, dyspnoea on exercise, and diffuse pulmonary nodules and cysts on chest imaging in smokers that may evolve to respiratory failure.
> - Smoking cessation should be obtained.
> - No medical therapy has demonstrated efficacy.

Imaging

Chest radiography is usually abnormal with micronodular and reticular opacities sparing the lower lobes. In advanced disease, the nodules are absent and chest radiography may suggest emphysema.

High-resolution computed tomography (HRCT) of the chest usually shows characteristic features in early disease with disseminated infracentimetric nodules, which may show cavitation and may further spontaneously disappear. The cavitated nodules may evolve to thick- then thin-walled cysts (figure 1). The cysts may then enlarge and become confluent with HRCT features resembling emphysema.

The differential diagnoses with other multiple cystic lung diseases on imaging comprise especially lymphangioleiomyomatosis, Birt–Hogg–Dubé and spontaneous familial pneumothorax related to *FLCN* mutations, Sjögren syndrome and nonamyloid immunoglobulin deposition disease. Pleural effusion and mediastinal lymphadenopathy is exceptional. Pulmonary artery enlargement is present in patients with pulmonary hypertension.

Lung function tests

Lung function tests may be normal or only mildly impaired in patients with nodular involvement. However transfer factor of the lung for carbon monoxide is usually decreased, even in patients with relatively few lesions on imaging. About one-third of patients develop airflow obstruction with inflation, which may progress to severe obstructive respiratory failure.

Diagnosis

The gold standard for diagnosis is lung biopsy showing the characteristic features described above. Surgical biopsy is often obtained during pleurodesis for refractory or relapsing pneumothorax. Because of the plurifocal distribution of the lesions in the lung, the yield of transbronchial lung biopsy is usually limited. Bronchoalveolar lavage (BAL) is currently considered of little if any value for diagnosis. It shows an increase in total cell counts with a large predominance of macrophages with possible slight increase in eosinophils. The CD4/CD8 lymphocyte ratio is decreased. The identification of Langerhans' cells in BAL with antibodies against CD1a has only poor sensitivity and specificity and their proportion is usually similar to that in smokers without LCH. Common laboratory tests are not contributive.

A presumptive diagnosis of pulmonary LCH may be accepted in patients with characteristic HRCT features and limited symptoms and impaired lung function. Lung biopsy is indicated in those patients with significant symptoms and deteriorated or deteriorating lung function who are considered for treatment. In patients with diffuse cystic lesions on HRCT with fixed lung function impairment, lung biopsy is of limited benefit especially as it may not show characteristic granulomatous lesions.

Evolution

About half of patients improve spontaneously or with corticosteroid treatment (which has not been evaluated). Poor outcome with respiratory failure may occur especially in older patients with systemic involvement and deteriorating lung function tests. Pulmonary hypertension, occasionally severe, is common in advanced disease. Lung cancer may develop resulting from smoking habits.

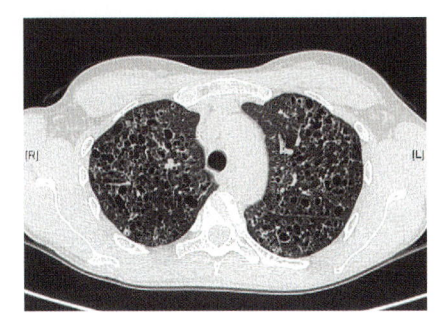

Figure 1. High-resolution computed tomography of the chest demonstrating numerous thin-walled cysts in a patient with LCH.

Treatment

Given the possibility of spontaneous recovery in a number of patients and the absence of controlled therapeutic trials, there is no evidence for efficacy of any treatment.

However, the strong association between pulmonary LCH and smoking suggests that smoking cessation should be obtained (at least to prevent further development of chronic obstructive pulmonary disease and/or lung cancer).

Corticosteroid treatment is often used in patients with symptomatic disease and worsening lung function, starting with prednisone 0.5-1 mg.kg^{-1} then tapered over 6-12 months. Whether improvement, when it occurs, results from treatment efficiency or is spontaneous cannot be established.

Cytotoxic agents (especially vinblastin) have occasionally been used with no conclusive efficiency. 2-chloro-deoxyadenosine (cladribin) has consistently been shown to be efficient in isolated cases, however it may be proposed and evaluated only in referral centres.

Pulmonary hypertension, when present, may be improved by pulmonary arterial hypertension treatment in some patients.

Lung transplantation (single- or double-lung, or heart–lung) may be considered in patients with end-stage disease. The majority of these present with moderate-to-severe pulmonary hypertension. Post-transplant survival is rather good with 10-yr survival >50%; however, pulmonary LCH may recur in about one-fifth of patients.

References

- Allen TC. Pulmonary Langerhans cell histiocytosis and other pulmonary histiocytic diseases. *Arch Pathol Lab Med* 2008; 132: 1171-1181.
- Caminati A, Harari S. Smoking-related interstitial pneumonias and pulmonary Langerhans cell histiocytosis. *Proc Am Thorac Soc* 2006; 3: 299-306.
- Dauriat G, *et al.* Lung transplantation for pulmonary Langerhans' cell histiocytosis : a multicenter analysis. *Transplantation* 2006; 81: 746-750.
- Fartoukh M, *et al.* Severe pulmonary hypertension in histiocytosis X. *Am J Respir Crit Care Med* 2000; 161: 216-223.
- Kiakouama L, *et al.* Severe pulmonary hypertension in histiocytosis X: long-term improvement with bosentan. *Eur Respir J* 2010; 36: 1-3.
- Lazor R, *et al.* Progressive diffuse pulmonary Langerhans cell histiocytosis improved by cladribine chemotherapy. *Thorax* 2009; 64: 274-275.
- Mendez JL, *et al.* Pneumothorax in pulmonary Langerhans cell histiocytosis. *Chest* 2004; 125: 1028-1032.
- Tazi A. Adult pulmonary Langerhans' cell histiocytosis. *Eur Respir J* 2006; 27: 1272-1285.
- Vassallo R, *et al.* Pulmonary Langerhans' cell histiocytosis. *N Engl J Med* 2000; 342: 1969-1978.

LYMPHANGIOLEIOMYOMATOSIS

J-F. Cordier and V. Cottin
National Reference Centre for Rare Pulmonary Diseases, Lyon, France
E-mail: jean-francois.cordier@chu-lyon.fr

Epidemiology and genetics

Lymphangioleiomyomatosis (LAM) is a rare (so-called orphan) lung disease affecting about 1 in 400,000 adult women (usually of childbearing age). It may be sporadic, or associated with tuberous sclerosis complex (TSC) where it affects 30–40% of adult women and, exceptionally, men.

TSC is associated with inherited mutations of the *TSC1* and *TSC2* genes, while acquired somatic mutations of *TSC2* are associated with sporadic LAM, resulting in constitutive activation of the kinase mammalian target of rapamycin (mTOR) signalling pathway.

Pathology

In LAM, the lung parenchyma is progressively replaced by cysts associated with a proliferation of immature smooth muscle cells and perivascular epithelioid cells (LAM cells). LAM cell proliferation usually develops around lymphatic vessels in the lung and possibly the axial lymphatics and the thoracic duct. LAM cells are stained with antibodies against smooth muscle actin, desmin, and HMB-45 (detecting characteristic pre-melanocyte proteins).

Clinical manifestations and lung function tests

Dyspnoea on exertion is the most common symptom, and pneumothorax the most common mode of presentation (often relapsing, and may be bilateral). Chylous effusion (chylothorax, chylous ascites) may be present.

Lung function tests are characterised by airflow obstruction and impaired gas transfer with decrease in transfer factor of the lung for carbon monoxide ($T_{L,CO}$). Exercise performance and maximal oxygen uptake are impaired. Hypoxaemia is present in advanced disease.

Imaging

Chest radiography shows reticular opacities and cysts, with further possible pleural effusion or pneumothorax.

High-resolution computed tomography (HRCT) of the chest has a major role in diagnosis. It shows characteristic multiple round cysts involving the whole parenchyma; these may progressively become confluent (fig. 1).

The differential diagnoses with the other multiple cystic lung diseases on imaging comprise especially Birt–Hogg–Dubé syndrome and spontaneous familial pneumothorax related to folliculin gene mutations, Langerhans' cell granulomatosis,

---

Key points

- LAM is a rare disease occurring in women of child-bearing age, characterised by dyspnoea on exertion, relapsing pneumothorax and numerous thin-walled cysts on chest imaging.
- Diagnostic criteria have been proposed recently.
- The disease may slowly progress to respiratory insufficiency.
- No effective therapy is available.

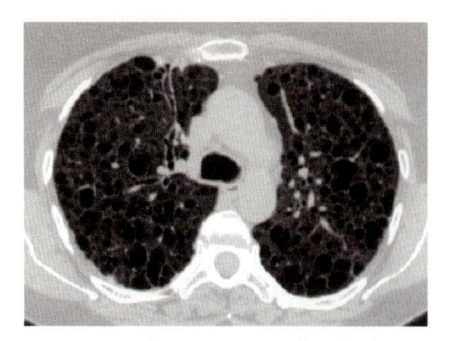

Figure 1. HRCT of the chest demonstrating numerous thin-walled cysts in a patient with LAM.

Sjögren syndrome and nonamyloid immunoglobulin deposition disease.

Cysts may be associated with some small nodules in TSC (corresponding to multifocal micronodular pneumocyte hyperplasia), pleural effusion or pneumothorax. The axial lymphatics in the thorax and the retroperitoneum may be dilated with lymphadenopathy, and abdominal cystic lymphatic collections called lymphangiomas (in up to 20% of patients) that may result in abdominal discomfort or compression.

Angiomyolipoma

Angiomyolipomas (AML) of the kidney (which are benign tumors composed of blood vessels, smooth muscle, and adipose tissue easily identified on HRCT) are associated with LAM in 50% of sporadic LAM and 80% of patients with TSC (where these are more often bilateral and larger). AML may enlarge with time and become prone to bleeding, especially when >4 cm in size (embolisation or nephron-sparing surgery is therefore indicated). Screening for AML in patients with LAM is recommended.

Diagnostic criteria

Diagnostic criteria for LAM have recently been proposed by a European Respiratory Society Task Force (table 1). The gold standard for diagnosis of LAM is lung biopsy fitting the pathological criteria for LAM. However, the association of characteristic HRCT features with AML or other characteristic features of LAM may obviate the need for biopsy. The differential diagnosis comprises other multiple cystic lung diseases including especially the Birt-Hogg-Dubé syndrome associated with mutations of the folliculin gene, familial

Table 1. European Respiratory Society diagnostic criteria for lymphangioleiomyomatosis (LAM)

Definite LAM
1. Characteristic[#] or compatible[#] lung HRCT and lung biopsy fitting the pathological criteria for LAM
OR
2. Characteristic[#] lung HRCT and any of the following:
   angiomyolipoma (kidney)[¶]
   thoracic or abdominal chylous effusion[+]
   lymphangioleiomyoma[§] or lymph-node involved by LAM[§]
   definite or probable TSC

Probable LAM
1. Characteristic[#] HRCT and compatible clinical history[ƒ]
OR
2. Compatible[#] HRCT and any of the following:
   angiomyolipoma (kidney)[¶]
   thoracic or abdominal chylous effusion[+]

Possible LAM
   Characteristic[#] or compatible[#] HRCT

[#]: characteristic: multiple thin-walled round well-defined air-filled cysts; compatible: only few multiple (>2 and ⩽10) <30-mm such cysts; [¶]: diagnosed by characteristic computed tomographic features and/or on pathological examination; [+]: based on visual and/or biochemical characteristics of the effusion; [§]: based on pathological examination; [ƒ]: compatible clinical features include pneumothorax (especially multiple and/or bilateral) and/or altered lung function tests as in LAM. Reproduced from Johnson et al. (2010).

isolated primary spontaneous pneumothorax (also associated with mutations of the same gene), cysts associated with lymphoid interstitial pneumonia, nonamyloid immunoglobulin deposition disease, *etc*. A diagnostic work-up for the preceding alternative causes of multiple cystic lung disease is mandatory in patients with probable and especially possible LAM.

Evolution and prognosis

Disease progression is variable with some patients remaining relatively stable for long periods whereas others deteriorate rapidly with ensuing respiratory insufficiency. Repeated measurement of forced expiratory volume in 1 s and $T_{L,CO}$ is used to assess disease progression with arterial oxygen measurement in advanced disease. Pulmonary hypertension, usually mild, may develop. 10-yr survival was about 70–90% in recent large series.

Management

As LAM occurs in women of childbearing age, oestrogens have been suspected to enhance and progestatives to prevent its development. However, hormonal interventions have not demonstrated significant advantages. Nevertheless, oestrogens (contraceptive pill, hormone replacement) should be avoided.

No effective treatment for LAM is available. The mTOR inhibitors, which transiently reduce the volume of AML, may mildly improve or stabilise pulmonary LAM; however, only limited evidence is currently available and tolerance may be poor.

There is a greater risk of pneumothorax and chylous effusion during pregnancy. To become pregnant is the patient's decision; however, pregnancy may be discouraged in patients with severe disease.

Influenzal and pneumococcal vaccination should be offered to patients with LAM. Inhaled bronchodilators should be prescribed to patients with airflow obstruction and continued if a response is observed.

In patients with end-stage disease LAM, transplantation (single or bilateral) is an efficient procedure with results comparing favourably with transplantation for other pulmonary diseases. As many LAM patients are rather young, lung transplantation may be proposed in most severe cases with poor prognosis. Recurrence of LAM on transplant is possible but does not affect survival.

References

- Avila NA, *et al*. Pulmonary lymphangioleiomyomatosis: correlation of ventilation-perfusion scintigraphy, chest radiography, and CT with pulmonary function tests. *Radiology* 2000; 214: 441–446.
- Avila NA, *et al*. Lymphangioleiomyomatosis: abdominopelvic CT and US findings. *Radiology* 2000; 216: 147–153.
- Benden C, *et al*. Lung transplantation for lymphangioleiomyomatosis: the European experience. *J Heart Lung Transplant* 2009; 28: 1–7.
- Bissler JJ, *et al*. Sirolimus for angiomyolipoma in tuberous sclerosis complex or lymphangioleiomyomatosis. *N Engl J Med* 2008; 358: 140–151.
- Johnson SR, *et al*. European Respiratory Society guidelines for the diagnosis and management of lymphangioleiomyomatosis. *Eur Respir J* 2010; 35: 14–26.
- Johnson SR, Tattersfield AE. Clinical experience of lymphangioleiomyomatosis in the UK. *Thorax* 2000; 55: 1052–1057.
- Moss J, *et al*. Prevalence and clinical characteristics of lymphangioleiomyomatosis (LAM) in patients with tuberous sclerosis complex. *Am J Respir Crit Care Med* 2001; 164: 669–671.
- Ryu JH, *et al*. The NHLBI Lymphangioleiomyomatosis Registry: characteristics of 230 patients at enrollment. *Am J Respir Crit Care Med* 2006; 173: 105–111.
- Urban T, *et al*. Pulmonary lymphangioleiomyomatosis. A study of 69 patients. Groupe d'Etudes et de Recherche sur les Maladies "Orphelines" Pulmonaires (GERM"O"P). *Medicine (Baltimore)* 1999; 78: 321–337.

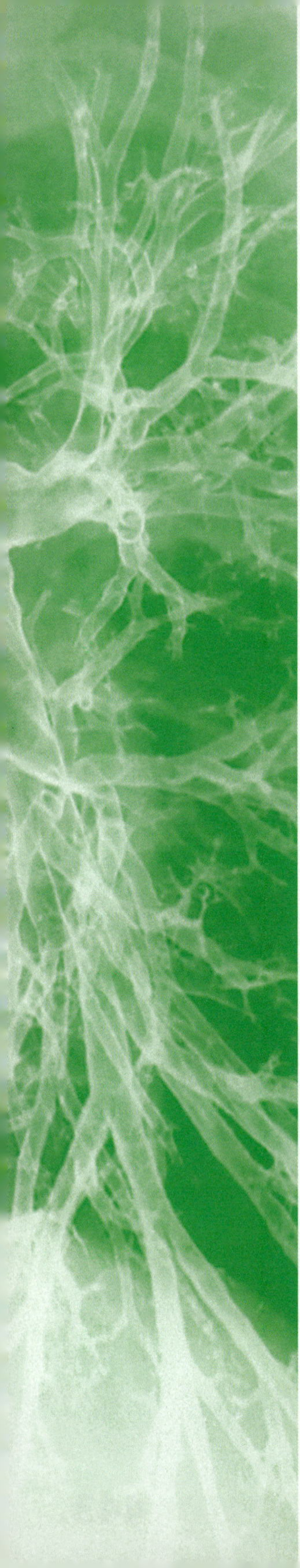

CHAPTER 17:

PULMONARY REHABILITATION

RESPIRATORY PHYSIOTHERAPY   **446**
J. Bott

PULMONARY REHABILITATION   **451**
T. Troosters, H. Van Remoortel, D. Langer and C. Burtin

RESPIRATORY PHYSIOTHERAPY

J. Bott
London, UK
E-mail: juliabott@aol.com

Respiratory physiotherapy spans a broad range of services, advice and nonpharmacological interventions used to help patients with a variety of respiratory conditions. Its use has been documented for over a century: postural drainage (PD) was reported for secretion removal in bronchiectasis in 1901 and, in 1915, breathing exercises and physical exercise for chest injuries.

General principles of physiotherapy

Physiotherapy is aimed at treating or alleviating problems rather than diseases. Strategies are used to restore, improve or maintain movement and/or function, and maximise participation in everyday life.

Key points

Physiotherapy is indicated in most respiratory conditions, both for groups and individuals, for:

- self-management advice and education on lifestyle modifications related to physiotherapy strategies
- breathlessness management
- improvement or maintenance of mobility and function
- airway clearance in well-defined cases
- prescription of exercise and exercise training
- prescription of walking aids

Physiotherapists are thus vital to the delivery of effective pulmonary rehabilitation (PR).

Physiotherapy is provided across all healthcare settings, from the patient's own home to the critical care unit. Physiotherapists are well qualified to provide assessment and monitoring of, for example, ventilatory function and cough effectiveness or exercise tolerance, including for ambulatory oxygen (O_2) assessment. Interestingly, there is wide variance in tasks undertaken by physiotherapists across countries.

Airway clearance

To help the patient better manage their secretions, a range of airway clearance techniques are available, including:

- independent techniques, *e.g.* the active cycle of breathing techniques, autogenic drainage
- mechanical or other devices, *e.g.* positive expiratory pressure (PEP)/oscillating PEP and high frequency chest wall oscillation
- PD or modified PD
- nebulised substances, *e.g.* hypertonic saline
- techniques for cough enhancement or support, *e.g.* maximum insufflation techniques and manually assisted coughing

Physiotherapists' physiological knowledge and practical skills means they are well placed to assist in the delivery of pharmacotherapy (inhalers) and their timing with respect to the physiotherapy intervention. Physiotherapists can also help in the delivery and correct application of O_2 therapy, including ambulatory O_2, as well as offering improvement of poor ventilatory function, including in the sedated and paralysed patients.

Strategies to enhance ventilation and gas exchange

Strategies to enhance ventilation and gas exchange include:

- positioning
- breathing techniques
- manual hyperinflation
- intermittent positive pressure breathing (IPPB)
- continuous positive airway pressure (CPAP)
- noninvasive ventilation (NIV)

Physiotherapists are considered by many to be invaluable in the delivery of an effective NIV service.

Physiotherapy is commonly helpful for postural problems and/or musculoskeletal dysfunction and pain as well as for improving continence. With an increased prevalence compared with that of nonrespiratory populations, this is especially warranted during coughing and forced expiratory manoeuvres.

Disease-specific physiotherapy

Chronic obstructive pulmonary disease (COPD)
Taking account of the altered mechanics of breathing in those with COPD is essential for effective breathlessness management and advice.

Breathlessness management includes:

- positioning to fix the shoulder girdle passively
- forward-leaning postures to improve the length tension ratio of the diaphragm

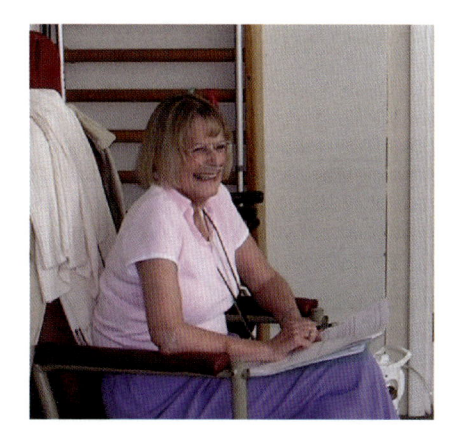

"Thank you for giving me my life back"

- breathing techniques to help the patient better control dyspnoea and panic, both at rest and during exertion

Physical activity and exercise should be encouraged throughout the course of the disease, including during hospital admission where possible and appropriate. When supervised and carried out at appropriate intensity these exercises are more effective. Exercise training programmes are indicated for patients who have symptoms and impaired physical activities in daily life.

Selected patients may benefit from inspiratory muscle training.

In both the acute and domiciliary settings:

- Wheeled walking aids (rollator frame) reduce the ventilatory requirements of ambulation.
- Wheeled walking aids are especially useful for those who are more disabled by breathlessness and those using ambulatory O_2.
- Patients severely disabled by breathlessness may find using a high gutter rollator frame allows some mobility.
- Along with occupational therapists, physiotherapists may promote energy conservation strategies to minimise the work of activities of daily living.

Airway clearance techniques should be used where indicated and IPPB may be considered in acute exacerbations of COPD for patients with retained secretions who are too weak or tired to generate an effective cough. NIV is now the first-line therapy for hypercapnic respiratory failure and both NIV and O_2 therapy should be delivered according to current guidance.

Asthma Some form of breathing retraining using reduced volume and/or frequency with relaxation is indicated to reduce symptoms and improve quality of life, along with prescribed medication. Several schools advocate specific techniques, but it is important to stress that these techniques are adjunctive to medication and not a replacement therapy.

Routine or regular airway clearance is rarely indicated in the asthmatic patient.

Disordered breathing (hyperventilation syndrome) Breathing exercises combined with relaxation (technique as for asthma) is an effective strategy to reduce symptoms once the diagnosis is confirmed.

Cystic fibrosis (CF) and non-CF-related bronchiectasis Physiotherapy is integral to the management of patients with bronchiectasis from any cause, including CF, with airway clearance and exercise central to this therapy. The acceptability of techniques and regimes, to enhance concordance with treatment, is vital to the success of therapy.

A variety of airway clearance techniques, including those with and without mechanical assistance if necessary, should be offered, in order to find one that is both acceptable and effective. The simplest technique that impinges the least on the patient's life is a good starting point.

Effective treatment might need to be supported by inhaled therapies, *e.g.* bronchodilators or hypertonic saline, O_2 and NIV or IPPB. These supportive therapies and PD to enhance airway clearance or exercise tolerance should be assessed for benefit on an individual basis. Regular review is advised to ensure continuing effectiveness and concordance with therapy; appropriate adjustment of treatment can be made if necessary.

- Physiotherapy for patients with CF should include assessment and treatment for musculoskeletal and postural disorders.
- Physiotherapists need to be scrupulous about hygiene for infection control in this population.
- For those with either CF or bronchiectasis continence problems should be identified and treated.
- For patients with bronchiectasis, PR is indicated when dyspnoea is impacting on exercise tolerance or functional activities.
- Exercise for the patient with CF must be undertaken individually to reduce risk of cross-infection.

Interstitial lung diseases There is little published evidence on physiotherapy for these conditions. Studies on the effectiveness of engaging in exercise training are emerging and patients with interstitial lung diseases can gain benefit from PR providing they are referred early in the disease process. Patients at a later stage of disease may benefit from wheeled walking aids, ambulatory O_2, breathlessness management and energy conservation strategies.

Community-acquired pneumonia (CAP) Traditional airway clearance techniques are rarely indicated.

For patients admitted to hospital with uncomplicated CAP:

- Regular use of PEP may reduce length of stay.
- Medical condition permitting, early mobilisation is indicated.
- Patients should be encouraged to sit out of bed for at least 20 min on the first day,

increasing the time and general mobility on each subsequent day.

CPAP may be helpful for patients in type I respiratory failure who remain hypoxaemic despite optimum medical therapy and O_2, and NIV may be an option for selected patients in type II respiratory failure, especially those with underlying COPD.

Chest wall disorders PR is indicated in a patient with chest wall deformity from any cause with reduced exercise capacity and/or breathlessness on exertion. The need for ambulatory O_2 or NIV should be assessed before undertaking exercise. Respiratory muscle training may have a role. It has yet to be established whether breathing or thoracic mobility exercises are helpful in this client group.

Neuromuscular disease and spinal cord injury (SCI) Respiratory problems are the commonest cause of morbidity and mortality for those with respiratory muscle weakness; physiotherapy therefore provides vital assistance with airway clearance. Difficulty clearing secretions may be due to inspiratory, expiratory and/or bulbar muscle weakness, depending on the underlying condition and stage of disease.

- Regular monitoring of O_2 saturation, vital capacity and peak cough flow can indicate impending problems with either ventilation or cough effectiveness.
- The use of respiratory aids when these measures fall may prevent or reduce complications.

O_2 therapy should be administered with great care in patients with neuromuscular disease because of the risk of increasing ventilation/perfusion mismatch and increasing hypercapnia. NIV should be considered in those at risk of developing hypercapnia. These actions are done together with the treating physician.

Traditional physiotherapy techniques are not useful in this client group.

Strategies to enhance maximal insufflation capacity are indicated and include:

- resuscitation bags
- NIV
- mechanical insufflation, and
- breath stacking *via* the above or
- glossopharyngeal (frog) breathing

The presence of severe bulbar dysfunction or paralysis renders breath stacking ineffective. Maximal insufflation capacity used regularly is also a means of maintaining range of movement to the lungs and chest wall. These techniques should be used along with strategies to enhance cough effectiveness: manually assisted coughing or mechanical insufflation–exsufflation.

Ventilatory function can be improved with careful positioning to optimise the effect of gravity on weak muscles, as can the use of abdominal binders for those with SCI.

In patients with SCI, exercise should be encouraged; respiratory muscle training and functional electrical stimulation may enhance muscle strength or vital capacity. Some patients with early neuromuscular disease may benefit from respiratory muscle training but caution is advised in Duchenne muscular dystrophy.

Patients with critical illness The principles of care remain the same; physiotherapists provide rehabilitation for the prevention and treatment of the common complications associated with prolonged bed rest, immobility and recumbency, including deconditioning, weakness and dyspnoea. Physiotherapy is also used to target specific respiratory problems, such as retained airway secretions, atelectasis and weaning failure.

References

- Bott J, *et al.* Guidelines for the physiotherapy management of the adult, medical, spontaneously breathing patient. *Thorax* 2009; 64: Suppl. 1, i1- i51. Available at www.brit-thoracic.org.uk/Portals/0/

Clinical%20Information/Physiotherapy/PhysiotherapyGuideline.
- Gosselink R, et al. Physiotherapy for adult patients with critical illness: recommendations of the European Respiratory Society and European Society of Intensive Care Medicine Task Force on Physiotherapy for Critically Ill Patients. *Intensive Care Med 2008; 34*, 7: 1188-1199.
- Langer D, et al. A clinical practice guideline for physiotherapists treating patients with chronic obstructive pulmonary disease based on a systematic review of available evidence. *Clin Rehabil* 2009; 23: 445-462.
- National Institute for Health and Clinical Excellence. NICE guideline 83: Rehabilitation after critical illness. www.nice.org.uk/CG83. Date last accessed: June 1, 2010.
- Nici L, et al. American Thoracic Society/European Respiratory Society statement on pulmonary rehabilitation. *Am J Respir Crit Care Med* 2006; 173: 1390-1413.

PULMONARY REHABILITATION

T. Troosters, H. Van Remoortel, D. Langer, C. Burtin,
M. Decramer and R. Gosselink
Respiratory Rehabilitation and Respiratory Division, University Hospital Leuven, and Faculty of Kinesiology and Rehabilitation Sciences, Department of Rehabilitation Sciences, Katholieke Universiteit Leuven, Leuven, Belgium
E-mail: Thierry.Troosters@med.kuleuven.be

Pulmonary rehabilitation is a recognised therapy for patients with respiratory diseases. The European Respiratory Society and the American Thoracic Society define pulmonary rehabilitation as *"an evidence-based, multidisciplinary, and comprehensive intervention for patients with chronic respiratory diseases who are symptomatic and often have decreased daily life activities. Integrated into the individualized treatment of the patient, pulmonary rehabilitation is designed to reduce symptoms, optimize functional status, increase participation, and reduce health care costs through stabilizing or reversing systemic manifestations of the disease"*. Although this is a long definition, it captures the core elements important in the selection and design of pulmonary rehabilitation. Importantly, pulmonary rehabilitation may be an integrated part of other care plans for chronic obstructive pulmonary disease (COPD) patients, such as self-management programmes, lung transplantation programmes, noninvasive ventilation or smoking cessation programmes.

The evidence base for pulmonary rehabilitation

Several reviews have summarised the evidence for pulmonary rehabilitation and practice guidelines are available. Briefly, pulmonary rehabilitation improves health-related quality of life and symptoms unequivocally and clinically significantly in patients with COPD, to a degree similar to or even larger than that obtained by pharmacotherapy. When exercise training is provided at adequate intensity, exercise tolerance is enhanced and functional exercise capacity improves. These improvements are also clinically relevant if an appropriate exercise stimulus is provided. Other improvements are also important but are to date less studied.

A significant proportion of patients referred for pulmonary rehabilitation suffer from psychiatric morbidity, most commonly anxiety and depression. A recent meta-analysis showed the potential small benefit of multidisciplinary pulmonary rehabilitation on mood status. The relatively small effect size may be a result of the dilution of depressed patients in the larger patient pool: effects on these variables can only be expected in patients with symptoms of depression and/or anxiety.

A less studied effect of rehabilitation is enhanced self-efficacy. Self-efficacy is the

Key points

- Pulmonary rehabilitation is an evidence-based treatment that improves health-related quality of life and symptoms in chronic obstructive pulmonary disease.
- Programmes should be tailored to the patient in terms of content, location, duration, frequency and exercise training.
- In order for the effects to be durable, patients' everyday activity should be higher after rehabilitation than before.

confidence patients have in their ability to carry out a specific task or manage a specific condition (*e.g.* breathlessness). Patients' confidence that they can manage dyspnoea improves after pulmonary rehabilitation, and one seminal study also showed an improvement in self-efficacy with walking. It is unclear to what extent this contributes to an effective change in behaviour after pulmonary rehabilitation.

The amount of activity patients carry out in daily life is an important outcome for rehabilitation. The systemic consequences of COPD, such as cardiovascular morbidity, muscle weakness and osteoporosis, originate largely – directly or indirectly – from an inactive lifestyle. When pulmonary rehabilitation aims at achieving a sustained effect, an inactive lifestyle after rehabilitation should be avoided. The effect of pulmonary rehabilitation programmes on physical activity levels is as yet unclear. Changing physical activity behaviour is a challenging task. Our research group showed that walking time in daily life changed only modestly after 3 months of pulmonary rehabilitation. After 6 months there was a more significant improvement in physical activity levels. Changing physical activity may not simply follow increased exercise capacity. Indeed, physical activity levels are a complex integration of exercise capacity and willingness to use that capacity. In recent years, appealing new strategies have been developed that may help to increase the effects of classical rehabilitation on physical activity. Providing real-time feedback with pedometers may, along with setting achievable goals, enhance daily activity levels in- or outside the context of pulmonary rehabilitation. Walking at home has been stimulated effectively using modern interfaces such as mobile phone technology, which included paced walking to the rhythm of music adapted to the capabilities of the patient. Future research should focus on further strategies that may help to lead to sustainable behavioural change.

An important spin-off of pulmonary rehabilitation may be a decrease in the use of healthcare resources, most importantly hospital admissions. There is a body of data suggesting that pulmonary rehabilitation reduces the number of hospital days. In more fragile patients, such as those recently admitted to hospital and at risk for readmission, a meta-analysis showed that the risk for readmission was reduced substantially following pulmonary rehabilitation.

Programme content and maintaining effects

As indicated above, programmes need to be individualised and aim at improving the systemic consequences (physiological and psychological) of the underlying disease, guiding patients and their families towards a long-term change in physical activity and self-management. Several options are possible in terms of programme content (the disciplines contributing), location, duration and frequency. These are summarised in table 1. Studies comparing different modalities of rehabilitation are scarce and no unequivocal preference has been reported. Studies comparing hospital-based outpatient rehabilitation to rehabilitation at home found no differences on short-term outcomes. More research is needed to evaluate the criteria for assigning patients to a specific form of rehabilitation. In addition, it remains unclear to what extent home rehabilitation results in more durable effects.

For the essential exercise training component, the programme needs to be individualised in terms of exercise modalities, specificity of training, training intensity and specific inspiratory muscle training. In order to obtain significant physiological improvements in skeletal muscle function it is important to train patients at an intensity that is high relative to their maximum capacity. In order to combine an effective training programme with patient comfort, clinicians have the choice of several exercise training modalities, including endurance, interval and resistance training. The duration of an exercise training programme is $\geqslant 8$ weeks and at least three sessions per week are needed. One of these sessions can be conducted outside the formally supervised setting, provided that the session is comparable in terms of duration and intensity to the supervised sessions.

There has been much debate as to whether the effects of a rehabilitation programme can be maintained. From earlier studies it is indeed difficult to claim durable effects for short-term (6–8 weeks) pulmonary rehabilitation programmes. Long-term studies (using up to 6 months of rehabilitation) did find more long-term effects.

Current understanding of the development of systemic consequences of COPD may help in the design of successful longer-term strategies to maintain the effects of pulmonary rehabilitation. First, efforts should be made to change the physical activity behaviour of patients. Physical inactivity is likely to be the most important contributor to the development of systemic consequences in COPD. If patients are not more active after the rehabilitation programme, it is likely that the effects of rehabilitation on enhanced exercise capacity and skeletal muscle force will be short lived. Longer programmes are more successful in achieving this goal than short-term programmes, but changes in the programme content, for example providing patients with direct feedback on their physical activity levels or using structured behavioural interventions, may yield results more rapidly. Secondly, exercise at home should be facilitated. This can be done using feedback on home exercises, or incentives. Such exercises need to be individually tailored to achieve effective intensity in order to provide a continued training stimulus. Ideally, exercises should be regularly supervised. Lastly, specific attention should probably go to patients who suffer from exacerbations, as these events acutely reduce muscle force and functional exercise capacity. Prevention of such events can be done in patients at risk by implementing self-management strategies and providing a case manager. There is currently little evidence for a short "booster" programme after a hospital admission to maintain the benefits of rehabilitation.

Examination of the strategies used to maintain the benefits of rehabilitation reveals that it is important to achieve a durable change in physical activity behaviour and that patients should continue to carry out planned exercises at high intensity to maintain the physiological benefits of rehabilitation. Interventions that are not regular or are less structured are not successful in maintaining the benefits of rehabilitation. More research is needed to identify optimal maintenance strategies after pulmonary rehabilitation.

Table 1. Choices to be made when prescribing pulmonary rehabilitation

Aspects to be individualised	Possible choices or options
Programme content	Disciplines typically involved: chest physician, physiotherapists, nurse, exercise specialist, occupational therapist, psychologist, social worker, dietician, general practitioner
Location	Rehabilitation centre: in-patient, out-patient, home based but supervised from a specialised centre Community based: out-patient in centre or primary care office Home based: supervised by primary care team
Duration	$\geq$8 weeks, but longer is typically more desired
Frequency	$\geq$3 sessions per week of which 2 are supervised
Exercise training component	Exercise modalities (walking, cycling, upper limbs, *etc.*) Exercise intensity Exercise type: interval, endurance, resistance Additional interventions: inspiratory muscle training, oxygen therapy, noninvasive mechanical ventilation, neuromuscular electrical stimulation

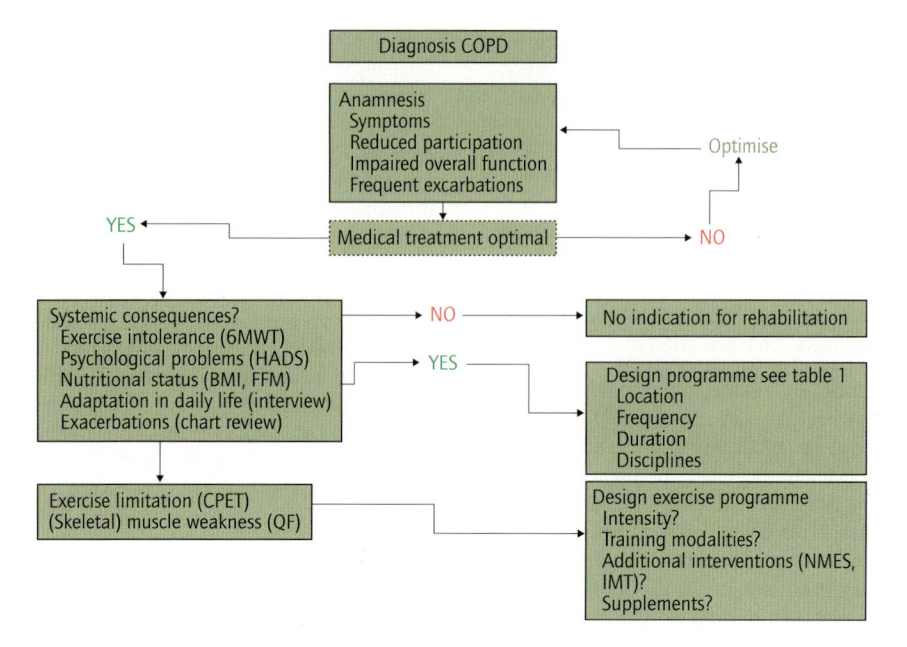

Figure 1. Flow chart for referral to pulmonary rehabilitation programmes. It should be emphasised that patients who are not candidates for pulmonary rehabilitation may still benefit from exercise training as an intervention to prevent morbidity.

Patient selection: patients with 'systemic consequences'

Extrapolating from the definition of pulmonary rehabilitation, the ideal candidate for rehabilitation is symptomatic, has impaired functional status and participation, is a heavy user of healthcare resources and should suffer from the "systemic consequences of COPD". Hence patient selection should not be based on lung function, but rather on the proper assessment of the extrapulmonary consequences of COPD found to be reversible with rehabilitation, symptoms, functional status, levels of participation in daily life and health-related quality of life. Other factors such as age, gender and smoking status are not important predictors of rehabilitation outcome. It is important that patients are screened for pulmonary rehabilitation after optimal pharmacotherapy is established. While being screened, patients can also be considered for other programmes such as a lung transplantation or lung volume reduction, a programme of noninvasive ventilatory support or oxygen therapy. Such programmes do not exclude pulmonary rehabilitation. On the contrary, pulmonary rehabilitation is often strongly recommended for these patients. Figure 1 gives an overview of the selection process and the design of the programme for patients with COPD.

Extrapulmonary consequences of COPD In the context of pulmonary rehabilitation, the most important "systemic consequence" of COPD is skeletal muscle dysfunction. In clinical practice, this can be assessed by skeletal muscle force or local skeletal muscle endurance, which is often even more affected. Approximately 70% of patients referred to an outpatient COPD clinic suffer from skeletal muscle weakness, and skeletal muscle force is acutely further reduced during acute exacerbations. Reversal of skeletal muscle dysfunction is an important goal of the exercise training component of a rehabilitation programme and hence patients suffering from skeletal muscle weakness are particularly good candidates for exercise training. Improving skeletal muscle strength can be done particularly effectively by including resistance training exercises in the exercise training sessions. When successful, muscle force increases and muscle oxidative capacity is enhanced.

More research is needed on pharmacological interventions that may assist pulmonary rehabilitation to restore muscle function more effectively. The short-term benefit of testosterone supplements in selected hypogonadal patients, in combination with resistance training, is an example of how pharmacotherapy and rehabilitation may have synergistic effects.

Impaired exercise tolerance and functional exercise capacity result from the pulmonary and systemic consequences of COPD. In the context of pulmonary rehabilitation, exercise tolerance is best formally assessed before the programme, using an incremental exercise test. This will help to guide the programme's intensity, training modalities and safety. Functional exercise capacity is best assessed using field tests such as the 6-min walking test, for which reference values exist and benchmark improvements for programme quality and clinical and statistical importance have been reported. When a patient's exercise tolerance is not abnormal, the indication for exercise training is questionable.

Another important extrapulmonary consequence of COPD is the derangement of body composition. It is important to pick up and treat both obesity and cachexia in pulmonary rehabilitation programmes. Obese patients may experience less dyspnoea than non-obese patients for a given oxygen consumption due to a favourable mechanical effect of obesity on operating lung volumes. Nevertheless, obesity (body mass index >30 kg·m^{-2}) limits the functional abilities of patients with limited ventilatory capacity as it increases the ventilatory needs for exercises against gravity. Cachexia, an involuntary loss of fat-free mass, leads inevitably to skeletal muscle weakness. It is a complex problem and its origin is not yet fully understood. The treatment of cachexia is an important aspect of rehabilitation in patients with COPD and requires individualised interventions by nutritional specialists. In order to appropriately assess this aspect, body composition should be assessed using DEXA-scan or bio-electrical impedance measures.

Symptoms The most disabling symptom in COPD is clearly shortness of breath. Patients report dyspnoea, particularly during exercise or activity, as a significant burden. Another important symptom is fatigue. Symptoms can be assessed during exercise using Borg symptom scores or during daily activities using specific questionnaires.

Physical activity Participation in daily activities is not easily assessed. Several questionnaires have been used, but increasingly activity monitors are preferred. In the future it is likely that benchmark values for physical activity will become available for patients with COPD. As indicated above, patients not meeting guidelines on healthy physical activity (30 min of moderate intense exercise on 5 days of the week) can be considered candidates for pulmonary rehabilitation.

Severe exacerbations Patients with COPD who have been hospitalised with an acute exacerbation are particularly good candidates for pulmonary rehabilitation programmes. These patients have lost muscle force and functional exercise tolerance and health-related quality of life acutely as the result of an exacerbation. Physical activity levels are also dramatically low during hospital admission and at least 1 month afterwards. Patients admitted to hospital for COPD are very likely to face new hospital admissions in the subsequent year. The risk of readmission is particularly high in patients who remain inactive after a hospitalisation. In these patients, the rehabilitation programme may need significant modification, with an emphasis on acquiring appropriate self-management skills to prevent subsequent admissions. Exercise training may need to be adapted to more severe ventilatory and/or skeletal muscle limitation, using resistance training or interval training at high intensities. A recent meta-analysis of a handful of studies showed that patients who suffered from exacerbations are very good candidates for pulmonary rehabilitation. Clearly these patients may impose a higher burden on the rehabilitation team and drop-out is a particularly important problem.

Summary

Pulmonary rehabilitation is an evidence-based intervention for patients with COPD. It is individually tailored to the needs of patients, both in terms of programme structure and its components. The aim of the rehabilitation programme is to reverse the systemic consequences of COPD, minimise healthcare use and lead to a durable change in physical activity and self-management behaviour. Although the short-term effects of rehabilitation are well known, the long-term effects are not always guaranteed. Further research should focus on the strategies to ensure the long-term benefits for patients with COPD. Further knowledge on the processes underlying a durable shift in lifestyle, as well as better understanding of the pathophysiological mechanisms leading to the systemic consequences of COPD and its treatments, may lead to major advances in the future.

D. Langer and C. Burtin are doctoral fellows of the Research Foundation Flanders. Supported by grant FWO G.0598.09N.

References

- Casaburi R, ZuWallack R. Pulmonary rehabilitation for management of chronic onbstructive pulmonary disease. *N Engl J Med* 2009; 26: 1329-1335.
- Clini EM, Ambrosino N. Nonpharmacological treatment and relief of symptoms in COPD. *Eur Respir J* 2008; 32: 218-228.
- Coventry PA, Hind D. Comprehensive pulmonary rehabilitation for anxiety and depression in adults with chronic obstructive pulmonary disease: systematic review and meta-analysis. *J Psychosom Res* 2007; 63: 551-565.
- Casaburi R, *et al.* Reductions in exercise lactic acidosis and ventilation as a result of exercise training in patients with obstructive lung disease. *Am Rev Respir Dis* 1991; 143: 9-18.
- Lacasse Y, *et al.* Pulmonary rehabilitation for chronic obstructive pulmonary disease. *Cochrane Database Syst Rev* 2006; 4: CD003793.
- Langer D, *et al.* A clinical practice guideline for physiotherapists treating patients with chronic obstructive pulmonary disease based on a systematic review of available evidence. *Clin Rehabil* 2009; 23: 445-462.
- Nici L, *et al.* American Thoracic Society/European Respiratory Society statement on pulmonary rehabilitation. *Am J Respir Crit Care Med* 2006; 173: 1390-1413.
- Pitta F, *et al.* Activity monitoring for assessment of physical activities of daily life in patients with COPD. *Arch Phys Med Rehabil* 2005; 86: 1979-1985.
- Puhan MA, *et al.* Interpretation of treatment changes in 6-minute walk distance in patients with COPD. *Eur Respir J* 2008; 32: 637-643.
- Puhan MA, *et al.* Interval *versus* continuous high-intensity exercise in chronic obstructive pulmonary disease: a randomized trial. *Ann Intern Med* 2006; 145: 816-825.
- Redelmeier DA, *et al.* Interpreting small differences in functional status: the six minute walk test in chronic lung disease patients. *Am J Respir Crit Care Med* 1997; 155: 1278-1282.
- Ries AL, *et al.* Effects of pulmonary rehabilitation on physiologic and psychosocial outcomes in patients with chronic obstructive pulmonary disease. *Ann Intern Med* 1995; 122: 823-832.
- Ries AL, *et al.* Maintenance after pulmonary rehabilitation in chronic lung disease: a randomized trial. *Am J Respir Crit Care Med* 2003; 167: 880-888.
- Ries AL, *et al.* Pulmonary rehabilitation: joint ACCP/AACVPR evidence-based clinical practice guidelines. *Chest* 2007; 131: 4S-42S.
- Spruit MA, *et al.* Resistance *versus* endurance training in patients with COPD and skeletal muscle weakness. *Eur Respir J* 2002; 19: 1072-1078.
- Troosters T, *et al.* Pulmonary rehabilitation in chronic obstructive pulmonary disease. *Am J Respir Crit Care Med* 2005; 172: 19-38.

SELF-ASSESSMENT

Further self-assessment questions and exclusive online content related to the ERS Handbook of Respiratory Medicine, can be found at www.ersnet.org/handbook. The code on the back cover of this book is your personal login.

The ERS Handbook of Respiratory Medicine is accredited by the European Board of Accreditation in Pneumology (EBAP) for CME credits.

European accreditation is granted by EBAP following the EACCME (European Accreditation Council for Continuing Medical Education) standards (D9908) in order to allow readers to validate the credits obtained through this activity in their home European country.

Each chapter has been afforded a maximum of 1 CME credit, which will be awarded once readers have successfully completed the CME questions relating to each chapter of the Handbook. A maximum of 17 CME credits for the whole book can be awarded. To take the CME test, please visit www.ersnet.org/handbook. In accordance with EBAP guidelines, all authors have declared potential conflicts of interest.

The questions presented here are purely for self-assessment purposes and are not CME accredited.

Notes on the questions
1. Always read the entire question and related answers carefully.
2. For **Type A questions** (in red), only one answer is correct.

   For **Type K' questions** (in blue), more than one answer may be correct.

Q1. Which of the following surfactant protein(s) play(s) an active role in innate immunity?
A. SP-A
B. SP-B
C. SP-C
D. SP-D

Q2. With regard to the anatomy of the respiratory system, which of the following statements is incorrect?
A. The right main bronchus is deep and measures about 20 mm in adults
B. The left main bronchus curves laterally and measures about 40 mm in adults
C. The right upper lobe always has three segments and has a tri-partite division at its origin
D. Each segment is a functional independent with its own blood supply and envelope by connective tissue that originates from the parietal pleura
E. The right middle lobe is a branch from the anterior portion of the right main bronchus

Q3. Why is alveolar dead space present at rest in young healthy subjects in the upright posture?
A. Alveoli at the base of the lung are small, and therefore poorly ventilated
B. Pulmonary capillaries at the base of the lung may collapse because of low intravascular pressures
C. Alveoli at the top of the lung are large, and therefore better ventilated
D. Pulmonary capillaries at the top of the lung may collapse because of low intravascular pressures

Q4. A 55-yr-old woman presents with a 2-yr history of paroxysms of dry cough when talking or bending. Which of the following investigations is mandatory at this stage?
A. Spirometry with reversibility
B. Chest radiography
C. Full blood count
D. Bronchoscopy
E. F_{eNO}

458

Q5. Which of the following is the most common nonrespiratory condition associated with chronic cough?
A. Sinusitis
B. Heartburn
C. Irritable bowel syndrome
D. Nasal polyposis
E. Congestive cardiac failure

Q6. Which of the following regarding examination of a patient with superior vena cava obstruction is/are true?
A. Giant 'V' waves are visible in the JVP
B. Peri-orbital oedema may be present
C. Dilated vessels are visible over the lower anterior abdominal wall
D. Signs and symptoms are more noticeable at the end of the day

Q7. Which of the following statement(s) is/are correct with regard to airway resistance measurements by whole-body plethysmography?
A. P_{box} provides an estimate of P_{alv}
B. P_{box} provides an estimate of P_{pl}
C. Inspiration increases P_{box}
D. Expiration decreases P_{box}

Q8. For which type of patients is medical thoracoscopy/pleuroscopy mainly indicated?
A. Patients with transudative pleural effusion of indeterminate origin
B. Patients with exudative pleural effusion of indeterminate origin
C. Patients with localised chest wall lesions
D. Patients with diffuse lung disease

Q9. The causes of exercise intolerance are best evaluated by the use of:
A. Walking tests
B. Cardiopulmonary exercise testing
C. Resting lung function measurements
D. All the above

Q10. The increase in functional residual capacity in airflow obstruction is the result of:
A. A decrease in lung elastic recoil
B. Dynamic mechanisms such as an increase in breathing frequency and/or expiratory flow limitation within the tidal breathing range
C. An increase in time constant of the respiratory system exceeding the expiratory time
D. A decrease in inspiratory muscle force

Q11. A 68-yr-old male with nonsmall cell lung cancer presents with increasing breathlessness. His chest radiograph shows complete collapse of the left lung and at bronchoscopy he has a polypoid tumour obstructing the left main bronchus. Which of the following is the most appropriate intervention?
A. Bronchoscopy and endobronchial sampling
B. Bronchoscopy with endobronchial tumour ablation with electrocautery or laser
C. Chemotherapy
D. Bronchsocopy with insertion of endobronchial stent
E. Treatment with antibiotics and steroids

Q12. Which of the following statement(s) regarding long-term oxygen therapy (LTOT) is/are true?
A. LTOT should be prescribed in all COPD patients with P_{a,O_2} in range 7.3-8.0 kPa
B. LTOT should be prescribed in a COPD patient with P_{a,O_2} 8.0 kPa and secondary polycythaemia
C. LTOT should be given during the daytime only
D. LTOT should be accompanied by ambulatory O_2 in active users

Q13. Which of the following statement(s) regarding home noninvasive ventilation is/are true?
A. It can be combined with cough assist devices in patients with neuromuscular disease and reduced cough efficacy
B. It increases survival in patients with COPD
C. It improves quality of life in COPD patients
D. It may reduce readmission in COPD patients with frequent hypercapnic exacerbations (revolving door admissions)

Q14. In which of the following patient(s) is/are the risk(s) of transition from latent tuberculosis infection to active tuberculosis increased?
A. Patients with end-stage renal disease
B. Patients after lung transplantation
C. Patients after cornea transplantation
D. Patients with Epstein–Barr virus infection

Q15. Which of the following diseases must be excluded before prolonged use of macrolides is considered?
A. Tuberculosis
B. Nontuberculous mycobacteria
C. *Pseudomonas aeruginosa*
D. *Aspergillus fumigatus*
E. HIV

Q16. A 60-yr-old farmer with moderate asbestos exposure 30 yrs ago presents with diffuse pulmonary fibrosis, predominantly basal, inspiratory crackles on chest examination, no plaques or pleural thickening on chest computed tomography and slowly deteriorating lung function. What is the likely diagnosis?
A. Asbestosis
B. Sarcoidosis
C. Idiopathic pulmonary fibrosis
D. Hypersensitivity pneumonitis
E. Nonspecific interstitial pneumonia

Q17. Which of the following statement(s) about occupational asthma (OA) is/are true?
A. Inhaled corticosteroids and bronchodilators are the preferred medications in symptomatic patients with OA
B. OA may occur in subjects without atopy
C. The diagnosis of OA cannot be excluded in a patient with pre-existing asthma
D. Twice daily peak-flow measurements are the most commonly used diagnostic test in OA

Q18. Which are the most investigated indoor pollution sources?
A. Fossil fuel
B. Biomass fuel, environmental tobacco smoke, mould/dampness
C. Environmental tobacco smoke
D. Furniture

Q19. Which is the most frequent aetiology of pleural effusions?
A. Infectious
B. Malignant
C. Immunological
D. Cardiac
E. Idiopathic

Q20. Which is the most common respiratory complication associated with neuromuscular disorders?
A. Obstructive sleep apnoea
B. Pulmonary embolism
C. Tracheal stenosis
D. Acute respiratory distress syndrome
E. Bronchial asthma

Q21. A 72-yr-old Caucasian male presents with chronic cough. He is a retired teacher, enjoys gardening, quit smoking 10 years ago, takes medications for hypertension and gastroesophageal reflux, and drinks 1–2 glasses of wine daily with dinner. Chest radiography shows a mass in the right upper lobe; a thorax computed tomography scan confirms the presence of a mass and shows that the subcarinal lymph nodes are enlarged. Biopsies obtained bronchoscopically show nonsmall cell lung cancer adenocarcinoma. Staging investigations reveal metastatic lesions in the liver. Which initial therapy would be most appropriate?
A. Neoadjuvant chemotherapy followed by lobectomy
B. Targeted therapy with erlotinib
C. Cisplatin-etoposide with concurrent radiation therapy
D. Cisplatin-pemetrexed chemotherapy

Q22. Metastatic pleural effusions are most frequently observed in:
A. Prostate cancer
B. Pancreatic cancer
C. Breast cancer
D. Kidney cancer
E. Lymphomas

Q23. Which of the following symptoms does not necessarily impede a radical treatment approach?
A. Liver metastasis
B. Bone metastasis
C. Vena cava superior syndrome
D. Brain metastasis
E. Axillar lymphadenopathy

Q24. Which of the following treatment options will most likely improve the left ventricular ejection fraction in a patient with congestive heart failure and Cheyne–Stokes respiration?
A. Nocturnal oxygen
B. Nocturnal CPAP
C. Acetazolamide
D. Nocturnal CO_2 inhalation
E. Theophylline

Q25. What has positively changed the natural history of cytomegalovirus infection post-bone-marrow transplant?
A. Immunosuppressive therapy
B. CMV prophylaxis or pre-emptive therapy
C. Extracorporeal photopheresis
D. Immunoglobulins
E. Antibiotic therapy

Answers

Q01. A,D
Q02. C
Q03. D
Q04. B
Q05. C
Q06. B
Q07. A,C,D
Q08. B
Q09. B
Q10. A,B,C
Q11. B
Q12. B,D
Q13. A,D
Q14. A,B
Q15. B
Q16. C
Q17. A,B,C
Q18. B
Q19. D
Q20. A
Q21. D
Q22. C
Q23. C
Q24. B
Q25. B

INDEX

A

abacavir 429
abscess, lung 189–190
N-acetylcysteine, idiopathic pulmonary fibrosis therapy 316–317
acid–base disorders 16, 80, 81
  arterial blood gas analysis 79, 80–81
acquired immune defence 28–29, 30
acreolin 36
acute bronchitis 240–241
acute chemical pneumonitis 274–276
acute cough 34
acute eosinophilic pneumonia 320
acute exacerbations of chronic obstructive pulmonary disease (AECOPD) 149–150
acute inhalation injury 273–277
  clinical presentation 273
    inhalational fever 273–274
    pneumonitis see toxic pneumonitis
  sequelae 277
acute interstitial pneumonia (AIP) 105, 311, 312
acute lung injury (ALI) 146–147
  drug-induced 325
  inhalation see acute inhalation injury
  radiation-induced 304
acute mountain sickness (AMS) 298–299, 300
acute-on-chronic respiratory failure 149, 150
acute oxygen therapy 151
acute respiratory distress syndrome (ARDS) 146–147
  diagnosis 105
  drug-induced 328
acute respiratory failure (ARF) 148–150
acute silico-proteinosis 276
acute thyroiditis 170
acute vasoreactivity testing, pulmonary arterial hypertension 343, 344
acute ventilatory support 152
adenocarcinoma, lung 373, 374–375
adenosine monophosphate (AMP) bronchial provocation testing 88, 89
adenotonsillectomy, obstructive sleep apnoea management 409
adjuvant chemotherapy
  definition 377
  nonsmall cell lung cancer 382
  small cell lung cancer 379
advanced lung disease
  gastro-oesophageal reflux 243–244
  see also specific diseases
air pollution 285–289
  asthma and 286, 287, 288, 289
  biological mechanisms 289
  children and 285, 286
  COPD and 248, 286, 287, 288
  indoor 287–289
  lung cancer and 286, 287–288
  outdoor 285–287
airway clearance techniques 446–447
  COPD 448
  neuromuscular disease 449

airway resistance 63–64
  measurement 64–65
airway stenosis
  impact of interventional bronchoscopy 120–121
  malignant, interventional pulmonology 118, 120–121
  pulmonary function tests 118–120
  upper see upper airway stenosis (UAS)
airway stenting 101, 120–121
airways, drug-induced disease 327
allergen bronchial provocation test 88, 89, 90
allergen immunotherapy, asthma 234–235
allergic alveolitis see hypersensitivity pneumonitis (HP)
allergic rhinitis 224–226
  asthma association 224, 226
  definition 224
  epidemiology 224
  pathophysiology 225–226
  treatment 225, 226
allergic rhinoconjunctivitis 170
allergy tests, asthma 230–231
  occupational 270
alveolar epithelium 8
alveolar haemorrhage, drug-induced 324, 325, 329
alveolar hypoventilation 20–21
  see also hypoventilation syndromes
alveolar macrophage pneumonia 312
alveolar macrophages (AMs) 27–28
alveolar pressure (P_{ALV}) 16, 17, 18, 19, 20
alveolar shunt 23
alveolar type I (ATI) cells 8
alveolar type II (ATII) cells 8
alveolar volume (V_A) 23
  measurement 69
  physiological influences 70, 71
amantadine 192
ambulatory oxygen therapy 151
American Society of Anesthesiologists (ASA), pre-operative risk classification 156, 157
amikacin therapy
  nontuberculous mycobacterial infections 220
  pulmonary tuberculosis 204, 205
amiodarone pulmonary toxicity (APT) 324, 325, 326, 327, 328
amoxicillin therapy, infectious COPD exacerbations 174, 175
amoxicillin-clavulanate therapy
  infectious COPD exacerbations 174, 175
  pulmonary tuberculosis 206
AMP (adenosine monophosphate) bronchial provocation testing 88, 89
amyloid A amyloidosis 433
amyloid light chain amyloidosis 433
amyloidosis 433–434
anaemia
  chemotherapy-induced 378
  dyspnoea and 43
anaesthesia, preoperative assessment 156–158
anatomical barriers 26
anatomy 11–14

see also individual anatomical structures
angina, dyspnoea and 42, 43
angio-oedema, drug-induced 323, 326, 327
angiomyolipoma (AML) 442
angioplastic pneumonectomy 386
angiotensin-converting enzyme (ACE), serum levels in sarcoidosis 5
angiotensin-converting enzyme (ACE) inhibitors, respiratory complications 323, 327
Annexin A11 (ANXA11) 3, 4, 5
antero-posterior (AP) radiograph 126
anti-inflammatory therapy
　rhinitis 225, 226
　see also corticosteroid therapy; nonsteroidal anti-inflammatory drugs (NSAIDs)
anti-tuberculosis drugs
　extrapulmonary tuberculosis 210
　latent tuberculosis 216
　nontuberculous mycobacterial infections 220
　pulmonary tuberculosis 204-208
　resistance 204, 206, 207-208
　　HIV association 427
antibiotic resistance
　anti-tuberculosis drugs *see* anti-tuberculosis drugs
　pneumonia pathogens 178
antibiotic therapy
　bronchiectasis exacerbations 253-254
　bronchitis 241
　community-acquired pneumonia 178-179
　cystic fibrosis 259, 262
　descending necrotising mediastinitis 359
　hospital-acquired pneumonia 182
　infectious chronic obstructive pulmonary disease exacerbations 174, 175
　lung abscess 189, 190
　pleural infections 188
　pulmonary tuberculosis 205
　purulent sputum and 38
　tuberculous meningitis 211
　upper respiratory tract infections 170
　see also specific antibiotics
anticholinergic therapy
　COPD 249
　rhinitis 225, 226
　vocal cord dysfunction 239
antigen-presenting cells (APCs) 28-29
antihistamines, rhinitis treatment 225, 226
antineutrophil cytoplasmic antibodies (ANCA) 336
α_1-antitrypsin (AT) deficiency *see* α_1-proteinase inhibitor (PI) deficiency
antiviral drugs
　cytomegalovirus infection prophylaxis, post-bone marrow transplantation 431
　oseltamivir 192-193
anxiety disorder, hyperventilation 42
apical parietal pleurectomy, pneumothorax management 355, 356
apnoea/hypopnoea index (AHI) 404, 405
Ardystil syndrome 276
arterial blood gas analysis 77-81
　acid-base status 79, 80-81
　asthma 230
　pulmonary gas exchange 77-80

arterial hypoxaemia *see* hypoxaemia
arterial oxygen desaturation 85
arterial pH 80
asbestos exposure 282-283
asbestos pleurisy 282-283
asbestosis 104, 283
Aspergillus pneumonia (AP) 184, 185
aspiration, pneumothorax 354
aspiration pneumonia 176, 178
aspirin, respiratory complications 327
assessment
　pre-operative 156-158
　　pulmonary resection 157-158
　see also physical examination
assisted coughing techniques, neuromuscular disease patients 364, 449
associated pulmonary arterial hypertension (APAH) 340-341, 344
asthma 227-235
　altitude effects 300-301
　comorbidities 234, 235
　　allergic rhinitis 224, 226
　　gastro-oesophageal reflux disease 234, 242, 243
　　vocal cord dysfunction 236, 237, 238, 239
　COPD vs. 229, 230, 232, 234
　diagnosis 227-234
　　allergy tests 230-231
　　arterial blood gas analysis 230
　　assessment of airway inflammation 232
　　bronchial provocation testing 90, 230
　　differential 229, 232, 234
　　exhaled breath analysis 94, 232
　　imaging 231-232
　　lung function tests 228-230
　　physical examination 228
　drug-induced 325, 327
　eosinophilic bronchitis vs. 319
　genetics 1, 5-6
　induced sputum biomarkers 93
　management
　　exacerbations 233, 235
　　pharmacological 231, 234-235
　　physiotherapy 448
　occupational *see* occupational asthma
　symptoms 227-228
　　cough 34, 35
　　dyspnoea 42, 44
　triggers 227, 228
　　air pollution 286, 287, 288, 289
　　exercise 228
　　mould exposure/dampness 288
　　smoking 292-293
　upper respiratory tract infection vs. 170
atovaquone, *Pneumocystis jirovecii* pneumonia management 425, 426
auscultation
　breath sounds 44-45, 54
　heart sounds 45
avian influenza 194
azathioprine therapy, idiopathic pulmonary fibrosis 316
azithromycin, *Pneumocystis jirovecii* pneumonia management 426

463

ERS Handbook: Respiratory Medicine

B

B-lymphocytes 29, 30
bacterial infections
　bronchiectasis 253
　bronchitis 240
　chronic obstructive pulmonary disease
　　exacerbations 172–173
　community-acquired pneumonia 177–178
　diagnosis see microbiological testing
　hospital-acquired pneumonia 181–182
　immunocompromised hosts 184
　　HIV-infected patients 423–424
　　with primary immunodeficiency 420, 421
　lung abscess 189
　pleural 186–187
　upper respiratory tract 169
　see also respiratory infections; specific bacteria; specific infections
bagassosis 280
balloon atrioseptostomy, pulmonary arterial hypertension 343
barotrauma, pulmonary 302–303
barriers, defence 26
bedside radiography 127
benzodiazepines, vocal cord dysfunction treatment 238
$β_2$-agonists, asthma management 234
beta-blocker-induced bronchospasm 326, 327
bevacizumab therapy, nonsmall cell lung cancer 380–381
biomass fuels, indoor air pollution 287, 288
biopsy
　lung see lung biopsy
　percutaneous fine-needle 110–111
　pleural 396
biplane fluoroscopy, fine-needle biopsy guidance 110
bird fancier's lung 278, 279, 280
bleb resection, pneumothorax management 355
bleeding
　alveolar, drug-induced 324, 325, 329
　thoracentesis-induced 117
blood culture 162, 163
body plethysmography 62, 64–65
bone
　metastases 390–391
　tuberculosis 211
bone marrow transplantation (BMT), pulmonary complications 430–431
　tuberculosis 212, 213, 431
bones, cystic fibrosis-related disease 262
Bordetella pertussis
　detection 166
　infection 169, 170
Borg scale 43, 44
Bornholm disease 50
bosentan, idiopathic pulmonary fibrosis therapy 317
botulinum toxin A (Botox), vocal cord dysfunction treatment 239
brachytherapy 101, 381
breast cancer, metastasis 388, 389, 390
breath sounds, auscultation 44–45, 54
breathing frequency 16, 19
breathing reserve (BR) 85
breathlessness see dyspnoea

bromhexine, bronchiectasis management 254
bronchi, anatomy 12–13
bronchial-associated lymphoid tissue (BALT) 26, 28
bronchial biopsy 100
bronchial brushings 100
bronchial carcinoma see lung cancer
bronchial clearance, bronchiectasis 254
bronchial provocation testing (BPT) 88–90
　clinical relevance 90
　　asthma diagnosis 230
　methods 88–90
bronchial responsiveness (BR), testing see bronchial provocation testing (BPT)
bronchial washings 100
bronchiectasis 252–254
　aetiology 252
　associated conditions 252
　　primary immunodeficiency 420, 421
　diagnosis 37, 252–253
　exacerbations 252
　　infective see infective exacerbations of bronchiectasis
　　management 253–254
　　prevention 254
　HIV-infected patients 424
　management 253–254
　　physiotherapy 448
　nodular 219
　symptoms 252
　　haemoptysis 38
bronchiolitis obliterans organising pneumonia (BOOP) 105, 312–313
　drug-induced 324, 327, 328
bronchiolitis obliterans syndrome (BOS) 244
　fume-related 276
　popcorn workers 277
bronchitis 240–241
　acute 240–241
　aetiology/risk factors 240
　chronic see chronic bronchitis
　definition 240
　diagnosis 241
　eosinophilic see eosinophilic bronchitis
　epidemiology 240
　prognosis 240–241
　symptoms 240
　treatment 241
bronchoalveolar lavage (BAL) 100, 103–108
　cell counts 107–108
　　nonsmokers vs. smokers 108
　complications 101
　cytological appearances 104–106, 108
　definition 103
　indications 103, 104–106, 108, 439
　procedure 103, 106–107
　sample processing 107
bronchodilator reversibility testing, asthma 229–230
bronchodilator therapy
　asthma 231, 234
　　exacerbations 233, 235
　bronchiectasis 254
　COPD 175, 249, 250

lymphangioleiomyomatosis 443
bronchogenic carcinoma see lung cancer
bronchoplastic lobectomy, nonsmall cell lung cancer 386
bronchopulmonary segments, anatomy 12
bronchoscopy 98-102
   advanced diagnostic procedures 101
   complications 100-101
   equipment 98
   fluorescence 101
   indications 98-99
      lung cancer diagnosis 98, 373
   interventional 101-102, 118, 120-121
   patient preparation 99
   procedure 99
   sampling techniques 99-100
bronchospasm
   drug-induced 323, 325, 326, 327
   dyspnoea 42
building dampness 288
bullae resection, pneumothorax management 355, 356
bupropion 296

C

cachexia, COPD patients 455
calcium channel blockers, pulmonary arterial hypertension management 343, 344
cancer
   genetics 3, 6
   lung see lung cancer
   see also tumours
cannabis smoke 292
capreomycin therapy, pulmonary tuberculosis 204, 205
capsaicin cough challenge 36, 37
carbon dioxide, ventilatory response to inhalation 72-74
carbon monoxide (CO)
   air pollution 285, 286, 288
   transfer factor see transfer factor of the lung for carbon monoxide ($T_{L,CO}$)
carboplatin chemotherapy 379
   nonsmall cell lung cancer 380
   small cell lung cancer 375, 378
cardiac chest pain 49, 50
cardiac disease see heart disease
cardiac risk assessment, peri-operative 157
   pulmonary resection 157-158
cardiopulmonary exercise testing see exercise testing
cardiovascular disease, as consequence of obstructive sleep apnoea 406, 407
cardiovascular response, exercise testing 86
catastrophic bronchospasm 323, 327
cavity lung disease 218-219
cefditoren therapy, infectious COPD exacerbations 175
cefuroxime therapy, infectious COPD exacerbations 175
central airway stenosis, impact of interventional pulmonology 120-121
central nervous system (CNS), tuberculosis 211
central sleep apnoea/hypopnoea (CSA) 410-413
   aetiology 410
   associated conditions 410, 412-413
   complex 412
   in heart failure patients 408, 410-412
   idiopathic 412
   management 408, 411-412, 413
   pathophysiology 410
   prevalence 410
cephalosporins
   community-acquired pneumonia management 178
   hospital-acquired pneumonia management 182
   infectious COPD exacerbation management 174, 175
cerebral oedema, high-altitude 299, 300
cervical lymph nodes, tuberculosis 210
cheese worker's lung 280
chemical pneumonitis see toxic pneumonitis
chemical worker's lung 280
chemokine production 29
chemopleurodesis, pneumothorax 355
chemoreceptor response
   carbon dioxide 72-74
   hypoxia 74-76
chemotherapy 377-381
   adjuvant see adjuvant chemotherapy
   administration routes 377
   Langerhans' cell histiocytosis 440
   malignant pleural mesothelioma 381, 397
   nonsmall cell lung cancer 374-375, 379-381, 382
   side-effects 378
      respiratory disease 322, 324, 325, 326, 328
   small cell lung cancer 375, 378-379
   see also specific chemotherapeutic agents
chemotherapy lung 328
chest
   bone metastases 390-391
   computed tomography indications 131, 132
   drains see chest tube drainage
   fluoroscopy 129
   pain 49-50
   percussion 52, 54
   physiotherapy see respiratory physiotherapy
chest physiotherapy see respiratory physiotherapy
chest radiography 126-129
   asthma 231-232
   basic techniques 126, 127
   bedside 127
   bronchiectasis 253
   chest pain investigation 50
   digital 127, 129
   drug-induced respiratory disease 324, 326-327
   indications 126, 128
   inspiratory-expiratory 127
   lung abscess 189
   lymphangioleiomyomatosis 441
   pleural infection 187, 188
   pneumonia 177
      eosinophilic 320
   pneumothorax 353, 354
   projections 126-127
   pulmonary alveolar proteinosis 435, 436
   pulmonary Langerhans' cell histiocytosis 439
   pulmonary tuberculosis 203
   sarcoidosis 309, 310
chest tube drainage
   lung abscess 190
   pleural infections 187, 188
   pneumothorax 354
chest wall compliance 66

chest wall disorders 366–368
  controversies 367
  hypoventilation and 417
  investigation, transthoracic ultrasonography 138–139
  management
    physiotherapy 449
    surgical 367, 368
  pathogenesis 366
  pectus carinatum 367
  pectus excavatum 366, 367
chest wall pain 49–50
chest wall tumours 392, 393
  clinical signs 393
  prognosis 393
  treatment 397
Cheyne–Stokes respiration (CSR) 410
  in heart failure patients 410–412
children
  air pollution hazards 285, 286
  influenza complications 193, 194
  Langerhans' cell histiocytosis 438
Chlamydophilia pneumoniae
  COPD exacerbations 173, 175
  detection methods 163, 165, 166
chronic beryllium disease (CBD)
  diagnosis 106
  genetics 2, 3, 5
chronic bronchitis 241, 246–247
  emphysema *vs.* 241
  see also chronic obstructive pulmonary disease (COPD)
chronic cough 34–36
  aetiology 34–35
  diagnosis 35
  epidemiology 34
  induced sputum biomarkers 93
  management 36–37
  risk factors 35, 36
    environmental tobacco smoke exposure 287
  sputum hypersecretion and 37–38
  see also cough
chronic eosinophilic pneumonia 320
chronic heart failure *see* heart failure patients
chronic lung disease (CLD), primary immunodeficiency-associated 420–421
chronic mountain sickness 300
chronic obstructive pulmonary disease (COPD)
  altitude effects 300
  asthma *vs.* 229, 230, 232, 234
  chronic bronchitis *see* chronic bronchitis
  emphysema *see* emphysema
  exacerbations *see* chronic obstructive pulmonary disease (COPD) exacerbations
  exercise intolerance 19, 83, 85, 455
  exercise testing 86, 87, 455
  exhaled breath analysis 94
  gastro-oesophageal reflux disease association 243
  genetics 248
  HIV association 428
  induced sputum biomarkers 93
  management *see* chronic obstructive pulmonary disease (COPD) management
  pathophysiology 246
  role of transforming growth factor-β 9–10
  physical activity levels 453, 455
    effects of pulmonary rehabilitation 452
    see also pulmonary rehabilitation
  risk factors 248, 249
    air pollution 248, 286, 287, 288
    smoking 241, 246, 248, 292–293
  secondary pneumothorax and 356, 357
  severity classification 247
  silicosis association 284
  symptoms 246, 455
    dyspnoea 41, 46, 455
    extrapulmonary 454–455
chronic obstructive pulmonary disease (COPD) exacerbations 42, 172–176, 246–250
  acute 149–150
  aetiology 172–173
    infectious *see* infective exacerbations of COPD
    noninfectious 172, 173
  definition 172
  frequency 172
  management 174–176, 249
    infective exacerbations *see under* infective exacerbations of COPD
    pulmonary rehabilitation 455–456
    see also chronic obstructive pulmonary disease (COPD) management
  outcomes 172, 173
chronic obstructive pulmonary disease (COPD) management 248–250
  bronchodilator therapy 249, 250
  corticosteroid therapy 249, 250
  influenza vaccination 250
  nutritional support 250
  oxygen therapy 151, 175, 250, 447, 448
  physiotherapy 447–448
  pulmonary rehabilitation 250, 447, 452, 453, 454–456
  ventilatory support 152
  see also under chronic obstructive pulmonary disease (COPD) exacerbations
chronic renal failure, tuberculosis 212, 213
chronic respiratory failure (CRF) 148
chronic rhinitis *see* rhinitis, chronic
chronic thromboembolic pulmonary hypertension (CTEPH) 341
  diagnosis 342
Churg–Strauss syndrome
  clinical presentation 337
  diagnosis 338
  epidemiology 336
  pathogenesis 336
  prognosis 338–339
  treatment 339
cigar smoke 291
cigarette smoke 291
cigarette smoking *see* smoking
ciprofloxacin therapy
  community-acquired pneumonia 178
  hospital-acquired pneumonia 182
  infectious COPD exacerbations 175
  pulmonary tuberculosis 205
cisplatin chemotherapy 379

malignant mesothelioma 381
   nonsmall cell lung cancer 374, 380
   small cell lung cancer 374, 375, 378
clarithromycin therapy
   nontuberculous mycobacterial infections 220
   pulmonary tuberculosis 206
cleft sternum 366
clofazimine therapy, pulmonary tuberculosis 206
co-trimoxazole, *Pneumocystis jirovecii* pneumonia management 425, 426
coal workers' pneumoconiosis (CWP) 283
colchicine, idiopathic pulmonary fibrosis therapy 316
colon, cystic fibrosis-related disease 261
combined antiretroviral therapy (CART) 423
   respiratory side-effects 428–429
   tuberculosis patients 427, 428
common cold 168, 169
community-acquired pleural infection 186
community-acquired pneumonia (CAP) 176–179
   clinical features 177
   definition 176
   diagnosis 177
      see also microbiological testing
   epidemiology 176
   management 178–179
      physiotherapy 448–449
   microbial aetiology 177
   microbial resistance 178
   severity assessment 178
complex sleep apnoea syndrome 412
compost lung 280
computed tomography (CT) 130–132
   chest, indications 131, 132
   descending necrotising mediastinitis 359
   drug-induced respiratory disease 324, 326
   fine-needle biopsy guidance 110
   high-resolution *see* high-resolution computed tomography (HRCT)
   lung abscess 189, 190
   magnetic resonance imaging *vs.* 130, 132
   malignant pleural mesothelioma 393
   pleural infection 187
   positron emission tomography and (PET/CT), lung cancer diagnosis 136, 137, 374
   sarcoidosis 309
   upper airway stenosis 119
computed tomography angiography (CTA), pulmonary embolism diagnosis 333–334, 335
congenital central hypoventilation syndrome 417
constant work rate (CWR) tests 84
continuous positive airway pressure (CPAP) therapy 152, 447
   central sleep apnoea 408, 411, 412
   community-acquired pneumonia 449
   obstructive sleep apnoea 407–408
continuous-volume computed tomography scanning 130, 131
controllers, asthma 234
conventional tube thoracostomy, pneumothorax 354–355
coronary artery disease (CAD), dyspnoea and 42, 43
corticosteroid therapy
   asthma 231, 234, 235

COPD exacerbations 175, 249, 250
drug-induced respiratory disease 323, 328
eosinophilic bronchitis 319
eosinophilic pneumonia 320
hypereosinophilic syndrome 321
hypersensitivity pneumonitis 281
idiopathic pulmonary fibrosis 315–316
Langerhans' cell histiocytosis 440
Pneumocystis jirovecii pneumonia 425
pulmonary vasculitis 339
rhinitis 225, 226
sarcoidosis 310
severe acute respiratory syndrome 196
costochondritis 49–50
cough 34
   acute 34
   assessment 51, 53
   asthmatic 34, 35
   bronchitis-associated 240
   chronic *see* chronic cough
cough challenge 36
cough peak expiratory flow (CPEP) measurement, neuromuscular disease patients 362
cough reflex 27
   capsaicin challenge 36, 37
   defective 34
   transient receptor potential 36, 37
cough suppression 37
coughing, manually assisted, neuromuscular disease patients 364, 449
counselling, smoking cessation 296
crackles 42, 45, 54
critically-ill patients
   respiratory intensive care 154–155
   respiratory physiotherapy 449
cryptogenic organising pneumonia (COP) 105, 312–313
   see also bronchiolitis obliterans organising pneumonia (BOOP)
CT *see* computed tomography (CT)
culture techniques 162–163, 164
   pulmonary tuberculosis diagnosis 203
CURB65 score 178
cyclophosphamide therapy
   idiopathic pulmonary fibrosis 316
   respiratory side-effects 325, 328
   Wegener's granulomatosis 339
cycloserine therapy, pulmonary tuberculosis 206
cyclosporine therapy, idiopathic pulmonary fibrosis 316
cystic fibrosis (CF) 256–264
   bronchiectasis 253
   clinical presentations 258
   diagnosis 258
   exercise intolerance 83
   exercise testing 86
   gastro-oesophageal reflux 242, 243–244
   genetics 2, 3–4, 256
   induced sputum biomarkers 93
   management 258–263
      gastrointestinal disease 261, 263
      lung disease 259–260, 261, 263
      novel therapies 263
      physiotherapy 448
   pathophysiology 256–257

prognosis 256
respiratory infections *see under* respiratory infections
cystic fibrosis transmembrane regulator (CFTR) 256
cytokine production 29
cytomegalovirus (CMV) infection, post-bone marrow transplantation 430, 431
cytomegalovirus pneumonia (CMVP) 185
post-bone marrow transplantation 431
cytosine methylation 3

D

D-dimer levels
idiopathic pulmonary fibrosis exacerbations 317
pulmonary embolism diagnosis 333
D-penicillamine, idiopathic pulmonary fibrosis therapy 316
dampness, exposure 288
dapsone, *Pneumocystis jirovecii* pneumonia management 425, 426
dasatinib, pleural injury 329
decompression stress 303
defence systems 26–30
acquired 28–29, 30
anatomical barriers 26
impairment/dysfunction 29
innate 8, 26, 27–28, 30
mucociliary clearance and fluid homeostasis 27
reflex mechanisms 26–27
"Dejours" hypoxia-withdrawal test 76
dendritic cells 28
descending necrotising mediastinitis (DNM) 358–360
clinical/radiological signs 359
diagnosis 358, 359
diffusion route 358
epidemiology 358
pathogens involved 359
treatment 359–360
desquamative interstitial pneumonia (DIP) 105, 312
development of respiratory system 14
dextromethorphan, bronchitis therapy 241
diabetes, dyspnoea 47–48
diacetyl-related bronchiolitis obliterans 277
diaphragm, anatomy 14
didanosine 429
diffuse alveolar damage (DAD), drug-induced 324, 325
diffuse alveolar haemorrhage, drug-induced 324, 325, 329
diffuse pleural thickening (DPT) 283
diffusion equilibrium 22
diffusion impairment 21–22
diffusion-weighted magnetic resonance imaging (DW MRI) 133
diffusive–perfusive conductance ratio 22
digital radiography (DR) 127, 129
direct immunofluorescence (DIF), respiratory virus detection 165
diving
pulmonary effects 303
pulmonary limitations at depth 302
diving-related disease 302–303
docetaxel chemotherapy 379
nonsmall cell lung cancer 375, 380
drug-induced respiratory disease (DIRD) 322–329

airways 327
clinical presentation 325–326
diagnosis 105, 323, 324, 326–327
HIV therapy-associated 428–429
methaemoglobinaemia 329
parenchymal 322, 327–329
pathophysiology 323–325
pleural 329
pulmonary vasculopathy 329
drug rash with eosinophilia and systemic symptoms (DRESS) 328
drug resistance
anti-tuberculosis drugs *see under* anti-tuberculosis drugs
oseltamivir 192–193
pneumonia pathogens 178
drug susceptibility testing (DST), anti-tuberculosis drugs 204, 206, 208
Duchenne muscular dystrophy 449
see also neuromuscular diseases (NMD), respiratory complications
dusts, inhalational injury
acute 273, 274
pneumoconiosis 282–284
dynamic hyperinflation 85
dyspnoea 41–48
aetiology 41–43
Borg scale 43, 44
as defence mechanism 27
definition 41
medical history 43–44
Medical Research Council scale 43, 44
pathophysiology 45–48
physical examination 44–45, 51, 53
see also specific diseases

E

echinacea 170
electrocardiography (ECG), cardiac chest pain investigation 50
embryology, respiratory system 14
emphysema 247
chronic bronchitis *vs.* 241
coal dust-associated 283
genetics 3, 4
silicosis association 284
see also chronic obstructive pulmonary disease (COPD)
empyema 187
chest radiograph 188
CT scan 189, 190
management 350
end-expiratory lung volume (EELV) 61–62
end-inspiratory lung volume (EILV) 62
endobronchial metastases 388, 389
endobronchial ultrasound-guided transbronchial fine needle aspiration (EBUS–TBNA) 101
endobronchial valves 101–102
endothelin-1 inhibitors, idiopathic pulmonary fibrosis therapy 317
endothelin receptor antagonist (ERA), pulmonary arterial hypertension management 343, 344
Enterobacteriaceae, as cause of hospital-acquired

pneumonia 181
environmental assessment, hypersensitivity pneumonitis 279
environmental tobacco smoke (ETS) 287–288
eosinophilic bronchitis 319
  chronic cough 35, 38, 319
eosinophilic diseases 105, 319–321
  see also specific diseases
eosinophilic pneumonia 320
  drug-induced 328
eosinophils 319
epidermal growth factor receptor (EGFR) 380
  mutations 375, 380
epidermal growth factor receptor (EGFR)-targeted therapies 375, 380
epigenetics 3
epiglottitis 169
epithelial barrier 26
Epworth Sleepiness Scale (ESS) 404, 405
equal pressure point (EPP) 19–20
equilibrium coefficient 22
ergots, pleural injury 329
erlotinib therapy, nonsmall cell lung cancer 380
etanercept therapy, idiopathic pulmonary fibrosis 317
ethambutol 205, 220
ethanol, cough challenge 36
ethionamide therapy, pulmonary tuberculosis 206
eucapnic voluntary hyperventilation (EVH) 89–90
exercise-induced asthma 228
exercise intolerance 83
  COPD 19, 83, 85, 455
exercise testing 83–87
  bronchial responsiveness 88, 89, 90
  COPD patients 86, 87, 455
  evaluation of therapeutic interventions 87
  indications 84
    pulmonary rehabilitation 455
  protocols 83–84
  response patterns 86
  variables and indexes 84–85
exercise tolerance, improvement
  bronchiectasis 254
  see also pulmonary rehabilitation
exercise training
  COPD management 250, 447
  see also pulmonary rehabilitation; respiratory physiotherapy
exhaled breath analysis 94–95, 229
exogenous lipoid pneumonitis 276
expiration 18–20, 63
expiratory flow limitation (EFL) 59
expiratory reserve volume 59, 61–62
extensively drug-resistant tuberculosis (XDR-TB) 204, 208
  HIV association 427
extracellular matrix (ECM) 7–8
extracorporeal membrane oxygenation (ECMO) 147
extrapulmonary tuberculosis (EPTB) 209–211
  diagnosis 210
  sites 209–211
  treatment 210
  WHO definition 209
  see also tuberculosis (TB)

F

familial pulmonary fibrosis 4, 5, 313
farmer's lung 278–279, 280
fatigue, chemotherapy-induced 378
FDG PET (2-[^{18}F]-fluoro-2-deoxy-D-glucose positron emission tomography)
  lung cancer diagnosis 136–137, 374
  pleural malignancies 394
FDG SUV (2-[^{18}F]-fluoro-2-deoxy-D-glucose standardised uptake value), lung cancer diagnosis 136, 137
female reproductive tract, cystic fibrosis-related disease 262
fever, inhalation 273–274
fibrosing mediastinitis 360
Fick's principle 15
  diffusion impairment 21
fine-needle aspiration biopsy
  percutaneous 110–111
  transbronchial *see* transbronchial fine-needle aspiration (TBNA)
flow-volume loop analysis, upper airway stenosis 118–119, 121
fluid homeostasis 27
fluorescence bronchoscopy 101
2-[^{18}F]-fluoro-2-deoxy-D-glucose positron emission tomography *see* FDG PET (2-[^{18}F]-fluoro-2-deoxy-D-glucose positron emission tomography)
2-[^{18}F]-fluoro-2-deoxy-D-glucose standardised uptake value (FDG SUV), lung cancer diagnosis 136
fluoroquinolones
  hospital-acquired pneumonia management 182
  pulmonary tuberculosis management 204, 205
  treatment of infectious COPD exacerbations 174, 175
fluoroscopy
  chest 129
  fine-needle biopsy guidance 110
fluticasone, bronchiectasis management 254
Forced Oscillation Technique 65
forced residual capacity (FRC) 16–17
foreign body inhalation 42
Framework Convention for Tobacco Control (FCTC) 295
functional residual capacity (FRC) 59, 61
fungal infections
  bronchiectasis 253
  immunocompromised hosts 184
    HIV-infected patients 424–426
    with primary immunodeficiency 421–422
  lung abscess 189
  see also specific fungal infections
"funnel chest" (pectus excavatum) 366, 367

G

gallium-67 scintigraphy 136
ganciclovir 431
gas dilution techniques 62
gas exchange *see* pulmonary gas exchange
gas microemboli, diving-associated 303
gas transfer factor *see* transfer factor of the lung for carbon monoxide ($T_{L,CO}$)
gases, inhalational injury *see* acute inhalation injury
gastro-oesophageal reflux disease (GORD) 242–245
  in advanced lung disease 242, 243–244

comorbidities
  asthma 234, 242, 243
  COPD 243
cough association *see* gastro-oesophageal reflux-induced cough
  management 244-245
  pathophysiology 242-243
  symptoms 242
  upper respiratory tract infections *vs.* 170
gastro-oesophageal reflux-induced cough 35, 242, 243
  management 37, 243
gastrointestinal disease, cystic fibrosis-related 261, 263
gefitinib therapy, nonsmall cell lung cancer 380
gemcitabine therapy 379
  malignant mesothelioma 381
  nonsmall cell lung cancer 374, 380
gene mutations 2-3
gene therapy, cystic fibrosis 263
genetics 2-6
  see also specific diseases
Geneva score 332
germ cell tumours 399-400
graft *versus* host disease (GVHD) 430-431
grain handler's lung 280
Gram stain, sputum 164
granulocyte macrophage-colony stimulating factor (GM-CSF) signalling, disruption in pulmonary alveolar proteinosis 8, 435
granulomatous lung diseases
  diagnosis, bronchoalveolar lavage 106
  see also specific diseases
group A streptococcal pharyngitis 169, 170

H

Haemophilus influenzae infection
  COPD exacerbations 173, 174, 175
  hospital-acquired pneumonia 181
Haemophilus influenzae type B (HiB) 169
  vaccination 170
haemoptysis 38
  fine-needle biopsy-induced 111
haemorrhage
  alveolar, drug-induced 324, 325, 329
  thoracentesis-induced 117
haemosiderosis, pulmonary 104
haemothorax 353-354
  laboratory investigations 350
  thoracentesis-induced 117
healthcare-associated pneumonia (HCAP) 180
  see also hospital-acquired pneumonia (HAP)
heart attack 42
heart catheterisation, pulmonary hypertension diagnosis 340, 343
heart disease
  as consequence of obstructive sleep apnoea 405-406, 407
  dyspnoea and 42, 43
  pulmonary hypertension and 341, 343
heart failure patients
  Cheyne-Stokes respiration/central sleep apnoea 408, 410-412
  dyspnoea 43, 47
heart rate reserve (HRR) 84-85

heart sounds, auscultation 45
helical computed tomography scanning 130, 131
heliox gas mixture, vocal cord dysfunction treatment 238
Henderson-Hasselbalch equation 16
heritable pulmonary arterial hypertension 340, 341, 343
high-altitude, physiological response 22, 298
high-altitude cerebral oedema (HACE) 299, 300
high-altitude disease 298-301, 413
high-altitude periodic breathing 298, 299, 413
high-altitude pulmonary oedema (HAPE) 299-300
high-dependency unit 154-155
high molecular weight (HMW) agents, occupational asthma 269, 270
high-resolution computed tomography (HRCT) 130-131
  bronchiectasis 253
  idiopathic pulmonary fibrosis 314
  lymphangioleiomyomatosis 441, 442
  pulmonary alveolar proteinosis 436
  pulmonary hypertension 342-343
  pulmonary Langerhans' cell histiocytosis 439
hila, anatomy 13
hilar amyloid lymphadenopathy 434
hilar lymph nodes, metastatic tumours 389-390
histamine bronchial provocation testing 88, 89, 90
histone modifications 3
HIV-related disease 423-429
  COPD 428
  infections 184, 423-427
    bacterial 423-424
    fungal 424
      see also Pneumocystis jirovecii pneumonia (PJP)
    tuberculosis 185, 201-202, 203, 212-213, 284, 426-427
  malignant conditions 427-428
  pneumonitis 428
  pneumothorax 428
  pulmonary arterial hypertension 428
  therapy-associated 428-429
  see also immunocompromised hosts
HIV therapy *see* combined antiretroviral therapy (CART)
home ventilatory support 152
Hoover's sign 44
hospital-acquired pleural infection 186, 187
hospital-acquired pneumonia (HAP) 176, 180-182
  definition 180
  diagnosis 177, 181, 182
  epidemiology 176, 180
  management 179, 182
  microbial aetiology 178, 181-182
  pathogenesis 181
  risk factors 181
  severity assessment 178
hot-tub lung 278, 280
hypercapnia 74, 78, 80, 81
hypercapnic respiratory failure 149, 150
  arterial blood gas analysis 78, 79
hypereosinophilic syndrome (HES) 320-321
hyperinflation, dynamic 85
hyperoxia, diving-associated 303
hyperoxic rebreathing method 72, 73-74

hypersensitivity pneumonitis (HP) 219, 278–281
  diagnosis 106, 279–280
    differential 281
  environmental assessment 279
  epidemiology 278
  host factors 279
  pathogenesis 279
  prognosis 281
  risk factors 278–279
  symptoms/findings 279
  treatment 280–281
  types 280
hypertension, pulmonary see pulmonary hypertension (PH)
hyperventilation syndrome 42, 45
  physiotherapy 448
hypocapnia 80
hypotension, thoracentesis-induced 117
hypoventilation syndromes 414–417
  aetiology 415–417
  clinical features 415
  diagnosis 415
  management 416–417
  pathophysiology 20–21, 414–415
hypoxaemia 16, 22, 23
  aetiology 15, 20–21, 22, 23, 24
  arterial blood gas analysis 77, 78
  oxygen therapy 151
hypoxaemic respiratory failure 148–149
  arterial blood gas analysis 77–78, 79
hypoxia, ventilatory response 74, 76
hypoxia-withdrawal test 76
hypoxic ventilatory decline 74, 75
hysteresis 60–61

I
iatrogenic pneumothorax 352, 353
idiopathic central sleep apnoea 412
idiopathic interstitial pneumonias (IIPs) 311–318
  classification 311, 312
  clinical features 311
  epidemiology 311
  management 311–312
  post-bone marrow transplantation 431
  see also specific forms
idiopathic pulmonary arterial hypertension 340, 341, 342, 343, 344
idiopathic pulmonary fibrosis (IPF) 311–312, 313–318
  clinical features 313–314
  diagnosis 105, 314
  exacerbations 314–315
  genetics 4, 5, 313
  management 315–318
  natural history 314
  pathogenesis 313
  physiology 313
Ig (immunoglobulin) production 29
IgA 29
IgG 29
IgM 29
IκBα kinase (IKK) 10
image-guided percutaneous drainage, lung abscess 190

imatinib therapy, hypereosinophilic syndrome 321
immune defence 26–30
  acquired 28–29, 30
  innate 26–28, 30
immune reconstitution disease (IRD) 428
immunocompromised hosts
  nontuberculous mycobacterial infections 219
  pneumonia 176, 177, 178, 183–185
  tuberculosis 184, 185, 201, 212–213
  see also HIV-related disease
immunodeficiency, primary, pulmonary diseases 420–422
immunoglobulin (Ig) production 29
immunosuppression
  infectious complications 184–185
  types 183, 184
  Wegener's granulomatosis management 339
immunotherapy, asthma 234–235
impulse oscillometry, vocal cord dysfunction diagnosis 237
indoor pollution 287–289
induced sputum see sputum induction
infective exacerbations of bronchiectasis 252, 253
  treatment 253–254
infective exacerbations of COPD 172–176
  diagnosis 173–174
  treatment 174–176
    antibiotic 174, 175
    nonantibiotic 174–176
inflammatory diseases
  diagnosis, gallium-67 scintigraphy 136
  see also specific diseases
influenza 170, 191–194
  chemoprophylaxis 192
  complications 177, 193, 194
  diagnosis 196–197
  pandemic 193–194
  seasonal 191–193
  treatment 170, 192
influenza vaccination 170, 192
  COPD patients 250
  lymphangioleiomyomatosis patients 443
influenza viruses 191
  detection 165
inhalation fever 273–274
  hypersensitivity pneumonitis vs. 281
inhalation injury, acute see acute inhalation injury
innate immune defence 8, 26, 27–28, 30
inspiration 17–18, 21, 63, 64
inspiratory capacity (IC) 59, 61
inspiratory-muscle pressure 16–17
inspiratory reserve volume 59, 61–62
inspiratory squeaks 45
inspiratory–expiratory radiography 127
insulin resistance (IR), obstructive sleep apnoea association 406, 407
intensive care unit 154–155
interferon-γ, lack of functional receptors 2–3
interferon-γ-1b, idiopathic pulmonary fibrosis therapy 316
interferon-γ release assays (IGRAs) 204, 213, 215, 216
interleukin-12, lack of functional receptors 2–3
interleukin-17 29

intermittent positive pressure breathing (IPPB) 447
  bronchiectasis management 448
  COPD management 448
interrupter technique 65
interstitial lung disease (ILD)
  diagnosis, bronchoalveolar lavage 103, 105
  drug-induced 322, 323, 327–329
  dyspnoea 43, 46–47
  exercise intolerance 83
  exercise testing 86
  genetics 4–5
  management, physiotherapy 448
  respiratory bronchiolitis associated 105, 312
  smoking and 293
interventional lung assist (ILA) 147
interventional pulmonology 118
  bronchoscopy 101–102, 118, 120–121
intraoperative interventions, pulmonary complications 157
intrapleural pressure (PIP) 16–17, 18, 19–20
isocapnic hypoxia 74–75
isoniazid therapy
  latent tuberculosis 216
  nontuberculous mycobacterial infections 220
  pulmonary tuberculosis 204, 205

J

Japanese summer-type hypersensitivity pneumonitis 280
joints
  cystic fibrosis-related disease 262
  tuberculosis 211

K

kanamycin therapy, pulmonary tuberculosis 204, 205
Kaposi sarcoma 427
"keel chest" (pectus carinatum) 367

L

lactate threshold 84
lactic acidosis, HIV therapy-associated 428–429
Lady Windemere's syndrome 219
Langerhans' cell histiocytosis (LCH)
  adult, pulmonary see pulmonary Langerhans' cell histiocytosis, adult
  in children 438
large cell carcinoma, lung 373
large cell neuroendocrine carcinoma (LCNEC), lung 373
laryngeal amyloidosis 434
laryngitis, symptoms and signs 169
laryngoscopy, vocal cord dysfunction diagnosis 237–238
latent tuberculosis infection (LTBI) 201, 215–217
  controversies 216–217
  detection 216
  immunocompromised hosts 213
    HIV-infected 427
  TB risk 215
  treatment 215–216
lateral chest radiograph 126, 127
lateral decubitus chest radiograph 126–127
Legionella spp.
  as cause of community-acquired pneumonia 177

detection methods 163, 164, 165, 166
Legionnaire's disease, diagnosis 164, 165
leukotriene antagonists, allergic rhinitis treatment 226
levofloxacin therapy
  community-acquired pneumonia 178
  hospital-acquired pneumonia 182
  infectious COPD exacerbations 174, 175
  pulmonary tuberculosis 205
Light's criteria 350
linezolid therapy, pulmonary tuberculosis 206
liver, cystic fibrosis-related disease 261
lobectomy, nonsmall cell lung cancer 383, 384, 385
  bronchoplastic 386
Löfgren's syndrome 308, 309, 310
long-acting β_2-agonists, asthma management 231, 234
long-term oxygen therapy (LTOT) 151–152
lordotic chest radiograph 127
low molecular weight (LMW) agents, occupational asthma 269, 270
lower respiratory tract infections (LRTIs)
  diagnosis
    bronchoalveolar lavage 104
    see also microbiological testing
  see also specific infections
lung(s)
  anatomy 11–12
  imaging
    computed tomography see computed tomography (CT)
    magnetic resonance imaging see magnetic resonance imaging (MRI)
    nuclear medicine scans 50, 135–137
      see also scintigraphy
    radiography see chest radiography
  molecular biology 7–10
lung abscess 189–190
lung biopsy
  bronchial 100
  percutaneous fine-needle 110–111
  pulmonary Langerhans' cell histiocytosis diagnosis 439
  sarcoidosis diagnosis 309
  transbronchial 100, 101
lung cancer 372–375
  classification 372–373
    see also specific histologic types
  diagnosis 373–374
    bronchoscopy 98, 373
    percutaneous fine-needle biopsy 111
    positron emission tomography 136–137, 374
  epidemiology 372
  functional assessment 374
    performance status see performance status (PS), lung cancer
  genetics 6, 372
  HIV association 428
  management see lung cancer treatment
  metastasis 388, 389, 390, 391
  non small cell see nonsmall cell lung cancer (NSCLC)
  risk factors 372
    air pollution 286, 287–288
    smoking 287–288, 292, 295, 372, 373

silicosis association 284
small cell *see* small cell lung cancer (SCLC)
staging 374, 375
   mediastinal lymph nodes 13-14, 374
   medical thoracoscopy/pleuroscopy (MT/P) 114
   transthoracic ultrasonography 141
symptoms 373
lung cancer treatment 374-375
  brachytherapy 101, 381
  chemotherapy *see* chemotherapy
  nonsmall cell lung cancer *see under* nonsmall cell lung cancer (NSCLC)
  palliative 381
  radiotherapy *see under* radiotherapy
  small cell lung cancer 375, 378-379
  surgical resection
    nonsmall cell lung cancer 374, 375, 382-386
    pre-operative assessment 157-158
    quality requirements 383
lung compliance 16-17, 65-66
  measurement 65-66
lung disease
  altitude effects 300-301
  transthoracic ultrasonography 141
  see also specific diseases
lung function
  impact of interventional bronchoscopy 120-121
  improvement, bronchiectasis 254
lung function testing
  asthma 228-230
  lymphangioleiomyomatosis 441
  neuromuscular diseases 361-362
  pulmonary Langerhans' cell histiocytosis 439
  upper airway stenosis 118-120
  see also specific tests
lung injury 146-147
  graft *versus* host disease 430-431
  inhalation *see* acute inhalation injury
  radiation-induced 304-305
lung transplant rejection, gastro-oesophageal reflux and 242, 244
lung transplantation
  idiopathic pulmonary fibrosis 317-318
  Langerhans' cell histiocytosis 440
  lymphangioleiomyomatosis 443
  pulmonary alveolar proteinosis 436
  pulmonary arterial hypertension 343
lung volumes 58-62
  measurement techniques 62
lupus, drug-induced 329
lymph nodes
  benign *vs.* malignant, transthoracic ultrasonography 138-139
  dissection, nonsmall cell lung cancer 385-386
  mediastinal *see* mediastinal lymph nodes
  metastatic tumours 389-390
  tuberculosis 210
lymphadenopathy, mediastinal *see* mediastinal lymphadenopathy
lymphangioleiomyomatosis (LAM) 441-443
  diagnosis 441-443
  disease progression 443
  epidemiology 441

  genetics 441
  management 443
  pathology 441
  prognosis 443
  symptoms 441
lymphatic drainage 11, 13
lymphoid interstitial pneumonia (LIP) 105, 311, 313
lymphoma 393, 399-400
  HIV-associated 427-428

M

macrolides
  bronchiectasis management 254
  community-acquired pneumonia management 178
macrophages, alveolar 27-28
magnetic resonance imaging (MRI) 132-133
  computed tomography *vs.* 130, 132
  diffusion-weighted 133
  indications 132
male reproductive tract, cystic fibrosis-related disease 262
malignant airway stenosis, interventional pulmonology 118, 120-121
malignant pericardial effusions 388
malignant pleural effusions (MPEs) 348, 349, 388, 392-393
  clinical signs 393
  diagnosis 393, 395-396
  management 350-351, 394, 397
  medical thoracoscopy/pleuroscopy (MT/P) 114
  transthoracic ultrasonography 139-140
malignant pleural mesothelioma (MPM) 392
  clinical signs 393
  diagnostic procedures 395-396
  imaging 133, 141, 393-394
  pre-treatment assessment 396
  prognosis 393
  staging 396
  treatment 381, 395, 396-397
malt worker's lung 280
mandibular advancement device (MAD) 408
mannitol
  bronchial provocation testing 89
  bronchiectasis management 254
manually assisted coughing (MAC), neuromuscular disease patients 364, 449
maple bark stripper's lung 280
matrix metalloproteinases (MMPs) 7-8
maxillomandibular advancement osteotomy, obstructive sleep apnoea management 409
maximal incremental exercise testing 83-84
maximal respiratory pressures, measurement 66
mechanical insufflation–exsufflation (MI-E), neuromuscular disease patients 364, 449
mechanical ventilation
  as cause of lung injury 146-147
  lung injury management 147
  measurement of respiratory mechanics 66
  neuromuscular disease patients 363-364
  noninvasive *see* noninvasive ventilation (NIV)
  respiratory failure management 150
  respiratory intensive care unit patients 154-155
mediastinal drainage 359-360

mediastinal lymph nodes 13–14
    metastatic tumours 389–390
mediastinal lymphadenopathy
    amyloid 434
    chest pain 49
mediastinal tumours 399–400
mediastinitis
    aetiology 358
    descending necrotising *see* descending necrotising mediastinitis (DNM)
    fibrosing 360
mediastinum, anatomy 13–14, 399
Medical Research Council (MRC) dyspnoea scale 43, 44
medical thoracoscopy/pleuroscopy (MT/P) 112–114
    contraindications 113
    indications 113–114
    techniques 112–113
    video-assisted thoracic surgery (VATS) *vs.* 112
meningitis, tuberculous 211
mepolizumab 321
mesothelioma *see* malignant pleural mesothelioma (MPM)
metabolic acidosis 80, 81
    HIV therapy-associated 428–429
metabolic alkalosis 80, 81
metabolic syndrome, obstructive sleep apnoea association 406, 407, 408
metacholine bronchial provocation testing 88, 89, 90
metal fume fever 273, 274
metal grinding, hypersensitivity pneumonitis 280
metastatic tumours 388–391
    bone 390–391
    hilar and mediastinal lymph nodes 389–390
    malignant pericardial effusions 388
    pleural *see* pleural metastases
    pulmonary 388–389
methaemoglobinaemia 329
methotrexate, Wegener's granulomatosis therapy 339
methotrexate lung 327–328
microbiological testing 162–167
    culture techniques 162–163, 164
        pulmonary tuberculosis diagnosis 203
    Gram stain 163–164
    nucleic acid amplification tests 163, 166–167
    rapid antigen tests 163, 164–165
    serology 165–166
    sputum samples 163–164
        pulmonary tuberculosis diagnosis 203
minocycline-induced eosinophilic pneumonia 323, 328
miRNAs 3
molecular biology, lung 7–10
mollusc-shell hypersensitivity 280
Moraxella catarrhalis, COPD exacerbations 173, 175
mould exposure 288
mountain sickness
    acute 298–299, 300
    chronic 300
moxifloxacin therapy
    infectious COPD exacerbations 174, 175
    nontuberculous mycobacterial infections 220
    pulmonary tuberculosis 206
mucociliary clearance 8, 27

multi-drug resistant tuberculosis (MDR-TB) 204, 206, 207–208
    HIV association 427
    treatment 207–208
mushroom worker's lung 280
myasthenia gravis 399
Mycobacterium abscessus 220
Mycobacterium avium complex (MAC) 219, 220
Mycobacterium kansasii 219, 220
Mycobacterium malmoense 220
Mycobacterium simiae 220
Mycobacterium szulgai 220
Mycobacterium tuberculosis 200
    infection *see* tuberculosis (TB)
Mycobacterium xenopi 220
Mycoplasma pneumoniae
    community-acquired pneumonia 177
    COPD exacerbations 173, 175
    detection methods 163, 165, 166
myocardial infarction 42

N

NAC (*N*-acetylcysteine), idiopathic pulmonary fibrosis therapy 316–317
nasal cilia 26
nasal continuous positive airway pressure (nCPAP)
    central sleep apnoea 408
    obstructive sleep apnoea 407–408
nasal mucosa 26
nausea, chemotherapy-induced 378
needles, percutaneous fine-needle biopsy 110–111
neuralgic pain 50
neuraminidase inhibitors 170, 192, 193
neuromuscular diseases (NMD), respiratory complications 361–364
    clinical evaluation 361
    dyspnoea 46, 47, 361
    hypoventilation 417
    management 363–364, 449
    pulmonary function testing 361–362
    sleep-disordered breathing 361, 362–363, 412–413
    sleep study 362–363
neuropathy, chemotherapy-induced 378
neuroventilatory dissociation (NVD) 46
neutropenia, chemotherapy-induced 378
neutrophils 27, 28
nicotine replacement therapy (NRT) 296
nitrogen dioxide (NO_2), air pollution 285, 286, 288, 289
nocturnal hypoventilation 414–415
nocturnal noninvasive ventilation 152
    obesity hypoventilation syndrome 415
nodular bronchiectasis 219
nonallergic rhinitis 225
    treatment 226
nonasthmatic eosinophilic bronchitis 319
noninvasive ventilation (NIV) 152
    bronchiectasis 448
    COPD 448
    neuromuscular disease patients 363–364, 449
    obesity hypoventilation syndrome 416–417
    respiratory intensive care unit patients 154, 155

see also continuous positive airway pressure (CPAP) therapy
nonsmall cell lung cancer (NSCLC) 373
  early-stage, definition 383
  staging 375, 383
  treatment 374–375
    chemotherapy 374–375, 379–381, 382
    radiotherapy 382
    surgical 374, 375, 382–386
    survival rates and 374, 375, 383, 384, 385–386
  see also lung cancer
nonspecific interstitial pneumonia (NSIP) 311–312, 313–318
  clinical features 313–314
  diagnosis 105, 314
  exacerbations 314–315
  management 315–318
  pathogenesis 313
nonsteroidal anti-inflammatory drugs (NSAIDs)
  respiratory complications 323, 327
  upper respiratory tract infection management 170
nontuberculous mycobacterial (NTM) infections 218–220
  epidemiology 218
  pathogenesis 218
  pulmonary 219–220
nosocomial pleural infection 186, 187
nosocomial pneumonia *see* hospital-acquired pneumonia (HAP)
nuclear factor-κB 10
nuclear medicine scans 50, 135–137
  see also scintigraphy
nucleic acid amplification tests (NAATs) 163, 166–167
Nuss technique 367
nutritional support, COPD 250

O

obesity
  COPD patients 455
  dyspnoea and 47
obesity hypoventilation syndrome (OHS) 415–417
oblique chest radiograph 127
obstructive lung disease
  dyspnoea 43
  hypoventilation 417
  lung volume changes 59, 61
  see also specific diseases
obstructive sleep apnoea/hypopnoea syndrome (OSAHS) 404–409, 414, 416
  altitude effects 301
  consequences 405–407
  definition 404
  diagnosis 405
  management 407–409
  pathophysiology 405, 406
  prevalence 405
  symptoms 404
occupational asthma 268–272
  associated occupations/industries 271
  diagnosis 269–270
  management 270–271
  sensitising/triggering agents 269, 270
  socioeconomic impact 271–272

symptoms 269
oesophagus, cystic fibrosis-related disease 261
opioid therapy, chronic, central sleep apnoea and 412
opsonins 27, 28
organic dust toxic syndrome (ODTS) 273, 274
  hypersensitivity pneumonitis *vs.* 281
oseltamivir 192–193
osteolytic metastases 390
otitis media 193, 194
outdoor pollution 285–287
ovarian cancer, metastasis 388, 390
oxidative stress, air pollution 289
oxygen pulse 84
oxygen therapy 151–152
  acute 151
  asthma exacerbations 233, 235
  COPD 151, 175, 250, 447, 448
  long-term 151–152
  neuromuscular disease patients 449
  physiotherapist's role 447
ozone, air pollution 285, 286, 289

P

paclitaxel chemotherapy 379
  nonsmall cell lung cancer 380
pain, chest 49–50
palliative treatments
  lung cancer 381
  malignant pleural mesothelioma 397
palpation 52
pancreas, cystic fibrosis-related disease 261, 262
pandemic influenza 193–194
paprika splitter's lung 280
paradoxical vocal cord movement (PVCM) 236, 238
parenchymal pulmonary amyloidosis 434
parietal pleurectomy, pneumothorax management 355, 356
particulate matter (PM), air pollution 285–287, 288, 289
passive smoking 293–294
peak expiratory flow (PEF) measurement, asthma 227, 228
  occupational 270
peak oxygen uptake 84
peat moss worker's lung 280
pectus carinatum (PC) 367
pectus excavatum (PE) 366, 367
pemetrexed chemotherapy 379
  malignant mesothelioma 381, 397
  nonsmall cell lung cancer 374, 375, 380
D-penicillamine, idiopathic pulmonary fibrosis therapy 316
penicillins
  community-acquired pneumonia management 178
  hospital-acquired pneumonia management 182
pentamidine, *Pneumocystis jirovecii* pneumonia management 425, 426
percutaneous drainage
  lung abscess 190
  see also chest tube drainage
percutaneous fine-needle biopsy (PFNB) 110–111
performance status (PS), lung cancer 374
  World Health Organization/Eastern Cooperative

Oncology Group (WHO/ECOG) scale 378, 379
perfusion lung scintigraphy (PLS)
    pulmonary embolism diagnosis 135-136, 334, 335
    pulmonary hypertension diagnosis 342-343
pericardial effusion
    dyspnoea and 42
    malignant 388
pericardium, tuberculosis 211
periodic breathing, high-altitude 298, 299, 413
PET (positron emission tomography), lung cancer diagnosis/staging 136-137, 374, 385
PET/CT (computed tomography/positron emission tomography), lung cancer diagnosis 136, 137, 374
pH, arterial 80
phagocytosis 27-28
pharyngeal specimens, antigen tests 164-165
pharyngitis 169, 170
phosphodiesterase type-5 inhibitors, pulmonary arterial hypertension management 343
phrenic nerve 14
physical examination 51-54
    auscultation 44-45, 54
    cough 51, 53
    dyspnoea 44-45, 51, 53
    inspection 52
    palpation 52
    percussion 52, 54
physiology *see* respiratory physiology
physiotherapy 446
    respiratory *see* respiratory physiotherapy
Pickwickian syndrome 415-416
picture archiving and communication systems (PACS) 129
pirfenidone, idiopathic pulmonary fibrosis therapy 316
Pisa score 332, 333
platinum-based chemotherapy 379
    malignant mesothelioma 381
    nonsmall cell lung cancer 374, 380
    small cell lung cancer 374, 375, 378
plethysmography, body 62, 64-65
pleura
    anatomy 11
    drug-induced disease 329
    pathology
        transthoracic ultrasonography 139-140
        see also specific diseases
pleural biopsy 396
pleural catheters 397
pleural cavity 11
pleural drainage, pleural effusions 350
pleural effusion 348-351
    aetiology 348
    definition 348
    diagnosis 349-350
        laboratory investigations 349-350
        medical thoracoscopy/pleuroscopy 113, 114, 349
        thoracentesis 115, 116, 349
        transthoracic ultrasonography 139-140, 141, 349
        transudate *vs.* exudate 350
    drug-induced 327
    exudative 349, 350
    malignant *see* malignant pleural effusions (MPEs)
    management 350-351
        thoracentesis 115, 116, 350, 351
    pathophysiology 348-349
    symptoms 349
        dyspnoea 43
    transudative 348
pleural fluid examination
    pleural effusion diagnosis 349-350
    pleural infections 187
pleural infection 186-189
    bacteriology 186-187
    clinical classification 187
    diagnosis 187, 188
    epidemiology 186
    management 187-188
    pathophysiology 186
    prognosis 188-189
    tuberculosis 210-211
pleural malignancies
    mesothelioma *see* malignant pleural mesothelioma (MPM)
    metastatic *see* pleural metastases
    transthoracic ultrasonography 141
pleural metastases 388, 392-393
    diagnosis 393, 395, 396
    prognosis 393
    treatment 397
    see also malignant pleural effusions (MPEs)
pleural pain 49
pleural plaques 282
pleural rubs 54
pleural tap *see* thoracentesis
pleurectomy, pneumothorax management 355, 356
pleurisy, asbestos 282-283
pleurodesis 397
pleuroscopy *see* medical thoracoscopy/pleuroscopy (MT/P)
pneumococcal vaccination 170, 179
    HIV-infected patients 424
    lymphangioleiomyomatosis patients 443
pneumoconiosis 282-284
Pneumocystis jirovecii pneumonia (PJP) 178, 184-185, 424-426
    management 184, 425-426
pneumomediastinum 353, 354
pneumonectomy, nonsmall cell lung cancer 383, 384
    alternatives 386
pneumonia
    Aspergillus 184, 185
    aspiration 176, 178
    clinical features 42, 177
    community-acquired *see* community-acquired pneumonia (CAP)
    cytomegalovirus *see* cytomegalovirus pneumonia (CMVP)
    eosinophilic *see* eosinophilic pneumonia
    epidemiology 176
    hospital-acquired *see* hospital-acquired pneumonia (HAP)
    idiopathic interstitial *see* idiopathic interstitial pneumonias (IIPs)
    in immunocompromised hosts 176, 177, 178, 183-185

HIV-infected patients 424
as influenza complication 177, 193, 194
investigations and diagnosis 177
see also microbiological testing
management 178-179
prevention 179
severity assessment 178
ventilator-associated 176, 177, 178, 180, 181
pneumonia severity index (PSI) 178
pneumonitis
chemical *see* toxic pneumonitis
HIV-associated 428
hypersensitivity *see* hypersensitivity pneumonitis (HP)
post-bone marrow transplantation 431
radiation 304, 305
pneumotachograph-shutter system, airway resistance measurement 65
pneumothorax 42
classification 352, 353
definition 352
HIV association 428
iatrogenic 352, 353
medical thoracoscopy/pleuroscopy 113, 114
spontaneous *see* spontaneous pneumothorax
traumatic *see* traumatic pneumothorax
Poland syndrome 366
polymer fume fever 273
polysomnography
central sleep apnoea assessment 411
neuromuscular disease patients 362-363
obstructive sleep apnoea assessment 405
popcorn worker's lung 277
positive end-expiratory pressure (PEEP), lung injury management 147
positron emission tomography (PET), lung cancer diagnosis/staging 136-137, 374, 385
positron emission tomography/computed tomography (PET/CT), lung cancer diagnosis 136, 137, 374
post-nasal drip syndrome 34
post-operative interventions, pulmonary complications 157
post-operative pulmonary complications
intraoperative interventions 157
post-operative interventions 157
pre-operative assessment 156-158
pulmonary resection 157-158
pre-operative interventions 157
risk factors 156-157
American Society of Anesthesiologists classification 156, 157
postero-anterior (PA) radiograph 126, 127
postural drainage (PD) 445
bronchiectasis 448
pre-operative assessment 156-158
pulmonary resection 157-158
pre-operative interventions, pulmonary complications 157
pregnant women
air pollution hazards 286
influenza complications risk 194
lymphangioleiomyomatosis 443

primary immunodeficiencies (PID), pulmonary diseases 420-422
primary progressive pulmonary tuberculosis 201
primary spontaneous pneumothorax 352-353, 352-355
primary viral pneumonia 193, 194
pro-motility agents 37
prophylactic cranial irradiation (PCI) 375, 379
Prospective Investigation of Pulmonary Embolism Diagnosis (PIOPED) study 332, 333, 334, 335
Prospective Investigative Study of Acute Pulmonary Embolism Diagnosis (PISA-PED) study 332, 333, 334
prostaglandins, pulmonary arterial hypertension management 343, 344
prostate cancer, metastasis 390
α_1-proteinase inhibitor (PI) deficiency 248
genetics 2, 4
proteinosis, pulmonary alveolar 8, 435-436
prothionamide therapy, pulmonary tuberculosis 206
proton pump inhibitors (PPIs), gastro-oesophageal reflux disease management 37, 243, 244
Pseudomonas aeruginosa infection
COPD exacerbations 173, 174
hospital-acquired pneumonia 181
psychotherapy, vocal cord dysfunction 239
pulmonary alveolar proteinosis (PAP) 8, 435-436
pulmonary amyloidosis 433-434
pulmonary arterial hypertension (PAH) 340
diagnosis 342-343
epidemiology 342
HIV association 428
prognosis 342
treatment 343-344
pulmonary barotrauma 302-303
pulmonary capillary haemangiomatosis 340-341
pulmonary complications, post-operative *see* post-operative pulmonary complications
pulmonary diffusive flux, impairment 21-22
pulmonary embolism (PE) 332
diagnosis 332-335
clinical probability assessment 332-333
computed tomography angiography 333-334, 335
D-dimer measurement 333
magnetic resonance imaging 132-133
perfusion lung scintigraphy 135-136, 334, 335
ventilation lung scintigraphy 135, 334
dyspnoea and 42
idiopathic pulmonary fibrosis patients 314, 317
pulmonary fibrosis
drug-induced 329
idiopathic *see* idiopathic pulmonary fibrosis (IPF)
radiation-induced 304-305
pulmonary function *see* lung function
pulmonary gas exchange 20
arterial blood gas analysis 77-80
enhancement strategies 447
exercise testing 86
impairments 20
see also transfer factor of the lung for carbon monoxide ($T_{L,CO}$)
pulmonary haemosiderosis 104
pulmonary hypertension (PH) 340-344

477

ERS Handbook: Respiratory Medicine

altitude effects 301
classification 340-342
diagnosis 342-343
drug-induced 329
epidemiology 342
pathologic features 341-342
prognosis 342
treatment 343-344
pulmonary Langerhans' cell histiocytosis, adult 438-440
diagnosis 104, 439
epidemiology 438
features 438
outcomes 439
treatment 440
pulmonary metastases 388-389
pulmonary oedema
drug-induced 324, 328
high-altitude 299-300
pulmonary rehabilitation 451-456
bronchiectasis 254, 448
chest wall disorders 449
COPD 250, 447, 452, 453, 454-456
severe exacerbations 455-456
definition 451
evidence base 451-452
maintaining effects 453
patient selection 454
programmes 452-454
see also respiratory physiotherapy
pulmonary resection
bronchiectasis 254
lung cancer see under lung cancer treatment
pre-operative assessment 156, 157-158
pulmonary surfactant see surfactant system
pulmonary tuberculosis 200-208
aetiology 200
clinical features 202
diagnosis 136, 203-204
epidemiology 201-202
pathogenesis 201
primary 202
secondary 202
treatment 204-208
see also anti-tuberculosis drugs
see also tuberculosis (TB)
pulmonary vascular disorders (PVD)
drug-induced 329
exercise intolerance 83
exercise testing 86
see also specific disorders
pulmonary vasculature, anatomy 13
pulmonary vasculitis 336-339
classification 337
clinical presentation 336-338
diagnosis 338
epidemiology 336
pathogenesis 336
prognosis 338-339
treatment 339
pulmonary veno-occlusive disease (PVOD) 340-341, 342-343
pulmonary ventilation see ventilation
pyrazinamide 204, 205, 220

R

radiation fibrosis (RF) 304-305
radiation-induced lung injury 304-305
radiation pneumonitis (RP) 304, 305
radiography see chest radiography
radiotherapy 304
lung cancer
nonsmall cell lung cancer 374, 382
palliative 381
small cell lung cancer 375, 379
malignant pleural mesothelioma 397
rapid-acting β_2-agonists, asthma management 231, 234, 235
rapid antigen tests 163, 164-165
rare lung diseases
diagnosis, bronchoalveolar lavage 104
see also specific diseases
Ravitch technique 367
reactive airway disease, dyspnoea 42
reactive airways dysfunction syndrome (RADS) 277
Read–Leigh rebreathing test 73-74
rebreathing test 72, 73-74
recoil pressure (PREC) 18, 19, 20
rectum, cystic fibrosis-related disease 261
reflex mechanisms, defensive 26-27
reflux cough 35, 36
see also gastro-oesophageal reflux-induced cough
regulatory genes 3
relaxation volume 58
relievers, asthma 234
reproductive tract, cystic fibrosis-related disease 262
residual volume (RV) 59-61
respiratory acidosis 80, 81
respiratory alkalosis 80, 81
respiratory bronchiolitis-associated interstitial lung disease 105, 312
respiratory exchange ratio (RER) 15, 20
respiratory failure (RF) 148-150
definition 148
hypercapnic see hypercapnic respiratory failure
hypoxaemic see hypoxaemic respiratory failure
idiopathic pulmonary fibrosis 313-314
management 150
neuromuscular disease patients 363-364
respiratory infections
bacterial see bacterial infections
cystic fibrosis 256, 258
management 259-260, 261, 263
HIV-related see under HIV-related disease
microbiological diagnosis see microbiological testing
post-bone marrow transplantation 431
primary immunodeficiency-associated 420-422
smoking association 293
see also specific infections; specific pathogens
respiratory intensive care unit (RICU) 154-155
respiratory mechanics 16-20, 63-66
expiration 18-20, 63
inspiration 17-18, 21, 63, 64
measurement in mechanical ventilation 66
respiratory muscle strength 66
respiratory-muscle work (W) 17-18
respiratory physiology 15-25

alveolar hypoventilation 20–21
diffusion impairment 21–22
pulmonary gas exchange 20
respiratory mechanics *see* respiratory mechanics
respiratory quotient *see* respiratory quotient (RQ)
ventilation–perfusion maldistribution 23–25
ventilatory requirements 15–16
respiratory physiotherapy 446–449
  airway clearance techniques 446–447
  bronchiectasis 448
  chest wall disorders 449
  community-acquired pneumonia 448–449
  COPD 447–448
  critically ill patients 449
  cystic fibrosis 448
  hyperventilation syndrome 448
  interstitial lung diseases 448
  neuromuscular disease 449
  spinal cord injury 449
  ventilation-/gas exchange-enhancing strategies 447
  see also pulmonary rehabilitation
respiratory polygraphy, neuromuscular disease patients 362–363
respiratory quotient (RQ) 15, 16
  reduced 20
respiratory syncytial virus (RSV), detection 165–166
respiratory system anatomy 11–14
respiratory viruses
  bronchitis-associated 240
  chronic obstructive pulmonary disease exacerbations 172, 173, 174
  detection methods 163
    antigen tests 164–165
    nucleic acid amplification tests 166–167
    serologic 165–166
  post-bone marrow transplant infections 431
  primary immunodeficiency-associated 421
  upper respiratory tract infections 169
restrictive lung disease
  dyspnoea 43
  lung volume changes 59, 61
  see also specific diseases
rhinitis, chronic 224–226
  asthma association 224, 226
  clinical aspects 224–225
  definition 224
  epidemiology 224
  pathophysiology 225–226
  treatment 225, 226
rhinoconjunctivitis, allergic 170
rhinosinusitis 169, 170
rifabutin therapy, pulmonary tuberculosis 206
rifampicin therapy
  latent tuberculosis 216
  nontuberculous mycobacterial infections 220
  pulmonary tuberculosis 204, 205
right-to-left shunt 22–23
rimantadine 192
Roughton–Forster equation 69–70

S

sarcoidosis 308–310
  clinical presentation 308–309
  diagnosis 5, 106, 309, 310
  epidemiology 308
  genetics 3, 4–5, 308
  induced sputum biomarkers 93
  natural history 309
  prognosis 309
  serum angiotensin-converting enzyme levels 5
  treatment 309–310
sarcoma, chest wall 393, 397
scintigraphy 50, 135–136
  gallium-67 136
  perfusion *see* perfusion lung scintigraphy (PLS)
  ventilation *see* ventilation lung scintigraphy (VLS)
seasonal influenza 191–193
secondary bacterial pneumonia 193, 194
secondary pneumothorax 353, 355–357
secretory IgA 29, 30
sedation, vocal cord dysfunction treatment 238
segmentectomy, nonsmall cell lung cancer 385
self-efficacy enhancement, pulmonary rehabilitation 451–452
serology 165–166
severe acute respiratory syndrome (SARS) 194–197
  clinical features 195–196
  diagnosis 196–197
  epidemiology 194–195
  management 196
  virology 196
silicosis 284
single breath (sb) technique 68
sinusitis 169, 170
Sjörgren's syndrome
  diagnosis 106
  lymphoid interstitial pneumonia association 313
skeletal muscle dysfunction, COPD 454–455
sleep-disordered breathing (SDB)
  neuromuscular disease patients 361, 362–363, 412–413
  see also central sleep apnoea/hypopnoea (CSA); obstructive sleep apnoea/hypopnoea syndrome (OSAHS)
sleep-induced hypoventilation 414–415
Smad proteins 8–9
small bowel, cystic fibrosis-related disease 261
small cell lung cancer (SCLC) 372–373
  genetics 6
  treatment 375, 378–379
  see also lung cancer
smoke inhalation 275, 276
smoking 295
  air pollution 287–288
  associated diseases *see* smoking-related diseases
  cessation *see* smoking cessation
  effect on bronchoalveolar lavage cell counts 108
  prevention 295–296
  protection against hypersensitivity pneumonitis 279
smoking cessation
  COPD management 248
  impact on survival 293, 294
  interventions 296–297
  Langerhans' cell histiocytosis management 440
  lung cancer patients 375
smoking-related diseases 291–294

asthma 234, 292–293
COPD 241, 246, 248, 292–293
desquamative interstitial pneumonia 312
in HIV-infected patients 428
interstitial lung diseases 293
Langerhans' cell histiocytosis 440
lung cancer 287–288, 292, 295, 372, 373
passive smoking-related 293–294
respiratory infections 293
pneumonia 179
sneezing 26–27
soluble mesothelin-related peptides (SMRPs) 396
speech therapy, vocal cord dysfunction 239
spinal cord injury (SCI)
hypoventilation 417
respiratory physiotherapy 449
spiral computed tomography scanning 130, 131
spirometry
asthma diagnosis 228–229
COPD severity classification 247
upper airway stenosis detection 119, 121
vocal cord dysfunction diagnosis 237
spontaneous pneumothorax 352–357
clinical features 352–353
complications 353–354
diagnosis 353
management 354–355, 356–357
primary 352–355
secondary 353, 355–357
sputum 37–38
bloody see haemoptysis
hypersecretion 37–38
microbiological testing 163–164
purulence 37, 38
sputum induction 92–94
disease biomarkers 93
procedure 92
pulmonary tuberculosis diagnosis 203
reproducibility and validity 93–94
safety issues 92–93
sputum reduction, bronchiectasis 254
sputum smear test, pulmonary tuberculosis diagnosis 204
squamous cell carcinoma, lung 373, 374
Staphylococcus, pleural infection 186, 187
Staphylococcus aureus infection
COPD exacerbations 173
hospital-acquired pneumonia 181
Starling resistor 405
stavudine 429
stenosis see airway stenosis
stenting, airway 101, 120–121
streptococcal pharyngitis 169, 170
Streptococcus milleri infection, pleural 186
Streptococcus pneumoniae infection
community-acquired pneumonia 177
COPD exacerbations 173, 174
detection methods 162, 163, 164
hospital-acquired pneumonia 181
pleural 186
streptomycin therapy, pulmonary tuberculosis 204, 205
stridor 44
subacute toxic pneumonitis 276–277

suberosis 280
sulphur dioxide (SO_2), air pollution 285, 286
superior vena cava obstruction 52, 54
surfactant system 8
abnormalities 8
pulmonary alveolar proteinosis 8, 435
surgeons, thoracic, qualifications 383
surgical thoracoscopy, medical thoracoscopy/pleuroscopy (MT/P) vs. 112
surgical treatment
bronchiectasis 254
chest wall disorders 367, 368
complications see post-operative pulmonary complications
lung abscess 190
lung cancer see lung cancer treatment
malignant pleural mesothelioma 396–397
mediastinal tumours 400
obstructive sleep apnoea 409
pleural infection 188
pneumothorax 355, 356
pre-operative assessment 156–158
pulmonary resection see pulmonary resection
see also video-assisted thoracic surgery (VATS)
sweat gland, cystic fibrosis-related disease 262
swine influenza 194
systemic amyloidosis 433
systemic sclerosis 106

T
T-lymphocytes 28, 29
talc pleurodesis 397
targeted therapies, nonsmall cell lung cancer 380–381
terizidone therapy, pulmonary tuberculosis 206
tetracycline therapy, infectious COPD exacerbations 174, 175
thiacetazone therapy, pulmonary tuberculosis 206
thoracentesis 115–117
complications 117
contraindications 116–117
diagnostic 115, 116, 349
procedure 115–116, 117
set 117
therapeutic 115, 116, 350, 351
thoracic surgeons, qualifications 383
thoracic surgery see surgical treatment
thoracoscopy 112
medical see medical thoracoscopy/pleuroscopy (MT/P)
surgical 112
see also video-assisted thoracic surgery (VATS)
thoracostomy
pneumothorax 354–355
see also chest tube drainage
thorax, normal appearance, transthoracic ultrasonography 138, 139
thymoma 399–400
thymus gland 13
thyroiditis, acute 170
tidal volume 18, 58, 59
Tietze's syndrome 49–50
tissue inhibitors of metalloproteinases (TIMPs) 7
tobacco dependence 295

prevention 295–296
treatment 296–297
see also smoking
tobacco smoke 291
tolerable limit of exercise (Tlim) 85
tonsillectomy, obstructive sleep apnoea management 409
total lung capacity (TLC) 16, 19, 58–60
toxic pneumonitis 274–277
  acute 274–276
  aetiology 274–275
  clinical presentation 275–276
  hypersensitivity pneumonitis *vs.* 281
  inhalation fever *vs.* 274
  management 276
  subacute 276–277
trachea, anatomy 12–13
tracheobronchial amyloidosis 434
tracheobronchitis 169
  chest pain 49
tracheostomy ventilation 152
  neuromuscular disease patients 363
traffic-related air pollution 286–287
transbronchial fine-needle aspiration (TBNA) 100
  endobronchial ultrasound-guided 101
transbronchial lung biopsy 101, 102
transfer coefficient of the lung for CO (K_{CO}) 69
  physiological influences 70, 71
transfer factor of the lung for carbon monoxide ($T_{L,CO}$) 21, 68–71
  calculation 68–70
  definition 68
  measurement technique 68
  physiological influences 70–71
transforming growth factor-β 8–10
transient lower oesophageal sphincter relaxations (TLOSRs) 242, 245
transient receptor potential (TRP) 36, 37
transplant patients, tuberculosis risk 212, 213
transplantation
  bone marrow *see* bone marrow transplantation (BMT)
  lung *see* lung transplantation
transthoracic fine-needle biopsy 110–111
transthoracic ultrasonography 138–141
  advantages 138
  appearance of normal thorax 138, 139
  chest wall pathology 138–139
  pleural pathology 139–141
  pulmonary pathology 141
  technical aspects 138
traumatic pneumothorax 352, 353
  fine-needle biopsy-induced 111
  thoracentesis-induced 117
tuberculin skin test 203, 213, 216
tuberculosis (TB) 200
  extrapulmonary *see* extrapulmonary tuberculosis (EPTB)
  in immunocompromised hosts 184, 185, 201, 212–213
    HIV-infected *see under* HIV-related disease
  latent *see* latent tuberculosis infection (LTBI)
  pulmonary *see* pulmonary tuberculosis
  silicosis association 284

tuberculous meningitis 211
tuberculous pleural effusion, diagnosis, medical thoracoscopy/pleuroscopy (MT/P) 113, 114
tuberous sclerosis complex (TSC) 443
tumour necrosis factor-α antagonists
  idiopathic pulmonary fibrosis therapy 317
  respiratory side-effects 326, 328–329
  tuberculosis risk and 212, 213
Tumour–Node–Metastasis (TNM) classification, lung tumours 137
tumours
  chest wall *see* chest wall tumours
  diagnosis, bronchoalveolar lavage 104
  HIV-associated 427–428
  lung *see* lung cancer
  mediastinal 399–400
  metastatic *see* metastatic tumours
  pleural
    mesothelioma *see* malignant pleural mesothelioma (MPM)
    metastatic *see* pleural metastases
    transthoracic ultrasonography 141
turbulent flow 17

U

ultrasound
  fine-needle biopsy guidance 110
  pleural infection 187
  transthoracic *see* transthoracic ultrasonography
upper airway, cystic fibrosis-related disease 262
upper airway collapse, obstructive sleep apnoea 405
upper airway stenosis (UAS)
  impact of interventional pulmonology 120–121
  pulmonary function testing 118–120
upper respiratory tract infections (URTIs) 168–170
  complications 169
  diagnosis 169–170
  HIV-infected patients 423–424
  pathogens 169
  predisposing conditions 168
  prevalence 168
  prevention 170
  symptoms and signs 168, 169
    cough 34
  transmission 168
  treatment 170
urinary antigen tests 164
usual interstitial pneumonia (UIP) 283, 312, 313–318
  clinical features 313–314
  diagnosis 314
  prognosis 313, 314
  see also idiopathic pulmonary fibrosis (IPF)
uvulopalatopharyngoplasty, obstructive sleep apnoea management 409

V

vaccination
  Haemophilus influenzae type B (HiB) 169
  influenza *see* influenza vaccination
  pneumococcal *see* pneumococcal vaccination
vagus nerve 14
valves, endobronchial 101–102
vapours, inhalational injury *see* acute inhalation injury

varenicline 296
vasculitis *see* pulmonary vasculitis
venous gas microemboli, diving-associated 303
ventilation
  control *see* ventilatory control
  enhancement strategies 447
  magnetic resonance imaging 133
ventilation lung scintigraphy (VLS)
  pulmonary embolism diagnosis 135, 334
  pulmonary hypertension diagnosis 342–343
ventilation–perfusion maldistribution 23–25
ventilator-associated pneumonia (VAP) 176, 177, 178, 180, 181
ventilator-dependent patients
  definition 155
  see also mechanical ventilation
ventilatory control 15–16, 72–76
  carbon dioxide responsiveness 72–74
  hypoxia responsiveness 74–76
ventilatory response
  to exercise 85
  see also ventilatory control
ventilatory support 152
  see also mechanical ventilation
video-assisted thoracic surgery (VATS)
  malignant pleural mesothelioma/pleural metastasis 396
  medical thoracoscopy/pleuroscopy (MT/P) *vs.* 112
  pleural infection management 188
  pneumothorax management 355
videobronchoscope 98, 99
  see also bronchoscopy
vinorelbine chemotherapy 379
  malignant mesothelioma 381
  nonsmall cell lung cancer 374, 378
viral pneumonia, primary 193, 194
viruses *see* respiratory viruses
vital capacity (VC) 61
vocal cord dysfunction (VCD) 236–239
  asthma association 236, 237, 238, 239
  clinical presentation 236–237
  diagnosis 237–238
  epidemiology 236, 237
  pathogenesis 236
  prognosis 239
  terminology 236
  treatment 238–239
vocal fremitus 52, 54
volatile organic compounds (VOCs), air pollution 288, 289
vomiting, chemotherapy-induced 378

W

walking tests 84
Wegener's granulomatosis 170, 336
  clinical presentation 337–338
  diagnosis 338
  epidemiology 336
  pathogenesis 336
  prognosis 338–339
  treatment 339
Wells score 332, 333
wheezing 42, 44, 54
whispering pectoriloquy (WP) 54
whole-body plethysmography 62, 64–65
whole-lung lavage (WLL), pulmonary alveolar proteinosis 436
whooping cough 169, 170
wood pulp worker's lung 280
wood trimmer's disease 280
work-exacerbated asthma (WEA) 268
work-related asthma (WRA) 268
  see also occupational asthma
World Health Organization (WHO)
  extrapulmonary tuberculosis definition 209
  lung tumour classification 372–373
  pulmonary tuberculosis treatment recommendations 204, 207
World Health Organization/Eastern Cooperative Oncology Group (WHO/ECOG) scale 378, 379

X

X-ray, chest *see* chest radiography

Z

zanamivir 192